COLUMBIA REVIEW

INTENSIVE PREPARATION FOR THE MCAT

COLUMBIA REVIEW

INTENSIVE PREPARATION FOR THE MCAT

Stephen D. Bresnick, M.D.

President and Director
Columbia Review, Inc.
Academic Physician
Stanford University Hospital
Stanford, California

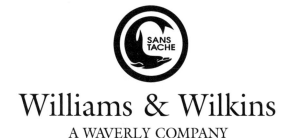

Williams & Wilkins

A WAVERLY COMPANY

BALTIMORE • PHILADELPHIA • LONDON • PARIS • BANGKOK
HONG KONG • MUNICH • SYDNEY • TOKYO • WROCLAW

Editor: Timothy S. Satterfield
Managing Editor: Amy G. Dinkel
Development Editors: Beth Goldner, Donna Siegfried
Production Coordinator: Danielle Santucci
Copy Editor: Catherine Nancarrow
Editorial Assistant: Carol Loyd
Designer: Ashley Pound
Illustrators: Patricia MacAllen, Hans & Cassady, Inc.
Typesetter: Graphic World, Inc.
Printer: Courier Companies, Inc.
Binder: Courier Companies, Inc.

351 West Camden Street
Baltimore, Maryland 21201-2436 USA

Rose Tree Corporate Center
1400 North Providence Road
Building II, Suite 5025
Media, Pennsylvania 19063-2043 USA

Printed in the United States of America

Library of Congress Cataloging in Publication Data

Bresnick, Stephen D.
    Columbia review intensive preparation for the MCAT/Stephen D. Bresnick.
        p. cm.
    ISBN 0-683-01027-1
    1. Medical colleges—United States—Entrance examinations—Study guides. I. Title.
        [DNLM: 1. Medicine—examination questions. W 18.2 B842c 1995]
    R838.5.B74 1995
    610'.76—dc20
    DNLM/DLC
    for Library of Congress   95-25627
                                                                              CIP

The Publishers have made every effort to trace the copyright holders for borrowed material. If they have inadvertently overlooked any, they will be pleased to make the necessary arrangements at the first opportunity.

96 97 98 99
1 2 3 4 5 6 7 8 9 10

Dedication

edication

This book is dedicated to all students who persevere, work hard, and aspire to enter one of the most important and gratifying professions—medicine. Best wishes in achieving your goals and fulfilling your dreams!

Contents

Contents

SECTION III   Preparation for the Biological Sciences

Preparation for Verbal Reasoning and the Writing Sample

Sample Full-Length MCAT with Solutions and Analysis

Preface

Preface

The MCAT is the most important test that you will ever take as a premedical student. Serious and intensive preparation is critical for MCAT success. Efficiency is also important. With this in mind, this book has been designed to be the most complete and intensive MCAT preparation book available, using materials from the national leader in intensive MCAT preparation.

It is becoming increasingly difficult to get into medical school, and a new approach is needed for many students to be able to compete for admission. We call this approach "Intensive MCAT Preparation," which focuses on an in-depth understanding of the MCAT, and includes an efficient study plan, excellent review and strategy materials, practice tests, quality study time, and a desire to succeed. **This book provides the needed information, strategies, and practice you will need to ace the MCAT.**

Columbia Review is a national MCAT preparation program, run by M.D.s, which specializes in MCAT preparation and medical school admissions assistance. The physicians directing our MCAT program have over 25 years of combined experience preparing students for the MCAT and have served on medical school admission committees. At Columbia Review, we focus all of our attention on the MCAT, and thus we are able to provide a focused, detailed, and efficient review. The live version of our program offers over 150 hours of classroom instruction. In addition to the classroom instruction program, Columbia Review offers a home-study MCAT review program. This book, authored by national MCAT experts and Director of Columbia Review, Stephen Bresnick, M.D., contains the finest MCAT study material available. You deserve nothing but the best!

Acknowledgments

ments

I would like to thank Dr. William Bresnick, physician, MCAT expert, and friend, whose collaboration and assistance with this book were appreciated. In addition, I would also like to thank Irene Bresnick, a superb educator and mentor, who taught me the importance of education and intensive study. Many thanks also to Frank Ospital and the staff of Columbia Review, whose caring dedication to premedical students is unparalleled.

Special acknowledgment to the following outstanding teaching staff of Columbia Review's Intensive MCAT Preparation Course: Chris Leptak, M.D., Ph.D., Lauren Yasuda, Ph.D., Dan Bender, Ph.D., Abby Parrill, Ph.D., Mark Sornson, M.D., Ph.D., Nori Kawahata, Ph.D., and George Hanson, Ph.D.

Finally, I would like to thank the staff of Williams & Wilkins for their dedication to creating a complete and thorough MCAT preparation book. I especially wish to thank Beth Goldner, Elizabeth Nieginski, Jane Velker, and Tim Satterfield for their valuable suggestions, assistance, and support for this monumental and important project.

Organization of this Book

This book is organized to focus on important skills and concepts you need to know for the MCAT. The structure of the book in many ways simulates the structure of the MCAT. Strategies are emphasized throughout the book.

The book consists of five sections. Section I discusses what the MCAT is all about, MCAT scoring, admission committees' evaluation of MCAT scores, exactly what is covered on the test, and key strategies for solving MCAT questions. Sections II and III offer a complete review of the Physical Sciences (physics and general chemistry) and the Biological Sciences (biology and organic chemistry), respectively. Following each science review, there are three timed practice tests in MCAT format. Many of these questions are similar in nature to recent MCAT questions. These practice tests, complete with solutions, allow you to solidify your understanding of the review material and focus on MCAT strategies. Section IV introduces the Verbal Reasoning and Writing Sample sections of the MCAT and provides strategic approaches for dealing with these two sections. Two Verbal Reasoning practice tests and sample student essays are provided. Section V offers a full-length practice MCAT, complete with detailed solutions and a computer analysis of your performance.

Features of this Book

- Outstanding MCAT preparation material from a top MCAT preparation course.
- Complete review of specific MCAT subjects: physics, general chemistry, biology, and organic chemistry
- Practice passage tests for each science, allowing you to test your understanding of the material, master timing and pacing, and practice MCAT problem solving strategies
- Over 800 practice questions, all in MCAT format—the equivalent of four full-length MCATs
- Verbal Reasoning strategies and practice tests with solutions
- Writing Sample strategies with sample scored essays and helpful critical analysis
- Challenging full-length practice MCAT with computer analyzed scoring. Predicted scoring was determined by administering this test to thousands of premedical students.

Good luck with your Intensive MCAT Preparation!

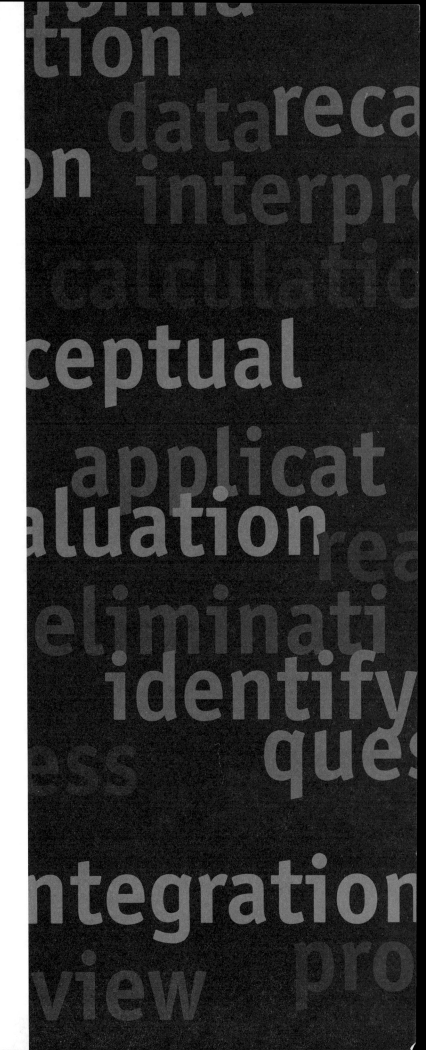

SECTION I

Introduction to the MCAT and Basic Strategies

....

A. Importance of the MCAT

B. Format and Content of the MCAT

C. MCAT Scores

D. How to Study for the MCAT: Basic Strategies

E. Strategies for Solving MCAT Science Passages

Importance of the MCAT

If you want to become a physician, the MCAT is the most important test that you take to begin reaching this goal. The MCAT is a prerequisite for admission to most medical schools in the United States. Your MCAT scores are carefully evaluated by medical school admissions committees. At many medical schools, your MCAT scores account for approximately 30% of your overall evaluation as an applicant. This is a large percentage, considering that the MCAT is only a one-day test. Although the test is completed in one day, many months of preparation are necessary for you to ace the MCAT. If you have significant weaknesses or remedial areas, you may need up to one year or more to prepare for the MCAT.

The MCAT may determine whether or not you gain admission to medical school, or the MCAT may determine which medical school you attend. State-supported medical schools are relatively inexpensive compared with private medical schools, and the difference in tuition between public and private medical schools can be more than $20,000 per year. A high score on the MCAT can make you competitive for a state-supported medical school and may save you tens of thousands of dollars in tuition. We strongly recommend that you take your preparation for the MCAT seriously because there is a great deal at stake, both professionally and financially.

Format and Content of the MCAT

Format

The MCAT is designed to assess your mastery of the basic skills that are a prerequisite for successful completion of medical school. The MCAT has been administered in its current format since April 1991. The MCAT is a 5 3/4-hour exam, divided into four general sections (Table B-1).

TABLE B-1. The Four Sections of the MCAT

Section	Number of Questions	Time (minutes)
Verbal Reasoning	65	85
Physical Sciences	77	100
(Lunch break)		60
Writing Sample	2	60
Biological Sciences	77	100

The **Verbal Reasoning** test is the first section of the MCAT and is designed to assess your ability to understand and evaluate information in arguments, which are contained in prose text (passages). The test consists of **9 passages, each 500–600 words in length.** The passages cover topics from the humanities, social sciences, and natural sciences. **Each passage is followed by 6–10 questions.** The questions are designed to measure performance in four areas: comprehension, evaluation, application, and incorporation of new information. Eighty five minutes is allotted for completion of this section, followed by a 10-minute break.

The second section of the MCAT is the **Physical Sciences** section. This section is composed of **77 multiple-choice questions** that test reasoning skills in **physics and general chemistry.** Sixty-two of the questions are based on problem sets (passages). Each problem set is approximately 250 words in length and describes a situation or scientific problem. The Physical Sciences section contains 11 passages, and each passage is followed by 5–8 questions. There are an additional 15 questions, which are independent of any passage or any other question. These questions are designed to test your knowledge in science and problem-solving abilities in physics and general chemistry. You are expected to be familiar with graphic and tabular analysis. There are four types of passages accompanying each problem set: informational presentation, problem solving, research study, or persuasive argument. You have 100 minutes allotted for answering all 77 questions. A 60-minute lunch break follows this section.

The **Writing Sample** section, which is administered following the lunch break, requires you to write **two essays;** you have 30 minutes allotted for each essay. The Writing Sample is designed to assess your skills in developing a central idea, synthesizing concepts, presenting ideas, and writing clearly with minimal errors in format. Each essay of the Writing Sample requires you to explain and interpret (with example) a statement of opinion, philosophy, or policy. Knowledge in any particular area is not expected. However, you are expected to explore the meaning of the essay statement and to discuss conflict resolution. You are scored on the degree in which you explain the meaning of the essay statement and the depth to which you explore examples and provide careful analysis. You are also scored on thoroughness, clarity, and form. A 10-minute break is given following this section.

The fourth and final section of the MCAT is the survey of the **Biological Sciences.** This section includes concepts from **biology and organic chemistry.** There are 62 multiple-choice questions that are based on passages and 15 multiple-choice questions that are independent of any passage or any other questions. The passage types are similar to those described for the Physical Sciences section. Again, a total of 100 minutes is allotted to answer all 77 Biological Sciences questions.

The MCAT is a challenging exam. You are probably not familiar with passage-type problems, which require you to analyze experimental data, research design, experimental apparatus, graphs, and information presented in tables and charts. The majority of the science questions on the MCAT present information in one of these formats. In addition, your college classes may not have covered all of the topics that are covered on the MCAT. This book will help you to review intensively the important MCAT testing areas and provide practice for solving MCAT passages and questions.

Content and Topics

The following MCAT content and topic listing has been assembled using information provided directly from the Association of American Medical Colleges (AAMC), the organization that authors the MCAT exam. Further discussion of the examination with sample test items is provided in the official AAMC publication: *The MCAT Student Manual.* The manual costs about $15.00 and is available at all major university bookstores or directly from the AAMC Publications Department (202-828-0416). In addition to the core subject areas listed below, you must be comfortable with the following mathematical concepts: basic math (simple calculations, proportion, ratio, percentage, and estimation of square root); exponentials and logarithms (natural and base ten); scientific notation; quadratic and simultaneous equations; graph nomenclature and interpretation (linear, semilog, and log–log); basic triangle relationships; basic principles of statistics; calculation of probability; vector math; and the right-hand rule. Luckily, there is no calculus on the MCAT.

The organization and topics reviewed in this book are based on the official MCAT topics that the AAMC compiles, so you should have confidence that you are reviewing the key material needed for MCAT success. As you review the topics listed in this section, you may want to cross off each science topic after you have thoroughly reviewed and mastered it.

PART I: VERBAL REASONING

Reading passages are drawn from subject material pertaining to three areas: humanities, social sciences, and natural sciences. (For further discussion, see Section IV: Preparation for Verbal Reasoning and the Writing Sample.) The subject topics for these three areas may include:

1. **Humanities:** architecture, art, art history, dance, ethics, literary criticism, music, philosophy, religion, theatre

2. **Social sciences:** anthropology, archaeology, business, economics, government, history, political science, psychology, sociology

3. **Natural sciences:** astronomy, botany, computer science, ecology, geology, meteorology, natural history, technology

PART II: PHYSICAL SCIENCES

The physical sciences test is composed of questions from two subject areas—inorganic chemistry and noncalculus physics. About half of the questions pertain to inorganic chemistry topics and about half of the questions pertain to physics topics. Questions are written to assess your **knowledge of basic physical science concepts** and your **ability to problem solve.** You should be fluent in your ability to read technical information, understand experiments (i.e., data tables, graphs, figures, diagrams, and charts) and solve basic scientific problems. Your ability to extract the needed information from the passages and answer questions quickly and correctly is extremely important. Recent MCATs have stressed information extraction (from the passage itself) and the understanding of basic principles and concepts. You are responsible for knowing and understanding key, basic formulas and equations. More complicated formulas are usually provided. You are responsible for a level of understanding of all MCAT science topics that is comparable to that of an entering first-year medical student. You are responsible for the following topics in inorganic chemistry and physics:

INORGANIC CHEMISTRY

1. **Stoichiometry,** including molecular weight, empirical and molecular formula, metric units, composition by percent mass, mole concept, Avogadro's number, density, oxidation number (common oxidizing–reducing agents, redox titration), and chemical–redox equations (conventions and balancing)

2. **Electronic structure and the periodic table**

    a. **Electronic structure,** including orbital structure of hydrogen, principal quantum number, number of electrons per orbital, ground–excited state, and electronic structure notation

    b. **Classification of elements by groups and rows,** including valence electrons of the common groups, first and second ionization energies and trends, electron affinity variation within groups and rows, and electronegativity

3. **Ionic and covalent bonds,** including Lewis electron dot formula, resonance structures, formal charge, Lewis acid-base, valence shell electron pair repulsion and the prediction of shapes of molecules, partial ionic character, role of electronegativity in determining charge distribution, dipole moment

4. **Phases and phase equilibria**

    a. **Gas phase,** including standard temperature and pressure, standard molar volume, ideal gas, ideal gas law, Boyle's and Charles' laws, kinetic molecular theory of gases, qualitative aspects of deviation of real gas behavior from ideal gas law, partial pressure, mole fraction, and Dalton's law of partial pressure

    b. **Liquid phase,** including hydrogen bonding, dipole interactions, and Van der Waals' forces

    c. **Phase equilibria,** including phase changes and diagrams, freezing, melting, and boiling points, molality, and colligative properties of vapor pressure lowering (Raoult's Law), boiling-point elevation, freezing-point depression, and osmotic pressure

5. **Solution chemistry**

   a. **Ions,** including cation, anion, and common nomenclature

   b. **Solubility,** including molarity, Ksp, common ion effect

6. **Acid-base equilibria**, including Bronsted acid-base, Kw, pH concept and calculations, conjugate acids and bases, strong and weak acids and bases, dissociation of weak acids and bases, hydrolysis of salts of weak acids and bases, K_a–K_b, pK_a–pK_b, buffers, and acid–base titration (indicators, neutralization, titration curves)

7. **Thermochemistry and thermodynamics**

   a. **Thermochemistry,** including thermodynamic system, state function, conservation of energy, endothermic and exothermic reactions (enthalpy, standard heats of reaction, Hess' law of heat summation), bond dissociation energy, calorimetry (heat capacity, specific heat), entropy, free energy, spontaneous reactions and standard free energy

   b. **Thermodynamics,** including First and Second Laws, energy units, temperature scales, heat transfer (conduction, convection, and radiation), coefficient of expansion, and heats of fusion and vaporization

8. **Kinetics and equilibrium**

   a. **Reaction rate,** including concentration effects, rate law, rate constant, and reaction order; rate-determining step, rate and temperature, activation energy (transition state, energy profile diagrams); kinetic and thermodynamic control of reaction, catalysts and enzymes, and reversible chemical reactions (law of mass action, equilibrium constant, Le Chatelier's principle)

   b. **Equilibrium constant** and **free energy relationship**

9. **Electrochemistry**

   a. **Electrolytic cell,** including electrolysis, anode–cathode, electrolytes, Faraday's law, electrode chemical processes, electron flow, and oxidation–reduction at electrodes

   b. **Galvanic cell,** including half-cell reactions, reduction potentials, cell potential, and direction of electron flow

   c. **Concentration cell,** including direction of electron flow

PHYSICS

1. **Translational motion,** including units and dimensions, scalars and vectors, speed and velocity, acceleration, uniformly accelerated motion, freely falling bodies, and projectiles

2. **Force, motion, and gravitation,** including mass, center of mass, weight, Newton's second and third laws, law of gravitation, uniform circular motion, centripetal force, friction, inclined plane, and pulley systems

3. **Equilibrium and momentum**

   a. **Equilibrium,** including translational and rotational equilibrium, torques, lever arms, Newton's first law, and inertia

   b. **Momentum,** including impulse, conservation of linear momentum, and elastic and inelastic collisions

4. **Work and energy,** including work, kinetic and potential energy, conservation of energy, conservative forces, power

5. **Solids and fluids**

   a. **Solids,** including density and elastic properties

   b. **Fluids,** including density, specific gravity, buoyancy (Archimedes' principle), hydrostatic pressure, viscosity, continuity principle (i.e., flow in equals flow out), Bernoulli's equation, turbulence, and surface tension

6. **Physical energy concepts,** including temperature, heat transfer mechanisms, thermodynamics, and calorimetry (i.e., heat gain equals heat loss in a closed system) [see General Chemistry Review Notes]

7. **Electrostatics and electromagnetism**

   a. **Electrostatics,** including charge, charge conservation, conductors, insulators, Coulomb's law, electric force, electric field (field lines, field due to charge distribution), absolute potential, potential difference, equipotential lines, and electric dipole

   b. **Electromagnetism,** including magnetic fields, electromagnetic spectrum, and x-rays

8. **Electric circuits,** including current; battery and voltage; resistor, resistance, and resistivity; capacitor, capacitance, and dielectrics; Ohm's law; series and parallel circuits [direct current (DC) circuits]; electric power; and root-mean-square current and voltage [alternating current (AC) circuits]

9. **Wave characteristics and periodic motion**

   a. **Wave characteristics,** including transverse and longitudinal motion, wavelength, frequency, wave velocity, amplitude, intensity, superposition of waves, phase, interference, wave addition, resonance, standing waves and nodes, and beats

   b. **Periodic motion,** including Hooke's law, simple harmonic motion, and pendulum motion

10. **Sound,** including sound production; relative speed in solids, liquids, and gases; intensity and pitch; Doppler effect; resonance in strings and pipes; and harmonics

11. **Light and geometrical optics,** including visual spectrum and color, polarization of light, reflection, mirrors, total internal reflection, refraction, refractive index, Snell's law, dispersion, thin lenses, combination of lenses, diopters, and lens aberrations

12. **Atomic and nuclear structure,** including atomic number and weight, neutrons, electrons, protons, isotopes, radioactive decay and half-life, quantized energy levels for electrons, and fluorescence (Some concepts in this section overlap with inorganic chemistry concepts.)

PART III: WRITING SAMPLE

The MCAT Writing Sample requires examinees to complete two independent 30-minute essays. Essay topics focus on interpretation of famous sayings, quotations, statements of policy, or social concern. Topics do not address science, medicine, the medical school application process, religion, or emotionally charged issues (see Section IV: Preparation for Verbal Reasoning and the Writing Sample).

PART IV: BIOLOGICAL SCIENCES

The biological sciences consists of questions relating to first-year, lower division biology and organic chemistry. The AAMC holds you responsible for knowing a large amount of biology! Some biology concepts are fairly advanced in nature (although fairly straightforward), so be sure to study all of the following topics. Although students tend to find the material covered in the organic chemistry section of the MCAT relatively straightforward, it is important that you master the tricky (and often tested) organic chemistry synthesis and research passage problems. You are responsible for the following topics in biology and organic chemistry:

BIOLOGY (This section focuses on the biology of vertebrates and microbes.)

1. **Molecular biology**

    a. **Enzymes and cellular metabolism,** including enzyme structure and function, control of enzyme activity, feedback inhibition, glycolysis (aerobic and anaerobic), Krebs cycle (citric acid cycle), electron transport chain, and oxidative phosphorylation

    b. **DNA and protein synthesis,** including DNA structure and function, DNA composition, the Watson-Crick model of DNA, the double helix, base-pair specificity, the genetic code, DNA replication, protein synthesis, transcription mechanism and regulation, and translation mechanism (codons, anticodons, mRNA, tRNA, rRNA, ribosome structure and function)

2. **Microbiology**

    a. **Viral structure and life history,** including DNA, RNA, and protein components, typical bacteriophage structure and function, relative size, and generalized phage and animal virus life cycles

    b. **Prokaryotic cells,** including structure, physiology, and bacterial life history

    c. **Fungi,** including major structural types, general life history, and physiology

3. **Generalized eukaryotic cell**

    a. Nucleus structure and function, including nucleolus, nuclear envelope, and nuclear pores

    b. **Structure and function of membrane-bound organelles,** including mitochondria, lysosomes, endoplasmic reticulum, and Golgi apparatus

    c. **Structure and function of the plasma membrane,** including protein and lipid components, fluid mosaic model, membrane traffic, osmosis, passive and active transport, endocytosis and exocytosis, membrane channels, the sodium–potassium pump, membrane potential, membrane receptors, and cellular adhesion

    d. **Structure and functions of the cytoskeleton,** including microfilaments, microtubules, intermediate filaments, cilia, flagella, and centrioles

    e. **Mitosis,** including mitotic process, phases of the cell cycle, centrioles, asters, spindles, chromatids, centromeres, telomeres, kinetochores, nuclear membrane breakdown and reorganization, and chromosome movement mechanisms

4. **Specialized eukaryotic cells and tissues**

    a. **Neural cells and tissues,** including cell body, axon, dendrites, Schwann cells and myelin sheath, nodes of Ranvier, synapse, and resting and action potentials

    b. **Contractile cells and tissues,** including striated, smooth, and cardiac muscle, sarcomere, and calcium regulation of contraction

c. **Epithelial cells and tissues,** including simple and stratified epithelium

d. **Connective cells and tissues,** including major cell and fiber types, loose and dense connective tissue, cartilage, and extracellular matrix

5. **Nervous and endocrine systems**

   a. **Nervous system structure and function,** including organization of the vertebrate nervous system, sensor and effector neurons, sympathetic and parasympathetic (autonomic) nervous systems

   b. **Sensory reception and processing,** including skin, proprioceptive, and somatic sensors, olfactory (smell) and gustatory (taste) systems, auditory (hearing), ear structure and hearing mechanism, and vision (eye structure and light receptors)

   c. **Endocrine systems,** including function, major endocrine glands and hormones, specificity, target tissues, cell mechanisms of hormone action, and hormone transport

6. **Circulatory, lymphatic, and immune systems**

   a. **Circulatory system,** including function, thermoregulation, the heart, pulmonary and systemic circulation, arterial, capillary, and venous systems, systolic and diastolic blood pressure, composition of blood, and the role of hemoglobin in oxygen transport

   b. **Lymphatic system,** including structure and function

   c. **Immune system,** including T and B lymphocytes, bone marrow, spleen, thymus, lymph nodes, antigens and antibodies, and antigen–antibody reactions

7. **Digestive and excretory systems**

   a. **Digestive system,** including ingestion, stomach, digestive glands (salivary glands, liver, pancreas), bile production, small and large intestines, muscular control of digestion

   b. **Excretory system,** including the role of the excretory system in body homeostasis, structure and function of the kidney, structure and function of the nephron, urine formation, and storage and elimination of wastes

8. **Muscle and skeletal systems**

   a. **Muscle system,** including functions, muscle types and locations, motor and sensory control, and voluntary and involuntary muscles

   b. **Skeletal system,** including function, bone structure (calcium and protein matrix), skeletal structure (bone types and joint structure), and structure and function of cartilage (ligaments and tendons)

9. **Respiratory and skin systems**

   a. **Respiratory system,** including gas exchange, role of alveoli, thermoregulation, mechanisms of protection against disease and particulate matter (immune and mucociliary systems), the diaphragm and rib cage, differential pressure (pleural space)

   b. **Skin system,** including structure and function (homeostasis, osmoregulation, thermoregulation, physical protection)

10. **Reproductive system and development**

    a. **Reproduction,** including male and female gonads, genitalia, gametes, gametogenesis (ovum and sperm) by meiosis, reproductive sequence, and structure and function of the placenta

b. **Embryogenesis,** including fertilization, cleavage, blastulation, gastrulation, neurulation, and major structures arising from the primary germ layers; developmental mechanism, including cell determination, cell differentiation, and induction

11. **Genetics and evolution**

a. **Genetics,** including mendelian concepts, Hardy-Weinberg principle and population genetics, meiosis and genetic variability, sex-linked characteristics, and mutations

b. **Evolution,** including natural selection, fitness, differential survival and reproduction, group selection, species and speciation concepts, origin of life, and chordate anatomic features and vertebrate body plan

ORGANIC CHEMISTRY

1. **Molecular structure of organic compounds**

a. **Sigma and pi bonds,** including hybrid orbitals; structural formulas for molecules involving H, C, N, O, F, S, P, Si, and Cl; and delocalized electrons and resonance

b. **Multiple bonding,** including the effect on bond length, energies, and rigidity in molecular structure

c. **Stereochemistry,** including structural, stereo, and conformational isomers, polarization of light, specific rotation, absolute and relative configuration, R/S conventions, and racemic mixtures

2. **Hydrocarbons**

a. **Alkanes,** including description, physical properties, important reactions (combustion–substitution reactions with halogens), free radical stability, chain reaction mechanisms (including inhibition), and ring strain in cyclic compounds

b. **Alkenes,** including structure, isomerization, physical properties, and electrophilic addition

c. **Benzene,** including description, and resonance stability (delocalization of electrons)

3. **Oxygen-containing compounds**

a. **Alcohols,** including dehydrations and carbocation formation, substitution $S_N(1/2)$ reactions, hydrogen bonding, and the effect of chain branching on physical properties

b. **Aldehydes and ketones,** including nucleophilic addition reaction, acetal/ketal/hemiacetal/hemiketal, imine/enamine, Aldol condensation, keto-enol tautomerism, the effect of substituents on carbonyl reactivity, steric hindrance, alpha-hydrogen acidity, carbanions, and alpha-beta unsaturated carbonyls

c. **Carboxylic acids,** including decarboxylation, esterification, H bonding, inductive effect of substituents, and carboxylate anion resonance stability

d. **Common acid derivatives,** including hydrolysis of fats and glycerides (saponification), hydrolysis of amides, relative reactivity of acid derivatives, and steric effects

e. **Ethers,** including cleavage by acid and weak basicity of ethers

f. **Phenols,** including effects of substituents on acidity and H bonding

4. **Amines**

   a. **Description,** including stereochemistry and physical properties

   b. **Major reactions,** including amide formation and alkylation; general principles, including basicity, carbocation stabilization, the effect of substituents on basicity of aromatic amines

   c. **Quaternary salts,** including solubility

5. **Biological molecules**

   a. **Amino acids and proteins,** including absolute configuration at the alpha-configuration, amino acids as dipolar ions, and acidic, basic, hydrophobic, and hydrophilic classification, reactions (cysteine and cystine sulfur linkage, peptide linkage, hydrolysis)

   b. **General principles,** including 1°, 2°, and 3° protein structures, 3° structure and proline, cystine, and H bonding, and isoelectric point

   c. **Carbohydrates,** including nomenclature, classification, common names, absolute configuration, hexose cyclic structure and conformations, epimers and anomers, monosaccharides oxidation, and hydrolysis of the glycoside linkage

   d. **Lipids,** including free fatty acids, triacylglycerols, and steroids

   e. **Phosphorus compounds,** including phosphoric acid

   f. **Chemistry and the structure of anhydrides and esters**

6. **Separations and purifications,** including extraction, chromatography (gas-liquid, thin-layer), distillation, recrystallization, solvents, and solubility

7. **Spectroscopy and structural identification**

   a. **Infrared region,** including intramolecular vibrations and rotations and absorption trends

   b. **NMR spectroscopy,** including protons in a magnetic field, equivalent protons, and spin–spin splitting

MCAT Scores

MCAT Scores

GENERAL INFORMATION

It is important to understand how MCAT scores are calculated and how they are weighed by medical school admissions committees. In addition, it is critical to understand your rights in controlling the release of these scores. Many students get themselves in trouble because they do not understand the importance of MCAT scores and how to release them to medical schools. This section helps you understand the important aspects of MCAT scoring, the meaning of MCAT scores, and how to release them to your greatest advantage. There is also a brief overview of how medical school admissions committees use MCAT scores for evaluating candidates.

You receive a separate score for each of the four sections of the MCAT. These four scores are always reported to you. If you wish, these scores can also be reported to designated medical schools as well as to your premedical advisor. Keep in mind that medical schools have access to a copy of your Writing Sample essays from the MCAT.

What should you aim for when taking the MCAT? The answer is simple. Aim for the highest score that you can. A good rule of thumb is that **double-digit MCAT scores make most students competitive for medical school.** A score of 10 or above in each section of the MCAT is high enough to allow most applicants to favorably compete in medical school admissions. Students with a lower-end grade point average (GPA) [less than 3.5] frequently need higher MCAT scores. The Verbal Reasoning section of the MCAT has become particularly difficult; thus, some applicants get by with a score of 9 in the Verbal Reasoning section if their Physical Sciences and Biological Sciences scores are particularly high.

IMPLICATIONS OF MCAT SCORES

MCAT scores should validate a good GPA. If you have good grades, your MCAT scores should be consistent with them. A mediocre MCAT performance may cast doubt on the validity of a high GPA. The admissions committee may believe that your grades are inflated or that the college you attended may have distributed high grades indiscriminately.

MCAT scores should suggest that your abilities are even better than your GPA reflects. If your GPA is below 3.5, there are many medical school applicants who will have better grades than you. You can increase your chances of admissions to medical school by making up for lower grades with high MCAT scores. For example, if you have a 3.3 GPA, a strong performance on the MCAT might show an admissions committee that you have good potential, and that perhaps your grades reflect the diversity of activities you were involved in as a college student (e.g., work, research, volunteer work).

MCAT scores should never cast doubt on your true abilities. If you have good grades, do not take the MCAT for granted. You are expected to perform at the same high level that you did in college. Do not take the MCAT without intensive preparation and serious studying.

HOW THE VERBAL REASONING, PHYSICAL SCIENCES, AND BIOLOGICAL SCIENCES SECTIONS ARE SCORED

In the Verbal Reasoning, Physical Sciences, and Biological Sciences sections, the number of correct answers determines your raw score. The MCAT graders convert your raw scores to scaled scores. The scaled scores used for reporting MCAT results theoretically range from the lowest score of 1 to the highest score of 15. Sometimes, when student scores are not well distributed, the MCAT grading center may limit score distribution to a smaller range. For example, on some Verbal Reasoning tests, a scale of 1–13 has been used.

When your MCAT scores arrive in the mail, you will see a numerical score, usually ranging from 1–15, for the Verbal Reasoning, Physical Sciences, and Biological Sciences sections. **A score of 8 in each of these sections is the approximate national mean.**

Keep in mind that the Verbal Reasoning, Physical Sciences, and Biological Sciences sections are scored by evaluating a bell-shaped curve of student performance. MCAT scores are not based on a simple arithmetic scale. In other words, an MCAT score of a 12 does not mean that you did poorly because you did not score a 15. An MCAT score of a 12 is an outstanding score, and it places a student in the top three percentile nationally.

Every 2 points above or below a score of 8 represents one standard deviation. For those of you not familiar with statistics, two thirds of students taking the test will fall between one standard deviation above and below the mean (**score of 8**). Thus, earning a score of 10 or above on an MCAT section places you approximately in the top twentieth percentile nationally. A score of **10 or above is known as a double-digit MCAT score.**

Ninety-five percent of students taking the test will fall between two standard deviations above and below the mean. Thus, a scaled score of 12 results in a top three percentile performance. An MCAT score of 15 in a section is a rare and exceptional score; only about 0.1% of students taking the test will score a 15. Because more than 60,000 students take the MCAT each year, approximately 60 students earn a score of 15 on any one section of the MCAT.

Figure C-1 shows a graph of typical curves for these three MCAT sections. Notice that the majority of students score a few points above and below an 8. As you look at MCAT scores of 10 and above, you can see that fewer students achieve these higher scores. Notice that the most common score given is an 8, which is an average score; for many students, a score of 8 is not high enough to make them competitive for medical school admissions.

FIGURE C-1.

Typical score distribution of the Verbal Reasoning, Physical Sciences, and Biological Sciences sections of the MCAT.

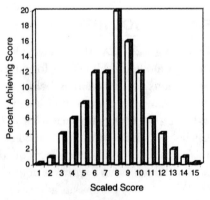

Figure C-1.

HOW THE WRITING SAMPLE IS SCORED

Figure C-2 shows the distribution of Writing Sample scores. To understand this graph, you need to understand how raw scores are determined. Your raw score on the Writing Sample is determined by two graders who assign each of your essays a score from 1 (lowest) to 6 (highest). The raw scores of your two essays are totalled, and this total number is converted to an alphabetic scale ranging from J (lowest) to T (highest).

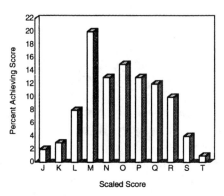

Figure C-2.

FIGURE C-2.
Typical score distribution of the Writing Sample section of the MCAT.

The same alphabetic score can result from different combinations of individual scores. For example, if you score a 4 and a 4 on the first essay, and a 4 and a 3 on the second essay, your total raw score is a 15. This raw score is assigned the same alphabetic score as if you had scored a 6 and a 5 on the first essay and a 2 and a 2 on the second essay. In both cases, the raw score is 15. A numerical score of 12–15 is in the average range and would probably earn you a letter score of N or O. As a general rule, **the letter score of N or O has been the national mean on the Writing Sample section.**

RELEASING YOUR MCAT SCORES

GENERAL INFORMATION

When you fill out the application to take the MCAT, you will be asked several questions. First, **the form will ask if you want your MCAT scores released to your premedical advisor.** If you say yes, a score report will be forwarded to the premedical advisor at your undergraduate institution. **Reporting your scores to your premedical advisor does not affect your application to medical school.** It is your decision whether or not to share your MCAT scores with your premedical advisor. Many students elect to tell their advisor about their MCAT scores verbally, and some students do not have active contact with an advisor.

You must not confuse the release of MCAT scores to your premedical advisor with the release of MCAT scores to medical schools. The MCAT application form **also asks whether or not you wish to release your MCAT scores to AAMC participating medical schools.** This is a critical question, and one that you must understand.

First, **you must decide to release or not release MCAT scores prior to taking the MCAT.** If you indicate that you wish to release your MCAT scores to medical schools, and complete the MCAT, the MCAT score you earn will be a part of your permanent record. In other words, **once you decide to release your scores, there is no way to eliminate this MCAT score from your record.**

When you apply to medical school, the AAMC will report all MCAT scores that you have agreed to release prior to each MCAT administration. For example, suppose you took the MCAT for the first time, released the scores, and did poorly on the test. You then retook the exam (having studied intensively and having released your scores) and did well on the test. When you apply to medical school, both MCAT scores are reported. The score you received the first time will not help you get into medical school!

If you indicate that you do not wish to release your MCAT scores to medical schools, your MCAT scores will only be sent to you. If you are satisfied with your scores, you can contact the AAMC and have the scores released. This is a great policy, because it allows you to preview your MCAT scores before deciding whether or not to release them to medical schools. If you wish to release your MCAT scores after receiving them in the mail, you can write or fax a letter to the AAMC requesting score release. It takes the AAMC about 4–6 weeks to process your request.

ADVICE FROM COLUMBIA REVIEW REGARDING THE RELEASE OF MCAT SCORES

Never take the MCAT for practice. The MCAT is not a test to underestimate. The MCAT is difficult. You are taking a great risk if you "check-out" the test without intensive preparation. Furthermore, **you can only take the MCAT three times.** You must petition the AAMC if you want to take the MCAT a fourth time. There are three released "real" MCAT tests available from the AAMC, and in this book, there is a fourth test with predictive MCAT scoring. Thus, you should only practice on released AAMC "real" MCATs or simulated full-length tests with accurate predictive scoring (similar to the sample MCAT in this book).

If you are taking the April MCAT, or taking the MCAT one year before you apply to medical school, we advise that you do not release your scores before seeing your results. Although it requires 4–6 weeks to release your scores after previewing them, this does not significantly slow down evaluation of your application to medical school. There is no disadvantage to seeing your MCAT scores before releasing them. Actually, this approach is strategic. If you do not release your scores and find that the MCAT did not go as well as you would have liked, you may retake the test and only have the second set of MCAT scores sent to the medical schools. Each MCAT has an independent score release. In other words, if you have taken the MCAT twice and withheld your scores on each of these tests, you can release the results of one test and not the other.

If you are taking the August MCAT and applying to medical school that same summer, we advise that you release your MCAT scores. It takes about 8 weeks after the test to receive your MCAT scores. Thus, August MCAT results come out at the end of October. If you did not release your scores, you have to contact the AAMC to release them (allowing 4–6 weeks for this release to be processed and for scores to reach the medical schools you are applying to). By this time, it may be as late as December and holiday season. Admissions committees may be on break, and your application may sit under the Christmas tree until after New Years! If you do not release your MCAT scores from an August MCAT the same summer you are applying to medical school, it greatly slows evaluation of your application and decreases your chances of getting admitted to medical school. If you do not release your scores at all, your application cannot be considered because the admissions committees will not have an MCAT score for their evaluation process.

ADDITIONAL CRITICAL INFORMATION ABOUT MCAT SCORES

Medical schools are told how many times you have attempted the MCAT. Schools are told the number of MCATs taken and given any of the scores that you have released. Thus, if you take the MCAT and never release the score, the medical schools still know that you have taken the test. This is not a serious problem, but you may be asked about the non-released MCAT scores in a medical school interview (which is another reason *not* to take the MCAT for practice).

Many medical schools average your released MCAT scores, while some schools only look at the most recent score. Most medical schools will not freely disclose their MCAT evaluation policies, so it is difficult for you to know which schools average MCAT scores and which schools only look at the most recent scores. **The majority of medical schools evaluate all MCAT scores on your record.** However, there is at least a subjective effect of a prior MCAT score at all medical schools. Thus, never take the MCAT without being totally prepared.

The Verbal Reasoning section of the MCAT is becoming more important. Some admissions committees heavily weigh the Verbal Reasoning section of the MCAT when evaluating an applicant. For example, the current admissions committee at a prestigious medical school in California believes that the Verbal Reasoning section is the most important section of the MCAT. To the surprise of many students, this committee weighs the MCAT Verbal Reasoning section more heavily than the science sections.

Admissions committees know that the grading of the Writing Sample is the most variable of all four sections. A copy of the essays that you write on the MCAT will be forwarded to the medical schools.

WHAT ADMISSIONS COMMITTEES DO WITH MCAT SCORES

As an applicant to medical school, MCAT scores are critical to your evaluation for admission. Because applicants are from all across the country and from hundreds of different undergraduate institutions, the MCAT provides a means for admissions committees to compare all applicants with a common measurement.

Most admissions committees use your MCAT scores and GPA in formulas, determining a total point value for you. Because there are often thousands of applicants to a medical school, a quantitative measurement of an applicant makes it easier for an admissions committee to rank an applicant. Some of the formulas used by medical schools link your science GPA with the science sections of the MCAT, and your nonscience or overall GPA may be linked with your Verbal Reasoning score. Each medical school uses a different system, but many schools **link your MCAT scores in a multiplicative way with your GPA,** which has very important implications. As you know, it is very difficult to raise your GPA to a significant degree in a short period of time. However, you can significantly raise your MCAT scores (and hence raise your "total points" on your admissions analysis) with intensive MCAT preparation over a short period of time. The importance of the MCAT cannot be stressed enough.

Based on a Columbia Review survey of United States medical schools, there are three factors that most admissions committees consider when evaluating applicants:

1. **GPA,** which accounts for about **40%** of your overall evaluation at many medical schools

2. **MCAT** scores, which account for about **30%** of your overall evaluation at many medical schools

3. **Other factors (e.g., personal statements, letters of recommendation, secondary application, interview, background),** which account for about **30%** of overall evaluation at many medical schools

Each of these categories carries a weight in your overall evaluation. Many medical schools assign the GPA a little more weight than the MCAT scores and other factors; however, the importance of the MCAT is clear. Because the background of applicants vary greatly, the MCAT offers the admissions committees a way to compare you with other premedical students. Make sure that you do well on the MCAT, so that you compare favorably with other applicants.

How to Study for the MCAT:
Basic Strategies

Overview

The MCAT is not a test of memorization. It is a test of reading comprehension, reasoning, and the application of science to problem solving. As you begin your MCAT preparation, there are some basic strategies that you should keep in mind. This section covers basic study strategies for the MCAT as well as specific, helpful test-taking strategies. Strategies for solving science passages are discussed in the last section of the introductory material (see Section I, Part E: Strategies for Solving MCAT Science Passages). Section IV: Preparation for Verbal Reasoning and the Writing Sample discusses specific strategies for those MCAT sections.

Before discussing specific strategies, the importance of relaxation cannot be overemphasized. **Relaxation is a key to success on the MCAT.** If you are too nervous, you will not be able to concentrate. It is normal to be moderately nervous about the MCAT. In fact, a reasonable amount of anxiety may increase your concentration and performance. However, it is important to control this anxiety and nervousness. You can control anxiety by keeping in mind that **relaxation comes with confidence.** If you have thoroughly prepared for the MCAT and worked harder than your competitors, you will be confident and relaxed. You must know the material well and be able to solve MCAT-style passages quickly and correctly.

The Basic Strategies

The key to mastering the material on the MCAT is to use three basic steps whenever you study: **preview, view,** and **review.** You will also use these basic steps when you actually take the MCAT.

THE PREVIEW STRATEGY

When you preview, you **skim and survey the material that you are going to study.** This first step requires very little time, yet provides a big return. Previewing allows you to make mental pictures of the information in a chapter or an MCAT passage. By understanding the organization of the material that you are studying or reading, you can focus on the difficult areas when you go through the material more carefully.

PREVIEWING WHEN STUDYING

When you are preparing for the MCAT, use the previewing strategy to skim the chapter(s) that you are studying. Some parts of a chapter may be easy for you because you are familiar with the material; these sections are not worth too much study time. Other parts of a chapter may be more difficult because either you never understood the material or it is unfamiliar to you. Previewing helps you designate and prioritize your study time.

PREVIEWING WHEN TAKING THE MCAT

You can use the previewing strategy successfully when you are taking the MCAT. The previewing strategy is great for planning your time use. For each section of the exam, quickly skim to see how many passages are on the science tests and the Verbal Reasoning test. Although the test has been consistent over the last several years with the number of passages per section, double-checking the number of passages can help you prevent disaster. For example, on the Verbal Reasoning test, quickly look to double-check that there are 9 passages. Because you have 85 minutes to complete this section, dividing 85 minutes by 9 passages leaves you with about 9 minutes per passage (with 4 minutes left over to check your work or finish a passage that was difficult for you). If you think previewing and time management are a waste of time, you are wrong! The biggest mistake that you can make on the MCAT is misjudging your time and not completing the test.

THE VIEWING STRATEGY

VIEWING WHEN STUDYING

After previewing, you must read through the material carefully, focusing on understanding the material. This process is time-consuming but very important. Comprehension is essential for maximizing the benefits of this step. As you probably know, it is very difficult to learn and recall material that you do not understand. Do not move on from one topic to the next unless you understand the material. The viewing step is the time to become compulsive and to strive for conceptual understanding of MCAT topics. Ask for help if you do not understand an area of study.

Condensation and integration of MCAT science topics are important strategies to know. Basically, this technique requires that you **go through MCAT review notes, college class notes, and reference books, and then recopy key MCAT information into a summary or outline format.** The science review notes in this book are very thorough and intensive, and they provide a basic information source. Creating condensed notes from the science review notes in this book and your college class notes is probably one of the best strategies for dealing with the overwhelming information pool in MCAT preparation.

Condensed review notes are important because (1) they provide you with an active learning process during the creation of the notes, (2) they allow you to assimilate and think about MCAT material, and (3) they provide a single, high-quality source of information in your own writing. The time-consuming part of this strategy is the preparation of quality notes. However, once you become skilled at making condensed notes, you can make them quickly and efficiently.

VIEWING WHEN TAKING THE MCAT

During the MCAT, you can use the viewing strategy to answer questions strategically. Remember that there is no penalty for guessing on the MCAT. When approaching a series of MCAT questions following a passage, address the easiest questions first or work the easiest problems first. Then, go back and answer the tougher questions and problems later (after you have answered all of the easier questions in that passage). **This approach is strategic because it gives you extra time to think about the difficult questions.** Also, **use brainstorming techniques to help figure out the hard questions.** For example, if you are asked to calculate the force on a particle, jot down all the expressions that you know which allow you to calculate force (e.g., $F = ma$, $F = qvB$). Having these expressions to look at may give you ideas for approaching or solving the problem. Remember, do not move on to the next passage without finally answering every question in the passage you are working on.

THE REVIEWING STRATEGY

REVIEWING WHEN STUDYING

When reviewing, **go over the material repetitively during your study time,** attempting to move the information that you are studying into your long-term memory. The following are some specific strategies for reviewing material during your preparation for the MCAT.

1. **Always review your weakest subject first.** Although you would probably like to put off studying the subject in which you feel least confident, your weakest subject should be attacked first. For example, if organic chemistry is a problem area, start studying organic chemistry first. Most likely, your weakness becomes a strength, because you have invested a considerable amount of extra time to relearn and review the material.

2. **Know your learning style.** You already know what study techniques work best for you. If you are a visual learner, create review notes in your own writing. These notes will be easy for you to visualize when you are trying to recall information. If you are a verbal learner, you may benefit most from attending review lectures that cover MCAT material. Use the techniques that worked for you in courses that you aced in college. Preparing for the MCAT is not the time to try new, unfamiliar study techniques.

3. **Use condensed notes and summary sheets to review material.** You may benefit from recopying key information contained in this book in your own writing. This process allows you to (1) think about the material when you initially compose condensed notes, (2) understand the material as you summarize it in written form, and (3) commit the material to memory as you continually skim over the material. When using condensed notes to review, you can go over material quickly and efficiently. Remember to be selective about what you put in the notes; try to concentrate on material that you are not familiar with or have trouble remembering.

4. **Do frequent, brief reviews.** Research clearly shows that students retain material most effectively when they do frequent, brief reviews. This process is more effective than infrequent, long reviews. You are better off studying for 2–3 hours at a time twice daily than studying 5–6 hours once daily.

5. **Use memory tricks when you review.** Experts have shown that you can lock something into your memory if you study it hard and recite it verbally. This process allows you to both *see* the material and *hear* the material, which better accesses the information into your long-term memory. Also, try to create mental pictures of the material.

6. **Use mnemonics when you study.** This strategy helps you recall the identity and relationships between items. For example, the mnemonic *AN OX, RED CAT* helps you remember key concepts from electrochemistry. *AN OX, RED CAT* means **ox**idation occurs at the **an**ode and involves the **an**ion, while **red**uction occurs at the **cat**hode and involves the **cat**ion. Look at all the infor-

mation you can recall with an easy-to-learn mnemonic!

ADDITIONAL TIPS FOR STUDYING

1. **Study at least 20 hours per week.** At Columbia Review, we have conducted informal surveys of premedical students. Students who study at least 20 hours per week do better on the MCAT than students who study less than 20 hours a week. Students who study *more* than 20 hours per week may still do better on the MCAT; however, the return is not as great proportionally. Remember, at a minimum, you must try to study at least 3–4 hours daily. If you skip 1 day, make up the lost time on another day. If you are remedial in one or more subject areas, you may need to allow yourself more study time per week. There are no excuses for putting in less than 100% effort!

2. **Create a study calendar.** MCAT success and getting into medical school must be priorities in your life. You must find time every day to study and practice MCAT-style passages. You can maintain balance in your life by scheduling in some time for relaxation, family, work, and school. Create a daily calendar and place your study periods on your daily schedule. You should begin scheduling your study periods at least 3–4 months before taking the MCAT.

3. **You must have a positive attitude when studying for the MCAT.** A positive attitude leads to constructive study periods. Tackling your weakest area first builds your confidence as the test draws near. Do not dwell on practice questions that you answer incorrectly. Learn from your mistakes and think about positive ways to avoid making the same mistakes on the actual MCAT.

4. **Never cram the night before the MCAT.** You should stop studying for the MCAT by early afternoon on the day before the test. Spend the later afternoon and evening relaxing. Go to a movie, hang out with friends, and get a good night's sleep. Whatever trivia you try to cram in the night before the test is unlikely to be of any value. Remember that the MCAT is a thinking and applications test. You are unlikely to be asked trivial questions. If you are stressed-out and tired on the day of the test, you may score lower than if you had relaxed the night before the test.

5. **Take as many practice tests as you can.** The best way to become skilled at solving MCAT passages is to practice as many MCAT questions as possible. You may want to take a preparation course to obtain more practice material. Columbia Review has both home study material and a live, intensive MCAT preparation course for your use if you feel you need them.

ADDITIONAL TIPS FOR TAKING THE MCAT

To perform well on the MCAT, you must have a good understanding of multiple-choice questions. Keep in mind the following strategies when taking the MCAT.

1. **Answer every question.** There is no penalty for guessing, so always answer every question.

2. **Look for questions containing qualifying words.** Qualifying words give you clues to what are the likely answers. Examples of qualifying words include *best*, *most likely*, *least*, and so on. Qualifying words are discussed in some detail in later sections of this book.

3. **Questions are not arranged by the level of difficulty.** The Scholastic Aptitude Test (SAT) is arranged by level of difficulty, but the MCAT is not arranged in this manner. Thus, there is no strategy for random guessing based on the position of the question (i.e., appearing at the beginning or the end of the test) on

the test.

4. **Look for absolute statements in the answer choices to multiple-choice questions.** Absolute statements are often answer choices that you may easily eliminate. As a general observation, absolute statements regarding MCAT passages are more likely incorrect than correct. These statements are frequently overgeneralizations and usually contain words such as *always, never, must,* and so on.

5. **Use the process of elimination on every question to arrive at the most likely answer.** Remember that there may be several correct statements as answer choices to a question, yet only one of the choices is the *best* choice. Select the best statement or choice for each question. It is a mistake to be impulsive by quickly choosing the first correct statement.

6. **Always use common sense.** Although this advice may seem obvious, under the stress of the MCAT and the difficulty of some of the passages, many students lose sight of basic common sense. If you know the material and seem to understand a passage, an answer choice that seems the most logical is probably correct.

7. **Transfer answers to the answer sheet in blocks after completing each passage.** It is better to transfer answers in groups after solving each passage than transferring each answer independently. Group answer transfer saves about 15 seconds per passage. This timesaving technique translates into several minutes over the course of one subtest. You may need every minute that you have. In addition, transferring answers in groups decreases the risk of accidentally misnumbering your answers.

8. **Test timing is a key to success.** Keep in mind that you have about 9 minutes for each Verbal Reasoning passage and about 8 minutes for each science passage. Bring a wristwatch that has a stopwatch mode with you to the MCAT. After completing 3 passages or so, check the elapsed time. These checks allow you to make timing adjustments as you are taking the MCAT, and it helps prevent you from not completing the test.

Strategies for Solving MCAT Science Passages

Introduction

Passage-based questions comprise 80% of the questions asked on the Physical Sciences and Biological Sciences sections of the MCAT. Remember that there are **77 questions total on each of these two sections,** 62 of which are based on passages. The remaining 20% of questions (15 questions) are independent, single-item multiple-choice questions. These questions are usually much easier to answer because they are less involved, more straightforward, and usually not based on data analysis.

These strategies for solving MCAT science passages present valuable information for improving your ability to tackle MCAT passages. It is highly recommended that you read this section several times, mastering the information presented and practicing these strategies on MCAT passages included in this book and on practice MCAT tests. Your goal is to learn to think like the people who write MCAT passages and questions. Familiarize yourself with the passage types, question types, and steps to follow in approaching passages.

Who writes MCAT passages? Believe it or not, basic science college instructors and professors write MCAT passages and questions. These test writers are biologists, chemists, and physicists, not M.D.s. It is important to understand where the test writers are coming from because it helps you understand their thought patterns.

As you are studying for the MCAT, do not spend too much time memorizing trivia. Important information you need to know for the MCAT is included in this book; however, being familiar with and understanding the material are more important than just memorizing the material. You must have a good knowledge base to answer questions; however, after efficiently reviewing a science, you should quickly move on to practicing passages.

We suggest budgeting at least as much time solving passage problems in a science as you spend reviewing that science. For example, if you spend 30 hours carefully reviewing physics, try to spend 30 hours solving physics passages.

Many of you will need to spend more time solving passages than reviewing. Successfully solving MCAT passages is a skill in itself, and you only get better at passages by practicing them.

Science Passages: Structure and Type

The Physical and Biological Sciences sections each contain about 11 passages, which describe a scientific problem. Some passages are fairly lengthy and wordy, especially the biology passages. Strong reading comprehension skills help you to quickly read and understand these wordy passages. You are not expected to have any medical knowledge, but you are expected to have a good knowledge of science. All of the information that you need to answer the question is either presented in the passage or is basic science information that you are responsible for and should know. Passages usually contain the following elements:

- 200–300 words of descriptive information
- A graph or table presenting data
- Statements presenting results of experiments or data
- A figure or experimental apparatus

There are four types of passages in the Physical and Biological Sciences sections of the MCAT:

- Information presentation passages
- Problem-solving passages
- Research study passages
- Persuasive argument passages

Information presentation passages look like textbook chapters or journal articles. These passages often contain new information of which you are not expected to have previous knowledge. These passages do not require you to have background knowledge in basic science. The questions that accompany the passages test your understanding and evaluation of the passages and test your ability to manipulate the information to solve problems.

Problem-solving passages present problems in science (physics, general chemistry, biology, and organic chemistry). Questions that accompany these passages require you to determine the probable causes of situations, events, or phenomena described. In addition, you are required to select appropriate methods for solving the problems.

Research study passages provide you with the rationale, method, and results of research projects. The questions that accompany these passages require you to interpret and understand the projects that are described. Data in the form of graphs and tables are often present.

Persuasive argument passages present you with two viewpoints on a particular topic. The passages may express single viewpoints or two opposing viewpoints. The questions that accompany these passages test your understanding of the arguments presented in the passages and require you to evaluate the validity of the arguments. This passage type is the least common type appearing on the MCAT.

Types of Questions

There are six types of questions that follow MCAT science passages:

- Information recall
- Data interpretation
- Simple calculation
- Conceptual understanding
- Application
- Evaluation

You should master this list of question types. Knowing the types of questions gives you a strategic advantage for approaching the questions. After you learn to recognize specific types of questions, you can save valuable time and be more efficient in solving them.

Information recall questions can be answered by drawing information directly from the passage. Believe it or not, many of these questions can be answered even if you do not have knowledge of the science on which the passage is based. The test writers are testing your ability to find information that is "buried" in a passage. These questions look very similar to the questions on the Verbal Reasoning section of the MCAT.

Data interpretation questions test your ability to interpret graphs, tables, and figures and to make sense of the data presented in them. These questions are common on the MCAT. Most premedical students have difficulty answering this type of question. People who have more experience with research and reading scientific papers are usually better at answering this type of question. If data interpretation is a weakness for you, focus on practicing with every passage you can get your hands on.

Simple calculation questions require that you work quickly and accurately with numbers. Strong math and analytical skills are required if you want to answer these questions correctly. Remember, no calculators are allowed when taking the MCAT.

Conceptual understanding questions test your understanding of basic scientific principles and are among the most common types of questions in the science sections.

Application questions require you to apply concepts or principles that you are supposed to know, or that are provided in a passage. You may be asked to apply the new idea or concept to a new situation. These questions test your ability to think flexibly and creatively.

Evaluation questions require you to evaluate arguments and information provided. You may be asked to draw conclusions from data or evaluate whether specific conclusions are justified. This type of question is usually linked to experimental data from which you are expected to be able to draw conclusions.

Strategies for Solving Science Passages

The MCAT experts at Columbia Review have carefully evaluated MCAT science passages and studied the best ways to approach them. We have arrived at what most students find to be an effective, strategic technique for passage solving.

First, keep in mind timing. We suggest that you spend the 8 minutes on any passage with this approximate breakdown:

1. Previewing for 30 seconds
2. Reading for 2 minutes
3. Answering questions for 5–5½ minutes

Second, keep in mind that any single MCAT question should take 1 minute or less to solve. If a question appears very difficult or time-consuming, it usually means that you do not know how to approach the question or you are not approaching the question correctly. Stop for a moment and rethink your approach.

Another basic rule to remember is that most MCAT questions that require a formula to solve a question only require the use of one formula. It is unusual to need multiple different formulas to solve a problem. Keep in mind that the test writers design questions to be answered in a minute or less; this fact will help you realize that the questions generally are not overly sophisticated and complex.

The Columbia Review Six-Step MCAT Attack Method (Step-by-Step Approach for Solving MCAT Science Passages)

STEP 1

Quickly read the question stems of each multiple-choice question following the passage (15 seconds). This strategy allows you to see exactly what is asked before you even read the passage. After skimming the question, you can focus on important information in the passages and find answers as you read.

STEP 2

Quickly look at any graph, table, or figure presented in the passage (15 seconds). If the author of the passage took the time to create a table or graph, you can predict that it is important. In addition, studies have shown that looking at a graphic representation of data more than once improves overall understanding and retention of information. A 15-second preview followed by a longer, more formal evaluation of the graph, table, or figure as you are reading the passage provides you with two opportunities to master the data presented.

STEP 3

Read the passage (2 minutes). **As you are reading, think about what type of passage it is and decide if the information presented is data, opinion, or fact.** Also, ask yourself if the passage is information presentation, problem solving, research study, or persuasive argument. Having a "feel" for the passage type gives you an idea as to the tone of the likely answers. Constantly ask yourself why the test writers provided the given information. If the information is data, think about its significance. If an opinion is presented, ask yourself if it is supported by the passage or data. Be sensitive to the tone of the passage. If a fact is given, ask yourself if it is questionable, or if it is contradicted by the passage.

STEP 4

Identify important points, formulas, and data. Underline, circle, and make notes in the margins any time you come across important points, formulas, or data. You should have an idea of what is important because you have already read the question stems. Following are some general rules about important points, formulas, and data.

- **Many of the formulas given in a passage are needed to answer the questions that follow the passage.** If you see a formula in a passage, circle it or rewrite it in the margin.

- **Any quantitative relationship you see spelled out in words should be written in symbols in the margin.** Many students read right over these relationships unless they write them out and put them in the margin. For example, suppose an MCAT physics passage stated: "The force experienced by a particle is equal to the product of the charge of the particle, the velocity of the particle, and the magnitude of the magnetic field that the particle is in." What would you do with this statement? You should write the relationship as a formula in the margin of the passage, so that you remember it and are ready to use it. You could write the statement like this: $F = qvB$.

- **You will frequently see the answers to information recall questions given in the text of a passage.** Underline or circle this information.

STEP 5

Begin answering questions. Always think about the type of question you are being asked. Thinking about question types can help you solve questions; it helps direct your time and effort effectively. Try to identify where in the passage a particular idea was developed. If possible, use associative reasoning to link various parts of the passage to various questions.

Also, remember that working backward is helpful for answering questions. Frequently you are asked a question that you really do not know how to answer. You can plug the choices back into the question and determine which choice fits the best. This strategy can help you identify correct answers.

STEP 6

Always arrive at an answer to a question by eliminating three choices. Always use the process of elimination. Even if you think you know the answer, eliminate the other choices before choosing an answer. There are only four choices for each question. If you eliminate a few choices, you have a much better chance of answering the question correctly.

Eliminate a choice if it violates the concept presented, tone of the passage, information given, basic principles, and so on. Also, you can eliminate choices that violate common sense or seem extreme. You may be able to eliminate choices that are simple manipulations of the numbers given in a problem. The test writers frequently write answer choices like this to attract test takers who do not know or understand the material.

For calculation questions, be mindful of units. Looking at the units of the answer choices can frequently help you work backward to solve the problem and eliminate answer choices.

Sample Passages with Strategic Analysis

The best way to understand the strategies presented in this section is to see application of these strategies to sample passages. The following biology and physics passages are very similar to recent MCAT passages, and they are followed by a detailed strategic analysis and discussion. First, read the passage; then, follow the step-by-step strategic approach.

EXAMPLE 1

A RECENTLY STUDIED genetic disorder in humans, named by research scientists Syndrome X, has been characterized by a range of birth defects. Children born with this disorder appear abnormal at birth, demonstrating syndactyly (webbing of the fingers), exophthalmos (protruding eyes), hypertelorism (eyes too far apart), and hypoplastic midface (small midfacial region). In addition, the skulls of children with Syndrome X do not develop normally, because the skull sutures fuse prematurely. Because of this fusion, the head grows into an abnormal shape. As a child with Syndrome X reaches several months of age, an obvious developmental delay is noted, because the normal developmental milestones are not reached. Many of these children are soon determined to be mentally retarded.

The mechanism for Syndrome X has been recently studied. Researchers have evaluated the chromosomes and genes of patients with this disorder. It has been found that one of the genes coding for a cell surface receptor found on all cells in the body demonstrates a mutation. This cell surface receptor is responsible for the binding of peptide molecules called growth factors, and is termed the growth factor receptor, or GFR. There is a family of similar, but distinct GFRs on each cell, so that a large variety of growth factors may each specifically bind to cellular receptors. Presence of the mutation makes it such that a specific growth factor does not bind to its receptor, and hence, cellular growth is affected. Growth factors are believed to affect cellular growth by binding to their receptors and stimulating an adenylate cyclase mechanism.

In a study conducted by researchers, two experiments were performed.

EXPERIMENT 1

The skull bones from patients with Syndrome X were studied. Researchers evaluated both fused and unfused skull bones from Syndrome X patients, and unfused skull bones from normal children. The level of GFRs in the skull bones was determined and is shown in Table 1.

more ▼

TABLE 1. Skull Bone Fusion and GFR Levels in Patients With and Without Syndrome X

Patient Group	Skull Bone	GFR Level (counts/mm^2)
Syndrome X	Fused	102*
Syndrome X	Unfused	156†
Normal	Unfused	234

*Significant decrease in GFR level from that of both Syndrome X (unfused) patients and normal patients.
†Significant decrease in GFR level from that of normal patients.
GFR = growth factor receptor.

EXPERIMENT 2

The hand skin from patients with Syndrome X was studied. Researchers evaluated both hand skin from webbed hands of Syndrome X patients and hand skin from children without Syndrome X with no webbing of the hands. The level of GFRs in the hand skin of patients was determined and is shown in Table 2.

TABLE 2. Hand Skin Webbing and GFR Levels in Patients With and Without Syndrome X

Patient Group	Hand Skin	GFR Level (counts/mm^2)
Syndrome X	Webbing	64*
Syndrome X	No Webbing	110†
Normal	No Webbing	189

*Significant decrease in GFR level from that of both Syndrome X (no webbing) patients and normal patients.
†Significant decrease in GFR level from that of normal patients.
GFR = growth factor receptor.

1. Which of the following terms best describes the abnormal development associated with Syndrome X?

    A. Differentiation

    B. Induction

    C. Morphogenesis

    D. Determination

2. According to the passage, the mutation associated with Syndrome X best affects:

    A. the DNA sequence at the chromosomal level, giving rise to variations in chromosomal number and function.

    B. the DNA sequence at the level of the gene coding for the growth factor.

    C. the gene coding for all cell surface receptors giving rise to cellular growth.

    D. the gene coding for a specific cell surface receptor.

3. Based on the data presented in the passage, which of the following statements is best supported?

more ▼

A. Patients with Syndrome X with skull fusion have significantly decreased levels of GFRs compared with patients with Syndrome X with unfused skulls or normal patients.

B. Patients with Syndrome X and unwebbed hands have significantly decreased levels of GFRs compared with patients with Syndrome X with webbed hands or normal patients.

C. Patients with Syndrome X with fused skulls have significantly decreased levels of GFRs compared with patients with Syndrome X with unfused skulls or patients with Syndrome X with webbed hands.

D. Patients without Syndrome X (normal patients) have significantly greater GFRs in body tissues than patients with Syndrome X.

4. What is the most likely mechanism by which the mutation causing Syndrome X acts?

A. The mutation causes a change in the primary sequence of the growth factor.

B. The mutation is most likely a nonsense mutation of the growth factor receptor (GFR) gene.

C. The mutation likely ultimately leads to the nonformation of the growth factor.

D. The mutation likely alters the three-dimensional conformation of the growth factor receptor.

5. Which of the following is the best explanation of the mechanism by which growth factors stimulate cellular growth?

A. The growth factor diffuses into the nucleus, where it binds its receptor and influences transcription.

B. The growth factor binds a receptor on the cell surface, stimulating a second messenger system within the cell.

C. The growth factor binds a receptor on the cell surface, and the complex moves into the cell, ultimately moving into the nucleus where transcription is affected.

D. The growth factors are direct stimulants of mitosis.

6. Which of the following statements is best supported by the information and data provided in the passage?

A. Both experiments suggest that there may be variable expression of the mutation causing Syndrome X.

B. Syndrome X is a common cause of skull fusion and webbing of the hands.

C. The mutation associated with Syndrome X is expressed in all cells of the body.

D. Syndrome X is caused by a rare mutation, and there is no data to analyze the expression of this mutation.

7. A man with Syndrome X marries a woman who does not have the mutation that causes Syndrome X. They have a daughter who has Syndrome X. Which of the following statements is correct?

I.   Autosomal dominant transmission is possible.

II. Autosomal recessive transmission is possible.

III. Sex-linked recessive transmission is possible.

    A.   I only

    B.   I and II only

    C.   II and III only

    D.   I, II, and III

Analysis and Discussion of Strategies for Example I

This is a research study passage in the Biological Sciences (biology) section. The information you need to answer the questions comes from the material in the passage, the data tables, and your understanding of biology concepts.

The Columbia Six-Step MCAT Attack Method discussed in this section is the best way to solve MCAT science passages. These steps are reviewed and discussed.

STEP I

Quickly read the question stems of each of the seven questions following the passage (15 seconds). Remember that the purpose of question stem skimming is to know what important information to recognize when reading the passage. Do not read the answer choices, because you will deal with them later. At this step, all you want is an overview of the questions that will be asked. The following is what you should extract from the question stems:

Question 1: Which term describes the development associated with Syndrome X? When you read the passage, think about what Syndrome X does to the individual.

Question 2: Look for what the mutation affects at the genetic level.

Question 3: Conclusions from data given in the passage are needed. This question lets you know that you must understand the data tables given in the passage.

Question 4: Look for how the mutation works.

Question 5: Look for information on how growth factors cause cellular growth.

Question 6: This question requires your having read the passage; it is an information recall question.

Question 7: It appears that all the data you need to answer this question is given. This is a conceptual question, somewhat independent of the passage.

STEP 2

Quickly look at any graph, table, or figure presented in the passage (15 seconds). Quickly look at the two tables given in the passage. This step helps you extract the important relationships that exist between variables and groups. Although you do not know what Syndrome X is at this stage, you can greatly benefit from a quick overview of the tables. By the end of this step, you should be no more than 30 seconds into the passage. The following is information that you should extract:

Table 1: Table 1 in Example 1 shows that the Syndrome X patients with skull fusion have lower growth factor receptor (GFR) levels than Syndrome X patients with unfused skulls or normal patients. It also shows that Syndrome X patients with unfused skulls have lower GFR levels than normal patients.

Table 2: Table 2 in Example 1 shows the same relationships as Table 1, except that skull fusion is replaced by hand skin webbing. Notice the similarities of the trends in both tables. GFR levels are highest in normal patients. Do not worry about details, just understand trends at this stage.

STEP 3

Read the passage (2 minutes). Notice that this passage is a research study passage. Reread the tables after finishing a careful reading of the passage. As you are reading, make sure that you follow Step 4.

STEP 4

Identify important points, formulas, and data. Always remember to underline, circle, and make notes in the margins every time you come across an important point or data that the question stems clued you into. This was the purpose of reading question stems first.

What should you have circled or noted as you were reading?

You should have noted in the margin next to the first paragraph that Syndrome X causes physical birth defects, which was asked about in the first question.

You should look for what the mutation affects at the genetic level. You should have underlined a key sentence in the second paragraph that gives you much of the answer: "It has been found that one of the genes coding for a cell surface receptor found on all cells in the body demonstrates a mutation."

You should have marked an important sentence in the second paragraph: "Presence of the mutation makes it such that a specific growth factor does not bind to its receptor, and hence, cellular growth is affected." This information gives you a clue about what the mutation does to the growth factor, which was asked about in Question 4.

You should have underlined, marked, or circled the last sentence in the second paragraph: "Growth factors are believed to affect cellular growth by binding to their receptors and stimulating an adenylate cyclase mechanism." This key sentence gives you a clue as to how growth factors work, which was asked about in Question 5.

Because several questions require your understanding of the differences among the groups in the experiments, focus on the trends that are repeated and what they mean. Notice that Syndrome X patients always have lower GFR levels than normal patients and that Syndrome X patients with skull fusion or webbed hand skin have lower GFR levels than Syndrome X patients without those findings.

STEP 5

Begin answering questions. Always think about the type of question you are being asked. Look for information recall questions, which have answers provided either directly or indirectly in the passage. You could spend a great deal of time trying to figure these questions out when the answer is printed in the passage! Question 2 is an information recall question, with the answer directly provided in the passage.

STEP 6

Always arrive at the best answer by eliminating three choices. Always use the process of elimination. You may have to work backward and try out each answer choice before determining the best answer. Also, remember that there may be more than one correct answer choice for each question. The only way to determine the best answer choice is to evaluate all the choices carefully. Let's go through each question using the process of elimination.

Answers and Explanations for Example 1

1. **C** This is a conceptual understanding question, which tests your understanding of some of the basic terms in development. These terms are discussed in the Biology Review Notes of this book. Note that the passage described some of the physical birth defects associated with Syndrome X. These are physical defects associated with the morphology of the individual. Morphogenesis is the development of physical structure. Induction (choice B) is the process in which the destiny of one tissue layer is affected by another tissue layer. An example is mesoderm inducing the overlying ectoderm to differentiate into a particular structure. This process is not discussed in the passage, so eliminate choice B. Determination (choice D) is a process in which cells become committed to form one particular cell type (e.g., heart cell, kidney cell, skin cell). This process is not discussed or supported in the passage, so eliminate choice D. Differentiation (choice A) refers to the maturation of cells. Frequently, this maturation is in a step-by-step process, which is not discussed or even implied in the passage; eliminate choice A.

2. **D** This is an information recall question, so look back to your markings in the margin of the passage or to areas that you have underlined or circled. As discussed earlier in this section, you should have marked the key sentences in this second paragraph based on your question stem reading. In the second paragraph of this passage, it is stated that one of the genes coding for a cell surface receptor found on all cells in the body demonstrates a mutation. The paragraph discusses that this cell surface receptor belongs to a family of receptors, each allowing specific binding of growth factors. Based on this information, you can eliminate choice A, because chromosomes are not discussed in the passage. Choice B attempts to confuse you, because it discusses gene coding for the growth factor and not the growth factor receptor (GFR); eliminate choice B. Choice C is incorrect because it discusses all cell surface receptors, whereas the passage refers to a mutation of a gene coding for a specific GFR. By process of elimination, choice D is the best answer.

3. **A** This is a data interpretation question, which requires that you understand the data tables that summarize the experiments. The best way to solve these questions is to work backward and determine which statements are correct. You can eliminate incorrect statements right away. Then see which statement is the best. Choice A is a correct statement because Table 1 shows that patients with Syndrome X and skull fusion have decreased levels of GFRs compared with the other patient groups. This comparison is mentioned in the legend below the table. Do not eliminate choice A. Keep evaluating the other choices to determine if any of them are better than choice A. Choice B is incorrect because the patients with Syndrome X that do not have webbed hands have greater GFR counts than with Syndrome X who have webbed hands; eliminate choice B. Choice C is incorrect because patients with Syndrome X with fused skulls have greater GFR counts than Syndrome X patients with webbed hands. It is also unclear if you can compare the two experiments with one another. Perhaps the experiments were conducted under different conditions. Finally, choice D can be eliminated because there is no data allowing you to make generalizations of this magnitude. The only data presented in this passage refer to skull tissue and hand tissue. Thus, choice A is the best choice.

4. **D** This is a conceptual understanding question, which requires you to utilize information presented in the passage. There is a key sentence from the second paragraph that can get you thinking in the right direction: "Presence of the mutation makes it such that a specific growth factor does not bind to its receptor, and hence, cellular growth is affected." Ask yourself how a mutation can interfere with the binding of a ligand to its receptor. Look at each of the choices

and use your conceptual understanding of biology and the process of elimination. The biology review notes in this book cover these concepts. Choice A is unlikely because the passage states that the mutation affects the gene coding for the growth factor receptor (GFR). Choice B is incorrect because a nonsense mutation creates a new stop codon, resulting in premature termination of a polypeptide chain. Choice C is incorrect because this choice also refers to a change at the level of the growth factor rather than at the level of the receptor. Choice D is the best answer choice because ligand binding to a receptor is dependent on the three-dimensional conformation of the receptor. Even a small mutation affecting the three-dimensional conformation of the receptor will interfere with growth factor binding. Because you know that the first three choices are poor or definitely incorrect, you can be confident that choice D is the best answer.

5. **B** This is a conceptual understanding question based on information presented in the passage. The last sentence of the second paragraph tells you that growth factors are believed to affect cellular growth by binding to receptors and stimulating an adenylate cyclase mechanism. The Biology Review Notes (see Section Three: Preparation for the Biological Sciences) review important ways that substances like growth factors (hormones) ultimately affect cells. Cells that utilize a cell surface receptor generally bind ligands (growth factors) on their surface, and this binding stimulates an adenylate cyclase enzyme which converts adenosine triphosphate (ATP) to cyclic adenosine monophosphate (cAMP). This results in protein kinase stimulation, protein phosphorylation, and multiple physiologic effects, including cellular growth. The cAMP system is known as a "second messenger" system, which choice B accurately describes. Look at the other choices. Choice A describes the way steroid hormones work. Generally, only lipid soluble substances can directly diffuse into a cell. Steroid hormones and thyroid hormones bind receptors in the cell cytoplasm or nucleus. The passage tells you that growth factors are peptides. Choice C is plausible, yet generally speaking, ligand–receptor complexes do not move into the cell. This is not the way the adenylate cyclase mechanism works. You can eliminate choice C because choice B is a better choice. Choice D is not supported by the passage. The passage does not state and does not imply that growth factors directly stimulate anything. Thus, choice B is the best answer to this question.

6. **A** This is an evaluation question, which asks you to evaluate statements and draw conclusions from data in the passage. Solve these questions by working backward and evaluating each choice. Start by looking at choice A. What is meant by variable expression? Recall from the passage that each patient with Syndrome X has a mutation for the growth factor receptor (GFR) gene. Why do some groups of these patients have skull stenosis, webbed hand skin, or both, and other groups of patients do not have these conditions? Perhaps variable expression is the expression of the genetic defect in some patients, but not in others. Evaluate choices B–D. Choice B is a poor choice because you are not given information about the other causes of skull fusion and hand skin webbing. You do not know that Syndrome X is a common cause for these problems. This is an overgeneralized statement, which is common among incorrect answer choices in MCAT passage questions. Choice C is contradicted by the data in the passage, which shows that some patients with Syndrome X do not express certain classic features (skull stenosis and webbing of the hands). Choice D is incorrect because the data tables provide you the data for evaluation.

7. **A** This is a conceptual understanding question that appears to be independent of the passage. These question types frequently appear on the MCAT. They are usually given when the test writer begins running out of things to ask about! To answer this question, you must know basic MCAT-level genetics. See the biol-

ogy review notes in this book for a review. Basically, a man with Syndrome X who marries a woman who does not possess the defective gene can only have a daughter with the condition if the trait is autosomal dominant. An autosomal recessive transmission would lead to the production of carrier children, but no children expressing the condition. If a sex-linked transmission occurred, all of the daughters would be carriers, and all the sons would be normal noncarriers. No expression of the trait would be seen. Thus, only statement I is true, and the best answer is A.

EXAMPLE 2

THE EXPERIMENTAL DETERMINATION of the mass of an electron can be performed by a mass spectrometer. This apparatus, shown in Figure 1, consists of a tiny filament heated by a small electric current. When the filament is red hot, it emits electrons. These electrons are attracted to a brass cone surrounding the filament. Within the cone, a high positive potential is set up. There is a significant potential difference within the cone, which acts on the electrons. The brass cone has a hole at its apex, allowing the electrons to emerge from the hole as a beam. The potential difference within the cone acts to accelerate the electrons and gives them kinetic energy as they emerge from the cone.

The electrons enter a magnetic field after leaving the cone. The magnetic field is directed into the field of the paper as shown in Figure 1. The field exerts a force on the electrons, pushing them into a circular path. This force obeys Newton's second law, which states that force equals mass times acceleration. Eventually, the electrons strike a detector at the end of the circular path.

There are a number of important equations that describe the physics of the mass spectrometer. First, the kinetic energy of an electron is equivalent to the product of its charge and the potential difference it is subjected to. Second, the force on electrons (F) is found to be $F = qvB$, where v is the electron velocity, and B is magnetic field strength.

The variable R is used to describe the radius of the curved path taken by electrons subjected to the magnetic field. The curved path, or arch, can be seen in the figure. The radius relates to the acceleration and velocity of the electron by following the following relationship: $a = v^2/R$.

FIGURE I.

The physics of the mass spectrometer.

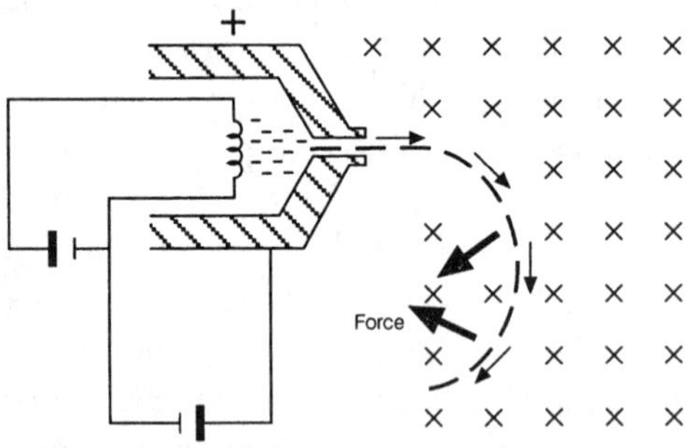

Figure I.

1. The most likely significance of the potential difference set up within the cone is:

   A. to impart force to the electrons.

   B. to transfer charge to the electrons.

   C. to accelerate the electrons.

   D. to impart additional mass to the electrons.

2. The kinetic energy of electrons leaving the hole of the cone is dependent on several factors. Which of the following LEAST relates to this kinetic energy?

   A. The mass of the electrons

   B. The velocity of the electrons

   C. The charge of the electrons

   D. The magnetic field direction shown in Figure 1

3. If you could triple the charge of an electron passing through this system, what would happen to the radius of the arch?

   A. It would increase by a factor of three.

   B. It would increase by a factor of nine.

   C. It would decrease by a factor of three.

   D. It would decrease by a factor of nine.

4. Which of the following particles would be LEAST likely to arch in the magnetic field shown in Figure 1?

   A. An electron

   B. A positron

   C. An ion

   D. A neutron

5. Which of the following particles would be expected to have the greatest R value?

   A. A particle with small mass

   B. A particle with large charge

   C. A particle with large velocity

   D. A particle with large acceleration

6. If the magnetic field magnitude was reduced, which of the following statements would be true?

   A. R would decrease

   B. R would increase

   C. F would increase

   D. Both R and F would decrease

Analysis and Discussion of Strategies for Example 2

This is an information presentation passage in the Physical Sciences (physics) section. The passage also has elements of a problem-solving passage as well. In this passage, you are introduced to a mass spectrometer. The apparatus is described in words, with formulas, and with a figure that demonstrates a mass spectrometer. This passage is very similar to an actual MCAT passage. It is also a great passage to illustrate basic strategies.

As discussed with Example 1, a step-by-step approach is the best way to approach science passages and the following reviews and discusses these steps.

STEP 1

Quickly read the question stems of each of the six questions following the passage. The following is what you should extract from the question stems:

Question 1: Find the significance of the potential difference.

Question 2: Find the factors relating to kinetic energy. These factors can be eliminated as potential answers.

Question 3: Look for a formula that allows you to predict the effect of doubling q and its effect on R.

Question 4: This is a basic conceptual question that you can probably answer right away.

Question 5: Look for formulas that maximize the value of R.

Question 6: Look for a formula(s) that relate B and either R or F.

Basically, from reading the question stems for this passage, you get an idea that formulas interrelating variables is very important for answering the questions. You can focus on quantitative relationships when you read the passage.

STEP 2

Quickly look at any graph, table, or figure presented in the passage. Spend 15 seconds looking at Figure 1 in Example 2, which shows a diagram of the mass spectrometer. Notice that negative charges appear to move through a cone-like exit and enter a magnetic field. The negative charges then curve back toward the spectrometer. This information is all you should get at this stage.

STEP 3

Read the passage. Spend no more than 2 minutes on this step.

STEP 4

Identify important points, formulas, and data. This passage is ideal to practice underlining important points and making notations in the margin. Always remember to recopy in the margin any formula you see given in the passage. In addition, write in symbols any relationship given in words. For example, if you see a formula written in the passage, write the formula with variables in the margin.

What should you have circled or noted as you were reading?

You should have underlined the last sentence in paragraph one. This sentence is the answer to the first question.

You may have wanted to note in the margin that the explanation of Figure 1 is in the second paragraph. It may have been helpful to look at Figure 1 as you were reading this paragraph to best understand the description of the apparatus.

You should have written in the margin of paragraph three: $KE = qV$, $F = qvB$, and $F = ma$. Note that the first and third formulas are spelled out in words in the passage.

Because you know that the variable R is asked about, write the formula containing R in the margin: $a = v^2/R$.

STEPS 5 AND 6

Begin answering questions. Always think about the type of question you are being asked. Always use the process of elimination to arrive at the best answer.

Answers and Explanations for Example 2

1. **C** This question is an information recall question. The answer is provided in the last sentence of the first paragraph. The passage states that the potential difference within the cone acts to accelerate the electrons, which is answer choice C. Choice A is not as accurate. Although electrons possess mass and the passage states that the potential difference acts to accelerate the electrons, the passage does not directly state that force is imparted to the electrons. The passage does directly state that acceleration occurs. It is plausible to select choice A because based on physics principles, it is not incorrect. You must always use the process of elimination to answer MCAT questions. Choice B is neither stated nor implied in the passage. Choice D is incorrect because additional mass can be added to electrons in this apparatus.

2. **D** The best way to answer this question is by looking at the expressions for kinetic energy (KE) that the passage provides. You should have written in the margin next to paragraph three: **KE = qV**. Also, write any other relationship you know for KE. Recall that **KE = ½ mv²**. Next, look at the answer choices. You are asked which choice least relates to KE. Choice A is incorrect because mass is directly related to KE. Velocity relates to KE as well. Finally, charge (q) relates to KE by the formula provided in the passage. By the process of elimination, choice D is the answer. Magnetic field direction does not relate to KE.

3. **C** Notice that this question asks you about several variables. Look to see if you have an equation that relates the two variables asked about. Unfortunately, you do not have a single formula that relates q and R. Therefore, take the formulas you do have and solve them for R in terms of q:

   $F = ma$ and $F = qvB$.
   Therefore, $ma = qvB$.
   Because $a = v^2/R$, you can substitute a with $m(v^2/R) = qvB$.
   Thus, $R = (mv^2)/qvB$.

   Because the question asks you what happens to R if you triple the charge (q), think about tripling the magnitude of the denominator. The value of R decreases by a factor of three when you do this. Thus, the best answer is C.

4. **D** This is a conceptual question that is not directly related to the passage. Look at the choices carefully. Notice that the question asks you about different particles and their behavior in a magnetic field. Only one of the particle types is uncharged. The uncharged particle, a neutron (choice D) would be least likely to arch in the presence of a magnetic field.

5. **C** This question also requires you to look at formulas and make predictions about the magnitudes of variables. Because the question asks you to maximize R, look at the formulas that you have for R that relate it to mass, charge, velocity, and acceleration. The formula derived in question 3 is most useful here: $R = (mv^2)/qvB$. This formula shows that small mass and large charge minimize the value of R. Thus, choices A and B are incorrect. Choice C is a true statement because a large velocity would maximize R. To evaluate choice D, use the formula for acceleration: $a = v^2/R$. This formula shows that a large value of acceleration occurs when R is minimized. Thus, choice C is the best answer.

6. **B** Again, this question tests your ability to quickly manipulate formulas. In this question, decrease the magnitude of B to determine the effects on R and F. Since $F = qvB$, when B decreases, F decreases. Thus, choice C must be incorrect. To determine the effect of decreasing B on R, find a formula that relates the two variables. You know from question 3, $R = (mv^2)/qvB$. Thus, if B decreases and other variables remain unchanged, R should increase. Therefore, choices A and D must be incorrect.

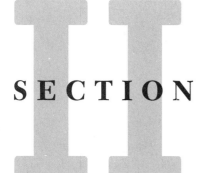

SECTION II

Preparation for the Physical Sciences

....

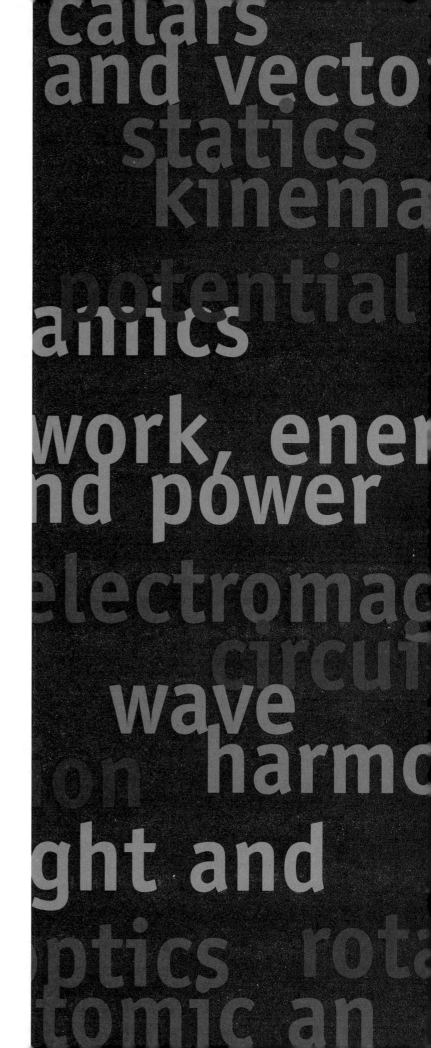

Physics

REVIEW NOTES

1

Scalars and Vectors

HIGH-YIELD TOPICS	**I.** Scalars
	II. Vectors
	III. Additional Points to Remember

To prepare for the physical sciences section, you need to review and master the basic terms, concepts, principles, laws, formulas, and problem-solving skills covered in a 1-year, noncalculus physics course. Studying physics for the MCAT is different, however, than studying physics for an examination in a physics course. Each MCAT physics question can be solved in about 1 minute or less. More than one half of the questions are conceptual. No calculators are allowed. In addition, you are not given all the formulas that you need to find the solutions.

The physics review notes provide a collection of the relationships and formulas that you need to know for the MCAT. It is important to understand these formulas and concepts; do not just memorize the material. **Success in physics requires conceptual understanding and the ability to apply knowledge to solve problems.**

I. Scalars

A scalar quantity measures only **magnitude.** Scalars are specified with a single number that has particular units. Scalars may be positive or negative and may be added together using simple arithmetic.

Common examples of scalar quantities include **mass, distance, volume, time, work, and power**.

II. Vectors

A vector quantity measures both **magnitude and direction.** These quantities are usually represented graphically by arrows, the heads of which point in the direction of the quantity and the length of which represents the magnitude of the quantity. Vector magnitude is always a positive number.

Common examples of vector quantities include **displacement, force, velocity, acceleration, momentum, gravity, E-fields, and B-fields.**

Two vectors are equal if they have the same magnitude and direction. They must point in the same direction and have equal arrow lengths.

The easiest way to add vectors is with the **graphic method.** Two vectors are added graphically by drawing the first vector and placing the tail of the second vector at the head of the first, keeping the same magnitude and direction. The sum of the two vectors is a vector that begins at the tail of the first and extends to the head of the second.

Figure 1-1 shows the addition of vector a and vector b to give the resultant vector c. Note that to generate vector c, the tail of vector b was placed at the head of vector a, maintaining magnitude and direction.

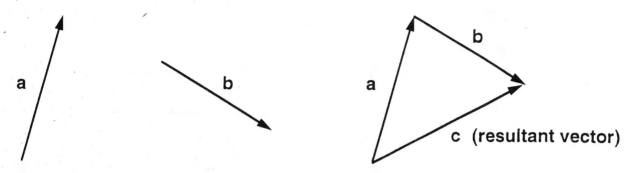

FIGURE 1-1.
Graphic addition of vectors.

The easiest way to solve a problem involving the subtraction of vectors is to change the direction of the vector being subtracted by 180° and then add the two vectors: a − b = a + (−b).

A second way to add vectors is to use the **component method,** which involves resolving each vector into its scalar components, adding the x and y components individually, and then using the Pythagorean theorem to find the magnitude of the resultant.

This technique is also useful when adding more than two vectors. To find the resultant force of several vectors, add the x components of the force vectors and add the y components of the force vectors. Then, use the formula:

$$F_R = (F_x^2 + F_y^2)^{1/2}$$

Once you find the magnitude of the resultant, you can find the direction of the resultant vector by using the following formula, in which θ is the number of degrees from the x-axis:

$$\tan \theta = (y \text{ component})/(x \text{ component})$$

FIND THE MAGNITUDE and direction of the sum of vectors A and B.

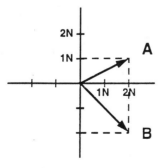

Figure 1-2.

EXAMPLE 1-1

FIGURE 1-2.
Two vectors added by the component method.

SOLUTION

In Figure 1-2, note that vector A has an x component of 2 N and a y component of 1 N. Vector B has an x component of 2 N and a y component of −2 N. The sum

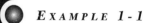

of the *x* components is 4 N and the sum of the *y* components is −1 N. Now use the Pythagorean theorem to find the resultant.

$$F = \{(4 \text{ N})^2 + (-1 \text{ N})^2\}^{1/2} = 4.1 \text{ N}$$
$$\tan \theta = y \text{ component}/x \text{ component} = -1 \text{ N}/4 \text{ N} = -0.250$$
$$\theta = \arctan (0.250) = -14° \text{ (Arctan values would be given on the MCAT)}$$

Thus, the resultant vector has a magnitude of 4.1 N and is directed 14° below the *x*-axis.

III. Additional Points to Remember

Some important relationships to commit to memory are those between the sides of right triangles (Table 1-1). Even if you forget the value of one of the sine or cosine values of the angles given in Table 1-1, you can always derive these values if you know the basic triangle relationships. Also included is the **3,4,5 triangle,** the sine and cosine values of which are often used in problems (Figure 1-3).

TABLE 1-1. Sine and Cosine Values of Right Triangle Relationships.

	Relationship	0°	30°	45°	60°	90°
Sin	opp/hypot	0	0.5 or 1/2	0.71 or $\sqrt{2}/2$	0.87 or $\sqrt{3}/2$	1
Cos	adj/hypot	1	0.87 or $\sqrt{3}/2$	0.71 or $\sqrt{2}/2$	0.5 or 1/2	0

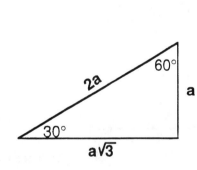 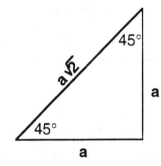 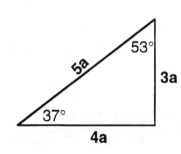

FIGURE 1-3.
Important triangle relationships.

2

Statics

Statics

I. Static Systems Without Rotation

II. Static Systems with Rotation—Torque

III. Center of Gravity and Center of Mass

HIGH-YIELD TOPICS

I. Static Systems Without Rotation

Static systems are not moving. The sum of the forces acting on the system **balance** such that the sum of the x components equals zero and the sum of the y components equals zero. Thus, in static systems:

$$\sum F_x = 0 \text{ and } \sum F_y = 0$$

Static systems require that forces be in equilibrium. The key to solving these problems is to pick a point at which all the forces on the system act.

A BLOCK HANGS at rest from wall surfaces A and B (Figure 2-1). The block is suspended by three weightless ropes. The tension in the rope attaching to wall A is 15 N and the angles the ropes make to the horizontal are 30° for A and 60° for B. Find the tension in the rope attaching to wall B and the weight of the block.

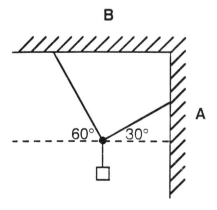

Figure 2-1.

E X A M P L E 2 - 1

FIGURE 2-1.
A block at rest, supported by three massless ropes.

more ▼

SOLUTION

Start by finding the point at which all the forces act. Note that all the ropes act at the intersection point; the rope suspending the block is counteracted by the ropes attached to the walls pulling up on the block. The system does not move because the forces in the x direction acting at this intersection point all sum to zero. Similarly, the forces acting in the y direction all sum to zero at this point. Draw a vector diagram showing the net forces (Figure 2-2).

FIGURE 2-2.
Vector diagram of net forces for Example 2-1.

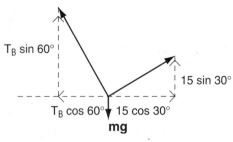

Figure 2-2.

You must sum all the x forces, which are vectors that have direction as well as magnitude. The magnitude of the forces are solved by components. If the vector points in the +x axis, give the magnitude a positive sign. If the vector points in the −x axis, give the magnitude a negative sign. The same principle applies for the +y and −y axis for up and down directions.
Therefore,

$$\Sigma F_x = 0. \qquad \Sigma F_x = 15(\cos 30°) + (-T_B\cos 60°) = 0$$
$$\Sigma F_x = 15(0.87) + -T_B(0.5) = 0$$
$$\text{so,} \qquad T_B \approx 26 \text{ N}$$

Because both of the ropes attached to the walls are pulling up on the intersection point, they will be added to the force associated with the rope pulling down on this point because of the weight of the block.
Now,

$$\Sigma F_y = 0$$
$$\Sigma F_y = 15(\sin 30°) + T_B(\sin 60°) - W = 0$$
$$\Sigma F_y = 15(0.5) + 26(0.87) - W = 0$$
$$W = 7.5 + 22.6$$
$$W \approx 30 \text{ N}$$

EXAMPLE 2-2

FIGURE 2-3.
Ropes supporting a block.

IN FIGURE 2-3, find the magnitude of the tension in ropes x and y.

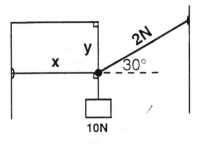

Figure 2-3.

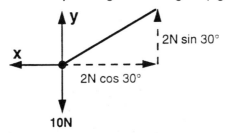
FIGURE 2-4.
Vector diagram for Example 2-2.

II. Static Systems with Rotation—Torque

Some static systems, when disturbed, want to rotate. Rotation occurs if forces act in such a way as to generate a net turning effect, or torque. This action may occur if a pulley or suspending rope is removed from a system with an axis of rotation.

Torque is a force multiplied by the perpendicular distance from the place where the force is applied to the axis of rotation. Torque is considered positive if it involves counterclockwise rotation and negative if rotation is clockwise. Taking the sine of the angle gives its component perpendicular to the lever arm. To find the torque of a body with the axis of rotation P, use the following:

Torque = (lever arm)(Force)(sin of angle between body and force)

or

Torque = rFsinθ

Figure 2-5 shows a nut being turned with a wrench. Assume the wrench is being pulled downward—a great example of applying torque. The axis of rotation, or point P, is at the nut. The radius is the distance from the nut to the hand. The force vector is in the direction of the forearm (down). The angle (θ) is the angle between r and F.

The lever arm is the distance from the place where the force is applied to the axis of rotation. Note that taking the sine of the angle described gives the perpendicular distance from the force to the axis of rotation.

Another way to calculate torque, if you do not want to memorize the equation for torque using the sine function, involves using basic trigonometry and triangle relationships to determine the perpendicular distance from the axis of rotation to the applied force. Torque is simply the product of the applied force and the magnitude of this perpendicular distance.

FIGURE 2-5.

Concept of torque. At left, torque is being applied to turn a nut with a wrench. At right, diagram showing F, r, and θ.

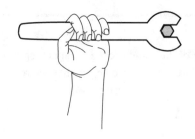
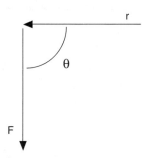

Figure 2-5.

For a potentially rotating system to be a static system, the the torques acting on the system must sum to zero. This concept is useful for solving two types of problems, namely, statics problems with a rotational component and center of gravity problems.

EXAMPLE 2-3

A 100-N WEIGHT hangs from the end of a massless rod (Figure 2-6). The rod makes a 60° angle with the wall. A cable, suspended from the wall at a 30° angle, attaches to the rod and aids in its suspension. The axis of rotation is where the rod contacts the wall. The length of the rod is *l* units long

1. Find the torque produced by the weight
2. Find the torque produced by the cable
3. Find the tension in the cable supporting the rod

FIGURE 2-6.

Torque problem in Example 2-3. Note that the block is suspended from a massless rod, which is in turn hinged to a supporting wall. A rope also connects the rod to a higher position on the wall.

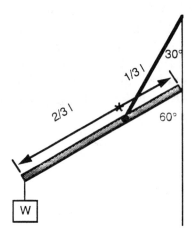

SOLUTION

This problem is somewhat difficult because the angles can be confusing. When calculating torque, picture in your mind what each applied force does in rotating the body. In this case, an applied weight makes the rod want to rotate counterclockwise about the axis of rotation (positive torque). The supporting cable applies a force (tension) pulling the rod upward and making it want to rotate clockwise about the axis of rotation (negative torque).

1. The torque related to the weight is found by using the equation provided previously in this chapter. Determining the magnitude of angle θ is difficult. Draw a line from the end of the rod back to the wall, making it perpendicular to the wall. Note that the angle between the rod and this line

is 30° and the angle between the weight and the line is 90°. Therefore, the angle between the rod and the weight is 120°.

$$\text{Torque} = rF\sin\theta = (l)(100N)(\sin 120°) = 87l$$

2. The key to solving this part is to know which angles are important. If you are to use the torque equation described previously, you need to use the angle between the F and r terms. The force that causes rotation is supplied by the cable. The "r" refers to the line between the axis of rotation and the point at which the cable attaches to the wall. The angle formed is 30°. Thus, the torque from the cable is $- (1/3\ l)(T)(\sin 30°) = -lT/6$

Notice that you are to leave the answer in terms of T. Also note that the rotation is clockwise, giving a negative torque.

3. Take the sum of the torques and set them equal to zero. Using the information from questions 1 and 2, the torque from the weight is 87l and the torque from the cable is $-lT/6$:

$$87l + (-lT/6) = 0$$
$$T = 522\ N,\ answer$$

CONCEPTUAL QUESTION

A plumber is trying to turn a bolt with a wrench, but it seems that the bolt is rusted in place. He tries to design a way to increase the torque applied to the bolt with his wrench. Which, if either, would you advise him to do: place a long piece of pipe on the handle of the wrench to lengthen the effective handle length, or tie a long rope to the end of the handle to give a longer line of force in which to help turn the wrench?

SOLUTION

The torque applied to the bolt depends on the force applied and the lever arm over which this force is applied. The bolt acts as a pivot point. Figure 2-5 showed the bolt/wrench system and the forces applied. The length of the wrench is the lever arm if the wrench is pulled at a right angle to the line of action of the applied force. Thus, torque can be increased by lengthening the wrench handle. Tying a rope to the end of the wrench to help turn the bolt may not increase the force applied to the lever arm.

III. Center of Gravity and Center of Mass

It is possible to use the concept of torques to find the center of gravity. The torque about any point produced by the weight of an object is equal to that from a concentrated object of the same weight placed at a point called the **center of gravity.** By definition, the center of gravity of an object is that point at which you may consider the total force of gravity to act.

The **center of mass** of an object is that point at which the total mass is concentrated. A suspended object always hangs so that its center of gravity is directly below the point of suspension. In this position, the torque resulting from the weight about that point is zero. It is intuitive that the center of gravity and the center of mass are usually located at the same point. The only instance in which they would not be equal is if the value of gravity varied over the volume of the object.

To calculate the center of mass, break up the object into small sections and take the center of mass of each section. The easiest way to find the center of mass of an object made up of two separate weights is to use the following formulas:

$$X = (x_1w_1 + x_2w_2)/w_{tot} \text{ or } X = (x_1m_1 + x_2m_2)/m_{tot}$$

in which X is the location of the center of gravity based on your chosen x-axis coordinate system, x_1 is the distance of the first weight from the chosen x-axis coordinate system, x_2 is the distance of the second weight from the chosen x-axis coordinate system, w_{tot} is the total weight of the object in question ($w_1 + w_2$), and m_{tot} is the total mass of the object in question ($m_1 + m_2$).

A similar formula can be set up for the y-axis. Just substitute y's for the x's in the preceding equation.

E X A M P L E   2 - 4

CONSIDER THE TWO-DIMENSIONAL shape in Figure 2-7 as having two halves. Each half has a point of mass concentration at the center of mass. Point A is located 2 cm above and 2 cm to the right of the lower left-hand corner of the shape. Point B is located 3 cm above and 8 cm to the right of the lower left-hand corner of the shape. Point A has a weight of 20 N, whereas point B has a weight of 30 N. Find the center of mass of the entire shape.

FIGURE 2-7.

Center of mass example.

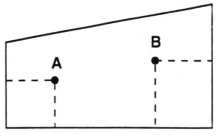

Figure 2-7.

SOLUTION

Use a coordinate system for the x-axis and y-axis, and suppose that the lower left-hand corner of the shape has the coordinates (0,0). Solve for the center of mass for the x-axis and y-axis independently.

$X = (x_1w_1 + x_2w_2)/w_{tot}$ $X = \{(2 \text{ cm})(20 \text{ N}) + (8 \text{ cm})(30 \text{ N})\}/(20 \text{ N} + 30 \text{ N}) =$
5.6 cm

$Y = (y_1w_1 + y_2w_2)/w_{tot}$ $Y = \{(2 \text{ cm})(20 \text{ N}) + (3 \text{ cm})(30 \text{ N})\}/(20 \text{ N} + 30 \text{ N}) =$
2.6 cm

Thus, the center of mass of this object is (5.6, 2.6) on the chosen coordinate system.

I. Basic Concepts	
II. Graphic Relations	**HIGH-YIELD TOPICS**
III. Kinematic Equations	

I. Basic Concepts

Kinematics is the study of the motion of objects and their path of travel. Some definitions are critical to your understanding of this subject.

The **displacement of an object** is the shortest straight line connecting its starting point and its ending point, no matter what its path. Displacement is a vector quantity, and shows both magnitude and direction. Do not confuse displacement with distance, which is a scalar quantity and describes the total length of travel, not the shortest path.

The **velocity** of a point is its net displacement divided by the time it takes the displacement to occur. It may also be written as:

$$v = (x_f - x_i)/\Delta t$$

in which x_f and x_i are final and initial positions, respectively.

The **average speed** of an object is its total distance traveled divided by the total elapsed time.

CONSIDER THE PATH followed by a boomerang that returns to its thrower. If the boomerang travels 10 m before returning to its thrower within 10 seconds, find the average speed and average velocity of the boomerang.

 EXAMPLE 3-1

SOLUTION
The average speed is the total distance divided by elapsed time.

Total distance = 20 m/10 sec = 2 m/sec

The average velocity is zero because there is no net displacement.

Constant speed is a constant change of distance covered over time. To say that an object traveled 20 m in 4 seconds at a uniform rate without mention of direction is to describe constant speed. **Constant velocity** infers travel at a constant rate in a constant direction, with zero acceleration.

Average acceleration is the change in velocity divided by the time required for the change to occur. **Instantaneous acceleration** is the average acceleration over a very short time interval.

$$a = \Delta v / \Delta t$$

Acceleration does not infer going faster or slower. It merely states that velocity is changing over time. An object may accelerate if its rate of travel is constant, yet its direction of velocity is changing. A prime example of this principle is discussed in Chapter 7 (Circular Motion).

II. Graphic Relations

To grasp the true meaning of the terms used in this chapter, study the following graphs. Clear understanding of the graphic representation of kinematic concepts is important.

The first graph (Figure 3-1) plots displacement over time. Each portion of this graph represents the following:

Section a: A period of rest, or no motion. Note that the displacement does not change over a period of time.

Section b: A forward velocity which appears constant as the slope of the line of displacement/time appears constant.

Section c: A second period of rest.

Section d: Acceleration. Note that the change in displacement/time appears to be an exponential function, and that the slope of lines tangential to points on the curve are increasing.

FIGURE 3-1.

Displacement versus time for an object. Slope = displacement/ time = velocity. If slope is constant, velocity is constant. If slope is not constant, velocity is not constant and there is acceleration.

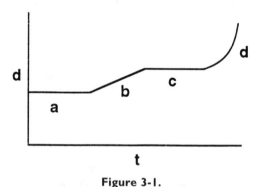

Figure 3-1.

Figure 3-2 shows velocity versus time. Each section of this graph represents the following:

Section a: Constant velocity (no acceleration).

Section b: Constant and negative acceleration (deceleration) or change in velocity divided by change in time.

Section c: Rest, because velocity is zero at this point.

Section d: Increasing acceleration or acceleration increasing over time.

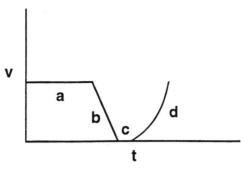

Figure 3-2.

III. Kinematic Equations

Several equations are useful for straight-line motion with constant acceleration.

$$x = 1/2(v_f + v_o)(t) \quad (1)$$

in which v_o and v_f are initial and final velocities, respectively. Equation 1 makes sense because the average velocity should approximate the average between initial and final velocities.

$$v_f^2 - v_o^2 = 2ax \quad (2)$$

in which x is the distance traveled. Equation 2 helps you find the final velocity if you know the initial velocity, the acceleration of the object, and the distance traveled.

$$x = v_o t + 1/2\, at^2 \quad (3)$$

One of the most useful for problem solving, equation 3 allows you to relate distance traveled with acceleration and time traveled. Remember to place a negative sign in front of the $1/2 at^2$ term if the acceleration is gravity (g). The value for g is -9.8 m/sec² or approximately -10 m/sec².

$$v_f = v_o + at \quad (4)$$

This formula is the definition of final velocity. Equation 4 makes sense because the initial velocity of the object is enhanced by the object's acceleration over a short unit of time.

Sample Problems

A CAR TRAVELING at a constant 100 m/sec for 10 seconds suddenly accelerates at 10 m/sec² for 10 seconds. How far does the car travel in the 20-second time period?

  E X A M P L E 3 - 2

SOLUTION
    For the **first 10 seconds:** x = vt = (100 m/sec)(10 sec) = 1000 m
    For the **second 10 seconds,** you must take acceleration into account:

        $x = v_o t + 1/2\, at^2$ (distance during the acceleration)
        x = (100 m/sec)(10 sec) + (1/2)(10 m/sec²)(10 sec)²
        x = 1500 m   (distance for acceleration period)
        Total distance covered = 1000 m + 1500 m = <u>2500 m</u>

EXAMPLE 3-3

A BULLET FIRED from a gun decelerates at 200 m/sec² in its first 1000 m of travel. If it covers this distance in 1.5 seconds and has a velocity of 500 m/sec at 1000 m, find the velocity at which the bullet left the gun.

SOLUTION

$$v_f^2 = v_o^2 - 2ax$$
$$(500 \text{ m/sec})^2 = v_o^2 - (2)(200)(1000)$$
$$250{,}000 = v_o^2 - 400{,}000$$
$$650{,}000 = v_o^2$$
$$v_o \approx 800 \text{ m/sec}$$

EXAMPLE 3-4

A PROJECTILE IS FIRED from the ground at an angle of 30° to the horizontal with an initial velocity of 10 m/sec.

1. What is the greatest height the projectile reaches?

2. How long is the projectile in the air?

3. How far from the firing site does the projectile land?

SOLUTION

Draw a vector diagram (Figure 3-3). You must find the x and y components of the initial velocity. Use the 30-60-90 triangle rule.

FIGURE 3-3.

Vector diagram for Example 3-4.

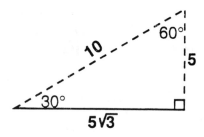

Figure 3-3.

1. To find the greatest height the projectile reaches, use the kinematic equation that has y as a variable.

$$v_{fy} = 0 \quad \text{(object is at rest at its highest point)}$$
$$v_{oy} = 10\sin 30° = 5 \text{ m/s} \quad (y \text{ component of initial velocity})$$
$$a_y = -10 \text{ m/sec}^2$$
$$v_{fy}^2 = v_{oy}^2 - 2ay$$
$$0^2 = (5 \text{ m/sec})^2 - (2)(10 \text{ m/sec}^2)(y)$$
$$y = 1.25 \text{ m}$$

2. Now find the time the projectile is in the air.

$$v_f = v_0 + at$$
$$0 = 5 \text{ m/sec} - (10 \text{ m/sec}^2)(t)$$
$$5 = 10 \, t$$
$$t = 0.5 \text{ sec}$$

more ▼

3. How far does the object travel in the horizontal direction? You know that the object reaches its highest point at 0.5 sec, so it again strikes the ground in another 0.5 sec. **The path is symmetric,** so the time it requires an object to reach its highest point when fired from the ground is equal to the time it requires to fall from the high point back to the ground. For this problem, total travel time is 1.0 sec. The horizontal distance traveled is the product of the x component of the initial velocity and the time in the air. Note that the x component of the initial velocity is constant throughout the travel of this projectile because there is no acceleration in the x-direction acting on the object.

$$x = (v_o)_x(t)$$
$$x = (5\sqrt{3} \text{ m/s})(1 \text{ sec}) = 5\sqrt{3} \text{ m}$$

The directions of the velocity and acceleration vectors in these problems differ. The velocity vector is tangent to the path the projectile travels while the acceleration vector is *down* (gravity).

Note: It cannot be overemphasized that the **horizontal travel of the projectile depends on the time the object is in the air and only the x component of its velocity.** The only acceleration acting on the projectile is gravity.

A STONE IS THROWN from the roof of a 10-m high building at an angle of 45° above the horizontal (Figure 3-4). If it strikes the ground 10 seconds later at a distance of 100 m from the base of the building, find:

EXAMPLE 3-5

FIGURE 3-4.
Diagram for Example 3-5.

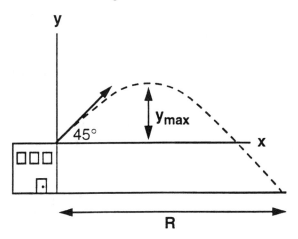

1. The initial velocity of the stone

2. The maximum height reached above the roof

SOLUTION

1. Find the x component of the initial velocity. Because the stone traveled 100 m in 10 seconds in the x-direction, $v_x = 10$ m/sec.

$$v_x = v_o \cos 45°$$
$$10 \text{ m/sec} = (v_o)(0.71)$$
$$v_0 = 14.1 \text{ m/sec}$$

2. Now find the vertical component of the initial velocity.
Recall that the final velocity in the y-direction at the highest point (y_{max}) is zero.

$$v_f^2 = v_o^2 + 2ay$$

Knowing that

$$v_{oy} = v_o \sin 45° = (14.1 \text{ m})(\sin 45°) = 10 \text{ m/sec},$$
$$0 = (10 \text{ m/sec})^2 + (2)(-10 \text{ m/sec}^2)(y)$$
$$y = 5 \text{ m}$$

Ex. 3-5 cont.

Conceptual Questions

1. As a ball rolls down a hill (Figure 3-5), how do its speed and acceleration change?

FIGURE 3-5.

Diagram for conceptual question 1.

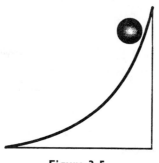

Figure 3-5.

Solution: The speed of the ball increases as it rolls down the hill. Acceleration, however, depends on how steep the hill is. Acceleration is the greatest at the top of the hill because the hill is steepest. As the ball rolls down the hill, the hill is less steep and the acceleration decreases. Thus, acceleration can decrease while speed increases.

2. You drop a small marble and a large bowling ball at the same time from the same height. Ignoring air resistance, why do both of these objects fall together with equal accelerations?

Solution: Ignoring air resistance, all free-falling objects fall with the same acceleration (-9.8 m/sec^2), given Newton's second law: $F = ma$ or $a = F/m$. Free-falling objects are subject to the force of gravity, which gives an object's weight. Thus, $a = W/m$. Because weight and mass are proportional, the relative increase in both of these values for large, heavy objects tends to cancel out in the $a = W/m$ expression. For example, a bowling ball that has 50 times the weight of a marble also has 50 times the mass. Because acceleration is the quotient of force (weight) and mass of falling objects, the effect of the greater weight and mass of the bowling ball compared to the marble cancels out, and both the bowling ball and marble fall with the same acceleration.

Dynamics

Dynamics

I. Force and Weight

II. Newton's Laws of Motion

III. Friction

IV. Incline Problems

V. Systems of Connected Bodies

HIGH-YIELD TOPICS

Dynamics is the study of how things move. This chapter offers a review of the basic concepts of dynamics, including force, Newton's laws of motion, and friction.

I. Force and Weight

Force is a mass times an acceleration. Force is what causes the acceleration of an object, commonly thought of as a "push" or a "pull." Newton's second law states:

$$F = ma$$

The terms of force in the SI system are a combination of base units of mass, length, and time, called the Newton (N). A Newton is force that imparts an acceleration of 1 meter per second to a 1-kg mass.

$$N = (kgm)/s^2$$

Weight is the downward force an object experiences on or near the surface of the earth. Weight is the product of the mass of the object and the acceleration of gravity.

$$W = mg$$

Remember that the weight of an object is exclusively the gravitational force exerted by the earth on an object. On different planets, an object will maintain the same mass, but may have different weights, because the value of g differs on other planets.

II. Newton's Laws of Motion

Newton's first law says that an isolated object at rest will remain at rest if no net force acts on it. If an isolated object is in motion, it will continue moving along a straight line at constant speed if no net force acts on it.

The first law emphasizes no net force. Several forces acting on an object that balance one another to produce zero net force are viewed the same as if no force is acting on the object at all.

Newton's second law says that if the sum of all forces on an object is not zero, then the object will be accelerated. The acceleration produced depends on the sum of the forces and on the mass of the object. Simply stated: F = ma.

Newton's third law says that for every force, there is an equal and opposite reaction force. If object A exerts a force on object B, then object B exerts an equal and opposite force on object A.

This law addresses the concept of normal force or N. A normal force is a reaction force that is perpendicular to the plane on which an object rests (Figure 4-1). If a block rests on a flat tabletop, normal force is directed straight up. If a block sits on a ramp, the normal force is directed perpendicular to the plane of the ramp.

FIGURE 4-1.

Normal force (N) is a reaction force directed perpendicular to the plane on which an object rests. Note the difference between the normal force and the weight (mg).

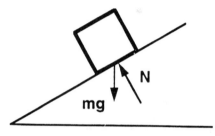

Figure 4-1.

III. Friction

As a block resting on a flat surface is subjected to force, the object usually slides along that surface. This movement occurs only if the force applied is greater than the friction force between the block and the surface. **Friction force** opposes the tendency to move when one object slides over another.

The friction force (f) is the coefficient of friction (μ) times the normal force.

$$f = \mu N$$

The coefficient of friction is a **property of the surfaces** that contact each other. The coefficient of static friction (μ_s) is involved if two or more objects have friction forces between them and no motion occurs between the surfaces. If motion occurs between the surfaces, it is known as the coefficient of kinetic friction (μ_k). **For a given pair of surfaces, the coefficient of kinetic friction is always less than the coefficient of static friction.**

Each of these friction coefficients is associated with a force. The force of **kinetic friction** is parallel to the surface of contact of the two objects, although the direction of the kinetic friction force is always opposite the velocity of the object. The **force of static friction** keeps an object from moving as a result of an applied force. The direction of this force is opposite the direction of the applied force. Figure 4-2 shows the direction of each of these friction forces.

By increasing the applied force on a block, you can overcome the force of static friction and start the block moving. In this case, the force of static friction disappears and the force of kinetic friction takes over.

If you are told that a surface is frictionless, ignore friction forces completely and concentrate on the applied forces. Consider the following examples of these concepts.

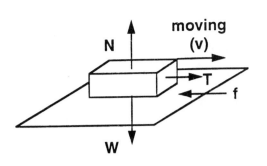
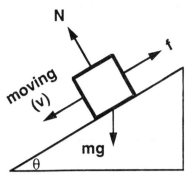

Figure 4-2.

FIGURE 4-2.

Forces acting on a block on a flat surface (left) and on an incline (right). For each situation showing a block with a velocity, note the direction of the normal force (N), weight (W or mg), and the friction force (f).

A 4-KG BLOCK rests on a frictionless surface and is subjected to a 10-Newton force to the right. Find the acceleration of the block.

EXAMPLE 4-1

SOLUTION

Start by drawing a diagram (Figure 4-3).

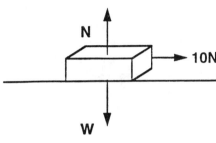

Figure 4-3.

FIGURE 4-3.

Diagram of relevant forces in Example 4-1.

The block has weight and a normal force, but no friction. Therefore, these forces do not affect the motion to the right.

$$\text{Newton's second law:} \quad F = ma$$
$$10 \text{ N} = (4 \text{ kg})(a)$$
$$a = 2.5 \text{ m/sec}^2$$

FOR THE PROBLEM detailed in example 4-1, find the acceleration of the block if the surface has a coefficient of kinetic friction of 0.2.

EXAMPLE 4-2

SOLUTION

Draw a diagram showing all the force vectors. Because this situation involves friction, remember to direct the friction force vector opposite to the applied force vector (Figure 4-4).

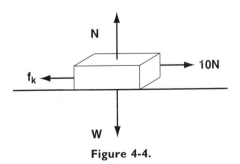

Figure 4-4.

FIGURE 4-4.

Diagram of relevant forces in Example 4-2.

more ▼

Newton's second law:

$$F = ma$$
$$F_{(applied)} - f_k = ma$$
$$10\ N - \mu N = (4)(a)$$
$$N_{(normal\ force)} = W, \quad because\ \Sigma F_y = 0.$$
$$10\ N - 0.2(40\ N) = (4)(a)$$
$$a = 0.5\ m/sec^2$$

EXAMPLE 4-3

A 40-KG BLOCK is pulled to the right by a massless rope with a force of 100 N at an angle of 45° to the horizontal. If the coefficient of kinetic friction is 0.2, find the acceleration of the block.

SOLUTION

Figure 4-5 is a vector diagram showing the relevant forces. The most important part of the problem is in the set-up. The upward pull of the rope decreases the friction of the block with the surface; it actually decreases the net normal force acting on the block. As shown in the following equation, the vertical component of the rope has been subtracted from the normal force. The horizontal component of the rope pull imparts the force that pulls the block to the right.

FIGURE 4-5.

Diagram of the relevant forces and both *x* and *y* components of the upward rope pull in Example 4-3.

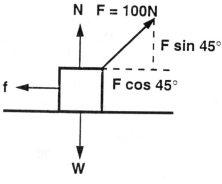

Figure 4-5.

$$F = ma$$
$$F\ (x\text{-component}) - \mu N = (40\ kg)(a)$$
$$N\ (normal\ force) = w - F sin\ 45°,\ because\ \Sigma F_y = 0.$$
$$100\ cos45° - (0.2)(mg - 100sin45°) = 40a$$
$$(100)(0.71) - (0.2)[400\ N - 100(0.71)] = 40a$$
$$a = 0.1\ m/sec^2$$

IV. Incline Problems

Problems that involve inclines or ramps are just variations of problems you have already reviewed. Figure 4-6 shows the derivation of the various force vectors based on similar triangles. Note that the force vector that is parallel to the plane of the ramp is the **mgsinθ** term, and the force vector that is perpendicular to the ramp is the **mgcosθ** term.

Solve problems involving incline planes in the same way you did those involving flat surfaces: with the principles of Newton's second law. Include all forces that act on the movement of the object and set these equal to mass times acceleration.

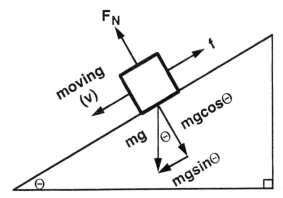

FIGURE 4-6.
Schematic incline plane
and its forces.

Figure 4-6.

A BLOCK OF MASS 10 kg slides down a 100-m long ramp that makes an angle of 30° to the horizontal. The ramp is frictionless. Find the acceleration of the block. Assume $g = 10$ m/sec^2.

SOLUTION

The only force acting on the block in the direction of motion is the force vector directed down the ramp, $mg\sin\theta$.

$$F = ma$$
$$mg\sin 30° = ma$$
$$(10 \text{ m/sec}^2)(0.5) = a$$
$$a = 5 \text{ m/sec}^2$$

EXAMPLE 4-4

A BLOCK OF UNKNOWN mass slides down a 100-m long ramp with a coefficient of kinetic friction of 0.1. The ramp makes a 30° angle to the horizontal. Assume $g = 10$ m/sec^2.

1. Find the acceleration of the block.
2. Find the velocity at the bottom of the ramp if the ramp becomes frictionless.

SOLUTION

1. Acceleration (a) of the block is as follows:

$$F = ma$$
$$mg\sin\theta - \mu N = ma$$
$$mg\sin\theta - (0.1)(mg\cos\theta) = ma$$
$$m(10 \text{ m/sec}^2)(\sin 30°) - (0.1)(m)(10 \text{ m/sec}^2)(\cos 30°) = ma$$
$$a = 4.13 \text{ m/sec}^2$$

Notice that the mass of the block is irrelevant in this problem. (The mass term cancels out in many problems of this type.)

EXAMPLE 4-5

more ▼

2. You can find the velocity assuming no friction in several ways. To apply a technique you have already learned, use the kinematic equations. Assume the block starts from rest, so $v_o = 0$.

$$v_f^2 - v_o^2 = 2ax \quad \text{or} \quad v_f = (2gh)^{1/2} = \sqrt{2gh}$$

Use gravity for the acceleration of the block and consider only the vertical distance the block falls as it moves down the ramp. Without friction, the path the block takes to cover this vertical fall is independent of the exact path. This equation relates to conservation of energy.

Use the 30-60-90 rule to find the height of the triangular ramp (Figure 4-7):

FIGURE 4-7.
Use of the 30-60-90 triangle to solve for an unknown length in Example 4-5.

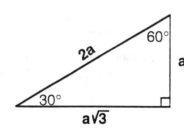
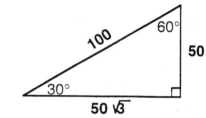

Figure 4-7.

Thus, $h = 50$ m and the acceleration is equal to g. Thus, the solution is:

$$v_f = \{(2)(10 \text{ m/sec}^2)(50 \text{ m})\}^{1/2} = 32 \text{ m/sec}$$

V. Systems of Connected Bodies

Newton's laws also apply to a group of objects that are connected to one another.

EXAMPLE 4-6

FIND THE ACCELERATION of the system in Figure 4-8. Assume that block m_1 has a mass of 2 kg, mass m_2 is 4 kg, and block m_3 is 5 kg. The pulleys and the table-top are frictionless.

FIGURE 4-8.
Diagram for Example 4-6.

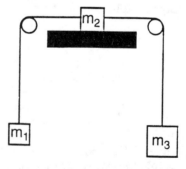

Figure 4-8.

SOLUTION
Draw a vector diagram that demonstrates the involved forces. Note the net movement to the right because $m_3 > m_1$ (Figure 4-9).

more ▼

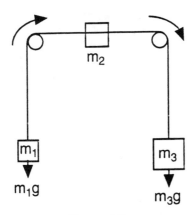

Figure 4-9.

You can see that the system will move to the right so that m_2 moves toward m_3. Set up an equation describing all the forces, and set it equal to the total system mass times system acceleration.

$$\text{(forces to the right)} - \text{(forces to the left)} = \text{(total system mass)(acceleration)}$$
$$m_3g - m_1g = (m_1 + m_2 + m_3)(a)$$
$$(5 \text{ kg})(10 \text{ m/sec}^2) - (2 \text{ kg})(10 \text{ m/sec}^2) = (11 \text{ kg})(a)$$
$$50 \text{ N} - (20\text{N}) = 11a$$
$$a = 2.7 \text{ m/sec}^2$$

How could you set up this problem if there was friction? Because the system moves to the right, friction force would act to the left. Simply add friction force to the (forces to the left) portion of the preceding equation.

Work, Energy and Power

HIGH-YIELD TOPICS	I. Work
	II. Conservation of Energy
	III. Power

This chapter is a review of the basic concepts, key definitions, and examples of work, energy, conservation of energy, efficiency, and power.

I. Work

Work is the product of the magnitude of a force and the distance over which the force acts. Work may also be thought of as the product of a force magnitude acting on an object and the object's displacement(s). There must be a net displacement of the object over which the force acts (Figure 5-1).

FIGURE 5-1.
Concept of work. If F_s is the component of F along s, then $F_s = F\cos\theta$. Work is then $W = Fs\cos\theta$.

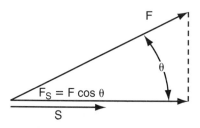

Figure 5-1.

To calculate work, multiply the component of the force that is parallel to the object's displacement(s) to the magnitude of the displacement.

If the force direction and the direction of displacement are not parallel or are in the same direction, simply use components. If the angle θ is the angle between the force vector and the direction of displacement, then $\cos\theta$ is the component of this angle that is parallel to these two vectors.

Thus, the definition of work is:

$$W = Fs \quad \text{or} \quad W = Fs\cos\theta$$

The unit of work in the SI system is the Newton-meter (Nm), which is also known as the joule (J). A joule is the work done when an object is moved 1 meter against an opposing force of 1 Newton. In the British system, the unit of work is the foot-pound (ft-lb).

EXAMPLE 5-1

A BOY IN A CART is pulled by a rope attached to the front of the cart. If the applied force is 10 N and the cart is pulled 10 m, answer the following questions:

1. Find the work done.

    Solution: $W = Fs = (10 \text{ N})(10 \text{ m}) = 100 \text{ J}$

2. Find the work done if the rope makes an angle to the front of the cart of 60° and the cart continues traveling straight ahead as in question 1.

    Solution: $W = Fs \cos\theta = (10 \text{ N})(10 \text{ m})(\cos 60°) = 50 \text{ J}$

3. Find the work done if the angle in question 2 becomes 90°.

    Solution: $W = Fs \cos\theta = (10 \text{ N})(10 \text{ m})(\cos 90°) = 0$

Note: This example shows that if the line of action of a force is at a right angle to the displacement, no work is done.

EXAMPLE 5-2

A MAN PERFORMS the following two actions with a book. Determine whether he does or does not perform work with respect to the book in each scenario given.

Scenario 1.   A man holds a book at the level of his waist and then lifts the book over his head.

Scenario 2.   A man holds a book at waist level while walking steadily.

SOLUTION

In each scenario, think about in what direction the applied force is directed. The man supports the book against the book's weight, and an upward force is applied on the book. In scenario 1, displacement of the book is in the same direction or parallel to this upward force. Thus, work is done.

In scenario 2, the displacement of the book is at a 90° angle to the upward force and no work is done. Note also that the man "is walking steadily," which suggests no acceleration. The fact that scenario 2 is not associated with work may be against your common sense because energy is expended in performing the actions described in this scenario. This question is only about work, however, and you must follow the conceptual definition of work to answer this and similar questions.

II. Conservation of Energy

A. Energy

Energy topics in physics usually relate to the storage of energy based on position or motion. Two basic types of energy are **potential and kinetic energy.**

Potential energy is the amount of work "stored" in an object based on its position, shape, or configuration relative to other objects. Several types of potential energy are defined as follows.

Gravitational potential energy relates to the "storage" of energy when an object is raised above an arbitrary reference point. The higher you raise an object, the greater its potential energy. To find the gravitational potential energy, use the equation:

$$PE = mgh$$

in which h is the height from the reference point.

A second type of potential energy is the potential energy of a spring. When a spring is stretched or compressed from its resting position, energy is stored in the form of elastic recoil. To calculate this potential energy, use the equation:

$$PE \text{ of spring} = 1/2 \ kx^2$$

in which k is the spring constant and x is the distance of the spring from its equilibrium or resting point.

The spring constant is a property of the spring. The stiffer a spring, the greater its spring constant. As shown in Figure 5-2, x is the additional stretch or compression of a spring from its equilibrium point. A stiffer spring has a higher value of k and more energy associated with it—and it is harder to compress. The greater the value of x, the greater the energy of recoil.

FIGURE 5-2.

A mass-spring system. Note that x is the distance a spring is displaced from its equilibrium or resting position.

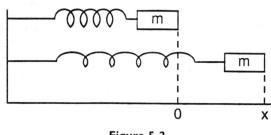

Figure 5-2.

Kinetic energy is that energy associated with the motion of an object. A moving object has the capacity to do work on another object, and this ability relates to the mass and velocity of the moving object.

$$KE = 1/2 \ mv^2$$

B. Conservation of Energy

Conservation of energy says that energy of a system cannot be created or destroyed, only converted from one kind to another. A ball raised above the level of the ground is gaining potential energy. When the ball is dropped, the potential energy is converted to kinetic energy. This kinetic energy is converted to heat as the ball is subjected to air friction and friction with the ground. All forms of energy are thus interconverted and not lost.

If friction is absent, the sum of the potential and kinetic energies of a system before an event will be equivalent to the sum of potential and kinetic energies after an event. Consider an example in which a cart is pushed up a hill. The energy during the push up the hill is primarily kinetic, yet the higher the cart goes up the hill, the more kinetic energy is converted to potential energy. Finally, when the cart is at the top of the hill, all the kinetic energy associated with the cart's movement has been converted to potential energy. The magnitude of the kinetic energy expended should ideally equal the potential energy stored if friction is absent.

A common sense expression for the conservation of energy follows:

$$\text{Conservation of Energy: } PE_a + KE_a = PE_b + KE_b$$

in which a and b represent two points (no friction).

EXAMPLE 5-3

A ROLLER COASTER CART starts at rest from the top of a crest 5 m high. Find the velocity of the cart at the base of the crest, assuming a frictionless surface.

SOLUTION
Use conservation of energy.

$$PE + KE \text{ (top)} = PE + KE \text{ (bottom)}$$
$$mgh + 0 = 0 + 1/2mv^2 \text{ (Note: masses cancel)}$$
$$(10 \text{ m/sec}^2)(5 \text{ m}) = (1/2)(v^2)$$
$$v = 10 \text{ m/sec}$$

III. POWER

Power is the rate at which work is done. The unit of power in the SI system is the watt (W). The watt equals 1 joule per second.

$$\text{Power} = \text{Work/time}$$

assuming applied force is constant.

A machine is a mechanical device that transmits changes in the magnitude or direction of an applied force. Common examples include pulleys, levers, incline planes, and gears.

Efficiency is work output of a machine divided by work input. This fraction is usually represented as a percent.

Mechanical advantage is the ratio of output force to input force.

EXAMPLE 5-4

A ROPE/PULLEY SYSTEM is used to hoist a block. The pulley system has an element of friction and, as a machine, acts with 80% efficiency. If 10 N of force is applied to the system and the rope is pulled 50 m, determine how much energy is lost as friction/heat.

SOLUTION
The key to this problem is to understand the conceptual principles. If the pulley system is 80% efficient, you can find the work associated with hoisting the block. The work associated with pulling on the rope, or work input, is W = Fs or (10 N)(50 m) = 500 J. Because the efficiency is 80% or 0.8, 0.8 = (work output)/500 J. Thus, work output must equal 400 J. Some energy is lost as friction, namely 500 J − 400 J = 100 J.

Conceptual Questions

1. A man walks up a steep, 500-m long hill. He decides to walk in a zigzag path, which is 500 m long. How does the energy he expends and the force he exerts for his zigzag path compare to the straight hill climb?

   Solution: The energy expended in each case is the same, because all paths to the top require the same energy output. Energy, in this case, is work: W = Fs. The work to get to the top of the hill is the same for both paths, but the distance is not the same for both paths. If the distance is doubled, the force is cut in half.

Thus, the zigzag path is associated with the same energy expenditure but only one half the force exerted.

2. A cart starting from rest rolls down a hill and reaches 10 m/sec at the bottom. If the same cart starts rolling down the hill from an initial speed of 5 m/sec, will its speed at the bottom be less than, equal to, or greater than 15 m/sec?

Solution: The final speed would be less than 15 m/sec. Rolling down the hill adds a certain amount of kinetic energy, but not a certain amount of speed. Speeds do not add in this problem because each cart spends a different amount of time on the hill in which to gain speed. When the cart starts at 5 m/sec, it spends less time on the hill and so picks up less speed going down. To make the calculations in this problem, convert speed to kinetic energy and add energy units.

6

Momentum and Impulse

I. Momentum and Impulse	**HIGH-YIELD TOPICS**
II. Conservation of Momentum	
III. Elastic and Inelastic Collisions	

Momentum is a conserved quantity. When two objects collide, the momentum of each may change, but the total momentum of the system remains constant. A clear understanding of this property is extremely useful.

I. Momentum and Impulse

A. Momentum (p)

Momentum is the product of the mass and velocity of an object. Momentum allows you to analyze motion in terms of the mass and velocity of an object rather than its force and acceleration. Momentum is a vector that has the same direction as the object's velocity.

$$p = mv$$

B. Impulse

Impulse is a force multiplied by the time during which the force acts. An impulse is the product of a force applied over a short time causing a change of momentum. A body receives momentum by the application of an impulse.

$$\text{Impulse} = Ft = \Delta mv$$

II. Conservation of Momentum

Conservation of momentum states that if the net force acting on a system is zero, the total linear momentum of the system will remain constant. Therefore, the momentum of the bodies before a collision equals the momentum of the bodies after the collision.

$$p_1 + p_2 = p_1 + p_2$$
$$\text{Before} = \text{After}$$

The momentum of a grenade before its explosion equals the sum of the momentum of all the fragments of the grenade after its explosion. The velocity vectors of the fragments cancel each other out when all the momentum vectors are added together.

III. Elastic and Inelastic Collisions

A. Elastic Collisions

Elastic collisions occur between two or more bodies in which no kinetic energy is lost and the total linear momentum is constant.

An example of an elastic collision is when two balls on a pool table strike one another. The sum of the momentum of the balls before the collision equals the momentum after the collision. Also, the sum of the kinetic energies of the balls before contact equals the sum after contact.

Elastic Collision = Momentum conserved, kinetic energy conserved

Problems requiring calculations for a two-particle elastic collision are unlikely to appear on the MCAT. Questions on this topic typically are conceptual.

B. Inelastic Collisions

Inelastic collisions occur between two or more bodies in which kinetic energy is lost because of transformation to heat, sound, and the like. Momentum of the bodies before and after the collision is constant. The collision is **completely inelastic** if the colliding particles stick together after the collision.

A good example of an inelastic collision is two cars colliding at high speed. The energy associated with the kinetic energy of the cars is transformed to heat deformation and sound as the cars collide. The smashed wreck of the two colliding cars has a momentum equal to the sum of the precrash momentum of the cars, assuming no friction with the ground.

Inelastic Collision = Momentum conserved, kinetic energy not conserved

E X A M P L E 6 - 1

A 1-KG BLOCK sits at rest on a frictionless surface. A smaller block, moving to the right with mass 0.5 kg, strikes the 1-kg block with a speed of 2 m/sec. Assuming a perfectly elastic collision without friction, find the velocities of the two blocks after the collision.

SOLUTION

Such a time-consuming problem will not likely appear on the MCAT, but you may be asked to identify a correct equation or to demonstrate an understanding of how to set up the conservation of momentum and conservation of energy equations.

In the following equations, the smaller block is given the subscript 1, and the larger block is given the subscript 2. Before collision is designated by "I" for initial, and after the collision is denoted by "f" for final.

The conservation of momentum equation is:

$$p_{1i} + p_{2i} = p_{1f} + p_{2f}$$
$$m_1 v_{1i} + 0 = m_1 v_{1f} + m_2 v_{2f}$$
$$(0.5 \text{ kg})(2 \text{ m/sec}) = (0.5 \text{ kg})(v_{1f}) + (1 \text{ kg})(v_{2f})$$
$$1 = 0.5 v_{1f} + v_{2f}$$

more ▼

This equation has two unknowns, which means the conservation of energy equation is as follows:

$$KE_i + PE_i = KE_f + PE_f$$

Given only KE in this problem:

$$1/2\ m_1(v_{1i})^2 = 1/2\ m_1(v_{1f})^2 + 1/2\ m_2(v_{2f})^2$$
$$1/2(0.5\ kg)(2\ m/sec)^2 = 1/2(0.5\ kg)(v_{1f})^2 + 1/2(1\ kg)(v_{2f})^2$$
$$1 = 1/4(v_{1f})^2 + 1/2(v_{2f})^2$$

To solve for the final velocities, take the final equations from the conservation of momentum and conservation of energy expressions and solve for the unknowns. You can use any algebraic method. If you solve these equations, you find that $v_{2f} =$ 4/3 m/sec and $v_{1f} = -2/3$ m/sec. The negative sign going with the final velocity of block 1 means that this block moves in the opposite direction from which it came. Thus, this block moves to the left after the collision.

A CANNON IS BOLTED to the floor of a closed railroad car (Figure 6-1). The railroad car sits on a frictionless track at rest and has a mass of 10,000 kg. A cannonball of mass 10 kg is fired from the cannon with a velocity of 100 m/sec to the right.

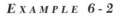

FIGURE 6-1.
Diagram for Example 6-2.

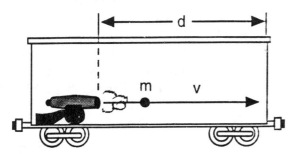

Figure 6-1.

1. Find the velocity and direction of any motion exerted on the railroad car.

2. When the cannonball strikes the far wall of the railroad car, it becomes embedded. What happens to the velocity of the railroad car when the cannonball strikes the wall?

SOLUTION

1. When the ball is fired to the right, the cannon is pushed to the left. Because the cannon is bolted to the floor of the railroad car, the entire cannon-railroad car complex is pushed to the left. Because the mass of this complex is great, its velocity of motion will be small. The momentum before the firing is zero, so after firing the momentum of the ball to the right must be equal in magnitude to that of the car and cannon to the left. Thus, mv = MV.

more ▼

$$V = mv/M$$

or

$$V = (10 \text{ kg})(100 \text{ m/sec})/(10,000 \text{ kg}) = -0.1 \text{ m/sec}$$

Note: The negative sign shows that the velocity vector of the railroad car is opposite that of the cannonball.

2. As the cannonball becomes embedded in the wall, it exerts a force on the wall to the right. The wall exerts an equal and opposite reaction force on the ball to the left. The ball and railroad car both stop moving because the net momentum is still zero. Thus, the railroad car will roll to the left while the ball is in the air. Once the ball strikes the wall, the car will stop moving.

EXAMPLE 6-3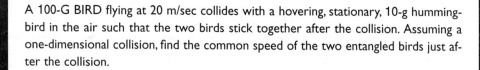

A 100-G BIRD flying at 20 m/sec collides with a hovering, stationary, 10-g hummingbird in the air such that the two birds stick together after the collision. Assuming a one-dimensional collision, find the common speed of the two entangled birds just after the collision.

SOLUTION

This problem illustrates an inelastic collision, albeit much simplified because only one dimension need be considered (no angles). If the birds were flying at angles to one another, you would have to figure out components of their velocities.

Conservation of momentum:

$$mv_i + mv_i = mv_f$$
$$(0.1 \text{ kg})(20 \text{ m/sec}) + (0.01 \text{kg})(0 \text{ m/sec}) = (0.11 \text{ kg})(v_f)$$
$$2 = 0.11 \ v_f$$
$$v_f = 18 \text{ m/sec}$$

Conceptual Questions:

1. A continuous force acts on an ice skater on a friction-free ice skating rink that causes her to accelerate. This applied force causes her speed to increase a certain amount. What would happen to the speed of the ice skater if: (a) the force and mass of the skater are unchanged but the time the force acts is tripled, and (b) the force is doubled while the mass and action time are unchanged?

   Solution: Consider this question conceptually. The force described increases the speed of the skater a certain amount each second it acts. Thus, if you triple the time the force acts, you must triple the increase in speed. The magnitude of the force applied also can increase the speed. Without applied force, no speed change occurs. A small force produces a small speed change. If you double the force, you double the speed change by doubling the acceleration.

   You can also think about this problem mathematically. $Ft = \Delta mv$, so $\Delta v = Ft/m$. Force and time vary directly, while mass varies inversely to Δv.

2. The physics of riot control are discussed in a police academy class. Suppose that rubber bullets bounce off people, whereas lead bullets penetrate.

Officers are told that rubber bullets are more effective than lead bullets in riot control because they are more likely to knock rioters to the ground and cause less tissue damage. On the basis of your understanding of basic mechanics, are both of these assertions correct if a rubber and a lead bullet have the same size, speed, and mass?

Solution: Yes, these assertions are correct. The equal momentum values of both bullets as they leave a gun change as soon as they make contact with a rioter. The impulse of the rubber bullet is greater because it bounces back, whereas the lead bullet penetrates. The rubber bullet contacts the rioter for significantly more time, and impulse equals the product of force and time. The impulse is greater for the rubber bullet because the rioter provides not only the impulse to stop the rubber bullet, but also the additional impulse to cause rebound of the bullet. Depending on the elasticity of the rebound, up to twice the impulse for the impact of the rubber bullet with the rioter occurs, and therefore up to twice the momentum is imparted to the rioter. Remember $Ft = m\Delta v$. Thus, the rubber bullet is more likely to knock over the rioter. The momentum of the lead bullet is completely transferred to the rioter, who supplies the necessary impulse to stop it.

Although the rubber bullet gives the rioter the most momentum, it does not give the most energy. When the rubber bullet bounces back, it keeps much of its kinetic energy. The lead bullet slows and stops, surrendering most or all of its kinetic energy as heat and deformation—tissue damage.

In conclusion, the rubber bullet puts much momentum but little energy into the collision with the rioter, whereas the lead bullet puts in little momentum but much energy into the collision.

7

Circular Motion and Gravitation

HIGH-YIELD TOPICS	
	I. Circular Motion
	II. Angular Velocity and Acceleration
	III. Centripetal Acceleration and Force
	IV. Conceptual Relationships in Circular Motion
	V. Gravitation

This first of two chapters concerning rotational systems is an overview of the basics of circular motion and its application to the study of gravitation. Chapter 8 provides a review of the physics of rotational dynamics, including inertia and torques. This material is confusing, so concentrate on the basic conceptual principles.

I. Circular Motion

Figure 7-1 illustrates a point that rotates around a circle from point A to point B. As the object rotates, it creates an angle θ measured at the center of the circle. **The magnitude of the angle θ through which the object passes is the angular displacement.** The quantities (r) and (s) represent the radius and arc length of the objects rotation, respectively.

FIGURE 7-1.
A unit circle. Note the radius (r), arc length (s), angular displacement (θ), and origin (O).

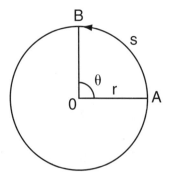

Figure 7-1.

Angular displacement can be represented in degrees, revolutions, or radians. Use the units of radians in situations in which both linear and circular quantities appear. By definition, **a radian is the angle the arc length of which equals the radius of the circle.** The important relationships between radius, arc length, and θ are as follows:

$$\theta = s/r \quad \text{or} \quad s = r\theta \quad (\theta \text{ in radians})$$

Suppose an object rotates along a unit circle (radius = 1) and does one complete rotation. A comparison of the units of rotation follows:

$$360 \text{ degrees} = 2\pi \text{ radians} = 1 \text{ revolution}$$

It is important to review some basic definitions and to understand the difference between the tangential and angular measurements.

Tangential velocity is the velocity of a mass moving through a particular point on a circular path. The direction of the velocity vector is **perpendicular** to the radius of the circle. Figure 7-2 shows the direction of a tangential velocity or tangential acceleration vector. Think about what happens if you swing a ball from the end of a string over your head and then suddenly let go. The ball and string heads off in a direction tangential or perpendicular to the original circular path.

v_t or a_t

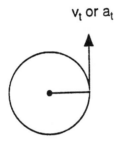

Figure 7-2.

FIGURE 7-2.
The tangential velocity or tangential acceleration for an object in a circular path is perpendicular to the radius of the circle.

Tangential acceleration is the acceleration associated with a mass moving through a particular point on a circular path. The direction of the acceleration vector is tangent to the circle and perpendicular to the radius.

Figure 7-3 shows that the direction of the angular velocity and acceleration of a rotating point are totally different than the tangential velocity and acceleration. **The angular velocity and angular acceleration vectors are directed upward/downward along the axis of rotation.** These directions were assigned based on the mathematics of circular motion, and are not directly intuitive.

ω, α

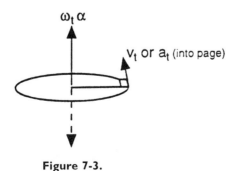

v_t or a_t (into page)

Figure 7-3.

FIGURE 7-3.
The direction of angular velocity and acceleration vectors are either upward or downward along the axis of rotation. Note that the tangential velocity or acceleration are directed tangent to the circle.

Where does tangential acceleration arise? Consider a mass rotating in a circular path. If the angular velocity increases, so then does the tangential speed. Changes in angular speed translate into changes in tangential acceleration.

II. Angular Velocity and Acceleration

The average angular velocity of an object (ω or omega) is the change in angular displacement of an object divided by time required for the displacement to occur. The units are in radians per second.

$$\omega = \Delta\theta / \Delta t$$

Angular velocity in units of radians per second can also be found as follows: $\omega = 2\pi f$, in which f is frequency in revolutions per second.

The average **angular acceleration** of an object (α or alpha) is the change in angular velocity of the object over the time interval during which this change takes place:

$$\alpha = \Delta\omega / \Delta t \qquad \text{or} \qquad \alpha = (\omega_f - \omega_o) / \Delta t$$

Linear velocity and accelerations can be converted into angular velocity and acceleration by dividing the linear quantities by the radius of rotation of the object:

$$\omega = v/r \qquad \text{and} \qquad \alpha = a_t/r$$

in which a_t is the tangential acceleration.

The vector directions of both angular velocity and acceleration were shown in Figure 7-3.

E X A M P L E   7 - 1

A BELT PASSES OVER a wheel with a radius of 25 cm. A point on the belt has a speed of 5 m/sec. Find the angular speed of the wheel.

SOLUTION

You are given the linear speed of the point on the belt (the units describe linear motion). Thus, $\omega = v/r$. $\omega = (5 \text{ m/sec})/(0.25 \text{ m}) = 20$ rad/sec. To convert radians per second into revolutions per second, multiply by the conversion factor:

$$(20 \text{ rad/sec})(1 \text{ rev})/(2\pi \text{ rad}) = 3.2 \text{ rev/sec.}$$

E X A M P L E   7 - 2

A ROPE WINDS AROUND a pulley with a radius of 5 cm. The pulley rotates at 30 revolutions per second and then slows uniformly to 20 revolutions per second over a time interval of 2 seconds. Answer the following questions.

1. Find the angular deceleration.

2. Find the number of revolutions associated with the two seconds of deceleration.

3. Find the length of rope that winds around the pulley in 2 seconds.

SOLUTION

1. $\alpha = (\omega_f - \omega_o) / \Delta t = (20 \text{ rev/sec} - 30 \text{ rev/sec})/2 \text{ sec} = -5 \text{ rev/sec}^2$

2. The number of revolutions should equal the average angular velocity multiplied by time.

$$\theta = (\omega_{ave})(t) = 1/2(\omega_f + \omega_o)(t) = 1/2(20 + 30)(2) = 50 \text{ revolutions}$$

more ▼

III. Centripetal Acceleration and Force

An object travels in a circular path at a constant rate. As the object rotates from A to B, its direction is constantly changing (i.e., the direction of its tangential travel). Objects naturally want to leave a circular rotation to travel tangentially. If you tie a weight to the end of a rope and begin rotating the rope and weight above your head in a circular path, you feel a force on your hand wanting to move the weight away from the circle. The force of your hand holding the rope resists the rope and weight leaving their circular orbit. If you let go of the rope, the weight would leave the circular orbit tangential to the spot on the circle from which it was released.

Study Figure 7-4. As a point rotates from A to B with constant speed, the direction of the tangential velocity vector changes. An acceleration is associated with this change because the velocity is changing over time. Velocity may change if direction changes and magnitude is constant. The acceleration associated with this velocity change is known as **centripetal acceleration** and is directed radially inward. **This acceleration is associated with the force holding the object in a circular path.**

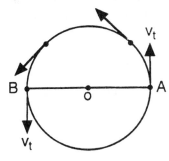

Figure 7-4.

FIGURE 7-4.
A point rotates in a circular path from A to B. Even at constant speed, the direction of the tangential velocity changes, which gives rise to a centripetal acceleration.

Two types of acceleration are shown in Figure 7-5. Tangential acceleration (a_t) is the acceleration of a rotating point tangent to the circle. Centripetal acceleration (a_c) is the acceleration associated with keeping an object rotating in a circular path and is directed inward. Use the following equation to find the magnitude of each type:

$$a_t = \alpha r$$

Centripetal acceleration: $\quad a_c = v^2/r \quad$ or $\quad a_c = \omega^2 r$

The force holding the rotating object in its circular path is the **centripetal force (F_c):**

$$F_c = ma_c = mv^2/r = m\omega^2 r$$

FIGURE 7-5.
Centripetal acceleration and
tangential acceleration vectors.

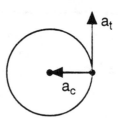

Figure 7-5.

$E\,X\,A\,M\,P\,L\,E\;\;7\,\text{-}\,3$

ANSWER THESE QUESTIONS.

1. A car drives on a circular flat track at constant speed. What are the forces that act on the car and the road?

    Solution: The weight of the car acts on the road, and an equal and opposite force is imparted to the car from the road. A small backward force on the car results from air resistance, and a forward force is exerted by the road on the tires. Finally, an inward-directed friction force is exerted on the tires by the road.

2. Which force keeps the car moving in a circular fashion and prevents it from flying off the track?

    Solution: The friction force between the tires and the road prevent the car from leaving the track. A centripetal acceleration results from a frictional force exerted on the tires by the road. This frictional force acts perpendicular to the motion of the car and is directed inward, as is the centripetal acceleration.

3. What would make the car fly off the track?

    Solution: If the driver tries to negotiate a curve too rapidly, the maximum frictional force will be exceeded and the car will skid. If the tires are bald, a smaller maximal frictional force is all that can be achieved, and the car is at increased risk to skid off the track. A wet track surface will also interfere with the friction between the tires and the road.

$E\,X\,A\,M\,P\,L\,E\;\;7\,\text{-}\,4$

WHY DO YOU THINK that good highways have banked curves rather than flat curves?

SOLUTION
Banked curves ensure that the normal force exerted by the road on the car has a horizontal component—the force the highway exerts against the vehicle. This horizontal component can provide part of or all the force needed to produce the centripetal acceleration, reducing the role of frictional force. The road becomes safer, especially when road surfaces are slippery.

IV. **Conceptual Relationships in Circular Motion**

Examine the relationships between v, a_c, and a_t in Figures 7-6, 7-7, and 7-8. In each circle, assume that a point is rotating with the conditions given. Note that a_c is associated with a change in direction, whereas a_t is associated with a change in magnitude.

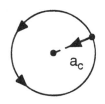

FIGURE 7-6.
Uniform circular motion with constant speed. Note an acceleration, namely a_c, but no a_t, at constant speed.

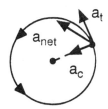

FIGURE 7-7.
Ever increasing speed. Note an acceleration tangentially as well as centripetally in this situation. The net acceleration vector, therefore, is a combination of these forces.

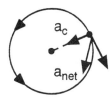

FIGURE 7-8.
Ever decreasing speed. A deceleration vector is directed opposite the direction of motion. Again, the net acceleration is the result of adding a_c and a_t.

V. Gravitation

Centuries ago, Newton described the law of universal gravitation, which states that every object in the universe, regardless of its mass, attracts every other object with a force that is proportional to the masses of the two objects and inversely proportional to the square of the distance between them:

$$F = G(m_1 m_2)/r^2$$
$$G = \text{universal constant } (6.67 \times 10^{-11} \text{ Nm}^2/\text{kg}^2)$$

The distance (r) is measured from the center of mass of one object to the center of mass of the other object.

Faraday developed the concept of a gravitational field, such that an object modifies the space surrounding it by establishing a gravitational field that extends outward in all directions. If a massless test point is placed near a second mass, such as the earth itself, you can derive the formula for the gravitational field of the earth (g):

$$g = GM/r^2$$

The gravitational field of a planet is related primarily to its mass. To find the value of g at the surface of a planet, simply use r = radius of the planet. For example, the value of g for the planet Jupiter would be:

$$g_{\text{Jupiter}} = G (M_{\text{Jupiter}} / r^2_{\text{Jupiter}})$$

Conceptual Questions:

1. Two identical objects rotate in circular paths of equal diameter. One object rotates twice as fast as the other. How does the centripetal force of the faster object compare to that of the slower object?

    Solution: The centripetal force varies as the square of the velocity or angular velocity. Thus, the centripetal force needed to keep the faster object rotating in a circular path is four times that needed for the slower object.

2. Two boys stand on opposite ends of a carousel that is turning clockwise. If one boy throws a ball directly toward the other, will the boy likely catch the ball?

Solution: Most likely, the ball will not be caught. When initially thrown, the ball might start going toward the recipient. Once the ball is in the air, however, the recipient and carousel turn clockwise and the ball will miss its target. The ball carries with it the velocity imparted by the ball thrower. The principle that explains the deflection of objects subjected to turning is the **Coriolis effect.**

8

Rotational Dynamics

dynamics dynan

| **I.** Moment of Inertia |
| **II.** Rotational Torque and Angular Momentum |
| **III.** Circular Applications of Kinematic Equations |

HIGH-YIELD TOPICS

Mass is the property of an object that resists acceleration. The moment of inertia takes the place of mass in rotational motion. **The moment of inertia is the quantitative angular measure of the property of an object that resists rotational acceleration.**

I. Moment of Inertia

The moment of inertia of a rigid body depends on the shape and axis of rotation of the body. Different formulas allow calculation of the moment of inertia of various different shapes (Table 8-1). The formula for a point mass is important to know.

TABLE 8-1. Moment of inertia formulas for common objects.

Shape	Formula
Point mass or thin ring	$I = mr^2$
Solid cylinder	$I = \frac{1}{2}mr^2$
Solid sphere	$I = \frac{2}{5}mr^2$

m = mass of the object; r = radius of the object.

II. Rotational Torque and Angular Momentum

Applying Newton's second law, $F = ma$, to rotational systems results in an expression for rotational torque (τ):

$$\tau = I\alpha$$

The rotational torque of an object is the moment of inertia times the angular acceleration. When compared to Newton's second law, the moment of inertia term replaces mass and the angular acceleration replaces linear acceleration.

The angular momentum (L) of a rotating object is similar to the expression for linear motion. Instead of mass, use moment of inertia (I) and instead of linear velocity, use angular velocity (ω).

$$L = I\omega$$

Just like with linear momentum, angular momentum is conserved if the external torque acting on the system is zero. Conservation of angular momentum says:

$$I\omega_{\text{(initial)}} = I\omega_{\text{(final)}}$$

EXAMPLE 8-1

What happens when you sit on a spinning bar stool with your legs folded, and then outspread them?

SOLUTION

The rate of spin decreases. In other words, your angular velocity decreases. This slowing occurs because the moment of inertia increases when your legs are outspread (radius increases) and because angular momentum is conserved, angular velocity must decrease.

EXAMPLE 8-2

Why does an ice skater in a spin turn faster when she pulls in her arms?

SOLUTION

This increase occurs because she is decreasing her moment of inertia (her radius decreases). Because angular momentum is conserved, her angular velocity increases.

Kinetic energy is associated with rotational motion. This type of energy is rotational kinetic energy. It is derived from the standard kinetic energy expression, although mass is replaced by moment of inertia and linear velocity is replaced by angular velocity.

$$\text{Rotational KE} = \tfrac{1}{2}I\omega^2$$

▌III. Circular Applications of Kinematic Equations

The kinematic equations reviewed in Chapter 3 can be fully applied to rotational systems by substituting the angular velocities and accelerations for the linear values. Distances are replaced with angle values. The rotational kinematic equations are presented in Table 8-2. If you know the linear forms of these equations, you need not memorize the rotational forms.

TABLE 8-2. Rotational kinematic equations.

Linear	Angular
$v = v_0 + at$	$\omega = \omega_0 + \alpha t$
$v_{\text{(ave)}} = \tfrac{1}{2}(v_i + v_f)$	$\omega_{\text{ave}} = \tfrac{1}{2}(\omega_i + \omega_f)$
$v_f^2 = v_0^2 + 2as$	$\omega^2 = \omega_0^2 + 2\alpha\theta$
$s = v_0 t + \tfrac{1}{2}at^2$	$\theta = \omega_0 t + \tfrac{1}{2}\alpha t^2$

A rotating disk, starting from rest, reaches a speed of 5 revolutions in 10 seconds. The moment of inertia of the disk is $I = \frac{1}{2} mr^2$, in which $m = 1$ kg and $r = 2$ m.

EXAMPLE 8-3

1. Find the angular acceleration of the disk.

2. Find the angular speed of the disk at $t = 11$ seconds.

3. Find the rotational torque of the disk.

SOLUTION

1. The angular acceleration $= \alpha = \Delta\omega/\Delta t = $ (5 rev/sec $-$ 0)/(10 sec) $=$ *0.5 rev/sec²*

2. The angular speed $\omega = \omega_o + \alpha t$; thus $\omega =$ (5 rev/sec)(2π rad/rev) $+$ (0.5 rev/sec)(2π rad/rev)(1sec) $= 10\pi$ rad/sec $+ 1\pi$ rad/sec $= 11\pi$ rad/sec $\approx$ *34 rad/sec*

Note that the initial angular speed was taken at $t = 10$ sec, so that at time 11 sec, only 1 sec had elapsed from the initial setting.

3. Rotational torque $= \tau = I\alpha = $ (1/2 mr²)(0.5 rev/sec)(2π rad/rev) $=$ *6.2 Nm*

9

Mechanical Properties

Mechanical Properties

HIGH-YIELD TOPICS	**I.** Important Terms
	II. Stress, Strain, and Moduli
	III. Surface Tension

The properties of solids are important topics in the health sciences, especially in such medical specialties as orthopedics and sports medicine. The key points in the following discussion are density, specific gravity, stress, strain, and elasticity.

I. Important Terms

The **density** of an object (ρ) equals its mass divided by its volume.

$$\rho = m/v \qquad \text{(units in SI system} = kg/m^3)$$

The specific gravity of an object is its density divided by a standard density. For gases, the density of air is used as the standard density. For liquids and solids, the density of water is used as the standard. Thus, the specific gravity is just a comparison of the density of an object to the density of a standard substance.

$$SG \text{ (liquid)} = \text{density of a particular liquid/density of } H_2O$$

The **elasticity** of an object is the property by which a body returns to its original size after deforming forces are removed.

II. Stress, Strain, and Moduli

A. Stress

Stress is a measure of the strength of an agent causing a deformation. A stress is a force applied over a unit area.

$$\text{Stress} = F/A \qquad \text{(units in SI system} = \text{Pascals (Pa) or } N/m^2)$$

Objects subjected to forces change their shape and may fracture. The fractional change in size or shape is the **strain,** and the force per unit area producing the deformation is the **stress.** For small applied forces or torques, the stress and strain in a material are usually linearly related. **The proportionality constant relating stress and strain is Young's modulus for tensile strain.**

B. Strain

Strain is the fractional deformation on an object resulting from a stress applied on the object.

$$\text{Strain} = \Delta \text{ dimension/original dimension (unitless)}$$

Three types of strain show dimensional changes as a result of an applied stress:

1. **Tensile strain:** The change in length of an object divided by the object's original length.

$$\Delta L/L_o$$

2. **Compressional strain:** The change in the volume of an object divided by the original volume of the object.

$$\Delta V/V_o$$

3. **Shear strain:** The distance a surface is sheared divided by the width of the object being sheared (Figure 9-1).

$$\Delta x/L$$

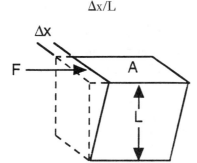

Figure 9-1.

FIGURE 9-1.
Shear strain. Note that a force causes the object to "shear" a distance (Δx). An example is pushing on the binding of a book. L represents the width of the object being sheared.

C. Moduli

The **elastic modulus** is the quotient of stress and strain. It is a measure of how hard it is to compress or stretch an object.

$$\text{Elastic modulus} = \text{Stress/strain}$$

Three types of moduli measure the fraction of stress over strain. The first type is **Young's modulus.** It is the ratio of stress and strain when an object stretches. The second type is **bulk modulus.** It is the ratio of stress to strain when the volume of an object changes. The third type is **shear modulus,** which is the ratio of stress to strain when an object is subject to shearing.

Young's modulus: Stretching stress/stretching strain = $F/A/_{\Delta L/Lo}$

Bulk modulus: Volume stress/volume strain = $\Delta P/_{-\Delta V/V}$

Shear modulus: Shearing stress/shearing strain = $F/A/_{\Delta x/L}$

III. Surface Tension

Surface tension is the amount of work (energy, or ΔE) required to expand the surface of a liquid by a given amount of area (ΔA).

$$\text{Surface tension} = \Delta E/\Delta A$$

Surface tension results from intermolecular attraction forces causing molecules on the surface of a liquid to be attracted to one another and to molecules below the surface. The molecules on the surface have a net attraction to the interior of the liquid, and try to form a surface that minimizes surface area. In Figure 9-2, notice that the surface of the liquid forms a "film" that minimizes surface area. An example is dewdrops you see early in the morning. These drops form spheres, which minimize the surface area for a given volume.

FIGURE 9-2.
Surface tension.

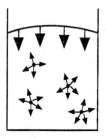

Figure 9-2.

Cohesive forces are forces that attract like particles. An example is water molecules attracting one another. **Adhesive forces** are the attractions between unlike particles, such as water molecules being attracted to the glass wall of a container. If cohesive forces are larger than the adhesive forces in a given liquid, such as mercury, the fluid in a glass container will contact the container with a downward slope (Figure 9-3). If adhesive forces are stronger than cohesive forces, the liquid becomes attracted to the container sides and will slope upward to the point of contact (see Figure 9-3).

FIGURE 9-3.
When cohesive forces are greater than adhesive forces, a downward sloping fluid may result, as in mercury (left). When adhesive forces are greater, an upward sloping fluid may result, as in water (right).

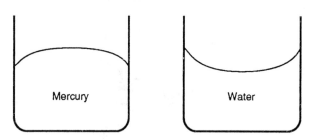

Mercury   Water

Figure 9-3.

10

Fluids

Fluids

I. Fluid Statics		**HIGH-YIELD**
II. Fluid Dynamics		**TOPICS**

Fluids are substances that have no rigidity, lack a fixed shape, and take the shape of the container that holds them. The focus of this chapter is on applying the laws of mechanics to fluids. Because a given mass of fluid does not have a fixed shape, the terms density and pressure are used instead of mass and force.

I. Fluid Statics

A. Basic Concepts

The **density** of a fluid (ρ) is the ratio of the mass of the fluid to its volume.

$$\rho = m/v \quad \text{(in kg/m}^3\text{)}$$

The **pressure** exerted on a fluid is the ratio of the force acting on the fluid to the surface area at which the force acts:

$$P = F/A$$

Pressure is a scalar quantity and is measured in the SI system in units of N/m^2, or Pascals (Pa).

The pressure in a container of fluid increases as one moves deeper below the surface. You have experienced this principle in a swimming pool; the pressure on your eardrums is greater at a deep region in the pool than in a shallow region.

The **pressure at any depth** below the surface of a fluid is proportional to the fluid density and depth. It also depends on the acceleration of gravity (g), because the pressure at any depth depends on the weight of fluid over any point below the fluid surface.

To calculate the pressure at a point below the surface of a fluid (Figure 10-1), you must first remember that atmospheric pressure acts at the surface of a fluid. **Thus, the pressure at a point below the surface of a fluid will be the sum of the atmospheric pressure at the surface and the weight of the water above the point.**

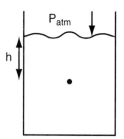

Figure 10-1.

FIGURE 10-1.

Pressure at a depth (h) below the surface of a fluid depends on the atmospheric pressure acting on the surface, the density of the fluid, the depth of the point of interest, and the acceleration of gravity.

Pressure at a depth (h) below the surface of a fluid:

$$P = P_{atm} + \rho gh$$

To find the pressure difference between two points in a fluid (Figure 10-2):

$$P_{diff} = \rho g \Delta h$$

FIGURE 10-2.

Difference in pressure between two points in a static fluid depends on the density of the fluid, the height difference between the two points, and the acceleration of gravity.

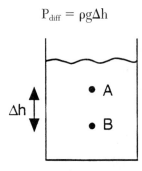

Figure 10-2.

in which Δh is the height difference between the two points.

B. Pascal's Principle

This basic law of fluids says that a change in pressure in a confined fluid is transmitted without change to all points in the fluid. Stated more simply, the pressure is the same at two places at the same depth in a fluid at rest. By Pascal's principle, points B, C, and D in Figure 10-3 are all subjected to the same pressure. Even if the container over point B was sealed at the fluid surface, the pressure at B would still equal that at C and D. Do not be tricked by the shape of the fluid container; the issue is the depth of the points in question.

FIGURE 10-3.

Pascal's principle. Pressure at points B, C, and D are equal.

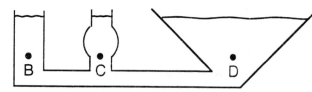

Figure 10-3.

The most common application of Pascal's principle is the **hydraulic lift** (Figure 10-4). A hydraulic lift contains an incompressible fluid. When a force is applied to the piston on one end of the lift, the pressure is transmitted through the liquid undiminished to the other piston on the opposite end of the lift. Therefore, a piston with small surface area transmitting a small force is effective in transmitting a large force to a large piston, because $P = F/A$ and the pressure is transmitted through the system unchanged. A similar situation occurs when you jack up your car. A force applied on a small surface-area piston generates pressure that is transmitted to the other end of the hydraulic jack. The pressure then acts on a larger surface-area piston, which, in turn, generates a larger force.

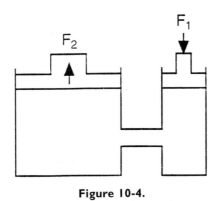

FIGURE 10-4.
Hydraulic lift.

Figure 10-4.

Thus, for hydraulic lifts or closed systems in which pressure is transmitted:

$F_1/A_1 = F_2/A_2$ or $F_2/F_1 = A_2/A_1$ where A_1 and A_2 are the areas of the pistons

C. Archimedes' Principle

An object that floats or is submerged in a fluid experiences an upward or buoyant force because of the fluid. The buoyant force is equal to the weight of fluid that the object displaces. **Archimedes' principle states that the buoyant force exerted on a body partly or completely immersed in a fluid is equal to the weight of the fluid displaced by the body.**

Figure 10-5 demonstrates that when an object with volume (V) is immersed in a fluid-filled container, several forces act on the object. The buoyant force (B) pulls the object to the surface of the fluid. The weight of the object (w_o) makes it sink in the fluid. Whether or not the object sinks or rises depends on the balance of these upward and downward forces.

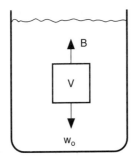

FIGURE 10-5.
Archimedes' principle.

Figure 10-5.

To find the **magnitude of the buoyant force,** use the following formula:

Buoyant force (B) $= mg = \rho Vg$

in which ρ is the density of the fluid, **V** is the volume of the object or the fluid volume displaced, and **g** is the acceleration of gravity.

If an object is suspended from a string into a fluid (Figure 10-6), you can find the **tension** on the string by diagramming the forces involved. The upward forces are tension and buoyant force. The downward force is weight. Tension will be (Weight) − (buoyant force).

FIGURE 10-6.

To find the tension on a
string for the diagram in
Figure 10-6, take the difference of the weight of
the block and the buoyant
force acting on the block.

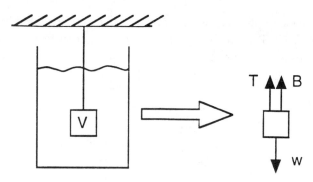

Figure 10-6.

E X A M P L E   1 0 - 1 ●

A GLASS IS FILLED with water and ice cubes. The water level reaches the rim of the glass and the ice cubes rise out of the water above the rim of the glass. What would you expect to happen when the ice melts?

SOLUTION

The water level will not change. Ice has a density far less than that of water, which is why it floats. The ice cubes will position themselves in the fluid based on the ratio of their density to that of the water. As the ice melts, it becomes water (more dense) and fills a smaller volume. The volume filled by the melted ice will equal the amount the water rose when the ice was first added.

A rule to remember when solving these conceptual problems is: **The ratio of the densities of an object to that of a fluid will equal the fraction of the volume submerged.** This idea makes sense because less dense objects should have less volume submerged and more of their volume floating.

E X A M P L E   1 0 - 2 ●

AN ICEBERG FLOATING in the Arctic Sea has a density of 920 kg/m³. Find the fraction of the iceberg that floats **above** the surface of the sea. Assume the density of sea water is 1025 kg/m³.

SOLUTION

Find the ratio of the densities:

(Density iceberg)/(density seawater) = 920/1025 = 0.90

Thus, 90% of the iceberg is submerged and 10% of the iceberg floats above the sea surface.

II. Fluid Dynamics

A. Continuity Equation

The **continuity equation** (Figure 10-7) says that the volume of fluid entering a pipe per unit time must equal the volume of fluid leaving the pipe per unit time, even if the diameter of the pipe changes:

$$A_1 v_1 = A_2 v_2$$

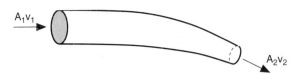

FIGURE 10-7.
Continuity equation.

Figure 10-7.

in which **A** is the cross-sectional area of the pipe and **v** is the velocity of fluid flow. This idea makes sense because what flows into a system must flow out. Because fluid is incompressible, the fluid flow rate through a large pipe and into a small pipe will increase in velocity. The product (A)(v) for the fluid will not change, however, which is the same as saying that the volume of fluid per unit time will not change.

Think about a garden hose. The flow of water from the end of the hose is the same whether or not you narrow the opening. When you do narrow the opening, you decrease the cross-sectional area of the hose, and the velocity of fluid flow increases.

B. Bernoulli's Principle (Figure 10-8)

This important principle says that the quantity: $P + 1/2\rho v^2 + \rho gh = $ **a constant** everywhere in a flow tube; **P** is pressure, **v** is velocity of fluid flow, and **h** is the height of the tube from a reference point.

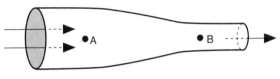

Figure 10-8.

Notice that the $1/2\rho v^2$ term resembles the kinetic energy expression, and describes the kinetic energy per unit volume of the fluid. The pgh term looks like the potential energy expression, and describes the potential energy per unit volume of the fluid. Thus, the **Bernoulli equation is simply a manipulated conservation of energy expression.**

The Bernoulli equation is useful in solving qualitative, conceptual questions. Suppose you are asked how the pressure will compare as fluid flows from a large rigid tube to a small rigid tube at the same height. To answer this question, realize that the velocity of fluid flow will increase from the large tube to the small tube (continuity equation).

$$P + 1/2\rho v^2 + \rho gh \text{ (large tube)} = P + 1/2\rho v^2 + \rho gh \text{ (small tube)}$$

Because the KE term of the small tube is greater than that of the large tube (because of a higher velocity), and because the heights are the same, the pressure of the small tube must be smaller. Thus, the pressure of fluid flow at point B (Figure 10-8) is less than at point A. This concept may seem anti-intuitive, but remember you are solving a fluid dynamics problem, not a fluids-at-rest problem.

C. Laminar Versus Turbulent Flow

Laminar flow or streamline flow is best thought of conceptually. If fluid travels in cylindric "sheets" through a tube, each "sheet" slides by its neighbor. In this way, the fluid flow in a tube is directed in one direction without disorganized turbulence.

When the properties of the fluid such as its density or velocity are increased, fluid flow tends to be **turbulent.** Consider an avalanche on a snow-covered mountain. Snow flows with disorganized turbulence, not in organized "sheets."

Fluid may flow in turbulent spiraling waves through a tube. **The Reynold's number** is a quantitative relationship that suggests whether flow will be turbulent or laminar/streamline. Values of the Reynold's number over 2000 suggest turbulent flow, whereas values less than 2000 suggest laminar flow.

$$\text{Reynold's number} = 2\rho vr/\eta$$

in which ρ is fluid density, v is velocity, r is radius of tube, and η is fluid viscosity.

D. Viscosity

Intuitively, viscosity depends on the "thickness" of a fluid. Syrup is considered viscous because it is "thick." To understand viscosity and how it is measured, consider **two flat plates separated by a thin fluid layer.** If the lower plate is fixed and a force is applied to the upper plate in an attempt to move it at constant speed, you could measure the force applied. **This force would be a measure of the viscous forces of the liquid. Viscosity is a measure of how fluid flows,** and is defined based on a relationship among an applied force to an area (flat plate), velocity (of upper plate), and separation (between plates).

$$\eta \text{ (viscosity)} = {}^{F/A}\!/_{v/l}$$

in which F is force applied, A is the area to which force is applied, v is velocity of the upper plate, and l is the distance between plates.

Conceptual Questions:

1. A man fills a "weightless" water balloon with water from a swimming pool. He ties a string to the end of the water balloon and lowers the balloon into the pool, suspended from the string, until it is completely submerged. What fraction of weight of the balloon (in air) must he exert to hold the balloon at a constant level in the pool?

    Solution: The man exerts no force. Because the fluid in the pool is the same as the fluid in the balloon, the weight of the water in the balloon equals the weight of the water displaced; i.e., the buoyancy of the surrounding water supports the water balloon.

    If the balloon contained a fluid that was twice as dense as the pool water, the man would have to pull up with a force equal to the apparent weight (weight submerged in the pool) of the balloon. To find the apparent weight of an object submerged, subtract the weight of the volume of pool water displaced from the weight in air of the fluid-filled balloon.

2. A fisherman sits on a pier and lowers a fishing line into the sea. On the end of the line is a spherical lead weight. When the weight is submerged halfway to the ocean floor, the fisherman estimates that he has to support only 5 pounds. As he lowers the weight still further, what happens to the force needed to support the weight?

    Solution: The force needed to support the weight does not change. The lead weight is buoyed by a force equal to the weight of the seawater displaced. This buoyant force does not depend on the depth submerged as long as the object is fully below the water surface and is not touching the ocean bottom.

3. Some swimming pools are constructed with concrete walls that are thicker at the bottom than toward the top because water pressure increases with depth. Pool A is 10×20 ft and 15 ft deep. Pool B is 30×50 ft and 10 ft deep. Which pool should be the stronger based on physics principles?

    Solution: The construction of Pool A, the deeper pool, should be the strongest. The walls of the pool are subjected to pressure that depends only on the depth of the pool and not on how much water it contains. Thus, the pressure on the walls of the pool is greater for the deeper pool.

(II)

Temperature and Heat

I. Temperature	
II. Thermal Expansion	**HIGH-YIELD**
III. Heat and Heat Transfer	**TOPICS**
IV. Conservation of Energy	

The basics of thermal energy are defined and discussed in terms of thermal energy, temperature, thermal expansion, heat, heat capacity, specific heat, heat transfer, and conservation of energy. Chapter 12 addresses the topics of calorimetry and thermodynamics.

I. Temperature

A. Thermal Energy

The thermal energy in a substance is the kinetic energy associated with the random motion of the atoms and/or molecules it contains. As the thermal energy status of a substance increases, so does the total kinetic energy associated with that substance. This kinetic energy allows for additional atom and/or molecule translation, rotation, and vibration.

B. Temperature

Temperature is an indicator of the average random kinetic energy of the atoms and/or molecules in a substance. Average random kinetic energy of substance atoms and/or molecules increases as temperature is increased. Although the term **thermal energy** corresponds to the total kinetic energy associated with a substance, **temperature** is a measure of the average thermal energy per atom and/or molecule.

Thermal energy is an **extensive property** (its value is proportional to the amount of substance present); temperature is an **intensive property** (does not depend on the amount of substance present). To make the distinction clear, compare a cup of tap water to a large lake, both with a temperature of 67°F. Although the two bodies of water have the same temperature (i.e., same average thermal energy per molecule), their thermal energies differ (i.e., total energy content).

Thermometers measure temperature. Classic thermometers measure temperature as a function of liquid mercury expansion and contraction. The details of thermometer design are of less importance, however, than a good understanding of **temperature scale.** A temperature scale is an arbitrary system used to quantify the temperature of a substance. The scale is constructed by assigning arbitrary values to points on the device associated with important thermodynamic events (usually the melting and freezing points of pure water at one atmosphere pressure) and dividing the spaces between these reference temperatures into equally spaced values.

The temperature associated with the freezing of water is the **freezing point,** and the temperature associated with the boiling of water is the **boiling point.** Unfortunately, the point (i.e., the value) on the temperature scale assigned to the melting or boiling of water varies according to which of three temperature scales is used.

The official (SI) unit of temperature is the **Kelvin,** abbreviated as K (not °K; no degree sign is used). The height of the liquid–mercury column at the time of water freezing is marked 273 K, and that associated with boiling is marked 373 K. Thus, a **temperature interval** (i.e., difference or delta) of 100 units exists between the two standard reference points.

The English system, or the "unofficial science language," defines the two reference points using the principle of "number simplicity;" the freezing point of water is zero degrees **Celsius** (0°C) and the boiling point is 100°C. Again, 100 units or degrees exist between the reference points of freezing and boiling.

Using the "American science language," the **Fahrenheit** temperature scale sets the freezing point at 32° Fahrenheit (32°F) and boiling at 212°F, creating a temperature interval between the two reference points of 180 units or degrees. Thus, it can be said that a one-unit temperature change in the Kelvin and Celsius systems is of a larger magnitude than one unit change in the Fahrenheit system. Another way of phrasing this same idea is that a change in one degree Fahrenheit (i.e., the American way) is "worth less" than a change in one degree of the systems used elsewhere. The key is that the differences in terminology are more than just semantics. The differences "between the languages" are the varying reference temperature values and intervals.

As shown in Figure 11-1, temperature scale conversions are straightforward. Computations to remember follow:

$$°C = K - 273$$
$$T_F = 9/5 \, T_C + 32$$
$$T_C = 5/9(T_F - 32)$$

FIGURE 11-1.
Three temperature scales.

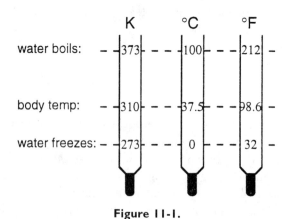

Figure 11-1.

Be aware that 0 K is a special temperature point and is referred to as **absolute zero** (i.e., the temperature at which all atoms and/or molecules possess zero kinetic energy).

Answer the following questions:

1. Can you calculate absolute zero in terms of °C and °F?

    Answer: −273°C and −460°F, respectively.

2.   Is there a temperature less than 0 K?

    Answer: No. Absolute zero is the "absolutely" lowest temperature and energy state possible.

II. Thermal Expansion

Both solids and fluids can experience changes in dimensions (linear and volume) that correlate directly with the amount of temperature change. Most substances expand as they are warmed and contract as they cool. Thermal expansion and contraction are a direct result of altered (increased and reduced, respectively) atom and/or molecule movement within the material. Residents of regions with cool temperatures witness the linear changes in sidewalk and road cement (buckling) that occur during summer heat waves. Temperature-induced changes in both linear and volume dimensions occur.

The amount of change in dimension logically is proportional to the initial dimension of the object (length [L] or volume [V]), the amount of temperature change ($\Delta T = T_{final} - T_{initial}$), and some coefficient indicative of how easily that material changes dimension (α or β). Two equations express this principle:

Linear change equation: $\Delta L = \alpha \, L_{initial} \, (\Delta T)$
Volumetric change equation: $\Delta V = \beta \, V_{initial} \, (\Delta T)$

Alpha (α) is the **coefficient of linear expansion.** The units of this term must be reciprocal Celsius degrees ($°C^{-1}$) in order for a unit of length to result. Beta (β) is the **coefficient of volume expansion** for both solids and fluids. For a solid, $\beta = 3\alpha$ (length, width, and height are changing).

Conceptually, it makes sense that gasoline vapors expand more easily than rubber > aluminum > steel > concrete > glass. What would be a good way to remove an aluminum lid that is tightly covering a glass jar? Heat the lid slightly, allowing the aluminum to expand. The glass does not expand as much as the aluminum per unit temperature change.

III. Heat and Heat Transfer

A. Heat

Heat is the amount of energy transferred from one object or body to another because of a difference in their temperatures. Heat (Q) is quantified in energy units of joules (J) according to SI conventions. Heat is commonly expressed in units of calories (cal), in which 1 calorie is the amount of heat required to increase the temperature of 1 g of water by 1 K or 1°C at room temperature (293 K). Note that **1 cal = 4.2 J.** When the term calorie is capitalized, it implies kilocalories. Thus, food companies and hospital dieticians use 5 Calories to mean what is really 5 kilocalories (5 kcal) or 5000 calories.

Heat capacity is the amount of heat energy needed to raise the temperature of a certain amount of substance by 1 K or 1°C. The amount of heat (Q) required to increase the temperature of a given substance from any initial temperature (T_i) to any final temperature (T_f) can be determined by knowing the heat equation:

$$Q \text{ (heat)} = m \, c \, \Delta T$$

in which m is the mass of the object, c is the specific heat capacity of that particular substance, and ΔT is the change in temperature.

The **specific heat capacity** of a substance is the heat capacity per unit mass (i.e., the amount of heat that must be added to 1 g of that substance to raise its temperature by 1 K or 1°C). **Specific heat is the amount of heat in *calories* required to raise the temperature of 1 g of a substance by 1°C.** It is important to know specific heat values of water and ice (1.0 and 0.5 cal/g°C, respectively). Sample problems are provided in Chapter 12.

B.   Heat Transfer Mechanisms

Heat is transferred from one region or body to another by the following basic mechanisms.

Convection involves the actual **movement** of part of the system from an area of high temperature to one of lower temperature. This process occurs in both gases and liquids. **Examples** of this process include movement of hot air pockets in a gas oven or in the sky.

Conduction involves thermal energy **transfer** without the macroscopic movement of the medium that carries the heat. Thus, like sound and electricity, heat conduction requires contact between neighboring molecules and molecule-to-molecule transfer of energy. Heat of conduction varies directly with surface area of the heat source and difference in temperature between the source and recipient locales. Heat of conduction varies inversely with distance from the source (i.e., the farther you are from the heat source, the less heat is transmitted to you). **Examples** include transfer of heat across a hot metal grill, around a cooking pan, or up the handle of a soup spoon.

Radiation involves the transfer of heat by **electromagnetic (EM) radiation.** Unlike convection and conduction, radiation can transmit heat energy through empty space. All forms of EM radiation have energy associated with them and, thus, heat energy. **Examples** include microwaves, ultraviolet light, x-rays, and deadly gamma rays. Remember: heat of radiation is proportional to the area (A) of the emitting surface, several constants (related to how good a radiator a particular object is), and to the fourth power of temperature (T) in units of Kelvin; heat of radiation is proportional to T^4 (where T is in units of K).

Question: What is the difference in the heat of radiation of Object A with a temperature of 1 K and Object B with a temperature of 2 K? **Answer:** Object B emits about 16 times more radiation than Object A if all other values are equal ($2^4 = 16$). Remember also that all objects above absolute zero (0K) emit radiation.

IV. Conservation of Energy

Energy is a **conserved** property (i.e., the total energy of a closed system is **constant**). Energy can be transferred between objects within a sealed system and/or can be converted to different forms. It makes sense that thermal energy (TE) change is one component of the energy conservation equation because energy in a system can exist as or be converted to thermal energy. Heat (Q) is also part of the energy conservation equation, because heat is a source of energy input into a system. If the total energy of a system is constant, then an expression that accounts for energy dynamics follows:

$$\text{Heat} + \text{Work (input/output)} =$$
$$\text{Sum of changes in different forms of energy (KE, PE, and TE)}$$

The **conservation of energy principle** states that what energy goes into or comes out of a system in the form of heat or work leads to a change in the various energy forms within the system (such as changes in kinetic energy, potential energy, and/or thermal energy).

Thermodynamics

Thermodyn

I. Thermodynamic Principles		
II. Calorimetry		**HIGH-YIELD**
III. Work		**TOPICS**
IV. Laws of Thermodynamics		

The goal of this review of thermodynamic principles, the science of heat and temperature, and the laws governing the conversion of heat into other forms of energy, is to ensure strong qualitative and quantitative understanding of thermodynamics.

I. Thermodynamic Principles

Before solving thermodynamic problems, it is important to understand certain terms. Figure 12-1 displays a sealed glass box that contains a solid metal ball. Given that the box and ball are our main interests, we call the inside of the box the **"system"** under study. The system therefore comprises: (1) the air inside the box, and (2) the metal ball itself. The area outside of the system, or outside the box in this example, is the **"surroundings."**

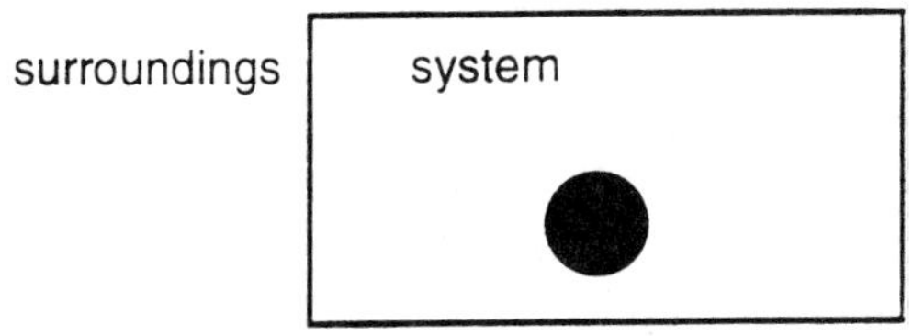

Figure 12-1.

FIGURE 12-1.
A system and surroundings.

   If the system is **"closed"** (i.e., sealed), the system does NOT interact or exchange energy with the surroundings. If no energy in the form of heat can enter or leave the system, the net change in the system's overall energy and heat content is zero. If the system is **"open,"** the system and surroundings are free to interact and exchange energy forms. Systems can be open or closed.

   Thermodynamic equilibrium exists if the measurable physical parameters of a system (e.g., temperature, volume, and pressure) are constant over time. **Thermal equilibrium** exists if two systems are in thermal contact and no heat flow between them occurs (their temperatures are equal).

If no change or net change in heat content occurs, then **Q = 0.** If a system gains energy in the form of heat, then the heat content increases [i.e., **Q is positive (+)**]. If a system releases heat, **Q is negative (−).** Recall the relationship: $Q = m\,c\,\Delta T$; Q is positive (+) if $T_{final} > T_{initial}$ and negative (−) if $T_f < T_i$.

The principle of **phase change** also warrants review. Many substances have the potential to exist in three states or phases: solid, liquid, and gas. The phase of a substance at any time (t) is related solely to its energy state at that particular time.

Figure 12-2 shows an experiment that involves the study of the phase changes experienced by water (H_2O) as it is heated. The H_2O used is pure (distilled) and is placed in a room at one atmosphere pressure. A hot Bunsen burner is placed below a 5-g block of ice (solid H_2O) with an initial temperature of −20°C (point **A** on the graph in Figure 12-2). As heat is supplied to the ice cube, the average random kinetic energy (KE) of the H_2O molecules increases, and they move more and more.

FIGURE 12-2.

Phase changes of water (H_2O).
s = solid, l = liquid, g = gas,
p = plasma.

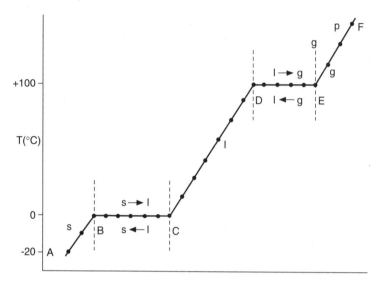

Time

Figure 12-2.

The ice is warmed until it reaches 0°C (point **B**), the **melting point** for pure H_2O at 1 atm pressure. Note that although the temperature of the entire ice cube is increasing, no change in phase has occurred (i.e., it does not melt at all). Not until **all** regions of the ice cube (both the inside and outside) reach the melting point (0°C) does a change in phase occur (i.e., melting of the ice cube begins). Then, energy supplied by the hot flame goes to melt the ice cube only, with no ΔT during the melting process. Not until every molecule changes phase (solid → liquid) does the temperature again begin to increase.

Point C represents newly formed water (the liquid form of H_2O) at 0°C. Heat from the flame then warms the water. The phase of the water does not change at all until every region of the flowing fluid reaches 100°C (point **D**), the official **boiling point** for pure water at 1 atm pressure. As heat is absorbed by the water, the energy level of the water molecules increases, leading to **vaporization** (molecules escaping the surface of the liquid because of their great energy level).

Figure 12-2 shows that temperature always remains constant during a phase change. Water at 100°C is converted to vapor at 100°C. As long as even one water molecule at 100°C is still around, the temperature of the steam will not rise above 100°C. Once all the liquid (i.e., water) at 100°C has been converted to gas (i.e., water vapor) at 100°C (point **E**), the temperature of the gas begins to rise.

The phase change from B → C is **melting** or **fusion;** the change from D → E is **evaporation.** If a hot object releases energy in the form of heat, it can move from E → D in a process termed **condensation.** If more energy is released from the object, it can move from C → B, which is termed **freezing.** The process involving the direct conversion of either the solid to the gas form (B → E) **or** gas to solid form (E → B), without going through the liquid phase, is **sublimation.** Gases, when exposed to extremely high energy, may decompose into hot charged particles referred to as **plasma** (occurs at point **F** on Figure 12-2; p, plasma phase of matter).

Physicists define the **heat of fusion (H_f)** of a substance as the amount of heat needed to transform 1 g of a substance from a solid to a liquid. The H_f of ice is 80 cal/g. The **heat of vaporization (H_v)** is the amount of heat required to convert 1 g of a liquid into a gas. The H_v for water is 540 cal/g. Clearly, it takes more energy per gram substance to vaporize than to melt (almost seven times as much energy per gram). Similarly, 1 g of steam undergoing condensation releases more energy than 1 g of water undergoing the freezing process (also about seven times more energy per gram given off). The heats associated with the two phase changes just mentioned can be calculated for any substance given the H_f and H_v values and the mass (m) of substance going through the phase change:

$$Q_{fusion} = mH_f \qquad Q_{vaporization} = mH_v$$
("interphase" heat equations)

In this chapter, the term **"interphase"** refers to the heat involved in the phase change occurring between two different phases. The preceding formulas are used **only** for "interphase" processes. To calculate the amount of heat needed to heat water from 20° to 30°C, or the amount of heat released when cooling water from say 30° to 20°C, use the **"intraphase"** (i.e., within a single phase) equation:

$$Q = m\,c\,\Delta T \qquad \text{("intraphase" heat equation)}$$

The specific heat capacity (c) of ice is 0.5 cal/g°C, whereas that of water is 1.0 cal/g°C. This equation is used to determine how much heat is required or released from $T_{initial}$ to T_{final}. Remember that ΔT is defined as the change in temperature ($T_{final} - T_{initial}$). (See the sample problems illustrating the use of these expressions in the Calorimetry section.)

II. Calorimetry

Calorimetry is the science of "counting calories." Calorimetry is often used when quantitating energy gained or lost during some chemical reaction, biologic process, or activity. Calorimetric techniques are based on principles of energy (thermal energy) conservation, which were discussed previously.

The **calorimeter** is a well-insulated device that allows for the creation of a closed (sealed) thermal system. Ideally, no transfer of heat should occur from the surroundings into the system or from the system into the surroundings. Such ideal conditions are realized by excellent calorimeter design and construction. The calorimeter consists of a durable metal, glass, or other strong container that usually is surrounded by a good insulator, such as styrofoam, which prevents heat transfer. The container is filled with a material of known composition, temperature, and thermal behavior. The test object, with an unknown thermal content, is then introduced into the container. Such a calorimetric setup is demonstrated in Figure 12-3.

If a researcher wants to know the amount of heat released by a chemical reaction, biologic process, or mass, he inserts the test object into the container. It is assumed that any change in the temperature and/or state of the fluid is related to the energy content of the test object. It is now possible to quantitate thermal processes, given that the heat energy gained by the colder object must equal that lost by the warmer object (i.e., **no net change**

FIGURE 12-3.

A calorimeter.

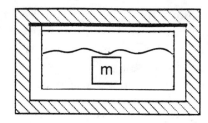

Figure 12-3.

in the heat content of the system). These statements are equivalent but can be expressed separately as equations:

$$Q_{gained} = Q_{lost} \quad \text{or} \quad \Delta Q = 0$$

which is equivalent to:

$$mc\,\Delta T_{gained} = mc\,\Delta T_{lost} \quad \text{or} \quad (mc\,\Delta T_{gained}) + (mc\,\Delta T_{lost}) = 0$$

Calorimetry can be used to determine any of the following variables found in the heat content equation if all others are known: final temperature of a mixture, specific heat capacity of some unknown material, and the mass of a material present in the container.

EXAMPLE 12-1

AS SHOWN IN FIGURE 12-3, a 25-g block of pure metal (unknown type) with a temperature of 100°C is placed into a well-insulated container filled with 50 g of water (c = 1.0 cal/g°C) at 20°C. The lid of the container is tightened to ensure total insulation. The metal is completely submerged in the water and the mixture is allowed to sit for 5 minutes. The thermometer that penetrates the lid shows the final temperature for the water bath is 24°C. What is the specific heat capacity of the metal?

SOLUTION

Taking into consideration that a "small hot" mass is immersed in a "moderate" volume of "cool" water, it is reasonable to expect the water to warm slightly as a result of thermal energy (heat) released by the hot metal. Determine c_{metal} using the principles discussed previously.

Using the formula $Q_{gain} = Q_{lost}$ is often a faster and safer way to calculate unknowns in calorimetry problems because you need not assign positive or negative signs to Q values. Be sure, however, that each quantity in the expression has a positive value (because you are summing values to be used for equivalency).

When final temperature is less than initial temperature, as is in the following example (*), the normal definition of ΔT ($T_f - T_i$) is reversed (changed to $T_i - T_f$) so that the quantity itself is positive. Because a phase change in this experiment is unlikely (given the numbers provided), it is possible to use the intraphase heat transfer expression: $Q = m\,c\,\Delta T$.

$$Q_{gained\ by\ the\ water} = Q_{lost\ by\ the\ metal\ block}$$
$$(m)(c)(T_f - T_i) = (m)(c)(T_i - T_f)*$$
$$(50\ g)(1.0\ cal/g°C)(24 - 20°C) = (25\ g)(c)(100 - 76°C)$$
$$200\ cal/(25\ g \times 76°C) = 0.1\ cal/g°C = c,\ answer$$

EXAMPLE 12-2

FIFTY GRAMS OF ICE at $-2°C$ is added to 10 g of steam at 100°C in a sealed chamber. What is the final temperature of the mixture if no heat can enter or leave the system?

SOLUTION

Keep in mind that the steam gives up heat energy to the ice, and the ice gains heat energy from the steam. The system reaches an equilibrium point (i.e., only one phase). Also, energy gained by the ice is equal to that lost by the steam. Start by predicting what happens to each substance as the experiment continues. You have 50 g of "slightly cold" ice (which needs only slight warming to reach a phase change location) and only 10 g of "very cold" steam (100°C is the lowest temperature at which pure steam can exist before cooling [condensing] to become liquid [water]).

Q_{gain}: i. Ice probably warms to 0°C, and then:

ii. Ice probably goes through a phase change (melting) to become water at 0°C, and then:

iii. Water at 0°C probably warms to some T_f that corresponds to the liquid temperature range.

Q_{lost}: iv. Steam already at 100°C probably goes through a phase change (condensation) to become water at 100°C, and then:

v. Newly formed hot water at 100°C probably cools to some T_f in the liquid temperature range.

To set up the quantitative expression and solve for T_f:

Heat gained by ice = Heat lost by steam

$$(mc\Delta T)_{ice} + (mH_f)_{ice \to water} + (mc\Delta T)_{water} = (mH_v)_{steam \to water} + (mc\Delta T)_{water}$$

$$(50 \text{ g})(0.5 \text{ cal/g°C})(0 - [-2]) + (50 \text{ g})(80 \text{ cal/g}) + (50 \text{ g})(1 \text{ cal/g°C})(T_f - 0)$$

$$= (10 \text{ g})(540 \text{ cal/g}) + (10 \text{ g})(1)(100 - T_f)*$$

$$50 \text{ cal} + 4000 \text{ cal} + 50T_f = 5400 \text{ cal} + (1000 - 10T_f)$$

$$60T_f = 2350$$

$$\mathbf{T_f} = 39°C \text{ (liquid phase)}$$

Note that each quantity on both the left and the right are positive; you are summing each side, assuming total heat acceptance or contribution.

Calorimetry techniques can be used to determine basal metabolic rate. A person is placed in a small, closed chamber filled with cool air of known mass (m), specific heat (c), and temperature (T). Energy in the form of heat leaves the warm person and heats the air circulating through the chamber. The amount of energy per unit time released from the subject is calculated by using equipment outside the chamber.

III. Work

The discussion of work in Chapter 5 dealt with mechanical work. The following section also addresses mechanical work but with the additional consideration of pressure–volume systems acting as energy sources.

A metal container has a piston-type lid that moves up and down depending on the pressure underneath it (Figure 12-4). The container is filled with gas molecules, which

FIGURE 12-4.

A Bunsen burner heating a piston system. As the kinetic energy of the gas molecules increases, pressure increases in
the piston system, which leads
to a volume increase.

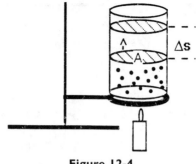

Figure 12-4.

when heated, tend to bump harder against the walls and lid of the container. As the gas molecules obtain greater and greater kinetic energy from heating, the pressure inside the container increases.

If the lid, with surface area A, rises a distance Δs, then the work done on the system (i.e., the container) by the surroundings (the Bunsen burner) can be derived by using the following concept: work is proportional to the force applied, the distance over which it is applied, and the angle between force and direction of travel [considered to be 0°, so ø = 1].

$$W = (F)(\Delta s) = (P \bullet A)(\Delta s) = (P)(\Delta V)$$

Thermodynamic work is equal to the pressure of a system times the change in volume produced as a result of a force. This simple expression assumes constant pressure conditions throughout the work process (more of a rarity in real life).

According to MCAT physics conventions, work done **by the system** is considered "positive" (+) work, whereas work done **by the surroundings** is "negative" (−) work. This designation is arbitrary and may disagree with the conventions used in many college chemistry and/or physics courses.

The logic behind the signs is better appreciated by knowing the corresponding official MCAT physics internal energy expression **(first law of thermodynamics),** which states that the change in the internal energy status of the system (ΔU or ΔE on the MCAT) is equal to the change in heat content of the system (ΔQ) **minus** the work done by the system:

$$\Delta U \text{ (or } \Delta E) = \Delta Q - W \text{ (First law of thermodynamics)}$$

It follows that if the system does work (W+), the overall internal energy status of the system is less (i.e., ΔU or ΔE is < 0) (see subsequent discussion in this chapter).

The PV work done by or on the system can be illustrated graphically. If pressure is plotted on the ordinate (y or vertical axis) and volume on the abscissa (x or horizontal axis) for several different times, a PV curve is generated (Figure 12-5). In this experiment, a piston is locked to compress the gas molecules residing within the chamber leading to a relatively low volume and high pressure state (point A on Figure 12-5). The process leading to a smaller volume and higher pressure is a **compression.**

FIGURE 12-5.

A representative PV diagram.

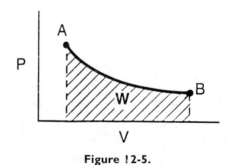

Figure 12-5.

The piston is allowed to move freely and the volume of the chamber expands, allowing the gas molecules to occupy more volume of the chamber and leading to lower total pressure (point B on Figure 12-5). The work associated with this **expansion** is positive and can be determined by measuring the area underneath the experimental PV curve.

The area under a complex PV curve can be difficult to approximate. Because the MCAT work definition holds true if P is constant, however, only those situations in which compression (a decrease in volume) or expansion (an increase in volume) occur with no or minimal change in system pressure require such an approximation.

A more typical PV diagram is shown in Figure 12-6. After studying this curve, answer the following questions: What process occurs as the piston moves from Point A to Point B? What are the units of work? How much work was done? Assume 1 atm ≈ 1 × 10⁵ Pa.

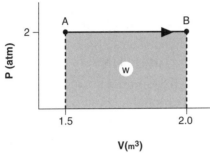

FIGURE 12-6.
Typical PV diagram. Note constant pressure.

Figure 12-6.

Solution: The process occurring from points A to B is an **isobaric** (in Latin, *iso* means same, *baric* refers to pressure) **expansion**. Units of work in the SI system are Pascals (pressure unit) and m³ (volume unit). The units of Pa and m³ multiply to yield joules. Because the graph in Figure 12-6 shows a pressure of 2 atm, the pressure in Pascals is $(2)(1 \times 10^5) = 2 \times 10^5$ Pa. The volume change is $(2.0 - 1.5) = 0.5$ m³. Thus, $W = P \, \Delta V = (2 \times 10^5 \text{ Pa})(0.5 \text{ m}^3) = \mathbf{1 \times 10^5 \text{ J}}$.

IV. Laws of Thermodynamics

A. First Law of Thermodynamics

$$\Delta U \text{ (or } \Delta E) = \Delta Q - W$$

The first law states that the **energy of an isolated system is constant.** The internal energy status of the system (ΔU or ΔE) varies with changes in heat content (ΔQ) and work status (W) of the system. The internal energy status of an isolated system decreases (ΔU −) if heat is lost and/or if the system does work on the surroundings. The internal energy status increases (ΔU +) if the system gains heat and/or had work done to it by the surroundings.

ΔU **and** ΔQ **are state functions; their values are independent of specific pathway.** Important facts are where they came from initially and where they are now. Common thermodynamic terms include:

Isothermal: temperature is constant, $\Delta U = 0$

Adiabatic: no change in heat content, $\Delta Q = 0$

Isobaric: pressure remains constant, $\Delta P = 0$

Isovolumetric: volume remains constant and so $W = 0$

In an isothermal process, the change in heat content equals the work done. In an adiabatic process, the change in internal energy status equals work done. In an isovolumetric process, the change in internal energy equals the change in heat content.

B. Second Law of Thermodynamics

$$\Delta S \geq 0$$

The second law states that **entropy (disorder) always tends to increase.** Consider the entropy of a gas > liquid > solid, or disorder in everyday life that never seems to decrease. Entropy is abbreviated S; **entropy change** (change in amount of disorder) is abbreviated ΔS.

The second law allows for the following processes:

1. $\Delta S > 0$, which represents the **spontaneous** and **irreversible** processes that happen in nature: (e.g., balls initially at rest rolling down a steep hill toward the center of gravity; a clump of ants dispersing throughout the environment; heat flow from a hotter to a cooler object). In these cases, ΔS is positive (+).

2. $\Delta S = 0$, which states that disorder is not changing now, but it will change soon. Such processes are **reversible,** because they can become spontaneous and irreversible at any moment: (e.g., a ball at rest on a mountain peak that stays at rest until "a natural phenomenon," such as a wind gust or earthquake gets the ball rolling).

A relationship exists between heat content (Q), entropy (S), and free energy of a system (G): $\Delta G = \Delta Q - T \Delta S$. If a spontaneous process (ΔS +) occurs in a sealed system ($\Delta Q = 0$), then the free energy of the system (ΔG) must be negative (−). Therefore, ΔG is negative and ΔS is positive if a process is spontaneous. (For more discussion of this topic, see the General Chemistry Review Notes.)

13

Electrostatics

rostatics

Electros

I. Charge and Related Topics	
II. Coulomb's Law and Electric Force	**HIGH-YIELD**
III. Electric Dipole	**TOPICS**
IV. Electric Fields	

The focus of this discussion is on fundamental concepts relating to electrically charged particles at rest, including the definition of "electrical charge" and how charges interact with each other and their environment. Subsequent chapters address the topic of moving charged particles, assuming familiarity with the basic physics of "stationary charges."

By learning and thinking about electrostatics in a new, simplistic way, reviewing basic mechanical principles in preceding chapters, and tying concepts together, you will gain a solid understanding, both conceptually and quantitatively, of static and dynamic electrical phenomena.

I. Charge and Related Topics

A. Charge

Electric **charge** can be a property of a particle, substance, object, or body. A net electric charge exists if, and only if, there is a net inequality in the number of **electrons** and **protons** in a given atom. Remember that the neutron, a third subatomic particle, lacks charge. Also, whereas the mass of an electron is only 1/2000 that of a proton, the magnitude of the charge on each is the same, 1.6×10^{-19} coulombs (SI unit of charge is the coulomb [C], the experimentally determined net charge of 6×10^{18} protons). The sign of the charge for the electron is negative $(-)$, whereas that of the proton is positive $(+)$. Thus, $|e-| = |p+| = e = 1.6 \times 10^{-19}$ C. As an illustration, the spark seen when touching a doorknob is about 50 nC, whereas the average lightning bolt discharges approximately 5 C. The most common letter abbreviation for the magnitude of a charge is **Q** or **q** (e.g., $Q = 2 \times 10^{-7}$ C).

Electrons and protons are the fundamental "players" in the charge game. An atom, by definition, has no net charge (is electrically neutral overall) because it has equal numbers of electrons and protons. Although materials with an equal number of electrons and protons are electrically **"neutral"** overall, regions of charge imbalance may exist. Materials with an unequal number of electrons and protons are said to be **"charged."** Figure 13-1 shows a positively charged object.

FIGURE 13-1.

A charged object.

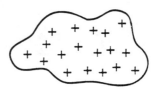

Figure 13-1.

Some atoms easily gain or lose an electron when interacting with other atoms. An atom that has lost an electron has a net positive charge (+e) and is called a **positive ion.** An atom that gains an electron has a net negative (−e) charge and is called a **negative ion.** Regions of a substance, object, and/or body can become charged by accumulating charged particles while remaining electrically neutral as a whole. Examples include common daily materials and tools, rocks, clouds, the human heart and nervous system, and the like.

B. Conductors, Semiconductors, and Insulators

Metal is a material that can accept and/or lose electrons easily and become electrically charged. Metals are generally referred to as **conductors** because they often are able to conduct electrical charge along their length. They may pass electrons from neighbor to neighbor, region to region, and end to end. Other good conductors include salt solutions, ionic compounds, and certain gases.

Insulators tend to prevent the flow of charge (electrons). Common electrical insulators include glass, rubber, wood, ceramic, and plastic. **Semiconductors** are materials that have a variable ability to conduct charge. The ability of a semiconductor to conduct charge varies with ambient temperature, becoming a better conductor (more electrons available) at higher temperatures and a poorer conductor (less free electrons) at lower temperatures. Frequently used semiconducting materials include silicon, carbon, and germanium.

Materials that are good thermal (heat) conductors tend to be good electrical conductors, whereas materials that are poor thermal conductors tend to be poor electrical conductors.

II. Coulomb's Law and Electric Force

If you place a small, positively charged metal ball (charge $+Q_1$) a short distance (r) to the left of a second positively charged metal ball (charge $+Q_2$) at rest (Figure 13-2), you would expect, based on experience with charged materials (e.g., magnets), that the two charges will move away from each other. It makes sense that the repulsion action allows for the production of an **"electric force"** that tends to push outward laterally from each ball (shown as arrows). This scenario has overtones relating to Newton's law of gravitation (see Chapter 7). The amount of force exerted on a ball is directly proportional to the magnitude of the charges involved (Q_1 and Q_2), inversely proportional to the square of the distance (r) separating the charges involved, and proportional to some constant (k). This deduction is the basic expression experimentally determined by Charles Coulomb in 1788:

Coulomb's law: $$F_{(of\ Q1\ on\ Q2)} = \frac{k\ |Q_1||Q_2|}{r^2}$$

FIGURE 13-2.

Forces associated with two positively charged objects.

F_2 on 1 ← (+Q_1) ←—— r ——→ (+Q_2) → F_1 on 2

Figure 13-2.

Coulomb's law determines the magnitude of electrostatic force between two charges at rest. Recall that units of force, charge, and distance are Newtons, coulombs, and meters, respectively. Can you deduce the proper units of k? (**Answer:** Nm²/C².)

As reviewed in Chapter 1, a force is a **vector** quantity, and thus, has both a magnitude and direction. Assuming the charges are static, it is possible to calculate the **magnitude** of the (electric) force that charge 1 places on charge 2, and vice versa. To recall the direction of any electric force, remember the saying: "likes repel, opposites attract." Similarly charged objects repel (move away from) one another, whereas oppositely charged objects attract (move toward) one another.

Question 13-1: Can you state the similarities and differences between gravitational and electrostatic forces?

Answer: Both of these forces are "real" forces between particles, vector quantities with both magnitude and direction, and inverse square laws; they obey Newton's third law, act through space, and must be added vectorially. These forces differ in that gravitational forces are "attractive" only and usually are weak, whereas electrical forces are attractive or repulsive and are strong (about $10^{40} \times F_{grav}$ on an atomic scale).

Figure 13-3 illustrates a more complicated problem involving **multiple** neighboring charges. In this coordinate system, Q_1 (+2 mC) is located 2 m to the left of Q_3 (+3 mC) and 1 m above Q_2 (−1 mC). Note that all three charges are within the same plane.

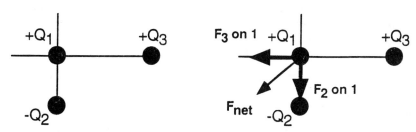

FIGURE 13-3.
Determining net forces involving multiple charges.

Figure 13-3.

Question 13-2: What is the net electric force experienced by Q_1 if k = 9 × 10^9 Nm²/C²? (**Remember:** "force" means both magnitude and direction relative to some reference point; also, mC means 10^{-6} C.)

Solution: Calculate the magnitude and direction of the net electric forces acting on charge 1. Using Coulomb's law, find that the force (F) of charge 3 on charge 1 equals $(k)(Q_3)(Q_1)/(r^2)$, which equals 0.014 N. The force (F) of charge 2 on charge 1 equals $(k)(Q_2)(Q_1)/(r_2)$, which equals 0.018 N.

Using techniques of vector summation, the resultant force $(F_R) = [(0.014 N)^2 + (0.018 N)^2]^{1/2} =$ **0.023 N.**

Because the direction of the electric force of charge 3 on charge 1 is toward the $-x$ direction and that of charge 2 is in the $-y$ direction, and because the magnitudes of the two forces are similar, the net direction is about midway between the negative horizontal and vertical axes. The exact angle below the horizontal can be determined by : $\tan \phi = (F_y/F_x)$ and thus, $\phi = $ arc tan $(F_y/F_x) = 52°$ below the $-x$-axis.

Question 13-3: What is the net electric force on a +5 mC point charge if it is surrounded symmetrically at a distance of 0.8 m by a metal hoop, the entire surface of which is covered with a charge −15 mC?

Answer: Because the sole positive charge is attracted to all points on the surrounding ring equally, the net electric force is **zero**—all points on the ring "enjoy" the presence of the positive charge equally.

III. Electric Dipole

In Figure 13-4, rod A is charged with a positive charge, and rod B is charged with electrons by rubbing rabbit fur across it several times. Two simple experiments are performed. In the first, as rod B moves toward a round metal ball, the positive charges within the metal ball move toward rod B because of electrical attraction. By lightly touching the rod to the ball (i.e., contact), **conduction** of electrical charge occurs. If in a second experiment, however, rod A is kept a slight distance from the metal ball, a special situation is created—**induction** of a dipole.

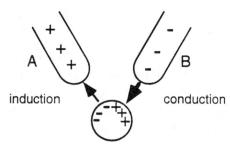

Figure 13-4.

An electric dipole is induced by the separation of oppositely charged particles (or regions) of equal magnitude—$+Q$ and $-Q$ are separated by a small distance (r). The electric dipole moment is a **vector** quantity. The magnitude of the electric dipole is expressed as follows:

$$\text{Electric dipole moment} = p = |Q|\, r$$

The direction (assigned by most physicists) is **from negative to positive charge** (i.e., $[-] \rightarrow [+]$). As detailed in the next section, this direction is exactly opposite to that of electric fields (E-fields), which, by convention, are directed from positive to negative charge (i.e., $[+] \rightarrow [-]$). Unfortunately, the direction of the dipole vector varies by specialty; chemists usually state that direction of a dipole is from the positively charged center of one atom to the negatively charged center of another. By normal "physics" conventions, the dipole moment is oriented from negative to positive charge (a dipole tends to align **with** the field).

IV. Electric Fields

A small positive test charge ($+q$, standard MCAT convention) is placed near a negatively charged metal ball ($-Q$) (Figure 13-5). What net effect will the metal ball have on the test charge?

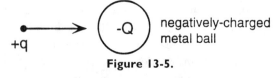

Figure 13-5.

The $+q$ will be attracted toward the metal ball, and thus experience a force (i.e., electric force) to the right. If you plot the relative force directions for a series of positive test charges ($+q$), you display **lines of force.** In actuality, lines of force are graphic representations of the **E-fields** produced around the positively charged metal ball. All charged particles, objects, and bodies set up an E-field around them. The density of lines drawn represents the relative magnitude of the E-field. The more lines per unit area, the greater the E-field strength. The line direction shows E-field direction.

To determine the lines of force (E-field) around any charge(s), determine the direction of the force experienced by a series of small test charges (+q) when placed in the vicinity of the charge(s) of interest. Figure 13-6 shows how test charges leave the region of +Q of a positively charged metal ball and head into the periphery.

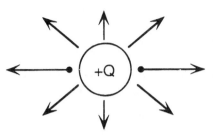

Figure 13-6.

Consider the situation of two equal magnitude charges positioned side by side. Figure 13-7 illustrates the E-fields around two oppositely charged objects (at right) and two positively charged objects (at left). As the E-field lines show, if you place a positive test charge in the vicinity of the oppositely charged objects, it is attracted to the negatively charged object and repelled by the positive. On the other hand, the positive test charge is repelled from both positively charged objects.

Note how the positive test charges minimize contact with positive charges while maximizing contact with negative charges. All charged objects in the world are surrounded by these amazing "invisible" E-fields.

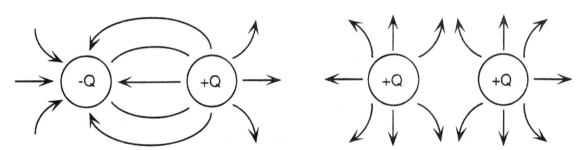

E-fields are vector quantities with a definite magnitude and direction. They are defined in terms of the force acting on a small, positive test charge placed in the field rather than in terms of the charges causing the field. The E-field, however, is solely determined by the charges causing the field, not the test charges. Thus, we use the concept of the test charge to find out what we want to know (i.e., the magnitude of an unknown E-field). The magnitude of a given E-field is calculated as follows:

$$E = \frac{F}{+q} = \frac{kQ}{r^2}$$

The E-field at a point in space is the ratio of the net electric force (F) acting on a small, positive test charge (+q) placed at that point, divided by the magnitude of that test charge.

Because $\mathbf{F} = kQq/r^2$, and $\mathbf{E} = \mathbf{F}/q$, then $\mathbf{E} = kQ/r^2$, which gives the magnitude of the E-field at a known distance (r) from a charge (Q). Be careful not to confuse this calculation with the expression for electrical potential (V = kQ/r; see Chapter 14).

The unit of E-field magnitude is N/C. The direction of the E-field, by convention, is from **(+)** → **(−)** (i.e., the direction a small [+] test charge would travel if placed in the vicinity of the charge[s] being studied).

To determine the net E-field at a location near two or more independent charges: (1) determine the magnitude of the E-field produced at that location by each charge; and then, (2) sum the individual E-fields using vector addition. To calculate the force a known charge (Q′) would experience if placed in an E-field of known magnitude (E), use the expression:

$$F = Q'E$$

CONCEPTUAL QUESTIONS

1. What is the magnitude and direction of the E-field at the center of a hollow metal sphere with a radius of 1 m and a surface charge of +4mC?

    Answer: No computation is required. By placing the positive test charge at the center of a circle, perfect symmetry exists; the test charge would not experience a net electric force. Opposing forces balance, and thus, E = 0 within the sphere.

2. What is true about the net E-field inside a hollow metal conductor that is placed within an external E-field?

    Answer: Most likely, the net E-field is zero. In Figure 13-8, note how the external charge rods set up an E-field directed to the right (from positive to negative terminals). Charges within the metal conducting plate are attracted toward the charged rods, creating an E-field directed to the left. Because E-fields are vector quantities, and the E-fields associated with the external charged rods and metal conducting plate oppose one another, the net (resultant) E-field is zero. The E-fields effectively cancel one another.

FIGURE 13-8.

Net E-field inside a hollow conductor placed within an external E-field is zero.

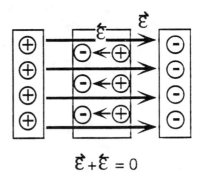

$$\vec{\mathcal{E}} + \overleftarrow{\mathcal{E}} = 0$$

Figure 13-8.

Remember these important points about E-fields:

1. E-fields exist around charged particles/objects/bodies (although they are "invisible").

2. E-fields have both magnitude and direction.

3. The density of field lines drawn correlates with the magnitude of the E-field (the more lines per area, the stronger the E-field).

4. The E-field, by convention, is oriented from positive to negative charge locales (because the direction is dictated by the direction of force on a positive test charge).

5. Units are N/C.

6. The net E-field inside a hollow conductor placed within an external E-field is zero.

7. The positive test charge used to determine E-field parameters must be small so it does not cause the charges under study to move in any way.

14

Electrical Potential

| **I.** Electrical Potential Energy |
| **II.** Electrical Potential Difference |
| **III.** Equipotential Lines |

HIGH-YIELD TOPICS

This chapter is a review of the basic concepts relating to electrical potential energy (PE_q). Understanding these concepts is made easier by familiarity with the gravitational potential energy (PE_g) concepts reviewed in other chapters. Learning by analogy is emphasized.

I. Electrical Potential Energy

Gravitational potential energy (PE_g) is created when a mass is lifted above the ground to the top of a "physical" hill (Figure 14-1**A**). As stated in Chapter 5, the amount of potential energy created depends on the magnitude of the mass, the magnitude of the parameter (g) causing the object to fall toward the ground, and the distance between the top of the hill and the ground surface. A "real" force (F_g) is created as the mass accelerates toward the ground surface. As discussed in Chapter 13, electrical charges also exert "real" force and, as shown subsequently, possess energy (i.e., electrical potential energy, PE_q) .

Electrical forces (F_q) are created when charges are placed near one another (Figure 14-1**B**). A small positive charge placed near a large fixed positive charge experiences a repulsive electrical force, which allows for the creation of a "potential" energy situation. When located near the fixed charge, the mobile charge is said to have maximal **electrical potential energy (PE_q).** As the mobile charge moves away from the fixed charge, the electrostatic force between the charges decreases, as does the induced PE_q. The reduction in PE_q, as the distance between the like charges increases, can be likened to the small charge falling down an "electrical" hill (Figure 14-1**C**).

FIGURE 14-1.
Basic concepts in electrical potential.

A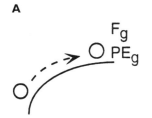

B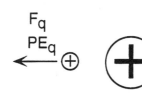

C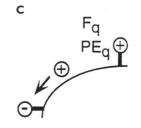

The **electrical potential (V)** existing at some point A is equal to the amount of work (W) required to bring a positive test charge (+q) from infinite distance away from the charge to point A, divided by the magnitude of the test charge.

$$V = W/q$$

The electric potential energy (EPE) is equal to the work (W) associated with this process.

$$EPE = W$$

Thus,

$$V = EPE/q$$

Figure 14-2 is a diagram of electrical potential (V). Note that the electrical potential at point A is equal to the work to bring the positive test charge from infinity to point A.

$$\infty \quad \oplus \quad\text{—}W\text{———}\rightarrow \bullet \ A$$

Figure 14-2.

FIGURE 14-2.
Electrical potential at point A is equal to the work required to bring a positive test charge from infinity to point A, divided by the magnitude of the test charge.

The potential at a distance r from an isolated point charge Q, or from the center of a uniformly charged sphere, is proportional to the magnitude of the charge (Q) and inversely proportional to the distance r (k, as previously, equals 9×10^9 N•m²/C²). The SI unit of electrical potential is the volt (V) =1 joule/coulomb (J/C). The derivation of the expression for potential is as follows:

$$V \text{ (potential)} = \frac{W}{^+q(\infty \to A)} = \frac{[(F)(s)]}{^+q} = \frac{[(k \bullet Q)(^+q) \quad (r)]}{(r^2) \quad ^+q} = \frac{k \ Q}{r}$$

This expression shows the potential associated with bringing a unit positive charge from an infinite distance up to a distance r from a point charge.

A charge's potential is defined in terms of **the amount of work required to move a small, positive test charge from a reference location infinite (∞) distance from the point of interest (with zero absolute potential) to some point at or near the charge of interest. Voltage is a scalar quantity,** having magnitude only.

▌II. Electrical Potential Difference

To compare the potential energy at two different points requires determining the amount of potential difference between two points, A and B.

The amount of electrical **potential difference** (also referred to as **voltage** or V_{AB} or **ΔV**) between points A and B is defined as the **work required to move a positive test charge ($^+$q) from point B to point A, divided by the magnitude of the test charge** (see Figure 14-2).

The potential difference (i.e., voltage) between points A and B is the magnitude of the potential at point B minus that at point A:

$$\text{Potential difference (voltage} = V_{AB} = \Delta V) = V_B - V_A = \frac{W}{^+q_{(B \to A)}}$$

$$_B\bullet \text{—}W\rightarrow \bullet_A$$

Therefore, the electrical potential energy difference (voltage) between points A to B is the change in electrical potential energy that occurs when a small positive test charge moves from position B to position A. Because potential difference (voltage) merely refers to a difference in potential, units are also **volts.** A volt is the amount of potential difference between two points if one joule of work is required to move one coulomb of charge from one point to the others.

Remember: Although both potential and potential difference units are expressed in volts, they differ in that potential refers to the amount of potential electrical energy relative to some zero potential reference point, whereas voltage refers to the difference in electrical potential energy between two points of interest of known electrical potential. Whereas electricians use potential difference and voltage interchangeably, a student of physics should use only the term potential difference, be it to describe electrical potential between points A and B, the intracellular and extracellular environments of a human muscle cell, or the microscopic regions between adjacent human neurons.

Potential difference allows for muscle contraction, nerve conduction, and ion transport in tissues. It is what makes a battery a "good" battery. The potential difference between the two terminals of a transistor radio battery is 9 volts. Therefore, the battery's voltage (i.e., difference in electrical potential between the two terminals) is 9 volts. The voltage is the electromotive force (EMF) that drives current (electrical charges) around the closed electrical circuit (see Chapter 16 for more discussion).

Figure 14-3 shows the analogy between gravitational and electrical potential energies. Note that pushing a positively charged ball toward another positively charged ball results in an increase in potential energy, similar to the action of pushing a metal ball up a steep hill. Potential energy is at a minimum as the positively charged ball moves to the left toward the negatively charged ball, as is the potential of a rolling ball at the bottom of a steep hill. In both scenarios, potential energy is a function of relative position (how close to other charged objects or vertical distance from the ground).

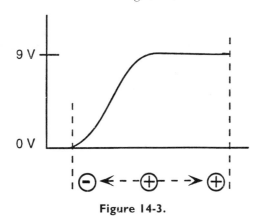

Figure 14-3.

FIGURE 14-3.
Analogy between gravitational and electrical potential energies.

The potential difference equation can be modified to allow calculation of the amount of work required to move a charge Q from some point A to B:

$$W = (Q)(\Delta V)$$

In a uniform electric field (E-field):

$$\Delta V = W/q = [(F)(d)]/q = (E)(d)$$

in which d is the distance between the two points of interest. Note that potential difference is a **scalar quantity.**

III. Equipotential Lines

The concepts of electrical potential and electrical potential difference (voltage) can be understood by using a pictorial example. A large, positively charged metal ball sits in the plane of this paper. If you place positive test charges around the ball, regions of similar electrical potential would exist around the ball at points equidistant from the ball's center.

If a region of 5 V potential exists at a radius 4 mm away from the ball's center on its left side, the same potential must exist at a radius of 4 mm from its right side, above it, and below it. Thus, **equipotential lines** or **rings** exist around the ball. Every point on a line or ring is of the same electrical potential. Because the metal ball is three dimensional (3-D), 3-D **equipotential surfaces** surround the ball like "rings of onion surrounding the onion core."

A bird's-eye view of a charged ball and the surrounding equipotential rings (i.e., lines) is provided in Figure 14-4. Remember that these rings (lines) are 3-D surfaces that symmetrically surround the charged object.

FIGURE 14-4.

Cross section of a positively charged ball surrounded in 3-D by equipotential rings.

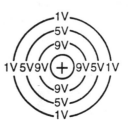

Figure 14-4.

Because equipotential lines (surfaces) are of the same electrical potential energy, **no work is required to move from one point on a line (surface) to any other point on that same line (surface).** As expected, work is required to move from a line (surface) of low potential to one of higher potential, just as work is required to move from the bottom to the top of a steep hill. Recall that W = (Q)(ΔV).

The E-field direction is found by seeing what happens to a positive test charge placed in the vicinity of the charges in question. In Figure 14-4, a positive test charge would be moved away from the ball, perpendicular to the equipotential rings. Thus, the E-field direction is perpendicular to equipotential surfaces.

Electromagnetism

HIGH-YIELD TOPICS

Qualitative and quantitative understanding of basic electromagnetic (EM) principles and phenomena is important in preparing for a career in basic science research or clinical medicine. The goal of this chapter is to review key elements of this straightforward and interesting topic that many students have described as "confusing, vague, nebulous, and boring."

I. Magnetic Properties

Some materials have magnetic properties (e.g., magnets) and some do not (i.e., notebook paper). It is the existence of **moving unpaired electrons** that ultimately is responsible for the creation of magnetic properties. Magnetism is a property of some materials composed of certain atoms the electrons of which produce tiny net magnetic fields (B-fields) because of their specific **orbital motion** and **intrinsic magnetic dipole moments.** An unpaired, orbiting electron is like a tiny bar magnet that creates a tiny B-field. Figure 15-1 shows a moving electron creating magnetic field lines like a tiny bar magnet. A standard magnet with its associated magnetic field lines is also shown.

FIGURE 15-1.

Magnetic properties of materials depend on moving unpaired electrons. At left, an electron moving in a circular orbit and the resulting magnetic field lines. At right, the magnetic field lines associated with a magnet.

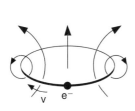

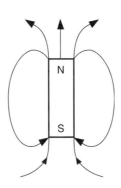

Materials can be classified as having one of three possible magnetic properties:

A. Nonmagnetic Material

Electron spin and orbital motion cancel, so this material has no magnetic properties: no B-field is produced and no alignment is seen when the material is placed into a preexisting external B-field.

B. Paramagnetic Material

Magnetic regions or "domains" exist in the material. The net B-field of the material is about zero, although alignment of "**magnetic domains**" is seen when the material is placed into an external B-field. A weak, temporary B-field exists when placed into a preexisting external B-field. Figure 15-2**A** shows an object that consists of many regions or domains, each with its own magnetic dipole moment. In Figure 15-2**B**, the B-fields of each domain tend, for the most part, to align with the direction of the external B-field while it is present. In Figure 15-2**C**, the near total domain alignment in Figure 15-2**B** is lost soon after the object is removed from the external field.

FIGURE 15-2.

An object consisting of domains, each with its own magnetic dipole moment. Note the effect of an external B-field on domain dipole alignment.

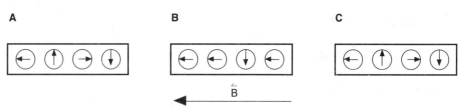

Thermal motion of unpaired electrons is responsible for destroying alignment of B-field domains. Most of the **transition metals** and their compounds in oxidation states involving incomplete inner electron subshells are paramagnetic.

C. Ferromagnetic Material

Materials consisting of magnetic "domains" retain their alignment after being removed from an external B-field. These materials subsequently have a net B-field associated with them; thus, they are, or can be, **permanently** "magnetized." Figure 15-3 illustrates how domains within ferromagnetic materials align with an external B-field and retain their alignment even after the external field is removed. Ferromagnetism can be considered an extreme form of paramagnetism. A critical interatomic distance (not too close, not to far) is required. These materials tend to consist of elements with incompletely filled d or f electron subshells. Materials composed of iron (Fe), cobalt (Co), nickel (Ni), and gadolinium (Gd) are ferromagnetic at room temperature.

FIGURE 15-3.

Alignment of domains within ferromagnetic materials due to an external B-field.

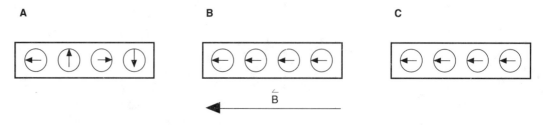

II. Magnetic Fields

A positive test charge exists in space. If you detect a force acting on this test charge when it is at rest, an electrostatic field is present. If the test charge is moving, it experiences a magnetic force and a magnetic field exists.

Magnetic fields (B-fields) are **real** fields (like gravitational and E-fields) that can be "emitted" from an object and create "forces" that cause objects nearby to move in an altered path. B-fields are either "intrinsic" properties of a material or object, or they can be induced by moving electric charges.

A. Intrinsic Property

Permanent magnets are an example. Magnets, such as those with which children play, have a net magnetic dipole moment associated with them. Electron orbital motion and intrinsic magnetic moment are ultimately responsible for the object "emitting" B-fields (Figure 15-4). Like gravitational (G) and electric (E) fields, B-fields have both magnitude and direction. **B-fields are vector quantities.** The magnitude can vary (the more lines per unit area, the greater the magnitude); **the direction is always from north to south poles.** As with charges, like poles repel, opposite poles attract.

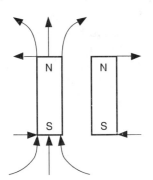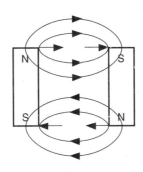

FIGURE 15-4.
Magnetic fields as an "intrinsic" property. Here, magnets "emit" B-fields. At left, two magnets with similar poles close together emit fields that oppose one another. At right, two magnets with poles attract one another.

B. Induced Property

Electrical wires are an example. Think of a segment of electrical wire as a substance (a metal) through which electrons travel. The electrons traveling along the length of wire are responsible for the creation (induction) of B-fields around the wire (Figure 15-5). B-fields emanate from the wire, just as sound waves emanate from a loud speaker, and "fade away" (decrease in magnitude) as one moves farther and farther from the source (the electrical wire). "Induced" B-fields are produced as a result of charge moving through a metal wire.

1. Magnitude

Figure 15-5 shows current (I) moving through a wire. The magnetic field produced encircles the wire. The magnitude (strength) of the B-field at some point near the electrical wire should **be directly proportional to the magnitude of the electrical current** (I) [i.e., the flow of charge] producing the field. The B-field strength **is inversely proportional to distance (r) from the wire.** The constant (m_o) is the permeability of free space and is not dependent on the material or wire.

FIGURE 15-5.
"Induced" magnetic field, produced by charge moving through a metal wire. "Circle" indicates the magnetic field comes out of the plane, while "X" indicates magnetic field goes into the plane.

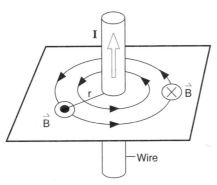

Like sound intensity, B-field magnitude is high when the source is "at a maximum"[2] (i.e., current running through the wire is high) and is close to the source (i.e., close to the wire). Magnitude can be expressed as:

$$B = \frac{u_o\, I}{2\pi r}$$

The SI unit of B-field magnitude is the **Tesla (T)** = Weber/m^2 = 10^4 gauss. The B-field produced by the common toy magnet is about 0.005 T; that produced by the planet Earth is about 5×10^{-5} T.

Magnets produce B-fields that can do many things. Strong B-fields erase credit cards or ATM cards. The magnets used in magnetic resonance imaging of the body produce a B-field of about 1 to 2 T.

The concept that current moving through an electrical wire sets up a surrounding B-field is important to understand because it holds true for wires of many shapes: linear (as just mentioned), loop-shaped (Figure 15-6, at left), and solenoid/coil (Figure 15-6, at right). **The magnitude of the B-field created around the wire is directly proportional to the amount of current and inversely proportional to the distance from the wire to the point of interest.** Therefore, the B-field experienced as a result of current travelling through a wire is maximum when I is maximum and distance from the wire is minimized.

FIGURE 15-6.

B-fields produced by current passing through a loop (left) and solenoid/coil (right).

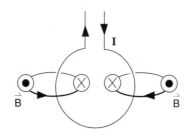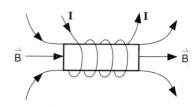

2. **Direction**

The location and direction of the B-field produced around an electrical wire can be determined by using the **Right Hand Rule Part I,** which says: **If you wrap the fingers of your right hand around the wire and point your thumb in the direction the electrical current (I) travels, your nonthumb fingers (on your right hand) curl in the direction of the induced B-field.** Review Figures 15-5 and 15-6 and make sure you agree with the direction of the B-fields shown by using the Right Hand Rule.

B-fields are real and "alive" in our world. They can be produced by some materials at all times (e.g., magnets) or produced (induced) by some materials (e.g., electrical wires, power lines, appliance cords, overhead lamps) when electrons run through them.

▌III. Magnetic Forces

A gravitational field is responsible for the production of a gravitational force, which, in turn, can cause objects to accelerate toward the ground. An electric field is responsible for the production of an electric force, which, in turn, can cause charged objects to move in some way. A magnetic field has the potential to produce a **magnetic force** (F_{mag}), which, in turn, can cause moving charged objects to deviate or deflect from their original course (Figure 15-7).

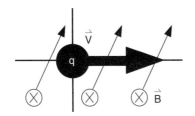

Magnetic forces are real forces, as they can exert an action force on moving charged particles or objects. A **magnetic force** is created and can act on an object **if and only if:**

1. The object of interest is electrically charged (with a charge **q**)

2. The object of interest is moving (with a speed **v**)

3. The object is in the vicinity of a magnetic field (of magnitude **B**)

4. The object is moving in such a way that:

    a. **its v vector is perpendicular (90°) to the B vector** *or*

    b. **a component of its v vector is perpendicular (90°) to the B vector**

A. Magnitude

The **magnitude** of the magnetic force (F$_{mag}$) can be determined using the expression:

$$Fmag = q\,v\,B \sin \emptyset$$

in which ø is the angle (0 to 180°) between the v and B vectors (Figure 15-8).

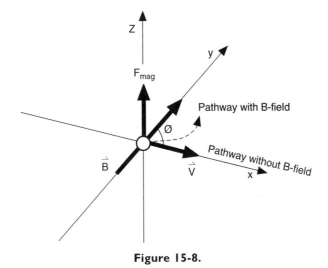

FIGURE 15-8.
Relationships between (F$_{mag}$), B, v, and ø. Deflection of a positively charged particle (+q) from its original path (along the x-axis) toward the vertical (x–z plane) is caused by F$_{mag}$. Note: +q at origin of the figure.

Figure 15-8.

The amount of force (deflection) experienced by a moving charge is proportional to:

1. How much charge is present

2. The speed at which the charge is moving

3. The amount of B-field ("pushing ability") present

4. The "push angle" (ø)

Thus, highly charged particles or objects that are moving quickly in a region of a strong B-field are set up for experiencing a strong magnetic (push) force. If all else is equal, F_{mag} is maximal when $ø = 90°$ ($90°$ is the best "push angle"). As shown in examples 2 and 3 of Figure 15-9, F_{mag} causes the moving charge to deviate from its linear original path along the x axis; the charge moves along the x axis but soon deflects vertically.

FIGURE 15-9.

Three examples showing the calculation of F_{mag}. A charge with a velocity and a B-field are shown in each case. Note the deflection of the charge in Examples 2 and 3 caused by F_{mag}.

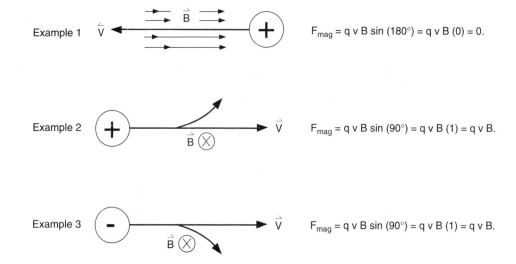

Example 1 $F_{mag} = q v B \sin(180°) = q v B (0) = 0.$

Example 2 $F_{mag} = q v B \sin(90°) = q v B (1) = q v B.$

Example 3 $F_{mag} = q v B \sin(90°) = q v B (1) = q v B.$

B. Direction

The **direction** of a magnetic force is determined by using the technique called the **Right Hand Rule Part II**, which says: **If you point your right thumb in the direction the charge travels (the direction of the v vector), and your remaining (straightened) right fingers in the direction of the B-field, your palm will face the direction of F_{mag} if the moving object is positively (+) charged. If the object of interest is negatively (−) charged, F_{mag} is simply the exact opposite direction or, simply, the direction the back of your hand faces.**

Be aware of symbols used to note relative direction: velocity and/or B-field vectors oriented into the plane of the paper are symbolized with a cross mark (the view of an arrow tail), and those oriented out of the plane of the paper (coming out directly at you) are symbolized with a bulls-eye mark (the view of an arrow tip coming toward your face).

In the examples in Figure 15-9, determine if an F_{mag} exists in each case.

If a charge moving at constant speed enters a B-field with its velocity perpendicular to the B-field, the charge will be deflected in a circular orbit. The radius of this orbit can be determined using the concept that magnetic force is converted to centripetal force:

$$F_{mag} = F_{centripetal}, \ qvB = (mv^2)/r, \ r = (mv)/qB$$

Remember, no magnetic force is created ($\mathbf{F_{mag}} = \mathbf{0}$) for the following:

1. Uncharged particles or objects
2. Charges at rest
3. Charges moving in a region with no B-field present
4. Charged particles moving parallel to the B-field

A magnetic force is produced **only** if the conditions are right—**a charged particle or object is moving through a B-field such that the v and B vectors have some perpendicular orientation to each other.** Note also that because the magnetic force vector is always perpendicular to the velocity/displacement vector ($\theta = 90°$), **no work is done by magnetic force on the moving charge (i.e., W = F s cos 90° = 0).**

C. Magnetic Forces Compared with Gravitational and Electrical Forces

Magnetic forces are fundamentally different from gravitational and electric forces. Although magnetic force is exerted only on objects that are moving, gravitational and electric forces are exerted on objects that are moving and on those at rest. Whereas magnetic force exists only if the direction (or a component) of the charge's motion is perpendicular to the B-field, gravitational and electric forces are independent of the direction in which the object moves.

More complicated scenarios involving magnetic force include:

1. The magnetohydrodynamic generator (E- and B-field balance)

2. The mass spectrometer (circular motion in a magnetic field)

3. The electric motor (wire loop magnetic torque principle)

No matter the scenario, moving charged particles or objects may be deflected from their original (usually linear) path on entering a region of uniform magnetic field. The direction of deflection is determined by the Right Hand Rule Part II [the right palm faces the direction of F_{mag} for positive (+) charges, the back of the hand faces the direction of F_{mag} for negative (−) charges].

IV. Magnetic Flux

A solitary loop of metal wire (Figure 15-10) initially has no electrical current or magnetic field running through it or any involvement with any outside process. A bar magnet with known B-field strength (B) is brought from the right toward the loop (North pole of the bar magnet facing the loop). B-fields from the magnet pass through the loop as the magnet approaches the loop. More and more B-field lines pass through the loop as the magnet is brought closer to the loop.

FIGURE 15-10.
Magnetic flux. Note the B-field lines as a magnet approaches a metal loop. The amount of magnetic field within the loop at a specific time is the magnetic flux.

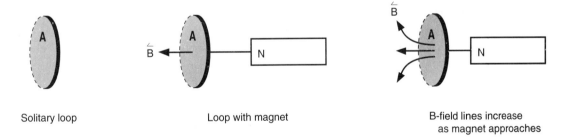

Solitary loop   Loop with magnet   B-field lines increase as magnet approaches

The amount of magnetic field within the loop at a specific time is called the **magnetic flux (F).** The magnetic flux through the loop is proportional to the amount of area inside the loop, the strength of the B-field within the loop, and the orientation of the loop in the field. A quantitative expression is:

$$\text{Magnetic flux } (\Phi) = A \ B \cos ø$$

in which A is the area inside the loop through which the external B-field passes, B is the magnitude of the magnetic field passing through the loop, and ø is the angle between B and a line perpendicular to the plane of the loop. Note that Φ is maximum when ø is zero degrees (i.e., the B-field lines fully transverse the area of the loop). Flux is zero when ø = 90° (because cos 90° = 0). These concepts are illustrated in Figure 15-11.

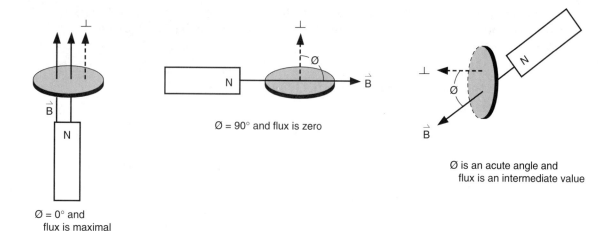

Ø = 90° and flux is zero

Ø = 0° and
flux is maximal

Ø is an acute angle and
flux is an intermediate value

FIGURE 15-11.

Magnetic flux with differing angles between B and a line perpendicular to the plane of the loop (differing ø values).

FIGURE 15-12.

Induction of a B-field by a loop ($B_{induced}$).

For purposes of understanding basic concepts, think of magnetic flux as a "bad" process, one that needs to be corrected (i.e., reversed). The external B-field ($B_{external}$) introduced disturbs the state of "homeostasis" in which the loop had been (it was used to having **no** magnetic fields present). A metal loop can return to its preflux state by counteracting the flux itself. The external B-field lines introduced by the magnet are negated or "neutralized" by the loop. The loop creates, or induces, its own B-field ($B_{induced}$) directed exactly **opposite to the change in the B-field** introduced by the magnet ($B_{external}$) (Figure 15-12).

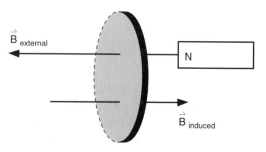

Figure 15-12.

Question: If you were a metal loop, how could you produce a B-field?

Answer: Produce your own. A B-field can be induced in a metal, conducting hoop by allowing current to run through it. Thus, a B-field can be induced by producing an **"induced" voltage (EMF$_{induced}$),** which in turn creates an **"induced" electrical current (I$_{induced}$);** it is $I_{induced}$ that is responsible for the creation of $B_{induced}$, which counters the B-field lines emanating from the external magnetic field **(B$_{external}$).**

The process by which voltage is induced by varying magnetic field inside a loop of wire is **electromagnetic induction;** it was discovered by Faraday in 1831. **Faraday's law says that the induced voltage (EMF) through a loop of wire equals the change of magnetic flux (ΔΦ) through the loop divided by the time (Δt) needed for that change in flux, or:**

$$\epsilon = -\Delta\Phi/\Delta t$$

SI units are as follows: 1 Wb/s = 1 V. The negative sign indicates that the induced voltage *opposes* the changing flux that caused that voltage.

Lenz's law states that the polarity of an induced voltage is such that it produces a current the magnetic field of which *opposes* the change in flux that caused the induced voltage. Electromagnetic induction can be viewed as a series of individual physical processes that "work together to solve a problem" (note the "negative feedback" loop—a term borrowed from the biological sciences) [Figure 15-13].

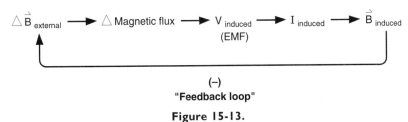

Figure 15-13.

A **change** in the flux "induces" this chain of events. A static loop in a constant B-field will **not** have an induced voltage. Only during the time the B-field, and therefore the flux, changes are an induced voltage, current, and B-field established.

You can use the Right Hand Rule Part I to determine the polarity (i.e., direction) of the induced current on the metal loop. Knowing that $B_{induced}$ should point in the direction to oppose the change in flux created as a result of some experimental procedure (e.g., pushing a bar magnet toward the loop, pulling the bar back through the loop, suddenly increasing or decreasing the magnitude of the $B_{external}$), curl your right fingers around the loop to curl in the direction of the required $B_{induced}$. The direction your right thumb points while grasping the loop (with fingers curling the needed $B_{induced}$) gives the direction of $I_{induced}$ on the wire loop.

Figure 15-14 offers the specifics for the example of magnetic flux in Figures 15-10 and 15-11. Note that $B_{induced}$ points toward the right to counter the $B_{external}$, which is directed to the left. Using Right Hand Rule Part I, have your right fingers curl and fingertips point toward the right. If you grasp the segment of the loop projecting out of the plane of the paper (sticking out at you), your right thumb points downward. Thus, $I_{induced}$ travels counterclockwise around the loop if you are an observer standing just to the right of the loop (see Figure 15-14).

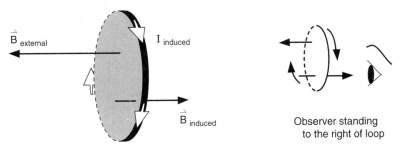

Observer standing
to the right of loop

Figure 15-14.

FIGURE 15-14.
The Right Hand Rule, Part I is used to find the direction of $I_{induced}$.

V. Electromagnetic Spectrum

An **electromagnetic (EM) wave** is an **electrical and magnetic disturbance** that moves through space (or a medium) at a definite speed. All waves move through space (a vacuum) at the speed of light (c, c = 300 million meters/second = 3×10^8 m/sec). Electromagnetic waves vary in energy content; wave energy depends on its **frequency (f)** of vibration (f is the number of complete vibrations per second of the field at a point along the path of the passing wave). Electromagnetic waves with "high" energy content (e.g., x-rays) vibrate more times per second than waves with "low" energy content (e.g., radio waves). The actual length of one wave (i.e., one complete vibration pattern) is the wave's **wavelength (λ). The following relationship holds true for all EM waves travelling in a vacuum.**

$$\text{Speed of EM wave travel (c)} = \text{Frequency of wave (f)} \times \text{wavelength of wave } (\lambda)$$
$$c = f\lambda$$

Electromagnetic waves are usually classified by frequency of vibration in a scheme called the **electromagnetic (EM) spectrum.** Examples of EM waves in increasing frequency/energy content and decreasing wavelength are: (1) AM and FM radio waves; (2) microwaves; (3) infrared light; (4) visible light; (5) ultraviolet light; (6) x-rays; and (7) gamma rays.

The EM wave is ultimately produced by an oscillating electric charge. Consider a radio station antenna (Figure 15-15). Electric fields (E-fields) and magnetic fields (B-fields) are **generated** then **radiate** from the antenna because of the continued movement of electrical charge up and down the length of the antenna. The moving charges in the antenna are responsible for producing both E-fields and B-fields that originate right next to the antenna. Fields at a specific location near the antenna have a specific magnitude and direction at some specific time. The magnitude (strength) of the fields is determined by the relative magnitude and location of the charge in the antenna. The polarity (i.e., direction) of the fields produced around the antenna varies in orientation (up [+] or down [−]) with the direction the charge moves within the antenna itself. The magnitude and polarity of the E- and B-fields existing at any one point near the antenna varies with respect to time. This variation (E- and B-field magnitude and polarity) over time is responsible for the production of the "wave" form. The waves move at a speed "v" away from the antenna. The combined electrical and magnetic field moving at speed c is an **electromagnetic wave.**

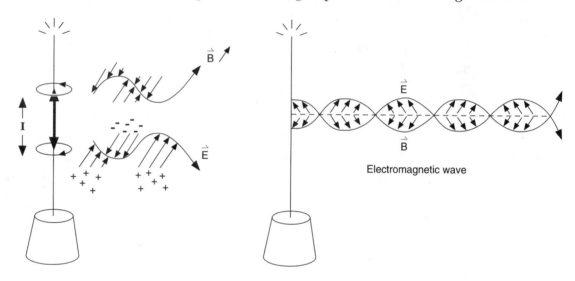

FIGURE 15-15.

Wave forms seen over time as charge moves up and down antenna.

DC Circuits

DC Circuits

DC Circuits

I. Terms and Concepts

II. Physics of the DC Circuit

This chapter brings electronic principles together. The DC circuit, a collection of various different separate entities, is defined and studied. Important topics include: batteries (the source of EMF that drives the circuit and creates voltage), current (the flow of electrical charge around the circuit), resistors (devices that resist the flow of electrical charge and consume voltage), capacitors (devices that store electrical charge, for possible later use), dielectrics (materials that allow capacitors to hold additional electrical charge), electric power (the rate at which electrical energy is converted to other forms of energy), and DC circuit physics.

I. Terms and Concepts

A. DC and AC Circuits

Direct current (DC) electric circuits are closed electrical systems in which the current (I, the flow of charge) and the voltage (V, the potential difference that allows charge to flow) are **constant** over time. A DC circuit is inside a transistor radio. A transistor radio battery produces a constant current and voltage. Another type of circuit—the **alternating current (AC)** circuit (see Chapter 18) differs from the DC circuit in that the current and voltage in AC circuits **vary** over time as a sinusoidal wave function (Figure 16-1). The electrical circuit in most homes is an example of an AC circuit.

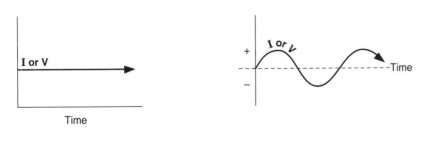

DC circuit   **AC circuit**

Figure 16-1.

FIGURE 16-1.
The DC (left) and AC (right) circuits.

B. Batteries

Batteries separate positive and negative charge, thus creating a **voltage** (potential difference) across them. Batteries are the source of **electromotive force (EMF)** that drives the circuit. Batteries convert chemical energy into useable electrical energy. "Good" batteries are able to separate charge, whereas "bad" batteries are unable to do so and should not be used because they can no longer drive a DC circuit. The common transistor battery has a voltage of 9 volts, which means the potential difference between the two battery terminals is 9 volts. The symbol for the battery is shown in Figure 16-2.

FIGURE 16-2.

The symbol for a battery.

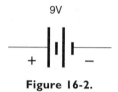

Figure 16-2.

C. Current

Current (I) refers to the rate at which charge flows past a point in the circuit:

$$I = \Delta Q / \Delta t$$

The unit of current is the ampere. **1 amp of current = 1 Coulomb of charge flowing past some point on the wire/1 second.** Current is really the flow of electrons through a conducting material such as a wire. Because of certain conventions, however, the direction of current is **not** considered the direction electrons flow, but rather, the direction that positive (+) charge flows. Thus, current is "**conceptualized" as being the direction positive (+) charge flows** (i.e., current always flows from a point of higher potential to a point of lower potential). Use this convention whenever dealing with both conceptual and mathematic problems related to current.

D. Resistance

Resistors are materials or deliberately designed devices that oppose the flow of electric current. They resist the flow of current by consuming voltage and releasing it in the form of **heat**. Resistors provide an example of how one form of energy (electrical potential energy) can be converted to another form (thermal energy). The unit of resistance is the ohm (Ω), named after the 19th century German electrical physicist Georg Ohm. The symbol for a resistor is ─␣␣␣─ .

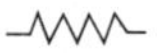

One **ohm is the electrical resistance of an object that will allow a 1-amp electrical current to flow when a 1-volt potential difference is placed across the object.** Resistance of a metal wire, or any body for that matter, depends on its length (L; the longer it is, the more resistance it has), cross-sectional area (A; the greater the area, the less resistance), and resistivity (r; an intrinsic measure of how well a material resists the flow of charge; the greater the value, the greater the resistance):

$$R = \rho \, (L/A)$$

E. Key Relationships

Ohm's law says that the three quantities just described (V, I, and R) are related as follows:

$$V = I \cdot R$$

This equation is used to calculate the voltage in a DC circuit if you know its total current and total resistance. Likewise, it is possible to determine the total current flowing through a DC circuit when the voltage of a battery (source of EMF) and total circuit resistance are known. In most test problems, the total circuit resistance is usually related to resistors. The wire itself might have a small amount of internal resistance, but usually the amount is so insignificant that it is not considered.

The electrical power used by a device can be determined by using the equation:

$$\text{Power} = IV = I^2R = V^2/R$$

Remember that one unit of electrical power, 1 watt (1 J/sec) = 1 volt-amp = 1 amp^2-ohm = 1 volt^2/ohm.

F. Capacitance

Capacitors are the fourth and final component of the DC circuit (the conducting metal wire, battery, and resistor are the first three components). **A capacitor is a pair of conductors: one conductor with a negative charge and the other with an equal positive charge. Capacitors store electric charge on their conducting surface.** The capacitor consists of two electrical conducting plates separated by a vacuum, air, or other nonconducting material (Figure 16-3). A capacitor does not allow electric current to pass through it.

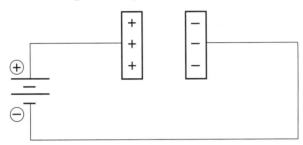

Figure 16-3.

The electronic camera flash device is an example of a capacitor at work; it stores a great deal of charge (the **charging** process often generates a high-pitched "whining" sound) and then releases it suddenly when you push the camera button. The **discharging** process provides a great deal of charge quickly that can be used by the flash light bulb to create a bright flash. The symbol for the capacitor is: ⊣⊢.

Capacitance (C) is the parameter that indicates how "good" a capacitor really is; that is, how much charge it can hold. The **better the capacitor, the higher its capacitance and the more charge it can hold on each of its two plates. Capacitance is defined as the charge on either conductor (plate) divided by the potential difference between the conductors:**

$$C = Q/V$$

When an insulating material is placed between the two conductors of a parallel plate capacitor, the capacitance increases. The insulating material is said to have a **dielectric constant K,** which is a measure of how much the insulating material increases the capacitance compared to when a vacuum exists between the capacitor plates:

$$K = C_{insulator}/C_{vac}$$

In short, dielectrics allow the plates to hold more charge; thus, the capacitance (i.e., the charge-storing ability) of the capacitor is increased. Dielectrics are made of polar compounds that tend to interact with the charge on the plates in a way that effectively "neutralizes" some of the charge on them, which allows more charge to be pushed by the battery onto the plates. Thus, the net or total capacitance (C_T) of a capacitor with an original capacitance (C_o) is increased by having a dielectric (with a $K > 1$) between its plates:

$$C_T = K \cdot C_o$$

Capacitance also depends on the surface area (A) of the conducting surfaces, the distance separating the two plate surfaces (d), the dielectric constant (K) of the material between the plates, and a constant (ϵ_o):

$$C = K \cdot \epsilon_o \cdot (A/d)$$

Note that capacitance is maximum for large plates that are close together but separated by a material with a large dielectric constant K, which allows for the storage of maximal electrical charge.

The unit of capacitance is the farad, named in honor of the English electrician Michael Faraday. 1 farad = 1 coulomb/volt. A 1-farad capacitor attached to a 1-volt battery would have a charge of +1 C on one plate and −1C on the other. Typical capacitors have a capacitance on the order of the microfarad $(\mu F = 10^{-6}$ F$)$.

The change in electrical potential energy that occurs when a capacitor (C) is charged with a charge (Q) from a battery with potential difference (V) is equal to:

$$1/2 \ QV = 1/2 \ CV^2 = 1/2 \ Q^2/C$$

II. Physics of the DC Circuit

The DC circuit is a collection of various electronic elements: conducting wire, battery, resistor(s), and/or capacitor(s). The backbone of the circuit is the metal conducting material (usually metal wire) connecting the various circuit components. The power horse of the circuit is the battery, the source of voltage (EMF). One or more resistors consume voltage so the circuit will function (the voltage produced by the battery **must** be consumed **fully** for a potential difference to exist between the two ends of the circuit). If the battery produces 9 volts, 9 volts **must** be consumed by the resistor(s) present.

Current, on the other hand, remains constant in a DC circuit, except where the circuit divides into two or more separate junctions. **The sum of the currents within each junction must add to give the total current that was present just before and after the junction.** Figure 16-4 illustrates a simple (series, i.e., no branching occurs) DC circuit composed of a 9-volt battery, a metal connecting wire, and a light bulb with a resistance (R) of 9 ohms.

FIGURE 16-4.

A simple series DC circuit.

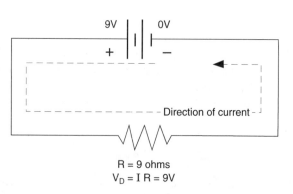

Note that a potential energy gain occurs across the battery terminals (0 volts exist at the negative terminal, 9 volts exist at the positive terminal). Recall that the direction positive charge follows is the direction of the current. Using Ohm's law, the current (I) produced in this circuit is:

$$I = V/R = 9 \text{ volts}/9 \text{ ohms} = 1 \text{ amp}$$

Voltage drop (V_D) across the bulb (a source of resistance, voltage is "consumed" and heat is produced) **must** be 9 volts because **all** 9 volts produced by the battery must be "consumed" by the time you get to the end of the circuit (i.e., the negative terminal) where V must equal zero. The current, 1 amp, is the same at every point in this series circuit.

Figure 16-5 shows a parallel type of connection in which the current reaches a **junction** (i.e., branching) point. The two resistors are said to be **parallel** (i.e., the charge travelling within the circuit must branch and travel to each separate circuit component). The current created by the battery breaks up at the junction in an **inverse ratio to the resistances of the resistors.** Thus, if the current sees two resistors in parallel, R_1 has a resistance of 2 Ω and R_2 has a resistance of 4 Ω (i.e., R_2 has twice as much resistance as R_1), the current splits in a way such that twice as much goes to the resistor of less resistance (R_1) than to the one of greater resistance (R_2).

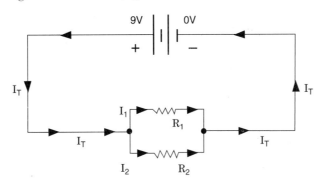

FIGURE 16-5.
A circuit with parallel resistors.

Summary:

$V = I_T \cdot R_T$; $I_T = I_1 + I_2$; $1/R_T = 1/R_1 + 1/R_2$; EMF = 9V = V_{DR1} = V_{DR2}.

FIGURE 16-6.
A circuit with multiple series resistors (left) and a circuit with multiple parallel resistors (right).

A circuit may include several resistors. Resistors connected end to end (Figure 16-6, at left) are said to be connected "in **series**," whereas those connected by a junction (Figure 16-6, at right) are said to be connected "in **parallel.**"

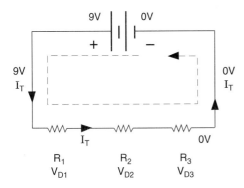

Summary:

$V = I_T \cdot R_T$; $R_T = R_1 + R_2 + R_3$;
EMF = 9V = $V_{DR1} + V_{DR2} + V_{DR3}$.

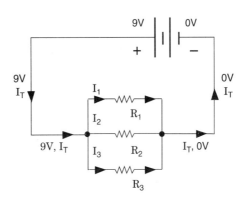

Summary:

$V = I_T \cdot R_T$; $I_T = I_1 + I_2 + I_3$;
$1/R_T = 1/R_1 + 1/R_2 + 1/R_3$;
EMF = 9V = V_{DR1} = V_{DR2} = V_{DR3}.

To determine the total resistance (R_T) of resistors in **series,** sum the individual values: $R_T = R_1 + R_2 + R_3 + \cdots$. To determine the total resistance of resistors in **parallel,** solve for R_T using the expression: $1/R_T = 1/R_1 + 1/R_2 + 1/R_3 + \cdots$. You must determine R_T if you want to know the V_T or I_T of a circuit, because Ohm's law says: $V_T = I_T \cdot R_T$.

The voltage drop across any resistor in a solely series circuit (V_{Dx}) is equal to the I travelling through that resistor (I_T) times the resistance of that resistor (R_x). The V_D across resistors in parallel with each other (within a single junction) **must** be equal, and can be determined using Ohm's law: V_D at a resistor in parallel connection is equal to the current (I) travelling through that resistor times the resistance (R) of that resistor.

In the series circuit on the left side of Figure 16-6, assume that EMF = 9 volts, I = 1 amp, and $R_1 = R_2 = R_3$ (R must be 3 ohms). The voltage drop across each resistor must be 3 volts ($V_{DR1} = V_{DR2} = V_{DR3} = 3$ volts), because EMF is "consumed" as it travels along the circuit from the positive terminal to the negative terminal (the EMF is 9 volts at the positive terminal and zero volts at the negative terminal). Simple mathematics confirms our findings: $V_{DR1} + V_{DR2} + V_{DR3} = 9$ volts. **Remember that for resistors in series connections: $V_{DR1} = I \cdot R_1$.**

The parallel circuit in Figure 16-6 gives three resistors (R_1, R_2, and R_3) in parallel within one junction. Knowing that: (1) the EMF in a DC circuit must be "consumed" by the resistors contained within the circuit (R_{1-3} are the only resistors present here), and (2) the V_D across resistors in parallel are the same, it follows that $V_{DR1} = V_{DR2} = V_{DR3} = 9$ volts (each voltage drop must be the same, and the junction as a whole must consume the entire 9 volts, by rule). **Note:** if 10 resistors are placed in parallel here, each would have a 9-volt voltage drop across it. Even if 50 resistors are placed in parallel here, each would have a 9-volt drop across it.

The equal voltage drop across resistors of different resistance in parallel can be appreciated by looking at Ohm's law: $V_{Dx} = I_x \cdot R_x$. V_D for resistors in parallel are equal because of a "compensation mechanism," i.e., I and R values have an inverse relationship in parallel connections. Think of an example: a resistor with 1 unit of resistance gets twice as much current running through it than a resistor of 2 units resistance; a resistor of 2 units resistance gets one-half the current running through it than a resistor of 1 unit resistance. Thus, V_D ($= I \cdot R$) is **conserved** for resistors in parallel because I and R vary inversely with each other.

Some circuits contain resistors in series and resistors in parallel. Calculations and concepts are straightforward if you understand the fundamentals of single series and single parallel circuit systems. To avoid confusion, think in terms of individual components first.

Remember that EMF (circuit voltage) is consumed entirely; current is **conserved,** i.e., current travels through resistors in series untouched (i.e., current . . . what goes in is what comes out), whereas current divides at a junction, a point in an inverse ratio to the resistances of the resistors contained within that particular parallel connection, and then recombines on emerging from the junction in its totality (i.e., current . . . what goes into a junction comes out); the voltage drop across any resistor can be determined by using Ohm's law: $V = I \cdot R$ (use I_T and R_x values for a resistor "x" in a series connection, and I_x and R_x for a resistor in a parallel circuit in which I_x is the amount of current travelling through the branch of the junction containing resistor x).

For a circuit containing a single resistor (R_1) in series with two resistors in parallel with each other (R_2 and R_3), calculate the voltage drop across R_1 ($V_{D\ R1} = I_T \cdot R_1$) and subtract this value from the EMF. This calculation gives the remaining voltage that **must** be consumed within the parallel connection (EMF $-\ V_{D\ R1}$). The voltage drops across both R_2 and R_3 are equal and must be equal to (EMF $-\ V_{D\ R1}$) because the voltage drop across **all** resistors in parallel is the same (assuming each parallel junction in question contains one resistor).

To determine the total capacitance (C_T) for capacitors in series, use the reciprocal relationship similar to that used for resistors in parallel. For capacitors in a series connection, solve for C_T using the expression: $1/C_T = 1/C_1 + 1/C_2 + 1/C_3$. For capacitors in parallel, use: $C_T = C_1 + C_2 + C_3$. Table 16-1 summarizes series versus parallel circuit variables.

TABLE 16-1. Series versus Parallel Circuit Variables.

	Series	Parallel
Resistance (R) for 3 resistors in:	$R_T = R_1 + R_2 + R_3$	$1/R_T = 1/R_1 + 1/R_2 + 1/R_3$
Capacitance (C) for 3 capacitors in:	$1/C_T = 1/C_1 + 1/C_2 + 1/C_3$	$C_T = C_1 + C_2 + C_3$
Voltage drop (V_D) across 3 resistors in:	$V_{DT} = V_{D1} + V_{D2} + V_{D3}$	$V_{DT} = V_{D1} = V_{D2} = V_{D3}$
Current (I) through resistors in:	**Same** I runs through each.	I runs through resistors in an **inverse** ratio of their R

Wave Characteristics

Wave
Characteristics

HIGH-YIELD TOPICS

I. Transverse and Longitudinal Motion

II. Wavelength, Frequency, Velocity, and Amplitude

III. Wave Superimposition, Phase, and Interference

IV. Resonance, Standing Waves, and Nodes

V. Beats and Beat Frequency

Waves are oscillations created by a disturbance. A mechanical wave is set in motion by a disturbance that causes a rapid displacement of a small section of a medium. The particles within the medium do not move with the wave, but create an oscillation so that the wave can move from one place to another. This chapter reviews the concepts and equations that describe both individual waves and repetitive oscillations.

I. Transverse and Longitudinal Motion

When a medium is disturbed, the particles that make up the medium can vibrate back and forth. If a truck tumbles off a bridge into the water below, the truck entering the water is a disturbance that causes the water molecules to start vibrating to and fro about an equilibrium point. The equilibrium point is the previous horizontal level of the water. Over time, the waves travel outward from the truck in concentric circles. This type of wave motion is known as transverse motion, because the water molecules move up and down, while the wave moves horizontally (Figure 17-1, at left). **The direction of motion of the particles is perpendicular to the direction of motion of the wave, resulting in a transverse wave.** Other examples of transverse waves are waves in a rope fixed at the ends, or electromagnetic waves, such as light.

Longitudinal waves are waves in which the oscillations of the particles are in the same direction as the direction of wave motion. A good example is a child's "slinky" toy (Figure 17-1, at right). A slinky is held along the floor by two children. If one child quickly moves a hand forward and then back, the slinky will respond with a compressed area of the coils, followed by a region of rarefaction (an area of rarefaction has wider spaced coils). These areas will then move toward the other child as a wave. Looking at one point on the slinky as the wave passes, you can see that the movement of the particles in the coils is first forward, then backward. Thus, in longitudinal waves, such as slinky waves and sound waves, waves are areas of alternating compression and rarefaction of the particles, caused by oscillations of the particles parallel to the direction of the wave.

A. Transverse wave   **B. Longitudinal wave**

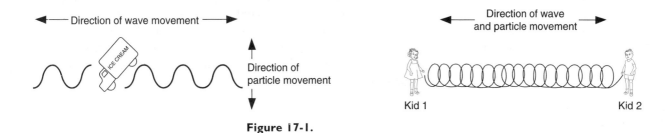

Figure 17-1.

II. Wavelength, Frequency, Velocity, and Amplitude

The diagram of a single cycle of a wave (Figure 17-2) shows that the wave consists of a variable that is changing with respect to time in a **sinusoidal** manner. Think of a string stretched from someone's hand to a wall. If the string is moved up and then down quickly, a pulse is generated that will travel the length of the string. If the string is moved up and down repeatedly, a train of waves will be generated that will travel down the string. The speed of the wave train travelling down the string is the same as the speed of a single pulse. These waves have a sinusoidal appearance. Figure 17-2 (at right) also presents a graphic display of the displacement of a certain point on the string versus time.

FIGURE 17-1.

Transverse **(A)** and longitudinal **(B)** waves.

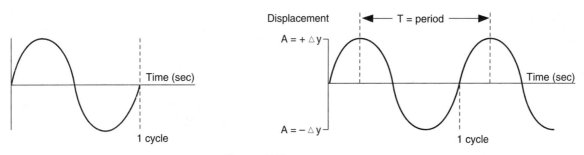

Figure 17-2.

The **frequency** is how many times per second a complete wave (cycle) passes at a certain point on the string (i.e., **the number of oscillations per unit time**). The frequency in the example in Figure 17-2 is 1 cycle per second.

The **amplitude** of the wave is the maximum displacement of the string. **Amplitude (A) in general refers to the magnitude of maximum displacement in the y direction.**

The **velocity (v)** is how fast the wave travels along the string. **The wavelength (λ) is the distance between two points that occupy the same relative position on a wave.** A wavelength is simply the length of one complete wave. In the example in Figure 17-2, the wavelength is the distance between two points on the string that have the same displacement and are moving in the same direction.

The period (T) of a wave is the time (seconds) required for one complete oscillation to pass a given point. Period is the inverse of frequency, which is measured in "per seconds," known as Hertz (1 cycle per second = 1 Hertz).

An important and particularly useful formula that relates frequency, velocity, and wavelength for all waves is:

$$v = f\lambda$$

FIGURE 17-2.

At left, a single cycle of a wave; at right, a plot showing the displacement of a single point on a string versus time.

If this formula is hard to remember, think about the units of the terms in the equation. Velocity is measured in meters per second, f in 1 per second, and wavelength in meters, so m/sec = (1/sec)(m).

III. Wave Superimposition, Phase, and Interference

If you send a pulse down the string in Figure 17-3, it will travel until it reaches the end of the string, where it will be **reflected.** The reflected pulse will **be inverted when compared to the incoming pulse, because of Newton's third law.** The incoming pulse pushes upward on the end point, causing an equal and opposite reaction force that pushes downward. The reaction force generates the reflected pulse, inverted because of the opposite orientation of the reaction force.

FIGURE 17-3.

At left, reflection of a wave causing an inverted wave; at right, constructive interference of waves.

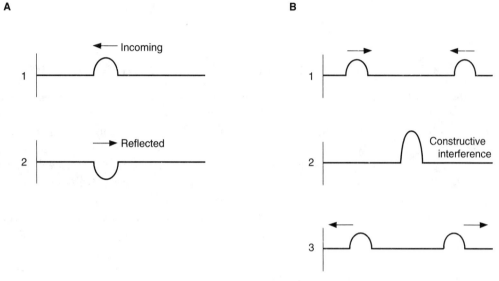

Figure 17-3.

If you send one pulse down from the held end of the string, and another pulse from the fixed end point, the pulses superpose when they meet in the middle of the string (Figure 17-3, at right). If the pulses have the same orientation, they interfere **constructively,** resulting in a **momentary wave of greater amplitude.**

If you send a pulse down the string, allow it to be reflected, and then send another pulse down the string to meet it as it returns, the two opposed pulses would interfere **destructively,** canceling each other.

Note that the amplitude of superposed waves is the sum of the amplitude of the individual waves; this is called the **principle of superposition:**

$$
\begin{aligned}
\text{Amplitude of} \quad &= \text{Amplitude of} \; + \; \text{Amplitude of} \\
\text{superposed wave} \quad &\quad\quad \text{wave 1} \quad\quad\quad \text{wave 2} \\
(y) \quad &= \quad\quad (y_1) \quad\quad + \quad\quad (y_2)
\end{aligned}
$$

Recall that the amplitude of a wave on a string is the maximum displacement of the string. Examining displacement as a function of time reveals it is a sinusoidal function. Remember the equation that describes the sinusoidal relationship:

$$\text{Displacement} = A \sin (2 \pi f t + \phi)$$

This equation allows the displacement to vary sinusoidally from the maximum positive displacement (A) and the maximum negative displacement ($-A$). Phi (ϕ) is the phase of the wave, a term to allow for the point to have an initial displacement at zero time. If the phase of the wave equals 90°, then the displacement at t = 0 is:

$$
\begin{aligned}
&= A \sin (2 \pi f t + \phi) \\
&= A \sin (\phi) = A \sin (90°) \\
&= A
\end{aligned}
$$

Note that although these concepts are related mainly to waves in strings in this discussion, they are equally applicable to other types of waves.

IV. Resonance, Standing Waves, and Nodes

Consider what would happen if you send a continuous train of waves down a string and let them interfere with their return waves. For most frequencies, the interference would be destructive, and no waves would be noticeable in the string. At certain frequencies, however, the incoming and return waves would interfere constructively. The interference effects produced by waves depend on their phases. If two waves reaching a point have their maxima at the same time, they are in phase and add constructively. If a maximum of one wave coincides with a minimum of the other, they are a half wavelength out of phase and interfere destructively. Figure 17-4 shows the constructive and destructive interference occurring between incoming and returning waves. (Note destructive interference illustrated in the middle diagram of Figure 17-4.)

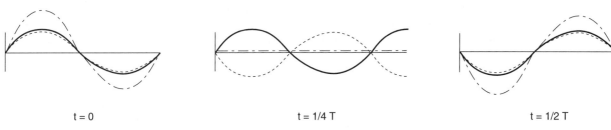

t = 0   t = 1/4 T   t = 1/2 T

Figure 17-4.

Standing waves result from the interference of two sine waves that have the same frequency and amplitude but are moving in opposite directions (Figure 17-5). Standing waves are observed when a string is vibrating so rapidly that the travelling waves are no longer observed and the string appears to have nonmoving waves.

FIGURE 17-4.
Summation of incoming waves (solid lines) and returning waves (dotted lines) to give a summation (dashed lines).

FIGURE 17-5.
Standing waves seen in a string fixed at each end.

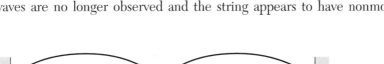

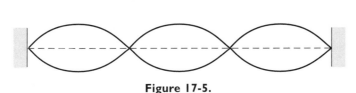

Figure 17-5.

To examine these ideas in more detail, think about a string tied at both ends, similar to a guitar or piano string (Figure 17-6). When the string is struck, it forms a standing waveform.

Question: What is the standing waveform with the longest wavelength?

Answer: The ends of the string are fixed and cannot move. The middle of the string can vibrate at maximum amplitude, which looks like one half of a sine wave. The wavelength of this waveform would be equal to twice the length of the string.

FIGURE 17-6.

Strings tied at both ends, similar to guitar or piano strings.
When these strings are struck,
standing waveforms result.

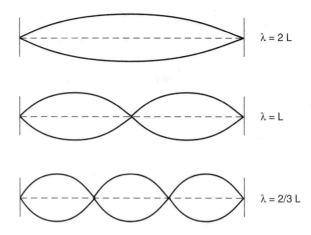

Other waveforms are also illustrated in Figure 17-6. In these standing waves, the points on the wave that always have zero displacement are known as **nodes,** and the points with maximum displacement are known as **antinodes.**

These standing waves demonstrate the idea of **resonance.** At certain frequencies, the incident and reflected waves from the ends of the string superpose constructively, resulting in a standing wave of large amplitude. When one of these standing waves is formed, the waves on the string are occurring at a resonance frequency of the string.

The best way to understand resonance is to think about forces. Energy is supplied most effectively to an oscillating system when an external force acts at the correct frequency. This correct frequency depends on the oscillating system. The optimal frequency causes the greatest amplitude and is known as the **resonant frequency.** If a boy on a swing has a friend apply force (pushing) from behind at just the right interval (correct frequency), the boy can attain the maximum height (amplitude) in the swing. The optimal frequency causing the maximum amplitude of the boy in the swing is the resonant frequency of this system.

The formula $\mathbf{v} = \lambda \mathbf{f}$ is important because **it describes the resonance frequency of the wave on the string,** associated with a wavelength and the velocity. **The velocity of waves along a string** can be described by the formula:

$$v = \sqrt{\frac{F}{m/l}}$$

in which v is the velocity of the wave along the string, F is the force of tension on the string, and m/l is the mass of the string per unit length.

This formula is useful when considering a guitar's strings. Some guitars strings are thick and massive per unit length, whereas others are thin. As the force of tension on the string increases, the velocity increases; as the mass/length increases, the velocity decreases. The wavelength of the possible standing waves is displayed in Figure 17-6. Given a fixed velocity on the string v, the resonance frequencies are:

$$f = \frac{nv}{2l}$$

in which l is the length of the string and n is the set of integers from 1 to infinity.

more ▼

TO TEST HOW standing waves on a string work, take a string that is pinned down at the ends and pinch the string at B (a ruler is given beneath for reference):

string

A   B   C   D

| ---------- | ---------- | ---------- | ---------- | ---------- | ---------- | ruler

1. Would the string have a lower frequency standing wave if it were plucked at A or C?

2. If the string were plucked at A, what would be the amplitude of the vibration at C?

3. If the string were plucked at A, what would be the amplitude of the vibration at D?

SOLUTION:

1. The frequency would be lower when the string is plucked at C, because the wavelength would be longer. Note that v is given by the formula

$$v = \sqrt{\frac{F}{m/l}}$$

so it is constant. Thus, the frequency varies inversely with wavelength, according to the relationship $v = \lambda f$.

2 and 3. The resulting standing wave would resemble that shown in Figure 17-7, with a standing wave that has nodes at B and C. Thus, the amplitude of vibration would be equal to zero at C and maximal at D.

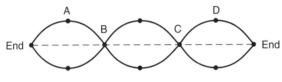

Figure 17-7.

FIGURE 17-7.
The standing wave that would result when the string is plucked at point A in Example 17-1.

V. Beats and Beat Frequency

If you add two travelling waves with slightly different wavelengths and frequencies, it is likely that the waves will add constructively in some regions and destructively in other regions. The resultant wave is likely a rapid oscillation that changes amplitude with time (Figure 17-8). You would expect to find places where the waves add to give a minimum or node as well as places where the waves would add to give maximum amplitudes. This phenomena is called **beating**.

The frequency at which the nodes of the resultant wave pass a given point on the x-axis is the beat frequency. A slightly different definition of beat frequency is **the frequency of the regular fluctuation of two superimposed waves of equal amplitude:**

$$f_{beat} = |f_1 - f_2|$$

FIGURE 17-8.
Resultant wave formed from the superimposition of two waves of equal amplitudes. Note that the resultant wave has a regular fluctuation in this graphic representation of beat frequency.

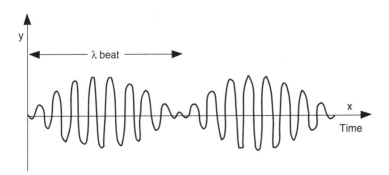

AC Circuits

AC Circuits

HIGH-YIELD TOPICS	**I. Alternating Current**
	II. Inductive and Capacitive Reactance
	III. Impedance
	IV. Voltage and Current Equations

This chapter provides a review of the properties of alternating current (AC) circuits, in which the voltage and current vary in a sinusoidal manner, as well as the concepts of inductance, reactance, and impedance.

I. Alternating Current

FIGURE 18-1.
Difference between DC and AC voltage and current.

In Figure 18-1, the currents and voltages of AC and DC circuits are graphically displayed versus time. In DC circuits, the voltage and current remain constant with respect to time. **In AC circuits, the voltage and current are always changing.** In terms of the actual movement of electrons within the wire, the electrons move in one direction, and then the other, driven by the continually changing electrical potential.

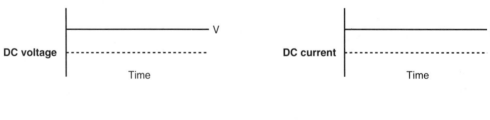

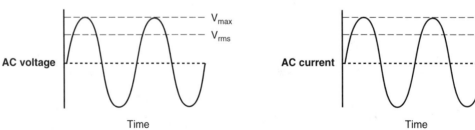

Because the current and voltage in the AC circuit are constantly changing, it is useful to have some terms to describe them that do not vary with time, such as I_{max} and V_{max}, which are the maximum current and voltage that occur (see Figure 18-1). Other important terms are **the Root-Mean-Squared (rms) current and voltage,** which define the "**effective**" current and voltage, and are a way of averaging the peaks and valleys. V_{rms} and I_{rms} are determined by the formulas:

$$V_{rms} = V_{max}/\sqrt{2} \text{ or } V_{rms} = 0.71 \ V_{max} \qquad I_{rms} = I_{max}/\sqrt{2} \text{ or } I_{rms} = 0.71 \ I_{max}$$

II. Capacitive and Inductive Reactance

Resistors, capacitors, and coils resist the flow of current through an AC circuit. A coil, also known as an **inductor,** consists of many loops of a wire. The opposition to current flow through coils and capacitors is termed **reactance (X),** to differentiate it from the resistance of resistors. Because the **reactance of a coil or capacitor in a circuit resists the flow of current,** reactances are also measured in ohms.

Figure 18-2 shows a coil connected to an AC generator. The type of reactance from the coil is inductive, which is given the symbol $\mathbf{X_L}$.

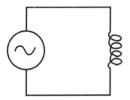 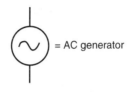 = AC generator

FIGURE 18-2.
An AC circuit containing a coil. This coil has an inductive reactance (X_L).

To identify the property of a coil that acts to resist current flow in an AC circuit, recall Faraday's law. The constantly changing current through the wire in the coil leads to a constantly changing magnetic flux in the center of the coil, which sets up an EMF that opposes the change in flux. Thus, it resists the change in the current. Think of energy being required to constantly change the flux in the coil. Work is done by the power supply's changing electric potential against the coil's induced EMF. This work becomes energy stored in the form of the coil's magnetic field. Because of this loss of energy across the coil, the current seems to encounter resistance.

The unit of measurement for a coil's strength (inductance) is the **Henry (H).** The **inductance** of the coil, given the symbol **L**, is proportional to the number of turns of the coil. The reactance of a coil in an AC circuit is described in terms of the inductance of the coil and the frequency of the current. As the frequency increases, the flux changes faster and faster, so the reactance increases:

$$X_L = 2 \ \pi \ f \ L$$

Capacitive reactance ($\mathbf{X_C}$), on the other hand, is caused by the charge storage features of capacitors. Assume that the capacitor in the circuit in Figure 18-3 has a low capacitance, i.e., for a given voltage difference across its plates, it holds little charge. When the generator puts voltage across the capacitor's plates, little current flows onto the capacitor for a given voltage; thus, a small capacitor allows little current flow in the circuit. In contrast, a high capacitance capacitor allows much current to flow for a given voltage difference across its plates, allowing more current flow within the circuit. **The capacitive reactance is thus inversely proportional to the capacitance of the capacitor.**

FIGURE 18-3.
A capacitor in an AC circuit.

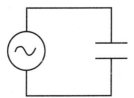

The frequency of the alternating current also affects capacitive reactance. With a low-frequency current, the voltage across the capacitor plates changes slowly with time, so not much current flows onto and off of the capacitor's plates. With a high-frequency current, the voltage changes quickly, allowing larger currents. Capacitive reactance is:

$$X_C = \frac{1}{2\pi f\,C}$$

III. Impedance

Because capacitors, coils, and resistors resist the flow of current within a circuit, their net (effective) resistance when combined within a circuit is **impedance (Z).** The equation for impedance in terms of resistance and reactance is:

$$Z = \sqrt{R^2 + (X_L - X_C)^2}$$

An important law relating current and voltage in AC and DC circuits is Ohm's law. In DC circuits, recall $V = IR$. The corresponding formulas for AC circuits are:

$$V_{rms} = (I_{rms})(Z)$$
$$V_{max} = (I_{max})(Z)$$

Question: In a given circuit (Figure 18-4), a coil and a capacitor are both connected in series to an AC generator. If the coil has an inductance of 1 Henry, and the capacitor has an inductance of 1 Farad, would there always be a reactance within the circuit?

Answer: The reactance of both the capacitor and the coil depends on the frequency of the generator. Therefore, a more general question would be: At some frequency of the generator, could the inductive and capacitive reactances cancel out? Yes, if the frequency was $\frac{1}{2\pi}$, then $X_L = X_C$, and the reactances would cancel.

FIGURE 18-4.

A circuit containing an AC generator (power source), a coil, and a capacitor.

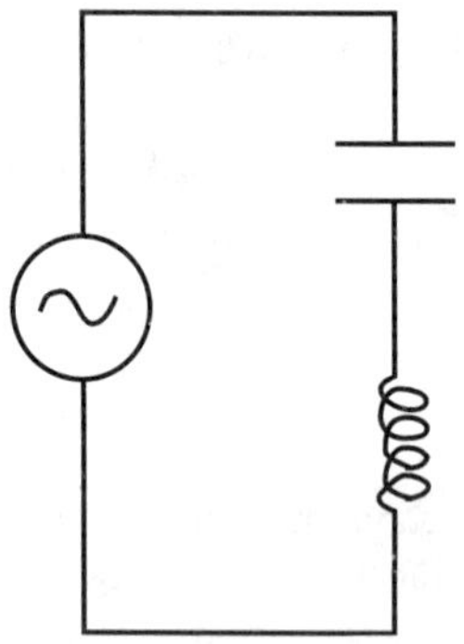

IV. Voltage and Current Equations

The function of resistors in AC circuits is similar to that in DC circuits: they resist the flow of current. In Figure 18-5, the voltage and current across a resistor are displayed graphically versus time. Note that the voltage and current always have the same phase.

Capacitors in DC circuits store charge when a voltage is placed across them. In an AC circuit, they act in the same way. When a capacitor is placed into a circuit with an AC generator, as in Figure 18-3, it experiences the potential difference established by the generator. This sinusoidal potential difference causes charge to flow onto and off of the capacitor.

Look at the AC potential drop (voltage) across the capacitor versus time in Figure 18-5. Note that at $t = 0$, point A, the voltage across the capacitor is increasing rapidly, causing a large current to flow onto the capacitor's plates. At point B, the potential drop across the capacitor has peaked, signifying the largest possible potential pushing charge onto the capacitor's plates. At point B, therefore, the capacitor stops charging, and I drops to zero. At point C, the voltage is sloping downward, meaning less potential pushing charge onto the capacitor's plates. Less charge causes the capacitor to discharge, sending the current in the opposite direction and leading to a negative I in the graph. Continuing to examine the movement of charges yields the two sine waves for V and I in Figure 18-5.

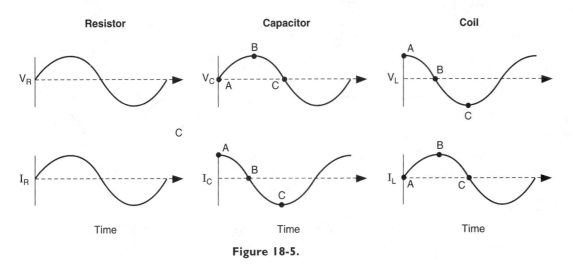

Figure 18-5.

Looking at the sinusoidal curves of V and I across the capacitor in the AC circuit reveals an important difference from a resistor AC circuit. In the resistor circuit, V and I vary in the same way with respect to time. In the capacitor circuit, the I sine wave leads the V sine wave by 90°; i.e., a phase difference of 90° exists between the two graphs. Thus, I_{max} precedes V_{max} by 90°.

In an AC circuit with a coil (inductor), the coil's properties also result in phase shifting between current and the potential drop across the coil versus time. Remember that the coil requires energy to constantly change the flux of its magnetic field, and this energy loss is seen as a voltage drop across the coil. Connecting the coil to an AC generator yields the V_L versus time and I_L versus time graphs in Figure 18-5.

As with the capacitor, compare the potential drop across the coil to the current flowing through the coil. Examine the current flowing through the coil, and use that knowledge plus Lenz's law to find the potential drop across the coil. At A in the I_L versus time graph, the current through the coil is zero, but it is increasing rapidly. To determine what will happen to the voltage drop, remember Lenz's law, which states $EMF = -\Delta\phi/\Delta t$. When the current increases rapidly, the flux will also increase rapidly, causing the large voltage drop across the coil seen in Figure 18-5. As the current stabilizes at the peak, the EMF induced in the coil falls to zero, because the flux is no longer changing, i.e., no voltage drop across the coil at this point. As the current moves in the opposite direction to point C, an EMF will oppose the change in flux, although the EMF will cause a negative potential drop across the coil. In effect, the coil is releasing the energy stored as the magnetic flux. Note that the voltage drops always oppose the changes in flux; thus, they lead the current wave by 90°.

Using a circuit such as that shown in Figure 18-6, you can show the voltage drops across each element of the circuit. The voltage drop of the resistor is always in phase with the current; as more current flows through the resistor, more heat dissipates and the voltage drop increases. The voltage drop across the capacitor follows the current by 90°; the capacitor has an increasing potential difference as charge flows onto it, and a decreasing potential difference as charge flows off. The voltage drop across the coil leads by 90°; Lenz's law states that the induced EMF (the potential difference across the coil) always opposes the change in flux versus time.

FIGURE 18-5.

Graphs of voltage and current over time for resistors, capacitors, and coils in AC circuits. (See text for detailed explanation.)

FIGURE 18-6.

An AC circuit containing a resistor, a capacitor, and a coil (left). A plot of current, and the voltage drops across each element in the circuit (right). Note the relationship between the voltage drop and current in each case. (See text for more discussion.)

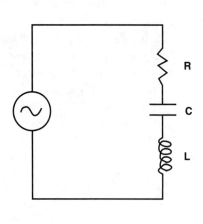

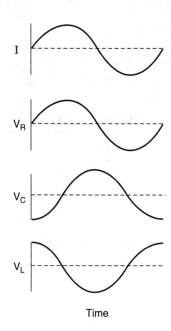

Figure 18-6.

The final concept to understand is the concept of power dissipation in an AC circuit. Power is dissipated in a resistor ($P = I^2R$), but no power is dissipated by capacitive and inductive circuit elements.

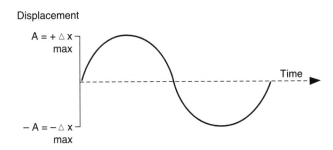

Simple Harmonic
Motion

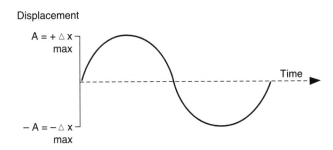
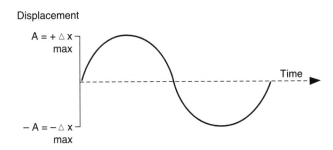

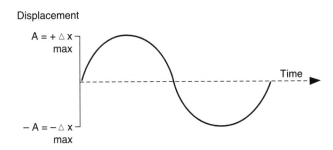19

I. **Periodic Motion and Hooke's Law**

II. **Kinetic Energy and Potential Energy of an Oscillating System**

HIGH-YIELD TOPICS

In simple harmonic motion, displacement varies in a sinusoidal manner with respect to time. The types of simple harmonic motion reviewed in this chapter involve pendulums and masses attached to springs. Concepts involving the energy of an oscillating system are also addressed.

I. **Periodic Motion and Hooke's Law**

In **simple harmonic motion,** a disturbance causes an object to vibrate about an equilibrium point. Figure 19-1 includes a graph of the displacement of the object versus time (sine wave) and the formula used to find the displacement of the object at any given time.

Displacement

$A = +\triangle x$ max

$-A = -\triangle x$ max

Time

Figure 19-1.

FIGURE 19-1.
Displacement of an object in simple harmonic motion described by formula and graphically. Displacement = A sin (2πft).

The formula in Figure 19-1 shows that displacement varies as a sine wave, multiplied by A, the maximum amplitude of the displacement. A pendulum swinging back and forth rapidly will have a high frequency, so $2\pi ft$ will increase rapidly with increasing time, and the displacement will move rapidly from A to −A. The frequency (f) is expressed in terms of cycles per second. Remember from previous discussion of circular motion that $2\pi f$ is ω, the angular frequency in radians per second, giving:

Displacement = A sin (ω t)

SECT. II
PHYSICS
REVIEW
NOTES

147

SPRINGS

In Figure 19-2, a spring is attached at one end to a wall and at the other end to a mass. The mass is resting on a frictionless surface at $\Delta X = 0$. Consider what would happen if you disturb the system. One way to disturb the system involves pulling the mass outward to the point $\Delta X = X_{max}$, but how much force would be required? The amount of force required depends on the properties of the spring; for example, it would be harder to pull the mass with a thick spring. It also depends on how far you stretch the spring. It makes sense that the farther you stretch the spring, the harder you will have to pull.

FIGURE 19-2.

A simple harmonic oscillating system: a spring attached to a mass and to a wall.

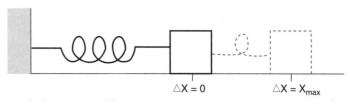

$\Delta X = 0$　　　$\Delta X = X_{max}$

Figure 19-2.

This reasoning leads to the following equation, called Hooke's Law:

$$F = -k\,\Delta x$$

which states that the force required will be equal to the displacement times k, the spring constant. The spring constant (k) reveals the stiffness of the spring. The right side of the equation is negative because Hooke's law actually tells how much force the spring will exert **against** any pull, so it is always directed against the direction of the displacement. A positive displacement will cause a negatively directed force from the spring. The force of the spring always being proportional to the displacement and directed opposite to the displacement is what defines simple harmonic motion. Using Newton's second law, $F = m\,a$, the acceleration of the mass will be:

$$a = -k\,\Delta x/m$$

Another formula that remains to be examined in the mass spring system involves what Hooke's law ($F = -k\,\Delta x$) can tell you about the frequency of the motion of the mass. Thinking intuitively, a strong spring will exert large forces on displacement, and it likely will pull the mass back fast, causing a higher frequency of vibration with a larger spring constant, k. If the mass is large, the acceleration caused by the force of a given spring would be relatively small, so you could guess that the frequency would decrease with increasing mass. Actually, when derived, the frequency and period can vary with the square roots of k and m. **The following formulas detailing the relationships between frequency, period, m, and k are important.** Remember that period (denoted T) $= 1/f$.

$$f = \frac{1}{2\pi}\sqrt{k/m}$$
$$T = 2\pi\sqrt{m/k}$$

SIMPLE PENDULUM

Another example of simple harmonic motion is the simple pendulum, in which a mass is suspended from a massless rod. When the pendulum swings back and forth with an angle of displacement $\theta < 10°$, it follows simple harmonic motion: the restoring force on the pendulum is proportional to the pendulum's angle of displacement. **The motion of the pendulum is described by the formulas:**

$$f = \frac{1}{2\pi}\sqrt{g/L}$$
$$T = 2\pi\sqrt{L/g}$$

A PENDULUM WITH A 5-kg ball and a length of 10 m is displaced by 10°. *EXAMPLE 19-1*

1. What is the frequency of its simple harmonic motion?

2. If the mass is doubled to 10 kg, what is the period of its simple harmonic motion?

SOLUTION:

1. Use the formula just provided to derive the frequency of the pendulum. L is given as 10 m; g was not given, and in such cases, it is assumed to be earth's gravity of 10 m/sec². Thus,

$$f = \frac{1}{2\pi} \sqrt{10/10}$$

= 1/2π cycles per second (Hz), **answer.**

2. The frequency and period of the pendulum do not depend on the mass of the pendulum. If you put a heavy mass on the end of the pendulum, gravity will pull it more strongly, but it will have a greater mass to accelerate. These effects cancel, causing the frequency to be independent of mass. To find the period, use the formula: $T = 2\pi \sqrt{L/g}$; **T = 2π seconds, answer.**

Note: More information was given than was required for solving the problem. It is important to be able to sort out what information given is required to solve the problem, and what information is unnecessary.

II. Kinetic Energy and Potential Energy of an Oscillating System

The kinetic energy (KE) of an oscillating system is expressed using the formula:

$$KE = 1/2\ mv^2$$

Because $v_{max} = \omega A$, the maximum kinetic energy of the oscillating system in terms of its amplitude and angular frequency is:

$$KE_{max} = 1/2\ m\omega^2 A^2$$

The potential energy (PE) of the oscillating mass spring system is:

$$PE = 1/2\ k\ \Delta x^2$$

in which Δx is the displacement from equilibrium. (Usually, x is defined as being = 0).

A MASS OF 4 kg resting on a frictionless surface is attached to a massless spring of spring constant k = 10 newtons per meter at rest. A ball of tape of 1 kg moving at 10 meters per second collides with the mass spring system and sticks. Using the diagram in Figure 19-3, determine the resulting amplitude of the simple harmonic motion. *EXAMPLE 19-2*

FIGURE 19-3.

A 1-kg tape ball moving at 10 m/sec collides with a mass spring system (see Example 19-2 for details).

Ex. 19-3 cont.

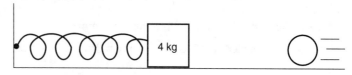

Figure 19-3.

SOLUTION:

This problem addresses two main concepts. The first part of the problem concerns the collision between the ball of tape and the mass attached to the spring. Because the ball of tape hits and sticks, it is a completely inelastic collision. During an inelastic collision, only conservation of momentum applies, because much energy is lost to deformation and heat. Considering conservation of momentum:

$$m_1 v_1 = (m_1 + m_2) v_f$$

$$v_f = \frac{m_1 v_1}{m_1 + m_2} \qquad v_f = \frac{(1)(10)}{1 + 4}$$

$$v_f = 2 \text{ m/sec, answer.}$$

Knowing the velocity of the tape ball and mass immediately after the collision, examine the conversion of kinetic to potential energy as the spring is pushed back toward the wall. Considering conservation of energy:

$$KE = PE$$
$$1/2 \ m_{total} \ v_f^2 = 1/2 \ k \ \Delta x^2$$
$$1/2 \cdot 5 \cdot 2^2 = 1/2 \cdot 10 \cdot \Delta x^2$$
$$\Delta x = \sqrt{2} \text{ m}$$

This problem is analogous to the "ballistic pendulum," in which a bullet strikes a hanging block. The same steps are taken in looking for the maximum height to which the pendulum + bullet rise: $PE = m_{(total)}gh$. If h is small compared to l (thus giving a small θ), then the resulting motion would be simple harmonic motion.

Sound

Sound

I. Basic Concepts		
II. Sound Intensity, Pitch, and the Decibel		**HIGH-YIELD TOPICS**
III. Doppler Effect		
IV. Resonance in Pipes and Strings		
V. Harmonics		

Simple vibrations of matter are responsible for the variety of sounds we hear, from the minute buzz of a mosquito's wings to the loud sounds of a rock concert. Sound can be transmitted through many types of matter. This chapter is a review of how sound travels in air, liquids and solids.

I. Basic Concepts

A. What is Sound?

Sound waves are longitudinal waves that can be transmitted through solids, liquids, or gases. Because they are longitudinal waves, the molecules vibrate in the **same direction** as the direction in which the wave travels. The frequency of the oscillations can vary greatly, giving rise to the wide variety of pitch in the sounds perceived. Perceptible sounds vary from 20 to 20,000 Hz. Sound waves are set up by a vibrating object or air column, and travel outward in three dimensions from the source.

B. Speed of Sound in Solids, Liquids, and Gases

What Determines the Speed of Sound in Solids and Liquids?

Think about a sound wave, which is **a pressure pulse travelling through a material.** A material has an area of compression and rarefaction that travels through it at a certain velocity. This area of compression and rarefaction is caused by the molecules first moving forward, then re-equilibrating by moving backward.

A factor that might affect the speed of sound is the stiffness of the material—its resistance to compression, also known as the bulk modulus, $\Delta V/V$. A stiff material cannot be compressed easily, which causes the sound wave to travel faster. Increasing the density of the material has the opposite effect. The pressure pulse of the sound wave must accelerate the substance, first forward and then backward, as it travels. **With a denser substance, these accelerations are slower.** Consider the quantitative formula:

$$v = \sqrt{BM/\rho}$$

which shows that the **velocity of a sound wave in a solid or liquid is proportional to the square root of the bulk modulus (BM) divided by the density.**

In air, the same ideas determine the speed of sound. One constant worth remembering is the speed of sound in air of normal composition at room temperature, 344 m/sec.

WHAT HAPPENS TO THE SPEED OF SOUND IN AIR AS THE TEMPERATURE INCREASES?

As temperature increases, the thermal motion of the molecules also increases, allowing the pressure pulse to travel faster. The velocity of sound in a gas is proportional to the square root of the absolute temperature in Kelvins.

C. Sound Intensity, Pitch, and the Decibel

Pitch is the perceived predominant frequency of a sound source. In the audible range, frequencies vary from 20 to 20000 Hz. Sounds with a frequency lower than 20 Hz are **infrasonic waves;** sounds with frequencies greater than 20000 Hz are **ultrasonic waves.** Note that in air, the wavelength of sound varies with frequency, $\lambda = v/f$, as the waves travel at a constant 344 m/sec.

When you hear a sound from a sound source, you are perceiving the pressure pulses. These pulses have energy that can be measured to determine their intensity. With a continuous sound, pressure pulses continue hitting with time, so they have power (remember P = energy/time). **Sound intensity is the amount of power (P) per unit area (A):**

$$I = P/A$$

Sound intensity falls off as $1/r^2$, in which r is the distance from the sound source. This relationship is similar to gravitational and electric fields, all of which expand in three dimensions. **The critical relationship between sound intensity and distance from the sound source is important to remember.**

EXAMPLE 20-1

A SOUND SOURCE MOVES from 2 m to 4 m away from a sound receiver. Explain how the sound intensity changes with this move.

SOLUTION:
Think of the sound intensity at 2 m as $1/2^2$, or 1/4. After the move, the intensity is $1/4^2$, or 1/16. Thus, when the distance from the source doubles, the sound intensity falls by a factor of 4 (from 1/4 to 1/16).

One way to understand sound intensity is to examine the differences between the intensities of certain sounds. The quietest sound that "good" ears can detect has a sound intensity of 10^{-12} watts/m². A quiet room has a sound intensity of approximately 10^{-9} watts/m². Normal conversation in a room produces a sound intensity of 10^{-6} watts/m². The front row of a heavy metal concert, on the other hand, has a sound intensity of approximately 1 watt/m².

It is difficult to portray such huge differences in sound intensity or even to think about a scale in which the numbers can vary by a factor of 10^{12} or more. To make the differences between sounds easier to write, and to provide a means to accurately describe the perceived loudness of sounds, the decibel scale was created. **The decibel scale is a logarithmic scale** in which zero dB was set equal to the quietest possible sound intensity, 10^{-12} watts/m². All other decibel levels were measured in terms of the reference point I_0, according to the formula:

$$\textbf{dB} = \textbf{10 log (I/I}_0\textbf{)} \text{ in which } I_0 = 10^{-12} \text{ watts/m}^2$$

When speaking about sound intensity in the decibel scale, the term **intensity level** is used. Note that the intensity level in dB is not a measurement of intensity, but is a comparison of the intensity of one sound to the intensity of the quietest sound that can be heard. In decibels, a quiet room is about 30 dB, normal conversation is about 60 dB, and a loud rock concert is in the range of 120 dB.

Because decibels are logarithmic measurements, you cannot directly add decibel units. If two people, each speaking at an intensity level of 50 dB, speak simultaneously, the total intensity level is not 100 dB. The addition of the intensity levels of these two speaking voices is about 53 dB. Thinking logically, if 10 voices at 50 dB speak simultaneously, a 10-dB increase in sound intensity level (in the decibel scale) will be heard, because a 10-dB increase corresponds to a 10-fold increase in the I values. Ten voices, each at 50 dB, give a total sound intensity level in decibels of 50 dB + 10 dB = 60 dB. Thus, the sound intensity level of two voices speaking simultaneously will predictably be less than 55 dB.

If you wish to calculate this log relationship, start by converting the decibel values to I values. Add the two I values and apply the decibel formula. Note the log 2 = 0.3.

THE SOUND INTENSITY at a distance of 1 m from a stereo speaker is 10^{-4} watts/m². Determine the approximate sound intensity level (in dB) at a distance of 3 m. *EXAMPLE 20-2*

SOLUTION:
Because sound intensity varies as $1/r^2$, the sound intensity at 3 m will be 1/9 that of 1 m. Thus, the intensity level will be approximately equal to 10 log [(1/9 • 10^{-4})/10^{-12}], or about 70 dB.

III. Doppler Effect

As cars go by during an Indianapolis 500 race, the frequency of the sounds seems to change. In Figure 20-1, one car is approaching a listener and one is receding from a listener. The cars are both emitting sound of the same frequency, but the sound waves of the car approaching the listener are compressed slightly because the car is moving closer each time a new wave is emitted. With the receding car, the waves are stretched slightly because the car moves away during each wave.

FIGURE 20-1.

A source approaching a listener (top) and a source receding from a listener (bottom) helps to understand the Doppler effect.

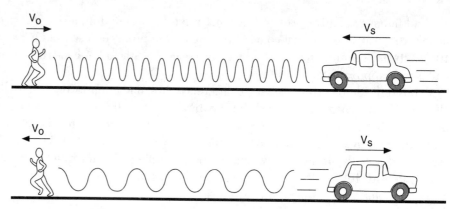

Figure 20-1.

The compression and stretching of the waves is perceived as a change in frequency, because the sound waves are still travelling at 344 m/sec, yet their wavelength has changed. (Remember $f = v/\lambda$.) An equation that describes the phenomenon follows:

$$f^1 = f\left(\frac{1 \pm v_0/v}{1 \mp v_s/v}\right)$$

in which v_o is the velocity of the observer, v_s is the velocity of the source, and v is the speed of sound. The + (numerator) and − (denominator) signs are used if the source is approaching the observer or the observer is approaching the source. The − (numerator) and + (denominator) signs are used if the source is fleeing from the observer or the observer is fleeing from the source.

Remember: the perceived frequency increases if the source or observer is approaching, and the perceived frequency decreases if the source or observer is receding.

IV. Resonance in Pipes and Strings

Chapter 17 of the Physics Review Notes provides a review of the introductory concepts of resonance in pipes and strings. Recall that a standing wave was created on a string by waves of certain frequencies undergoing constructive interference with the return waves from the end points.

On a string, nodes are always at the ends, because string movement is confined by being tied. The fundamental wave (lowest frequency, longest wavelength) has an antinode in the exact center. Other waveforms can be drawn by putting additional nodes and anti nodes on the string. Because the velocity is constant, the wavelength and frequency are related by:

$$v = f\lambda$$

Another example of standing waves is the vibration of air within a pipe. Waves on a string are transverse waves; the air within the pipe has longitudinal waves. **Three different types of pipes to remember are: closed at both ends, closed at one end, or open at both ends.**

A standing waveform for a pipe that is closed at both ends (Figure 20-2) is similar to a string's waveform. The nodes at each end are caused by the closed ends; the air is unable to move back and forth because its movement is stopped by the lack of movement of the end. In the center of the pipe, the air at the antinode is able to freely move back and forth. In the pipe with two open ends, the air at the ends is able to move freely, so there are antinodes at each end. The wavelength of the fundamental wave for an open ended pipe would be equal to 2L, as a complete wave would be twice as long as the pipe.

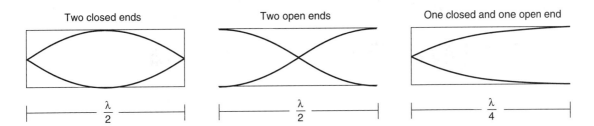

| Two closed ends | Two open ends | One closed and one open end |

The pipe with one closed and one open end has somewhat different properties (see Figure 20-2). Like the other pipes, the closed end has a node and the open end has an antinode. Unlike the other pipes, the wavelength of this fundamental wave would be four times as long as the length of the pipe.

FIGURE 20-2 caption

FIGURE 20-2.
Waveforms in pipes with closed ends (left), open ends (center), and one closed end, one open end (right).

V. Harmonics

Harmonics are resonance frequencies that are multiples of the fundamental frequency, including the fundamental frequency itself. They are numbered consecutively, with the fundamental being the first harmonic.

Figure 20-3 illustrates the harmonic frequencies for each of the types of pipe. The second harmonic wave has an additional node within the pipe; the third harmonic wave has an additional two nodes. The open and closed ends of the pipes have the same nodes and antinodes as the fundamental. The second harmonic is also called the **first overtone** (first tone "over" the fundamental), the third harmonic is also known as the **second overtone**, and so on.

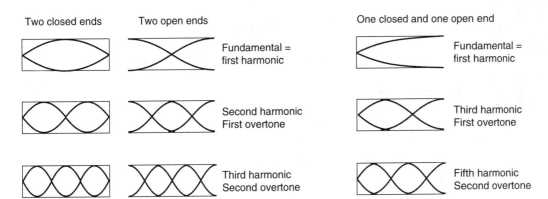

| Two closed ends | Two open ends | One closed and one open end |

Fundamental =
first harmonic

Fundamental =
first harmonic

Second harmonic
First overtone

Third harmonic
First overtone

Third harmonic
Second overtone

Fifth harmonic
Second overtone

The frequencies associated with the various harmonics with the different types of pipes are as follows. **The "both end closed or open" pipes have the same frequencies as a string, according to the formula:**

$$f = v/\lambda = (v)(n)/2L$$

The various frequencies are found by substituting for n any positive integer (1,2,3 . . .) and also substituting the length of the pipe, L.

The "open at one end and closed at one end" pipe is slightly different. Use the following formula for its resonance frequencies:

$$f = v/\lambda = (v)(n)/4L$$

in which n is the set of positive odd integers (1,3,5 . . .). These formulas, which arise from the familiar $f = v/\lambda$ formula, are found by deducing the possible values for the wavelength in terms of L, as shown in Figure 20-3. It is important to understand these formulas, and to be able to draw waveforms for the various pipes.

FIGURE 20-3.
The first harmonic frequency (fundamental frequency), and additional harmonic frequencies for the three different pipe types. Note the nodes, antinodes, and the difference between the different pipe types based on their open and closed ends. (See text for explanation.)

Light and Optics

This chapter provides a review of electromagnetic waves and the concepts and components of visible light.

I. Electromagnetic Waves and the Visual Spectrum

An **electromagnetic wave** is an electromagnetic disturbance that travels through space at a speed of 3×10^8 meters per second. As shown in Figure 21-1, **the electromagnetic wave is a transverse wave;** the electric and magnetic fields (on the x and y axes) vibrate **perpendicular** to the direction of the propagation of the wave (along the z axis).

FIGURE 21-1.

The electromagnetic wave is a transverse wave, with electric and magnetic fields oscillating in phase perpendicular to each other. Note the direction of travel of the electromagnetic wave.

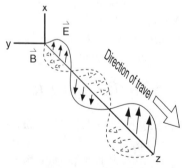

Figure 21-1.

Electromagnetic waves have a constant velocity in a vacuum, and their frequency and wavelength are inversely proportional. The properties of electromagnetic waves vary with frequency and wavelength, giving rise to the electromagnetic spectrum. The waves with the longest wavelength are radio waves, commonly used in AM, FM, and television broadcasting. At the shortest wavelength are gamma rays, the most energetic electromagnetic waves. The complete electromagnetic spectrum (Figure 21-2), with an expanded view of visible light, ranges from a wavelength of 700 nm for red to 400 nm for blue.

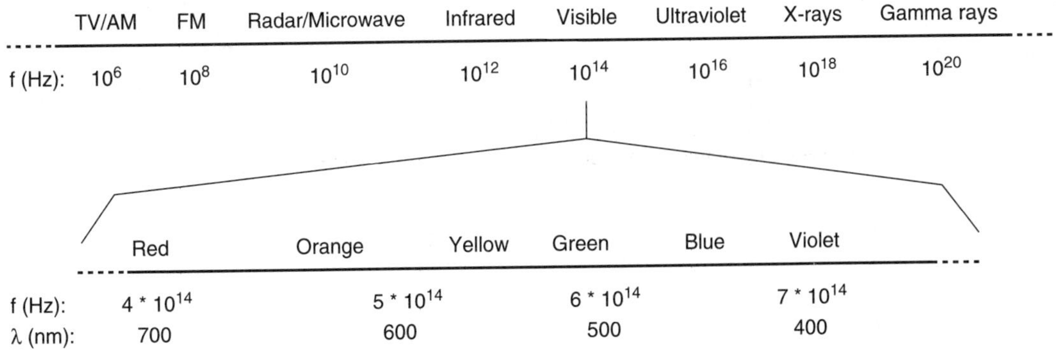

	TV/AM	FM	Radar/Microwave	Infrared	Visible	Ultraviolet	X-rays	Gamma rays
f (Hz):	10^6	10^8	10^{10}	10^{12}	10^{14}	10^{16}	10^{18}	10^{20}

	Red	Orange	Yellow	Green	Blue	Violet
f (Hz):	$4 * 10^{14}$	$5 * 10^{14}$		$6 * 10^{14}$		$7 * 10^{14}$
λ (nm):	700	600		500		400

II. Polarization of Light

Light from most sources is unpolarized, meaning that the direction of the E- and B-fields are at random, even when the light is moving in the same direction (same z axis). In polarized light, the waves have aligned electric and aligned magnetic fields (Figure 21-3).

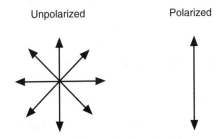

Unpolarized   Polarized

One of many ways for light to become polarized is for it to pass through a polarizing filter. Polarizing filters are plastic sheets with millions of aligned, long linear molecules. When light passes through the polarizing filter, those light waves with electric fields parallel to the molecules set up currents within the molecules and are thus absorbed. Light waves that have electric fields perpendicular to the molecules are not absorbed.

When two perfectly made polarizing filters are placed at right angles to one another, all of the incident light will be absorbed.

III. Refraction of Light and Snell's Law

When light strikes an interface between two media, part of the light is reflected and part is transmitted. The transmitted light is refracted at the interface, meaning that the light waves bend. Refraction leads to several important ideas within physics, and is the underlying mechanism behind the function of lenses and prisms.

When light waves enter a transparent medium other than a vacuum, such as glass, they *slow*, travelling at less than 3×10^8 m/sec. This concept is the basis for the **index of refraction, n,** of a medium, given by the formula:

$$n = c/v$$

in which **c** is 3×10^8 **m/sec,** the speed of light in a vacuum, and v is the speed of light in the medium where it is slowed. Thus, **for a vacuum, n = 1, and for other media, n > 1.**

FIGURE 21-2.
The electromagnetic spectrum. Note the expanded view of the visible light frequencies.

FIGURE 21-3.
Unpolarized versus polarized light as viewed looking down the z-axis at the E-field alone.

If the light wave enters a new medium perpendicular to the surface (Figure 21-4, at left), it will continue in the same direction. Should the light wave enter at an angle, however, it will **bend toward the normal vector (to the surface that it encountered) if the n value of that new medium is greater than the medium from which it came.** (The normal vector is a vector perpendicular to a given surface.)

These concepts should help you understand the diagram in Figure 21-4. The incident ray hitting a surface with $n > 1$ forms an angle θ_1 to the normal vector. The refracted ray forms an angle θ_2 that is less than θ_1.

FIGURE 21-4.

Light striking perpendicular to a surface with an index of refraction (n) greater than 1 (at left); light striking an interface with an incident angle, and bending toward the normal when n is greater than 1 (at right).

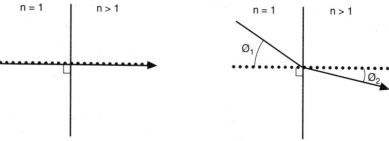

Note that as v slows, the ray bends toward the normal vector, and if v accelerates, the ray bends away from the normal vector. Thus, when a ray goes from a material with a low index of refraction to a high index of refraction ($n_{incident} < n_{refracted}$), it will bend toward the normal. If the ray goes from a material with a high index of refraction to a low index of refraction material ($n_{incident} > n_{refracted}$), it will bend away from the normal.

The angles are in all cases the **angles between the rays and the normal vector of the surface.** The exact relationship between θ_1 and θ_2 is expressed by **Snell's law:**

$$n_1 \sin \theta_1 = n_2 \sin \theta_2$$
or
$$v_2 \sin \theta_1 = v_1 \sin \theta_2 \text{ (since } n = c/v)$$

E X A M P L E 2 1 - 1

AS A CHILD is about to put a quarter into a machine to buy food for fish in a small pond, he drops the quarter and it rolls into the water. The coin seems to be close to the surface and easy to reach. Explain why the quarter might not be as near the surface as it appears to be.

SOLUTION:

As shown in Figure 21-5, the eyes sense depth by noticing the angle at which they converge in order to focus on an object. Because the quarter is under water, however, rays from the quarter reach the surface and then are bent away from the normal. The eyes interpret the bent rays as showing that the quarter is at depth d_2 instead of d_1.

FIGURE 21-5.

Explanation of how a submerged coin may appear close to the surface (see Example 21-1 for details).

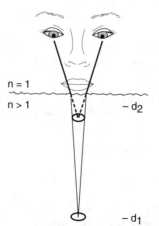

IV. Reflection and Total Internal Reflection

Reflection is a familiar concept. You expect light waves to "bounce off" of objects. When a light ray strikes a surface, part or all of the incident light is reflected at an angle θ_r, called the **reflected angle.** Figure 21-6 illustrates the concept of reflection.

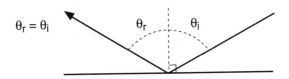

$$\theta_r = \theta_i$$

FIGURE 21-6.
Incident light reflects off a surface such that $\theta_i = \theta_r$.

The concept of total internal reflection is important. An incident ray from within a substance with $n > 1$ approaches an interface to a substance, air, or vacuum with a smaller n. As shown by the ray 1 in Figure 21-7, the ray will be refracted away from the normal vector. As the angle θ_i increases, you reach ray 2, and the refracted ray starts coming closer and closer to being parallel to the interface. Note that at ray 3, at the incident angle θ_c, the refracted ray actually skims the interface surface. **This angle is the critical angle,** because if θ_i increases still farther, none of the incident light will be refracted, and all will be reflected. This phenomenon is labeled **total internal reflection.** Where $\theta_i = \theta_c$, then $\theta_r = 90°$. Another way to derive the relationship between the indices of refraction and the critical angle follows:

$$n_i \sin \theta_i = n_r \sin \theta_r$$
$$\sin \theta_i / \sin \theta_r = n_r / n_i$$

Because $\sin \theta_r = 1$ when $\theta_i = \theta_c$, then

$$\mathbf{\sin \theta_c = n_r/n_i \text{ and } \theta_c = \arcsin(n_r/n_i)}$$

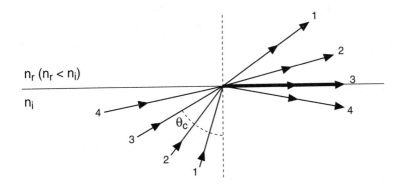

FIGURE 21-7.
The concept of the critical angle.

Total internal reflection can only happen when the light rays are coming from within the higher index of refraction material. **It does not occur when rays pass from a low n to a high n.**

The idea of the critical angle is behind the use of fiber optics in medicine. In fiber optics, thousands of extremely thin glass fibers are fused into a rod. Light incident at one end of the rod is transmitted through the rod via total internal reflection and can be seen at the other end. Many medical procedures such as endoscopy, colonoscopy, and laparoscopy depend on the concept of total internal reflection.

In total internal reflection, the index of refraction outside the transmitting substance (e.g., fiber optic rods) is less than the index of refraction of the transmitting medium.

Recall that it is possible to produce polarized light by using polarized filters. **Another way in which to polarize light is to reflect light off of a surface with a greater index of refraction,** such that the reflected and refracted rays make an angle of 90° (Figure 21-8). Angle θ_B in Figure 21-8 is known as **Brewster's angle.** To determine

Brewster's angle for a given interface between two media, use the formula:

$$\theta_B = \arctan{(n_r/n_i)}$$

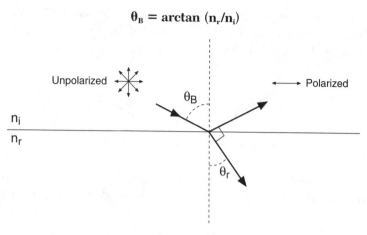

Figure 21-8.

FIGURE 21-8.

Production of polarized light by reflecting light off a surface with a greater index of refraction such that the reflected and refracted rays make a 90° angle.

Light incident on an interface will be partially reflected and partially refracted. If the incident light makes an angle equivalent to Brewster's angle with the normal vector to the surface, the reflected light will be totally polarized parallel to the interface between the two media.

V. Lenses and Mirrors

A. Lenses

CONVERGING (CONVEX) LENS

Lenses work by the property of refraction. When incident light rays encounter the lens, they are bent toward the normal vector. When the rays leave the lens, they are bent away from the normal vector. Because the normal vectors change across the lens and from one side of the lens to the other, the lens is able to **focus or diverge** light rays. To simplify the equations presented, all lenses in this discussion are thin lenses, implying that the thickness of the lens is less than the distance between the lens and the object on which it is focused.

Certain terms are used in a discussion of the function of lenses. The **object** is the item being examined with the lens or mirror. The **image** is the image of the object that is formed by light rays from the lens or mirror. **Object distances,** known as "p" and **image distances,** known as "q," are the perpendicular distances from the object or image to the lens or mirror.

Images can be **real or virtual.** A real image has light rays actually going through it, similar to the image formed by a slide projector. A virtual image, on the other hand, has no actual light rays travelling through it. It can be seen as the apparent location and size of the object when viewed via the lens or mirror creating the virtual image.

The **focal length** of a lens or mirror is the image distance if the object were held infinitely far away. In the ray diagrams that follow, solid arrows represent the object and dotted arrows represent the image. The **lens axis** is a line perpendicular to the surface of a lens and through its center.

To start ray tracing, choose the lens with which you have had the most experience—the convex (converging) lens, such as a magnifying glass. Just how it is possible to examine objects with this tool and have them appear bigger is illustrated in the ray tracing in Figure 21-9. The object is located at an object distance **p,** the image is located at the image distance **q,** and the focal points of the lens are marked with **f.** (The labels d_o for the object distance and d_i for the image distance are also common.)

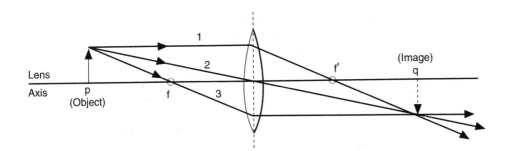

FIGURE 21-9.
Ray diagram for a convex lens.

In ray tracing, you draw light rays originating from the object and find out how the lens bends them. The intersection point of the traced rays identifies the position, orientation, and height of the image.

With the converging lens, you can draw three light rays. To start, it is important to realize that light rays from infinity are focused at f by a convex lens. Light rays from infinity are perpendicular to the plane of the lens, which makes them parallel to the lens axis.

The rays to draw:

1. A ray from the object that is parallel to the lens axis, refracted toward the focal point.

2. A ray travelling through the exact center of the lens. This ray will not encounter a net refraction as it passes through the lens, as the angle of the interface will not change after it passes through. To this ray, the lens is like a flat sheet of glass.

3. If needed, this ray is from the object passing through f on the same side of the lens as the object, refracted parallel to the lens axis.

Note that the intersection of these refracted rays gives you the location and height of the image. It is a real image because you have actual light rays that can come from the source to form the image. Another important characteristic is that a **converging lens is defined as having a positive focal length.**

DIVERGING (CONCAVE) LENS

When tracing rays from a concave (diverging) lens (Figure 21-10), you have the same goal of tracing multiple rays from the object through the lens and seeing where they intersect. Again, the intersection point gives you the location and height of the image. The image of this ray tracing is different, however, because it is the image from which the light rays appear to be coming.

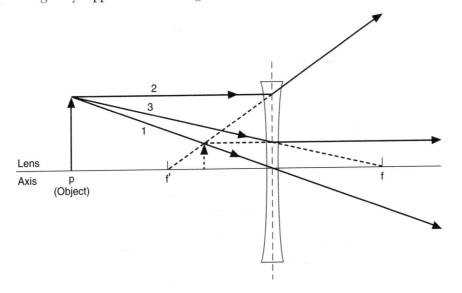

FIGURE 21-10.
Ray diagram for a diverging lens.

The rays to draw:

1. A ray goes straight through the center of the lens and is not refracted in any way. This ray can be treated in the same way as the unrefracted ray in the example of the converging lens.

2. A ray that is parallel to the lens axis hits the lens and diverges outward on a path that originates from the focal point f′.

3. A ray is aimed at the f point behind the lens and emerges from the other side of the lens as parallel.

The term f′ is the focal point of the diverging lens, and it is defined to be negative for a diverging lens. f′ is the point at which rays from infinity would seem to originate if an observer was looking from the other side of the lens.

If you draw rays 1 and 2 as just described and they do not intersect, think of this problem intuitively. The image is the point from which the diverged rays seem to be coming when viewed from the other side of the lens. So, draw the dotted line back from the refracted diverged ray back to f′. **The intersection of this dotted imaginary ray with the ray through the center gives you the location of the image.** In this diagram, as with that for the convex lens, the object distance is denoted p, and the image distance is denoted q. **The focal length f′ is a negative number.**

The image from a diverging lens is always Upright and Virtual. Virtual means it has no real light rays passing through it—it could not form an image on a screen. A good example of a virtual image is your reflection within a planar mirror; although it seems to be "behind" the mirror, no light waves are passing through that point.

B. Mirrors

FIGURE 21-11.

Ray diagrams for planar, concave (converging), and convex (diverging) mirrors.

In lenses, rays are bent toward and away from the normal by **refraction,** allowing the ray to be bent when it passes through a medium of n > 1 with nonparallel surfaces. In mirrors, the light rays are bent during **reflection,** and the law of reflection determines their path. Planar, concave, and convex mirrors are shown in Figure 21-11.

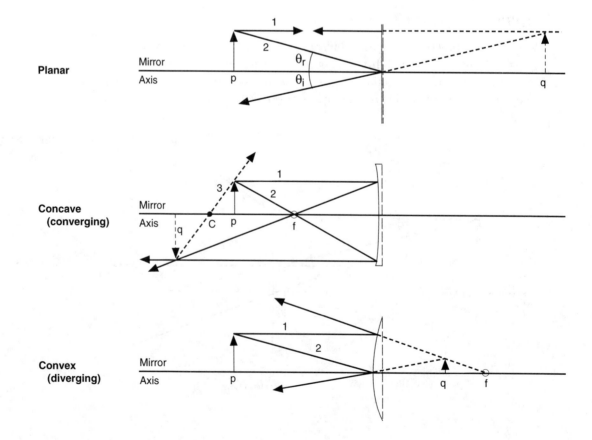

PLANAR MIRROR

The planar mirror can be approached by ray tracing using the law of reflection.

The rays to draw:
1. A ray from the object that is parallel to the mirror axis (perpendicular to the plane of the mirror) and reflected directly backward.
2. A ray that hits the mirror at the lens axis and is reflected at an angle $\theta_r = \theta_i$, causing it to reflect downward.

Tracing these rays back using the dotted lines demonstrates where the rays appear to originate, which is the location of the image. Note that in a planar mirror, **the image is of equal height to the object and it is located the same distance away from the mirror** ($q = p$).

The **magnification** is the height of the image divided by the height of the object, and is **equal to one** for a planar mirror.

CONCAVE (CONVERGING) MIRROR

A concave mirror acts to converge rays (see Figure 21-11, at center). An important new term for curved mirrors is the **radius of curvature (C).** By definition, $C = 2f$. A line from C to the mirror is always perpendicular to the mirror.

When a light ray hits the mirror, the incident angle, θ_i, and the reflected angle, θ_r, are both measured relative to the normal to the plane of the mirror; however, the normal to the plane of the mirror is also the line from **C** to the mirror. The focal point of a concave mirror is at 1/2 C, and it is the point to which a light ray parallel to the mirror axis is reflected.

The rays to draw:
1. A ray from the object parallel to the mirror axis, reflected through the focal point (1/2 C).
2. A ray from the object through the focal point, reflected back parallel to the mirror axis.
3. A ray from the object through the center of curvature. You may need to extend backward to find the image, especially when the object distance is greater than C.

Using these rays, it is possible to determine the location of the image (see Figure 21-11).

CONVEX (DIVERGING) MIRROR

A convex mirror acts to diverge rays. With a convex mirror, C and f are on the other side of the mirror from the object.

The rays to draw:
1. A light ray parallel to the axis of the mirror, reflected along a line originating at f. This ray can be traced back using the dotted line as shown.
2. A ray reflected across the mirror axis, which can also traced back. The intersection of the two traced back rays demonstrates the location of the image.

Similar to the diverging lens, the diverging (convex) mirror has a **D**iminished, **U**pright, **V**irtual (DUV) image.

VI. Thin-Lens and Lens Maker's Equations

Ray tracing diagrams are a conceptual representation of what lenses and mirrors do. A simple equation describes the formation of images by mirrors and lenses. The **thin-lens equation** follows:

$$\frac{1}{p} + \frac{1}{q} = \frac{1}{f}$$

Remember that p is the object distance from the lens or mirror and q is the image distance from the lens or mirror. This valuable equation is used to find any object or image distance and any focal length if two of the three variables in the equation are known.

E X A M P L E   2 1 - 2

A CONVEX (CONVERGING) lens with a focal length of 10 cm is placed 0.5 m from an object. Find the location of the image. State whether the image is real or virtual.

SOLUTION:
Recall the thin-lens equation. Always remember that distances are in units of meters. Thus, $f = 0.1$ m and $p = 0.5$ m. Fill in the known values in the thin-lens equation: $1/0.5 + 1/q = 1/0.1$. Solving the equation gives $2 + 1/q = 10$; $1/q = 8$; $q = 0.125$ m. Note that q is positive, corresponding to a real image. A real image would be found on the opposite side of the lens as the object.

Another critical formula is the **magnification equation:**

$$m = \frac{-q}{p}$$

which can be used to find the magnification of an image (**m**) if q and p are known.

The thin lens equation is valid when the following rules are observed:

For lenses:

> **p** + always
>
> **q** + means the image is a real image, on the opposite side of the lens as the object
>
>   − means the image is a virtual image, on the same side of the lens as the object
>
> **f** + for a converging lens (convex)
>
>   − for a diverging lens (concave)

For mirrors:

> **p** + always
>
> **q** + means the image is a real image in front of the mirror (on the same side as the object)
>
>   − means the image is a virtual image behind the mirror (on the opposite side as the object)
>
> **f** + for a converging mirror (concave)
>
>   − for a diverging mirror (convex)

The following outline clarifies the relationships between the image and the object with different lenses and mirrors.

I. With a diverging lens (concave) or mirror (convex):

A.   f is negative

B.   The image is DUV (diminished, upright, and virtual), and q is negative

(The image for convex mirrors is always diminished. For diverging lenses, the image is usually diminished).

II. With a converging lens (convex) or mirror (concave)

A. f is positive

B. If p > f, the image is real, inverted, and q is positive

C. If p < f, the image is BUV (bigger, upright, and virtual), and q is negative

To find the focal point of a lens, knowing just the index of refraction and the physical dimensions of the lens, use the **lens maker's equation:**

$$\frac{1}{f} = (n - 1)\left(\frac{1}{R_1} + \frac{1}{R_2}\right)$$

in which f is the focal length of the lens, n is the index of refraction of the material of the lens, and R_1 and R_2 are the radii of curvature of the two sides of the lens. Note that the definition of a radius of curvature for a concave side of a lens is negative, which allows a diverging concave lens to have a negative focal length. Also, it is possible to use this equation to find the focal length of a lens that has one convex and one concave side, such as lenses found in eyeglasses.

A FISH IN A fish tank swims by the bubbler, and takes a glance at his companion through one of the bubbles. Would the light rays from the companion be:

A. diverged as they pass through the bubble?

B. converged as they pass through the bubble?

C. unaffected as they pass through the bubble?

SOLUTION:

The light rays would be diverged as they pass through the bubble. The ray is bent away from the normal as it passes from the n > 1 water into the n = 1 air. Then, the ray is bent toward the normal as it passes from the n = 1 air into the n > 1 water again. Because the plane of the surface has changed, however, both of these effects act to diverge the light rays (Figure 21-12).

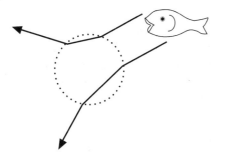

Figure 21-12.

EXAMPLE 21-3

FIGURE 21-12.
Concepts of light divergence through bubbles as discussed in Example 21-3.

YOU AND A FRIEND decide to invent a new way of seeing underwater. Instead of using a diving mask, which allows the cornea to converge light rays by providing an air interface, you devise different lenses to correct the diver's vision. You make a lens from glass with n = 1.4. Your friend shapes two thin glass plates, seals them, and then fills them with air.

EXAMPLE 21-4

1. Assuming that water has an index of refraction n = 1.33, whose design requires the greater radii of curvature?

2. What would be the shapes of the two lenses?

SOLUTION:

1. The ability of the lenses to bend light will depend on the ratio of their indices of refraction. From Snell's law, $n_1 \sin \theta_1 = n_2 \sin \theta_2$, the ratio of n_1 to n_2 describes the ability of the lens to bend light on entering and exiting the lens. Because of a greater percentage difference between the indices of refraction for air and water than for water and glass, the air-filled lens will bend light more effectively, and would not have to have as great a radius of curvature. Similarly, a glass lens is less powerful under water than it is in air because it is not able to bend light rays as well. The cornea acts as the most effective refractor of light rays (**not** the lens) because of the large ratio difference between n_{cornea} and n_{air}.

2. An air-filled lens under water functions in the opposite manner as a glass lens in air: a convex, air-filled lens under water diverges light rays and a concave, air-filled lens under water converges light rays. Thus, to counteract the diminished function of the cornea, you need a concave, air-filled lens.

Because its index of refraction is greater than that of water, the glass lens would function under water in the same manner as it would in air, albeit not as effectively. Thus, you would need a convex lens in order to converge the light rays.

VII Combinations of Lenses and Diopters

Combinations of lenses can be examined by using both equations and ray tracing. Ray tracing of combinations of lenses can be accomplished by using the image formed by one lens as the object of the other lens. For practice, combine the two lenses given in the ray tracing exercises in the preceding section on lenses. Draw the converging lens with the convex lens p being 2f, and place the diverging lens so that the image formed by the convex lens is at 2f'.

An important concept of lenses in day to day life is **power. The power of a lens is simply the reciprocal of its focal length, 1/f.** Thus, the lens maker's equation gives the power of the lens on the lefthand side of the equation. Power is measured in **diopters** (equal to **1/meter,** because f is measured in meters). **The powers of lenses in combination are additive,** with the total power of the combined lenses being equal to the sum of the individual powers:

$$1/f_t = 1/f_1 + 1/f_2$$

This equation can be combined with the thin lens equation for each lens to allow the calculation of p or q for either lens, if given all other variables.

VIII. Dispersion

Dispersion is the property of a prism that allows it to scatter light of different frequencies. In a vacuum, light waves of all frequencies travel with the same speed. When they enter a medium with n > 1, however, light waves of different frequencies travel with slightly different speeds, varying by approximately 1 to 2% across the visual spectrum. The higher frequency waves tend to travel slower; therefore, the index of refraction of the prism for blue waves is slightly higher, and they will bend more on entering and exiting the prism. With the triangular cross section of the prism, separation of light of different frequencies results (Figure 21-13).

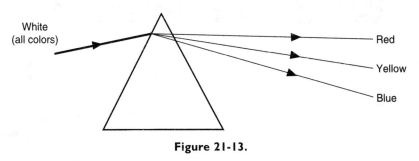

Figure 21-13.

FIGURE 21-13.
A prism separating light into its component colors (wavelengths).

Dispersion is responsible for a prism separating light into its component colors (wavelengths) and for rainbows, in which water droplets are acting as the "prisms."

Atomic and Nuclear Structure

The focus of this chapter is on the atom—its nucleus and the forces that bind it together. Other topics include radioactive decay and the photoelectric effect.

I. Basic Concepts

A. Atomic Number and Atomic Weight

The physicist's basic view of the atom follows:

A = Atomic weight (4 in this example)
  = Number of protons + number of neutrons

Z = Atomic number (2 in this example)
  = Number of protons

$$^{4}_{2}\text{He}$$

In this diagram, the atomic weight (A) is shown as the superscript over the element. It is the number of protons and neutrons in the atom. The atomic number (Z) is shown as the subscript under the element. It is the number of protons in the atom. $A - Z$ is therefore equal to the number of neutrons in the atom.

B. Neutrons, Protons, and Isotopes

Neutrons and protons are both nucleons, relatively large particles that make up the nucleus. Their weight is commonly measured in terms of atomic mass units, with

1 **amu** being equal to 1/12 the weight of a ^{12}C atom (carbon with 6p, 6n, and 6e); 1 amu = 1.66×10^{-27} kg. A proton weighs 1.0073 amu, and the neutron is slightly heavier, at 1.0087 amu. Electrons are lighter, at 5.48×10^{-4} amu.

Neutrons are neutral; they have no electric charge. Protons have a positive charge of +e, 1.6×10^{-19} Coulombs. Electrons have a negative charge of −e. The typical radius of an atom, including its electron cloud, is about 10^{-10} m.

In **isotopes** of an element, the number of protons remains the same, but the number of neutrons differs. Thus, different isotopes of an element have the same atomic number, but different atomic weights.

II. Radioactive Decay

Radioactive decay is the process in which a nucleus emits particles and energy, decomposing into another particle or particles. The three types of radioactive decay are described.

1. In the first type, alpha (α) particles, which are helium nuclei, are released during radioactive decay. Their chemical symbol is:

$$^{4}_{2}He^{+2}$$

They are relatively large and slow, and do not penetrate matter easily. Because paper shielding can stop alpha particles, they do not represent an external radiation hazard, but they can be hazardous if taken internally.

2. In the second type, beta (β) particles are released electrons (−e charge) or positrons (+e charge). They are stopped by shielding with approximately 1 cm of Lucite.

3. In the third type, gamma (γ) photons are released. These photons represent high energy, electromagnetic massless particles. Nuclei can emit gamma ray photons during radioactive decay. They penetrate matter easily, and require lead bricks as shielding.

Radioactive decay is examined in terms of the half life of a radioactive substance. **The half life ($t_{1/2}$) is the amount of time required for one-half of the nuclei in any sample of a given isotope to decay.** A graph of the number of radioactive nuclei with respect to time is presented in Figure 22-1. Note that the rate of radioactive decay is an exponential function.

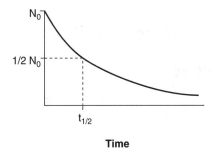

Time

Figure 22-1.

FIGURE 22-1.
The initial number of nuclei of radioactive isotope (N_o) versus time. The half-life is the time required for ½ of the initial number of nuclei to decay.

The decay rate is the number of nuclei that decay per unit of time. N is the number of nuclei, and λ is the **radioactive decay constant**, which is related to the half-life. Thus, the change in the number of nuclei with respect to time is given by:

$$\frac{\Delta N}{\Delta t} = -\lambda N$$

A more important equation relates the decay constant and the half-life:

$$\lambda = 0.693\ /t_{1/2}$$

III. Quantized Energy Levels for Electrons

This subject is addressed in the general chemistry review notes. As a brief overview, electrons circling a nucleus are confined to certain values (i.e., they are **quantized**). The energy level of an electron is determined by the principle quantum number, **n.** When an electron is taken away from the atom through ionization, the electron has been excited to the principle quantum number of n = infinity. Should the electron be excited by enough energy to change its principle quantum number, it will be held less tightly by the atom, but it will not be taken away.

IV. Mass Defect Principle and Nuclear Binding Energy

The mass defect principle states that the mass of every nucleus is less than the mass of the nucleons that make up that atom. Thus, the nucleus has a mass defect (Δm). The mass defect acts as a sort of a nuclear glue that gives stability to the atomic nucleus, preventing the protons' positive charge from pulling the nucleus apart.

The mass defect of carbon-12 is found from the atomic composition as follows: 6 protons (6 × 1.0073 amu) + 6 electrons (6 × 0.005 amu) + 6 neutrons (6 × 1.0087 amu) gives a total mass of 12.099 amu. Since carbon-12 has an atomic mass of 12.000 amu, there is a mass defect (Δm) of 0.099 amu.

The nuclear binding energy is the energy equivalent of the mass defect. It is found by using Einstein's formula:

$$E = (\Delta m)c^2$$

in which E is measured in Joules, m in kilograms, and c, the speed of light, in meters per second. The energy of 1 amu according to this formula is: (Note 1 eV = 1.6×10^{-19} J).

$$
\begin{aligned}
E &= 1\ \text{amu} \times c^2 \\
&= (1.66 \times 10^{-27}\ \text{kg})(3 \times 10^8\ \text{m/sec}) \\
&= 1.49 \times 10^{-10}\ \text{J} \\
&= 1.49 \times 10^{-10}\ \text{J}/1.6 \times 10^{-19}\ \text{J} = 9.3 \times 10^8\ \text{eV}
\end{aligned}
$$

The binding energy per nucleon gives a good idea of the stability of the nucleus. It shows how much "glue" is spread across each nucleon.

V. Photoelectric Effect and Fluorescence

A. Photoelectric Effect

A photon is a massless bundle of electromagnetic energy. The energy of a single photon can be described by the formula:

$$E = hf$$

in which E is the energy, h is a constant called Planck's constant, and f is the frequency. Thus, the energy of photons varies with frequency.

The photoelectric effect occurs when electrons eject from the surface of a metal when it is irradiated with electromagnetic radiation. For this effect, light of one frequency and wavelength (**monochromatic** light) strikes a metal plate. If an electron in the metal absorbs enough energy from the photons of light, it can escape the metal's surface. The electrons moving from the plate can be detected by a collector, thus illustrating a photoelectric current. The kinetic energy of the emitted electrons would be equal to:

$$1/2mv^2 = hf - \phi$$

in which ϕ, the work function, is the minimum amount of energy needed to escape the surface of the metal. All of the rest of the energy obtained from the photon is translated into the kinetic energy of the photon.

B. Fluorescence

Fluorescence is the property that allows electrons to emit light as they lose energy falling from an excited state to a less excited state or the unexcited ground state.

Physics

PRACTICE TESTS

Time: 50 minutes

Directions: This test contains as many physics passages as you may encounter on the MCAT. The time allotted approximates the time allowed to solve the given number of questions. Choose one best answer for each question.

Passage I (Questions 1-8)

The concept of using a lever to gain mechanical advantage is illustrated in Figure 1. A person standing at left applies a downward force to a pry bar in an attempt to lift a rock. In this situation, the lever acts as a force multiplier. The work done by the person is equal to the work done in lifting the rock. Although energy is conserved, the force on the rock is greater than that applied by the person pushing down on the pry bar. Note that $W = \mathbf{F}\Delta\mathbf{s}$, in which s is the displacement vector. Although the force applied by the person is less than that pushing up on the rock, the displacement Δs, through which that force is applied, is greater.

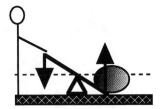

Figure 1. Lever as a force multiplier.

A different type of lever is depicted in Figure 2. The human arm is a velocity multiplier rather than a force multiplier. During bicep curls (lifting weights using the bicep muscles only), the bicep must exert a force **greater** than the weight being lifted. The mechanical advantage gained here is one of speed of forearm movement.

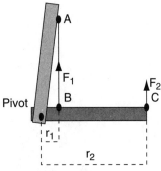

Figure 2. Lever as a velocity multiplier.

1. If the bicep attachment to the forearm (Figure 2, point B) is moved further away from the elbow (pivot) and closer to the wrist (point C), i.e., the ratio r_1/r_2 is increased, then:

    A. F_2/F_1 increases.
    B. F_2/F_1 decreases.
    C. F_2/F_1 remains unchanged.
    D. $F_2/F_1 = 1$.

2. Two people are doing bicep curls on a weight machine. One individual has longer arms than the other, yet they lift the same amount of weight to the same height. Which of the following statements is true?

    I.   The individual with shorter arms is doing more work.
    II. The individual with shorter arms is doing less work.
    III. The two people are doing the same amount of work.

    A. I only
    B. II only
    C. III only
    D. None of the above

3. The individual in Figure 1 applies a force F_1 on the pry bar in an attempt to move a rock of mass M. If the force on the rock (F_2) is insufficient to move the rock ($F_2 < Mg$), what is the work done by the individual?

    A. Mg
    B. Mg/2
    C. $(F_1/F_2)Mg$
    D. zero

4. A weight of mass M is suspended from point C in Figure 2. If the weight is lifted 0.1 m, how much work is done by the "arm"?

   I. Mg (0.1 m)
  II. F_2 (0.1 m)
 III. $F_1(r_1/r_2)$(0.1 m)

A. I only
B. II only
C. III only
D. I, II, and III (they are equivalent)

5. What is the torque on the arm (about the pivot) in Figure 2?

   I. $F_1 r_1$
  II. $F_2 r_2$
 III. $(F_2 - F_1)/(r_2 - r_1)$

A. I only
B. II only
C. I and II only
D. III only

6. In Figure 1, assume that:

W_1 = the work done by the individual.
F_1 = the force applied by the individual.
ΔS_1 = the displacement of the pry bar handle.
W_2 = the work done on the rock.
F_2 = the force applied to the rock.
ΔS_2 = the displacement of the rock.

Which of the following statements are true?

A. $F_1 > F_2$
B. $W_1 = W_2$
C. $\Delta S_1 = \Delta S_2$
D. All of the above

7. When the "bicep" in Figure 2 is contracting, which of the following statements are true?

   I. The displacement of point C exceeds that of point B.
  II. The angular speed of point C exceeds that of point B.
 III. The linear speed of point C exceeds that of point B.

A. I only
B. II only
C. I and III only
D. I, II, and III

8. Which of the following are vectors?

   I. Speed
  II. Velocity
 III. Force

A. I and II only
B. II and III only
C. III only
D. I, II, and III

Passage II (Questions 9-16)

Sublimation is the process whereby a solid converts directly into a vapor without passing through the liquid phase. The sublimation of dry ice (solid CO_2) is a familiar example. The heat of sublimation, L_s, is the latent heat associated with the phase change from solid to vapor. The first law of thermodynamics states: $Q = \Delta U + P\Delta V$. In sublimation, $Q = mL_s$, where L_s is the latent heat of sublimation per kilogram, and ΔU is the change in internal energy of the material as it converts from solid to vapor. ΔU is the energy required to break all bonds of an atom located at the surface. In general, a surface atom has half as many bonds to neighboring atoms as an atom located in the bulk of the material. Measuring L_s is a way to assess the strength of the interatomic bonds in the solid.

Figure 3 is a phase or P-T diagram for CO_2. The solid lines show where two or more phases exist in equilibrium. At the triple point (T = 216.6 K and P = 5.1 atm.), the three phases, solid, liquid, and gas, exist simultaneously. The straight line above the triple point is the melting curve, the positive slope of which indicates that CO_2 expands on melting.

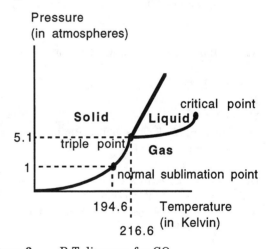

Figure 3. P-T diagram for CO_2.

9. When dry ice sublimes, what happens to the entropy, S, of the CO_2?

A. S increases
B. S decreases
C. S remains unchanged
D. Cannot say without specifying a value for P

10. Ice (frozen water) sublimes slowly at atmospheric pressure, which explains why ice cubes left in a freezer gradually diminish in size. As ice sublimes, it:

A. removes heat from its surroundings.
B. adds heat to its surroundings.
C. has no affect on the surroundings because Q_{in} is exactly balanced by Q_{out}.
D. is not possible to determine an affect without specifying a value for P.

11. The latent heat of sublimation, L_s, is an intrinsic property of a material and therefore does not depend on temperature or pressure. If you put dry ice in a hyperbaric chamber with P = 2 atmospheres, the sublimation rate will:

A. increase.
B. decrease.
C. remain unchanged.
D. It is not possible to determine without specifying a value for ΔV.

12. Water expands on freezing, i.e., solid water (ice) is actually less dense than liquid water. Pure silicon is another substance that expands on freezing. On a P-T diagram, the slope of the melting curve for both water and silicon must be:

A. negative.
B. positive.
C. zero.
D. It is not possible to determine without knowing the heat of sublimation.

13. At T = 100 K and P = 2 atm, CO_2 is a:

A. solid.
B. liquid.
C. gas.
D. mixture of all three phases that exists in equilibrium.

14. One liter of CO_2 is in a cylinder with a piston that maintains a constant pressure of 1 atm. What happens when you cool the CO_2 from room temperature (300 K) to 100 K?

I. Gaseous CO_2 condenses to liquid CO_2.
II. Liquid CO_2 solidifies to dry ice.
III. The CO_2 releases heat, Q, to its surroundings.

A. I only
B. II only
C. III only
D. II and III only

15. The heat of sublimation of silicon (Si) is 4.76×10^{-20} J per atom and the heat of sublimation of copper (Cu) is 7.44×10^{-20} J per atom. Each Cu atom in solid Cu

has 12 bonds to neighboring atoms, whereas each Si atom in solid Si has only four bonds to neighboring atoms. Therefore:

I. Si has stronger interatomic bonds.
II. Cu has stronger interatomic bonds.
III. More heat is required to sublimate Cu.

A. I only
B. II only
C. I and III only
D. II and III only

16. At the triple point (P = 5.1 atm and T = 216.6 K), CO_2 exists as a:

A. solid.
B. liquid.
C. gas.
D. mixture of all three phases that exists in equilibrium.

Passage III (Questions 17-24)

In an insulator, such as glass or asphalt, each electron is bound to a particular atom. In conductors (metals), however, one or more electrons per atom are free to migrate through the bulk of the conductor. The electrostatic consequences of this property are given by three observations.

Observation 1:

$\mathbf{E} = 0$ inside a conductor (Figure 4). Because electrons are free to flow in a metal, they are able to move in response to an external field. The resulting charge separation gives rise to a field of equal magnitude but opposite direction, resulting in a net field of zero **inside** the conductor. Outside the conductor, $\mathbf{E_o}$ and $\mathbf{E_1}$ do not cancel, and so the net field is **not** zero.

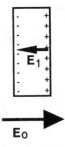

Figure 4. The relationship between E_0 and E_1 for a conductor.

Observation 2:

The charge density, ρ, is zero inside a conductor. Any net charge on a conductor resides on the surface.

Observation 3:

Just outside a conductor, **E,** if any, is perpendicular to the surface (Figure 5). If **E** were not perpendicular, electrons would flow along the surface until the tangential component of **E** was exactly canceled. The electrons are bound to the metal and are not free to leave the surface; therefore, they cannot respond to a perpendicular field outside the conductor.

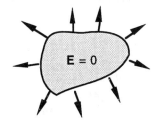

Figure 5. Inside a conductor, E = 0. Outside a conductor, E is perpendicular to the surface.

Observation 4:

The potential, V, is the same everywhere throughout a conductor.

17. An electromagnetic wave (light) is incident on a conductor. Just outside the conductor:

    I. **B** is parallel to the surface of the conductor.
    II. **B** is perpendicular to the surface of the conductor.
    III. **E** = 0.

    A. I and III only
    B. II and III only
    C. I only
    D. II only

18. A charge, q, is brought close to a neutral conducting sphere. Knowing that a charge gives rise to an electric field,

    $$E = \frac{1}{4\pi\epsilon_\circ} \frac{q}{r^2}$$

    which of the illustrations describe this scenario?

    (a) +q

    (b) +q

    (c) -q

A. a and c
B. b and c
C. b only
D. c only

19. If the electric field in a region is zero, the potential is:

    A. zero.
    B. constant.
    C. proportional to r.
    D. proportional to q.

20. The circuit shown below consists of a battery, a resistor, and a connection to ground. Which of the following statements are true?

    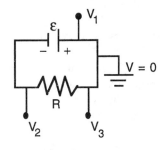

    I. $V_2 = 0$
    II. $V_1 = V_2$
    III. $V_3 = V_2(R/\epsilon)$

    A. I and II only
    B. II and III only
    C. I and III only
    D. None of the above

21. A net charge on the conductor in Figure 5 is equal to +q. What is the charge density (ρ = charge per unit volume) at the center of the conductor?

    A. $\rho = +q/V$
    B. $\rho = -q/V$
    C. $\rho = 0$
    D. None of the above

22. Referring to the conductors in Figures 4 and 5, which of the following statements are true?

    I. The net charge, if any, resides on the surface of the conductor.
    II. There is no net charge inside the conductor.
    III. The electric field just **outside** the conductor is zero.

A. I and II only
B. II and III only
C. I and III only
D. I, II, and III

23. In a metal, some electrons are free to move about in the bulk of the material and:

   I. there are at least as many "free" electrons as atoms.
   II. the "free" electrons are bound to the metal, i.e., they are not easily removed from the surface.
   III. the "free" electrons are attracted to one another.

   A. I and II only
   B. II and III only
   C. I and III only
   D. I, II, and III

24. Which of the following are vectors?

   A. Charge and potential
   B. Potential and resistance
   C. Resistance and current
   D. None are vectors

Passage IV (Questions 25-32)

Porous wax applied to the base of waxable cross-country skis interacts with crystallites in the snow to provide a relatively high coefficient of static friction, μ_s, and a low coefficient of kinetic friction, μ_k. The snow crystals catch in the pores of the wax when weight is transferred to the ski and the ski is briefly stationary with respect to the snow. The snow crystals do not catch in the wax pores when the ski is moving. In Figure 6, a cross-country skier is following a cross-country ski course. Five points along the course are shown, as is ϕ, the angle each point makes with the x-axis.

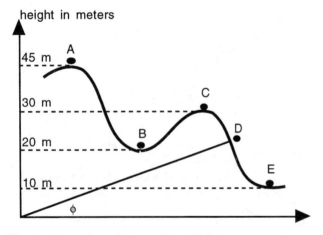

Figure 6. Sample cross-country skiing course.

25. A cross-country skier is following the course in Figure 6. If her mass, M, equals 50 kg, what is her acceleration at point D?

   A. $Mg[\sin(\phi)]$
   B. $g[\sin(\phi)]$
   C. $Mg[\cos(\phi)]$
   D. $g[\cos(\phi)]$

26. What is the frictional force on her skis as she passes point D?

   A. $\mu_k Mg[\sin(\phi)]$
   B. $\mu_s g[\sin(\phi)]$
   C. $\mu_s Mg[\cos(\phi)]$
   D. $\mu_k g[\cos(\phi)]$

27. If the skier is at rest at point A, what is the value of the frictional force she must overcome to begin moving forward?

   A. $\mu_k Mg$
   B. $\mu_s g[\sin(\phi)]$
   C. $\mu_s Mg$
   D. $\mu_k g[\cos(\phi)]$

28. Ignoring friction, what is the work done by gravity in moving the skier from point A to point E?

   A. 1.7×10^4 J
   B. Mgh (h = 35 m)
   C. 1.7×10^4 Newton-meters
   D. All of the above

29. The skier starts at rest at point C. Ignoring friction, what is her *kinetic* energy as she passes point E?

   A. 9.8×10^3 J
   B. Mg(30 m)
   C. Mv/2
   D. All of the above

30. The skier is at rest at point D. What condition must be satisfied to allow her to remain stationary on the slope?

   A. $Mg(20 \text{ m}) < Mg[\cos(\phi)]$
   B. $Mg[\sin(\phi)] < \mu_s$
   C. $\mu_k < 1/[g\cos(\phi)]$
   D. $\mu_s \tan(\phi) > 1$

31. If the surface of the snow could be made perfectly frictionless, which statement best describes what happens as the skier skis down the slope?

A. Energy (of the skier) is conserved.
B. Momentum (of the skier) is conserved.
C. Both energy and momentum are conserved.
D. Neither energy nor momentum are conserved.

32. Given that snow does produce friction against the base of the skis, which statement best describes what occurs as the skier travels down the slope?

A. Energy (of the skier) is conserved.
B. Momentum (of the skier) is conserved.
C. Both energy and momentum are conserved.
D. Neither energy nor momentum are conserved.

Passage V (Questions 33-40)

Surface waves on water (e.g., ocean waves) have a transverse and a longitudinal component. Elements of water move in a circular motion (Figure 7).

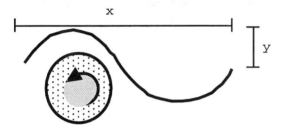

Figure 7. Circular motion of water during wave movement.

Although a wave moves across the ocean surface, water itself is not transported with the wave; its only movement is the circular motion that occurs as the wave passes by. All waves are caused by a displacement (ocean water gets pushed by surface winds) accompanied by a restoring force (which opposes the displacement and grows with increasing displacement, such as the spring force). Water is subject to two restoring forces: gravity and surface tension.

Two characteristic measurements associated with water waves are the depth of the water (h) and the wavelength of the surface waves (λ). When the depth is less than the wavelength, shallow water waves result, the speed of which is expressed as:

$$v = \sqrt{gh}$$

(for h < λ)

in which g is the acceleration due to gravity. When the depth of the water is greater than the wavelength, deep water waves result, the speed of which is expressed as:

$$v = \sqrt{\frac{g\lambda}{2\pi} + \frac{2\pi S}{\rho\lambda}}$$

(for h > λ)

in which S is surface tension and ρ is the density of the water.

33. Which of the following is true for long wavelength deep water waves? (Hint: long wavelength means $\lambda >> 2\pi S/\rho$.)

I. The dominant restoring force is gravity.
II. The propagation speed is proportional to the square root of the wavelength.
III. Increasing the density (e.g., by increasing the salinity) has little effect on the propagation speed.

A. I and II only
B. II and III only
C. III only
D. I, II, and III

34. Media that allow all wavelengths to propagate at the same speed are **nondispersive.** Visible light propagating in air is not dispersed into its constituent colors because all wavelengths (or frequencies) propagate at the same speed. Which of the following statements are true for surface waves on water?

I. Shallow water is nondispersive.
II. Deep water is dispersive.
III. Shallow water is dispersive.

A. I and II only
B. II and III only
C. I and III only
D. I only

35. If pollution from an industrial plant cut the surface tension of the water in a lake by one half, which of the following would be true?

I. The speed of short wavelength, shallow water waves would be unaffected.
II. The speed of long wavelength, shallow water waves would be unaffected.
III. The speed of long wavelength, deep water waves would be unaffected.

A. I and III only
B. II and III only
C. III only
D. I, II, and III

36. Referring to Figure 7, which of the following statements are correct?

I. x is the wavelength.
II. y is the wavelength.
III. The wavelength is expressed as $\lambda = \sqrt{x^2 + y^2}$

A. I only
B. II only
C. III only
D. None of the above

37. The energy carried by water waves is proportional to the:

A. wavelength squared.
B. amplitude squared.
C. square root of the wavelength.
D. square root of the amplitude.

38. Referring to Figure 7, which of the following statements are correct?

I. x is the amplitude.
II. y is the amplitude.
III. The amplitude is expressed as $A = \sqrt{x^2 + y^2}$

A. I only
B. II only
C. III only
D. None of the above

39. One way to characterize the frequency, f, of a wave is to count the number of wave crests that pass a given point in a fixed time interval. Which of the following statements are true for shallow water waves?

(Note: f = frequency; λ = wavelength; v = propagation speed.)

I. f is proportional to $1/\lambda$.
II. f is proportional to v.
III. f decreases as the depth of the water, h, decreases

A. I and III only
B. II and III only
C. I, II, and III
D. None of the above

40. Although the relationship between the wavelength and the frequency for deep water waves is complex, both characteristics can be measured. Suppose you have measured the density of a solution in a beaker. A fan that blows air across the surface of the solution excites waves of a single wavelength. The wavelength, λ, is less than the depth of the beaker. By measuring the wavelength and the frequency, you can determine the:

I. viscosity of the solution.
II. surface tension of the solution.
III. temperature of the solution.

A. I and III only
B. II and III only
C. I and II only
D. II only

180

Answers and Explanations to Physics Practice Test 1

1. **A** Recall that torque equals the product of the force and lever arm. Figure 2 shows two forces and two lever arms. Because the torques about the pivot at points B and C are the same: set $F_1 r_1 = F_2 r_2$. By rearrangement, $F_2/F_1 = r_1/r_2$, so if r_1/r_2 increases, then F_2/F_1 must increase.

2. **C** These individuals move the same amount of mass ($W = mgh$) to the same height. Thus, work (energy) is conserved. Because the lengths of their forearms differ, the force exerted by their biceps muscles and the velocity with which they move the weight will likely differ.

3. **D** You must have displacement to have work ($W = F\Delta s$). Because $\Delta s = 0$, $W = 0$. No calculation is required.

4. **D** Several different expressions allow you to calculate work. Using energy conservation, $W = mgh$ in which $h = 0.1$ m. Also, $W = F\Delta s$ because the angle between F and Δs is zero. In this problem, $\Delta s = 0.1$ m. The force acting on the mass is labeled F_2 in the diagram, but $F_2 = F_1(r_1/r_2)$. Therefore statements I, II, and III are equivalent.

5. **C** Two torques, at points B and C, cause rotation on the pivot point. Because $\tau = r \times F = rF$ when the angle between r and F is 90°, statements I and II are correct. Given the selection of possible answers, i.e., none include all three statements, no evaluation of statement III is necessary.

6. **B** Work (energy) is conserved and is the same on both sides of the pry bar. F_1 is actually **less** than F_2, which is the reason why a pry bar is used. In order that $F_1 < F_2$ and W be conserved, ΔS_1 must be greater than ΔS_2.

7. **D** Recalling the basic definitions of each of these terms, you see that displacement (Δs), angular speed ($\omega = \Delta\theta/\Delta t = \Delta s/r$), and linear speed ($v = \Delta s/\Delta t$) are all greater at point C than at point B.

8. **B** Speed is the **magnitude** of the velocity vector. Speed is a scalar. It does not indicate direction. Therefore, statement I is incorrect and choices A and D are incorrect. Both velocity and force are vectors, and so B is the best answer.

9. **A** Recall that entropy is a measure of disorder. Gaseous CO_2 is less ordered than crystalline CO_2. Therefore, the entropy of the CO_2 increases as it sublimes.

10. **A** When ice sublimes in a freezer, for example, P is constant but U and V both increase. Therefore, to satisfy the first law of thermodynamics, heat (Q) must be absorbed from the external environment.

11. **B** Increasing the pressure moves the system up on the P-T diagram into the region where the equilibrium phase is the solid phase and sublimation is suppressed. This change tends to decrease the sublimation rate, which eliminates choices A and C. Choice D is incorrect because the graphical data provide enough information to make statements about the sublimation rate.

12.	**A**	The passage states that a melting curve with a positive slope indicates that the material expands on melting (i.e., contracts on freezing). Because water contracts on melting and expands on freezing, its melting curve must have a negative slope.
13.	**A**	At $T = 100$ K and $P = 2$ atm, the system is clearly in the region where the solid phase is the equilibrium phase.
14.	**C**	Moving downward in temperature from $T = 300$ K along the $P = 1$ line, you see that CO_2 converts directly from a gas to a solid. Therefore, statements I and II are incorrect. Also, as the CO_2 solidifies, both U and V decrease, whereas P is held constant by the piston. Therefore, Q must decrease and heat is released to the external surroundings.
15.	**C**	Si has stronger interatomic bonds (U/bond = 4.76×10^{-20} J/4 = 1.19×10^{-20} J, whereas for Cu, U/bond = 7.44×10^{-20} J/12 = 6.2×10^{-19} J), but each Cu atom has more bonds to break to escape from the solid. The heat of sublimation for Cu turns out to be higher. Thus, statements I and III are correct and statement II is incorrect. Although choice A is true, choice C is the better answer.
16.	**D**	At the triple point on the P-T diagram, all three phases are in equilibrium.

PASSAGE III

17.	**C**	Just outside the conductor, E is perpendicular to the surface. In an electromagnetic wave, B is always perpendicular to E. Therefore, B must be parallel to the surface of the conductor.
18.	**C**	An external charge causes a charge separation on the surface of a conductor. Because unlike charges attract, an external charge induces a surface charge of the opposite sign.
19.	**B**	A potential is defined as the negative of the work done by an electric field in moving a positive unit charge a distance. Since we have no E-field, the potential at any one point is constant compared to any other point. If the question asked for the potential difference between two points, the answer would have been zero.
20.	**D**	V_2 cannot equal zero because of the resistor between it and ground ($V = 0$). V_1 does equal zero and, therefore, cannot be equal to V_2. The left side of statement III has dimensions of potential (volts), whereas the right side has dimensions of resistance (ohms).
21.	**C**	Read the passage carefully. All charge on a conductor resides at the surface. With no free charge in the interior of the conductor, the charge density there is zero.
22.	**A**	All charge resides on the surface of a conductor, i.e., no charge in the interior. There is no restriction on the magnitude of the electric field just outside the conductor (it depends on external fields, if any, and the charge on the conductor). Only the direction of the field is restricted. Thus, statements I and II are correct and statement III is incorrect.
23.	**A**	Electrons are negatively charged and repel one another. Thus, statement III is false. By eliminating any choice that contains statement III, the best answer is choice A.
24.	**D**	Recall which quantities are vectors. Electric and magnetic fields are good examples.

25. **D**   Review the concepts of dynamics and incline motion. The acceleration due to gravity is g. The component of g parallel to the ski slope is gcos(ϕ).

26. **A**   The frictional force, F_f is given by the coefficient of friction (in this case, kinetic) times the force normal to the surface. The normal force (component of gravity perpendicular to the ski slope) is given by Mg[sin(ϕ)]. So $F_f = \mu_k$Mg[sin(ϕ)].

27. **C**   The slope is horizontal and the normal force is simply equal to Mg. The skier starts at rest so she must overcome static friction. Thus, the best answer is the product of the coefficient of static friction and Mg, μ_sMg.

28. **D**   The work done by gravity is Mg times the difference in height between points A and E. g = 9.8 m/sec². So Mgh = (50 kg)(9.8 m/sec²)(35 m) = 17,150 kgm²/sec²). **Note:** A Newton is given by N = kgm/sec² and a Joule is given by J = kgm²/sec² = Nm.

29. **A**   The skier starts at rest, so her kinetic energy is equal to the potential energy she has lost in skiing from point C to point E. W = Mgh = (50 kg)(9.8 m/sec²)(20 m) = 9800 J.

30. **D**   The frictional force must exceed the component of the gravitational force parallel to the slope. Therefore, μ_sMg[sin(ϕ)] > Mg[cos(ϕ)]. Dividing both sides by Mg[cos(ϕ)] leads to $\mu_s$tan(ϕ) > 1.

31. **C**   In the absence of dissipative forces (in this case, friction), both energy and momentum are conserved. Choices A and B are true statements, but they are not complete.

32. **D**   Both energy and momentum are lost to friction and, in reality, neither is strictly conserved.

33. **D**   When the wavelength is long, then $\frac{2\pi S}{\rho\lambda} \approx 0$ and $v \approx \sqrt{\frac{g\lambda}{2\pi}}$. The restoring force is gravity. The speed is proportional to the square root of the wavelength and is independent of density. Therefore, all statements are correct.

34. **A**   The speed of shallow water waves is independent of the wavelength, so these waves propagate nondispersively. The speed of deep water waves depends on the wavelength, so these waves propagate dispersively. Therefore, statements I and II are correct.

35. **D**   The speed of shallow water waves is independent of surface tension (S). The speed of deep water waves does depend on surface tension, but when the wavelength is long, the surface tension term is zero. When the wavelength is short, the speed of deep water waves is proportional to the square root of the surface tension. So decreasing the surface tension causes the wave propagation speed to decrease.

36. **A**   The wavelength is the distance between equivalent points on the wave train, such as the peak to peak distance or, as in the figure, the trough to trough distance.

37. **B**   The energy of a mechanical wave is proportional to the square of its amplitude.

38. **B**   The amplitude of a wave is the height of the wave crest. x is the wavelength of the wave.

39. **C**   Velocity equals the product of frequency and wavelength. Frequency is inversely proportional to wavelength and proportional to velocity. Therefore, statements I and II are correct. Statement III is also correct, because as h decreases, velocity decreases. If velocity decreases, frequency decreases because it is proportional to velocity.

40. **D**   Viscosity and temperature are not variables in the second equation in the passage. Thus, statements I and III are not supported. Statement II is supported by the second equation in the passage.

Time: 50 minutes

Directions: This test contains as many physics passages as you may encounter on the MCAT. The time allotted approximates the time allowed to solve the given number of questions. Choose one best answer for each question.

Passage I (Questions 1-8)

Scientists have attempted to deploy a tethered satellite from the space shuttle. Investigative efforts in tether research have been directed toward generating electricity using the orbital momentum of the shuttle itself. This process is best understood by recalling theoretic and conceptual principles of electromagnetism.

The iron core of the earth generates a dipole magnetic field (Figure 1). A satellite in equatorial orbit sees approximately straight lines of magnetic induction (Figure 2).

Figure 1. Dipole magnetic field created by the iron core of the earth.

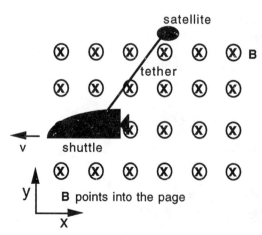

Figure 2. Relationship of the shuttle, satellite, tether, B field, and velocity vector. A coordinate axis is also shown for reference.

If the tether is made of a conducting material, such as aluminum, it becomes wirelike. Consider the tether to behave as a simple cable or wire. The motion of the tether through the earth's magnetic field will cause acceleration of the electrons in the conductor by the Lorentz force: $\mathbf{F} = q\mathbf{v} \times \mathbf{B}$, which provides a source of electrical energy. Recall that when v and B are parallel, the magnitude of the Lorentz force is zero.

Angular momentum is expressed by $L = I\omega$, in which I is the moment of inertia and ω is the angular velocity of the particular craft about the center of the earth ($\omega = v/r$). The distance from each craft to the center of the earth, r, is large relative to the dimensions of the craft, so they can be treated as point masses. Therefore, $I = mr^2$.

1. Along which direction are the electrons in the tether accelerated in Figure 2?

   A. x + y
   B. x
   C. y
   D. x − y

2. The electrons are constrained to move along the conducting tether. What is the magnitude of the component of acceleration (parallel to the tether) of an electron, assuming the tether forms a 45° angle to the x-axis? The mass of an electron is represented by m_e.

   A. $F[\sin(45°)]/m_e$
   B. $F[\cos(45°)]/m_e$
   C. $F[\tan(45°)]/m_e$
   D. $F/\{[\sin(45°)]m_e\}$

3. The linear speed of an object in orbit about the earth is expressed by:

$$v = \sqrt{\frac{GM}{r}}$$

184

M is the mass of the earth

G is the gravitational constant

r is the distance from the center of the earth to the orbiting object

If 10 kilojoules of energy is generated from the tether and stored in batteries on the shuttle, the shuttle-satellite system will:

A. slow down and descend to a lower orbit.
B. speed up and ascend to a higher orbit.
C. slow down and ascend to a higher orbit.
D. speed up and descend to a lower orbit.

4. What happens if we use a generator to force 10 kilojoules of electrical energy back through the tether (i.e., push electrons through the tether in the direction that is opposite to that in which they are accelerated by the motion of the tether through the earth's magnetic field)?

   I. The shuttle-satellite system will speed up and descend to a lower orbit.
   II. Some of the energy will dissipate as heat because of the resistance of the tether.
   III. The momentum and orbital position of the shuttle-satellite system will remain unchanged, but the tether will heat up.

A. I and II only
B. II and III only
C. I only
D. II only

5. If the tether is severed, the shuttle and the satellite will remain in their respective orbits, but their velocities will change in accordance with those orbits (the velocity of the shuttle-satellite system corresponds to the orbital position of their common center of mass). If the tether in Figure 2 is severed, which craft will travel faster?

A. The shuttle
B. The satellite
C. Neither; they will continue to travel at the same speed.
D. Not enough information is provided to determine

6. The linear velocities of a shuttle and a satellite coupled by a tether are identical. If two shuttles (of identical mass) are tethered as shown, which has the larger angular momentum about the center of the earth?

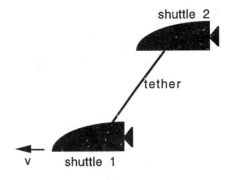

earth down below

A. Shuttle 1
B. Shuttle 2
C. Neither; the angular momentum is the same
D. Not enough information is provided to determine

7. A tethered satellite is deployed from the space shuttle. The resistance of the tether is 0.005 ohms. If 100 A is flowing through the tether, how much power is being radiated away as heat?

A. 0.0025 watts
B. 50 watts
C. 2.5 watts
D. 5 watts

8. A shuttle launched in polar orbit deploys a tethered satellite. As shown below, the lines of magnetic induction, **B**, are parallel to the linear velocity of the shuttle. Assuming that the tether forms a 45° angle with the x-axis, what is the magnitude and direction of the acceleration on an electron in the tether?

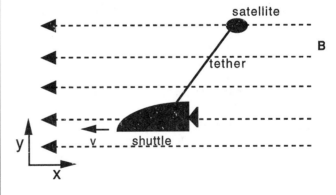

A. $[F/m_e](-\mathbf{x})$
B. $[F/m_e](\mathbf{x} + \mathbf{y})$
C. $\{F[\sin(45°)]/m_e\}(\mathbf{x} + \mathbf{y})$
D. Acceleration is zero

Passage II (Questions 9-17)

Surface diffusion on solids is a well-known example of a thermally activated process in which the diffusion rate is an exponential function of temperature. Surface diffusion obeys an equation (Arrhenius equation) of the form:

$$D = D_o \exp(-Q/kT)$$

in which k is the Boltzmann constant, T is the temperature, Q is a constant with units of energy (the same units as kT), and D_o is the diffusion constant, which has units of length. The constant Q is the activation energy; it is the average energy a surface atom must acquire from thermal fluctuations to move from one site on the surface to another.

Figure 3 graphically depicts surface self-diffusion on Cu (Cu atoms migrating over the surface of a Cu film). The distance a mobile atom migrates during a fixed time interval is plotted against 1000/T. Two different sets of data are shown (R = 0.1 and R = 10). Note that the x axis is linear and the y axis is logarithmic. By choosing this scaling, we create a linear expression of the Arrhenius equation.

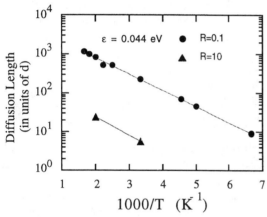

Figure 3.   Surface self-diffusion on Cu.

Take the log (base 10) of both sides of the Arrhenius equation:

$$\begin{aligned} \log_{10}(D) &= \log_{10}[D_o \exp(-Q/kT)] \\ &= \log_{10}(D_o) + 0.43(-Q/kT) \\ &= \log_{10}(D_o) - 4.3 \times 10^{-4}(Q/k)(1000/T) \end{aligned}$$

which has the same form as the equation for a straight line: y = a + bx, in which b is the slope of the line and a is the y-intercept.

9.   Consider the data set for which R = 0.1. What is the diffusion length when T = 500 K?

   A.   15 d
   B.   200 d
   C.   50 d
   D.   980 d

10.   The activation energy is proportional to:

   A.   slope.
   B.   y-intercept.
   C.   x-intercept.
   D.   the largest value of the diffusion length.

11.   Which of the following statements are true?

   I.   The diffusion constant, D_o, is the same for both data sets (R = 0.1 and R = 10).
   II.   The activation energy, Q, is the same for both data sets (R = 0.1 and R = 10).
   III. The diffusion constant is smaller for R = 10.

   A.   I and II only
   B.   II and III only
   C.   I only
   D.   III only

12.   Both sets of data show that:

   A.   the diffusion length increases with temperature.
   B.   the diffusion length decreases with temperature.
   C.   the activation energy increases with temperature.
   D.   the activation energy decreases with temperature.

13.   For the data set R = 0.1, which of the following statements are true?

   I.   In a given time interval, a surface atom is able to migrate about twenty times farther when the temperature is 500 K than when it is 200 K, i.e., D(T = 500 K)/D(200K) ≈ 20.
   II.   At 150 K, the diffusion length is about 10 d.
   III. The highest temperature for which data are shown is less than 1000 K.

   A.   I and II only
   B.   II and III only
   C.   I, II, III
   D.   None are true

14.   Given that the Boltzmann constant, k, is equal to 8.6×10^{-5} eV/K and the slope of both lines is equal to −1, what is the activation energy for surface self-diffusion on Cu?

   A.   5 eV
   B.   0.5 eV
   C.   2 eV
   D.   0.2 eV

15. When plotting data for surface self-diffusion on Ni, with the y-axis scaled logarithmically as shown in graph below, the data fall roughly on a straight line with a slope equal to approximately −2 (Figure 3 also displays R = 0.1 data for Cu). Which of the following statements is true?

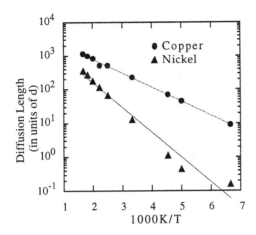

I. The activation for surface self-diffusion on nickel is higher than that for copper.
II. The activation for surface self-diffusion on nickel is lower than that for copper.
III. The activation for surface self-diffusion on nickel is the same as that for copper.

A. I only
B. II only
C. III only
D. Not enough information is provided to determine.

16. For nickel, which temperature best corresponds to a diffusion length of 100 d?

A. 500 K
B. 100 K
C. 1000 K
D. 10 K

17. If the y-intercept is greater for the nickel line than it is for the copper line, what does this tell you about the relative values of D_o for Ni and Cu?

A. Nothing, because the y-intercept is not related to D_o
B. D_o is greater for Ni than it is for Cu
C. D_o is greater for Cu than it is for Ni
D. D_o is the same for both metals

Passage III (Questions 18-25)

Since the break-up of the former Soviet Union, it has come to light that the Russian Republic and other former Soviet republics are littered with radioactive waste from nuclear power and nuclear weapons programs. One site near Chelyabinsk contains an estimated 1.2 billion curies (Ci) of plutonium 239 (^{239}Pu). By way of comparison, the Chernobyl disaster released a total of 50 million curies of radioactive products of all types and the Three Mile Island accident released about 14 curies.

A curie is a unit of "activity"; 1 Ci = 3.70×10^{10} disintegrations per second. ^{239}Pu is an alpha emitter with a half-life of 2.44×10^4 year. The three different categories of ionizing radiation are alpha particles, beta particles, and gamma rays. Alpha particles are helium nuclei (two protons and two neutrons) and are relatively heavy and slow moving (about 10^4 km/sec). As such, they are stopped easily by a piece of paper. Alpha emitters are **extremely** dangerous. When ingested or inhaled, the alpha emitter ejects alpha particles toward tissue with no intervening barrier. These heavy particles have a great deal of momentum (p = mv) and the effect on a DNA molecule is akin to shooting cannonballs at a building. Beta particles are electrons ejected from a radioactive nucleus at a rate that is close to the speed of light. Gamma rays consist of electromagnetic radiation that is more energetic than x-rays.

The decay of 1 Ci of ^{239}Pu is plotted on both a log-log and a semi-log plot in Figure 4. Radioactive decay is described by the following equation:

$$a = a_o \exp(-\lambda t)$$

in which a is activity, a_o is activity at t = 0, and λ is the decay constant (units of 1/time).

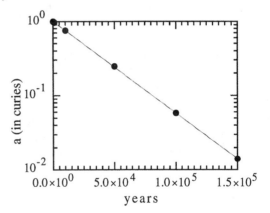

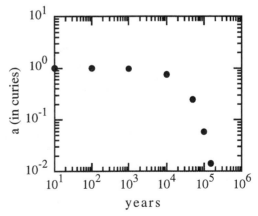

Figure 4. Log-log and semi-log plots of decay of 1 Ci of ^{239}Pu.

187

In the semi-log plot (y-axis logarithmic scale; x-axis linear), the decay equation is displayed linearly:

$$\log_{10}(a) = \log_{10}[a_o\exp(-\lambda t)]$$

$$= \log_{10}(a_o) + \log_{10}[\exp(-\lambda t)]$$

$$= \log_{10}(a_o) - \lambda t/\lambda n(10)$$

$$= \log_{10}(a_o) - (0.43\lambda)t$$

using the following relationship:

$$\log_{10}[\exp(-\lambda t)] = -\lambda t/\lambda n(10)$$

The log-log plot displays a better visual representation of the exponential decay, showing the persistence of activity over time in a long half-life material.

18. In units of activity, how much more radioactive material is stored at Chelyabinsk than was released at Chernobyl?

    A. About 25 times as much
    B. About 250 times as much
    C. About 2,500 times as much
    D. About 25,000 times as much

19. For an alpha emitter such as ^{239}Pu, 1 disintegration corresponds to the emission of 1 alpha particle. Which number most closely matches the number of alpha particles emitted in 1 year at Chelyabinsk (1 year = 3.15×10^7 sec)?

    A. The number of molecules in one thousand moles
    B. The number of seconds in ten thousand centuries
    C. The number of cells in the human body
    D. The number of electrons in a uranium atom

20. What fraction of the 1.2 billion curies of ^{239}Pu at Chelyabinsk will still be there ten thousand years from now?

    A. Over 99%
    B. Around 75%
    C. Around 40%
    D. Less than 10%

21. Given that neutrons and protons are about 2000 times more massive than electrons, how many beta particles traveling at two thirds the speed of light ($c = 3 \times 10^8$ m/sec) would it take to equal the momentum of a typical alpha particle (ignoring relativistic effects)?

    A. About 1000
    B. About 400
    C. About 10
    D. One

22. The atomic number of plutonium is 94. Which of the following statements are true?

    I. ^{239}Pu has 94 electrons
    II. ^{239}Pu has 94 protons
    III. ^{239}Pu has 145 neutrons

    A. I and II only
    B. II and III only
    C. II only
    D. I, II, and III

23. Which is the most likely reaction product after one ^{239}Pu (atomic number = 94) atom emits an alpha particle?

    A. ^{235}U (atomic number = 92)
    B. ^{237}Np (atomic number = 93)
    C. ^{243}Am (atomic number = 95)
    D. ^{236}Pu (atomic number = 94)

24. Which of the following statements are true?

    I. Gamma rays have a shorter wavelength than x-rays
    II. Gamma rays have no mass
    III. Gamma rays travel at the speed of light

    A. I and II only
    B. II and III only
    C. I, II, and III
    D. None are true

25. How much ^{239}Pu would be present after 9.8×10^4 years if 1 g of ^{239}Pu decayed spontaneously?

    A. 1/2 g
    B. 1/4 g
    C. 1/16 g
    D. 1/32 g

Passage IV (Questions 26-33)

The greenhouse effect is the action of certain atmospheric components in reflecting back toward the earth some of the heat that is radiated from the surface. Gases such as CO_2, which absorb strongly in the infrared (IR), re-emit this radiation in all directions (Figure 5). The net effect is that nearly half of the absorbed energy is reflected back toward the surface of the earth.

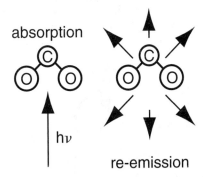

Figure 5. Gases that absorb strongly in infrared re-emit this radiation in all directions.

Molecules that are strong IR absorbers tend to be asymmetric and have appreciable dipole moments. Synthetic greenhouse gases such as dichloro-difluoro-methane (freon) are less potent IR absorbers, but they tend to absorb and re-emit in portions of the electromagnetic—spectrum where naturally occurring greenhouse gases are not active. Thus, the danger of freon is that it could close an atmospheric window in the electromagnetic spectrum through which terrestrial heat escapes. H_2O is one of the most active greenhouse gases known.

Initial concerns were that warming caused by the buildup of CO_2 and freon would cause enhanced evaporation of ocean water in the equatorial regions and lead to the so-called runaway greenhouse effect. In this scenario, global warming leads to increased cloud formation in the tropics, which in turn traps more heat. This positive feedback mechanism would lead to runaway warming because more water vapor leads to more warming, which in turn generates more water vapor.

In fact, the cycle is self-limiting. Clouds are reflective, and when they become sufficiently dense, they partially shield the earth from the heating effects of the sun. This protective effect is a perfect example of the way in which the physical properties of water regulate our climate and allow life to exist. The enormous heat capacity of water (C = 4.19 kJ/kg°C) and the large latent heats of fusion (melting; 334 kJ/kg) and vaporization (2260 kJ/kg) damp out thermal fluctuations. If the temperature of the earth decreases slightly, more ice forms at the poles, releasing large amounts of heat. Likewise, if the average temperature of the earth increases, the polar ice caps melt slightly and evaporation from the ocean surface increases; both processes remove heat from the surrounding environment.

26. Which of the following molecules would be the most active IR absorber?

A.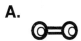

B.

C.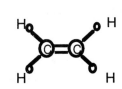

D.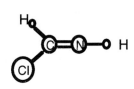

27. Which type of electromagnetic radiation has the longest wavelength?

   A. IR
   B. UV
   C. Microwaves
   D. x-rays

28. Which form of water has the lowest entropy?

   A. Ice
   B. Liquid
   C. Vapor
   D. Liquid and vapor together

29. Which process absorbs more heat?

   A. Raising the temperature of 10^3 kg of liquid water by 10°C
   B. Melting 100 kg of ice
   C. Evaporating 10 kg of water
   D. Freezing 10 kg of water

30. How much heat is required to convert 1 kg of ice at zero degrees celcius entirely into vapor?

   A. 2594 kJ
   B. 3013 kJ
   C. 2325 kJ
   D. 2679 kJ

189

31. One kilogram of water vapor in a cloud at 100°C condenses and falls as rain. Which of the following statements is true?

    A. 2260 kJ of heat is released to the surrounding environment

    B. 2260 kJ of heat is removed from the surrounding environment

    C. 334 kJ of heat is released to the surrounding environment

    D. 334 kJ of heat is removed from the surrounding environment

32. An electric dipole is formed when two equal and opposite charges, +q and −q, are separated by a small distance, L. An electric dipole moment is characterized by a vector, **p**, which points from the negative charge to the positive charge. **p** is the electric dipole moment, defined by: **p** = qL. Which of the following best represents the dipole moment of H_2O?

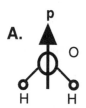

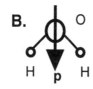

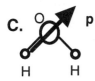

33. On a winter camping trip, you need water and are low on fuel. A river nearby is mostly frozen, but it does have some flowing water (water freezes at 0°C). To use the river water, you must boil it before drinking it (water boils at 100°C). On the other hand, there is plenty of snow around to melt. What is the best strategy to obtain water with the minimum expenditure of fuel?

    I. Melt snow

    II. Boil river water

    III. Either of the above methods, because they require the same amount of heat input

    A. I only

    B. II only

    C. III only

    D. Not enough information is provided to determine.

Passage V (Questions 34–40)

Two masses are connected by a massless cable on a pulley (Figure 6). The cable does not slip on the pulley, so if the cable moves, the pulley rotates accordingly. Assume that the pulley bearing is frictionless and that the drawing is not to scale.

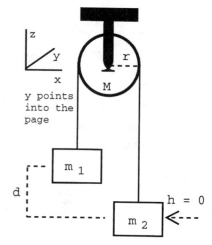

Figure 6. Two masses connected by a massless cable over a frictionless pulley.

The moment of inertia of the pulley is given by $I = (Mr^2)/2$, $m_1 > m_2$, and the pulley is held stationary (with a brake) in the configuration shown. Define the zero point of gravitational potential energy as the initial position of m_2.

34. The brake is released and the two suspended masses pass each other. What is the potential energy of the system at the point at which the two masses are at the same height? (g = the acceleration due to gravity)

    A. $U = (m_1+m_2+M/2)gd$

    B. $U = (m_1+m_2)gd$

    C. $U = (m_1+m_2+M/2)gd/2$

    D. $U = (m_1+m_2)gd/2$

35. v is the speed at which m_1 descends as the two masses pass each other. What is the kinetic energy of the system at this point?

    A. $KE = (m_1+m_2+M/2)v$

    B. $KE = (m_1+m_2-M)v^2/2$

    C. $KE = (m_1+m_2+M)v^2/2$

    D. $KE = (m_1+m_2+M/2)v^2/2$

36. The brake is released and the system is allowed to move. Which of the following statements are true?

I. Kinetic energy (KE) is converted into gravitational potential energy (U).

II. Gravitational potential energy is converted into kinetic energy.

III. The sum of U + KE remains unchanged.

A. I and III only

B. II and III only

C. III only

D. I only

37. a_1 is the acceleration of m_1 after the brake is released. If the pulley is replaced with a heavier one (mass 2 M), the acceleration of m_1 after the brake is released with the new pulley is denoted by a_2. Which of the following is true?

A. $a_2 > a_1$

B. $a_2 = a_1$

C. $a_2 < a_1$

D. None of the above

38. When the brake is applied, what is the tension in the cable?

A. $(m_1 + m_2)g$

B. $(m_1 + m_2)gd$

C. $(m_1 + m_2 + M/2)g$

D. $m_1 gd$

39. Torque is defined by: $\tau = \mathbf{r}\mathbf{F}$, in which $\mathbf{r}$ points radially outward from the center of the pulley. When the brake is released, along which direction is τ oriented?

A. $-z$

B. $-y$

C. z

D. x

40. In $\tau = \mathbf{r}\mathbf{F}$, $\mathbf{r}$ points radially from the center of the pulley. Assume τ_o is the magnitude of the torque. If the pulley of mass M is replaced by a heavier one (mass 2 M), the magnitude of the torque on the pulley when the brake is released will be equal to:

A. τ_o

B. $\tau_o/2$

C. $2\tau_o$

D. $\tau_o/4$

answers

Answers and Explanations to Physics Practice Test 2

PASSAGE I

1. **C** To determine if the electrons move more vertically or horizontally (x or y axis), use the right hand rule. Point the non-thumb fingers of your right hand in the direction of the B-field with the fingers wrapped around the wire (tether). Your thumb will show you the direction of the current (downward), which then indicates the direction of the electrons. Recall that the electrons flow opposite (180°) the direction of the current, which would be up or along the +y axis.

2. **A** You can rearrange Newton's second law, $F = ma$, to yield an expression for acceleration → $a = F/m$. The component along the tether is given by $a = F\sin$ of the given angle.

3. **C** 10 kJ of kinetic energy has been converted into electricity. Therefore, the shuttle satellite system has slowed down. Given that $v = (GM/r)^{1/2}$, in which G and M are constants, if v decreases, then r must increase.

4. **A** Pushing electrical energy back through the tether increases the orbital momentum of the shuttle-satellite system; harnessing of the orbital momentum of this system is what generates the electrical energy in the first place. In addition, resistive losses of energy routinely occur when electricity is conducted through standard metal conductors. Thus, both statements I and II are correct. Because the first part of statement III is incorrect, the best answer is choice A.

5. **A** Because the r value is less for the shuttle, it follows that the velocity of the shuttle must be greater. Note that the passage states that $v = \sqrt{Gm/r}$.

6. **B** Use the angular momentum formula: $L = I\omega = mr^2v/r = mvr$. m and v are the same for both ships, but r is greater for shuttle 2. Thus, the angular momentum is greater for shuttle 2.

7. **B** Recall the definition for power. $V = IR$ and $P = IV$, so $P = I^2R = (100 \text{ A})^2(0.005 \text{ ohms}) = 50 \text{ w}$.

8. **D** Refer to the equation for Lorentz force. When the velocity (**v**) and B-field (**B**) vectors are parallel, there is no force: $\mathbf{F = qvB} = 0$. Recall that $F = ma$; if there is no force, there is no acceleration.

PASSAGE II

9. **D** Look carefully at the units of the x-axis in Figure 3. The x-axis plots 1000/T. Thus, when T = 500 K, x = 2 and the corresponding data point is almost at y = 1000. The closest answer is choice D.

10. **A** This passage attempts to confuse you by showing derivations of graphical data. Simply see what Q represents. Use the information that $y = a + bx$ and the given data to choose the best option. $x = 1000/T$ and $y = \log(D_o)$, so the slope (b) $= -Q(4.3 \times 10^{-4})/k$. The best choice is A.

11. **B** The slope is the same for both sets of data and slope is proportional to Q; the y-intercept is smaller for R = 10 and the y-intercept is $\log(D_o)$. Statements II and III are correct. Statement I is incorrect, so the best choice is B.

12. **A** Look at the data sets carefully. As the temperature goes up, the value of $1000/T$ goes down, giving rise to a greater diffusion length. Thus, the diffusion length is higher for higher values of T (lower values of $1000/T$).

13. **C** Trying each of the statements will help you eliminate answer choices. Also, use estimation quickly and efficiently. At $T = 500$ K, $x = 2$ and y is about 1000. At $T = 200$ K, $x = 5$ and y is about 50, so $D(T = 500)/D(T = 200)$ is about 20. At $T = 150$, x is almost 7 and the corresponding data point is at about $y = 10$. There are no data for $T = 1000$ K or higher. All the statements appear to be correct, and so the best answer is C.

14. **D** This question is difficult. Compare $y = a + bx$ to $\log_{10}(D) = \log_{10}(D_o) - 4.3 \times 10^{-4}(Q/k)(1000/T)$ and identify slope as $b = -4.3 \times 10^{-4}$ $(Q/k)K^{-1}$; $b = -1$, so $Q = k/(4.3 \times 10^{-4}) = (8.6 \times 10^{-5}$ eV$)/(4.3 \times 10^{-4})K = 0.2$ eV.

15. **B** Q is proportional to the slope of the graphs in Question 15. A steeper slope means higher Q. Notice that the slopes are negative. The smaller negative number is the greater slope. Thus, copper has a greater Q value than nickel.

16. **A** In the graph from Question 15, for $y = 100$, $x = 2$; $T = 1000/x = 500$ K.

17. **B** The y-intercept is $\log_{10}(D_o)$. A greater y-intercept means a greater value of D_o. Because Ni has a greater y-intercept than Cu, the best answer is choice B.

18. **A** This passage prompts questions that evaluate your ability to sift through quantitative information and data. All that is required to answer this question is to divide two curie values provided: 1.2×10^9 Ci$/5 \times 10^7$ Ci $= 24$. The closest answer is choice A.

19. **A** A simple calculation is required: $(1.2 \times 10^9$ Ci$)(3.7 \times 10^{10}$ sec$^{-1}/1$ Ci$)(3.15 \times 10^7$ sec$) = 1.4 \times 10^{27}$. Avogadro's number = the number of particles in 1 mole of a substance $= 6 \times 10^{23}$. Therefore, $1.4 \times 10^{27}/6 \times 10^{23} =$ about 2000. The closest answer is choice A.

20. **B** Do not spend time on a complex calculation. Look at the log-log plot in Figure 4. Note that when $x = 10^4$, $y = 0.75$, which corresponds to choice B.

21. **B** Recall that mv (alpha particles) = mv (beta particles). Therefore: $(2000)(4$ particles total: 2 protons + 2 neutrons$)(10^4$ km/sec$)(1000$ m/1 km$) = (1)(2 \times 10^8$ m/sec$)(\#$ beta particles$) = 400$ beta particles.

22. **D** Atomic weight $= 239 = \#$ of protons $+ \#$ of neutrons. The atomic number $= \#$ of protons $= \#$ of electrons. Atomic weight $-$ atomic number $= \#$ of neutrons. Thus, all the statements are true.

23. **A** Alpha particles consist of two neutrons and two protons. Therefore, the atomic number must go down by two and the atomic weight must go down by four.

24. **C** The passage states that gamma rays are electromagnetic (EM) radiation that is more energetic than x-rays. Recall that higher energy means shorter wavelength. All EM radiation is massless; all EM radiation propagates at the speed of light. Thus, all the statements are correct.

25. **C** Think about this situation conceptually. Consider how many half-lives of this radioactive compound have passed over the time given in the question by dividing as follows: 9.8×10^4 yr$/2.44 \times 10^4$ yr $= 4$ half-lives. Thus, the 1 g starting mass will decay to $(1/2)^4 = 1/16$ of its original mass.

26. **D** You are told that molecules that are asymmetric and have appreciable dipole moments are the best IR absorbers. Choices A–C can be eliminated because of their symmetry and lack of electronegative atoms. Choice D has an electronegative atom (Cl is highly electronegative), is the least symmetric of the choices and thus would be the most active IR absorber.

27. **C** At the shortest wavelength are the gamma waves and x-rays, the more energetic waves. Eliminate choice D. At intermediate wavelengths are the IR, visible, and UV waves. Eliminate choices A and B. At the longer wavelengths are radio waves, radar, and microwaves. Thus, the best answer is choice C.

28. **A**   Recall that low entropy means high degree of order. Vapor has the greatest disorder and entropy. Ice is the most ordered form of water, and therefore would have the lowest entropy of the choices.

29. **A**   Basic calculations are required. For A: (4.19 kJ/kg°C)(1000 kg)(10°C) = <u>41,900 kJ</u>. For B: (334 kJ/kg)(100 kg) = <u>33,400 kJ</u>. For C: (2,260 kJ/kg)(10 kg) = <u>22,600 kJ</u>. For D: freezing water **releases** heat. The process in choice A absorbs the greatest amount of heat.

30. **B**   Remember that the ice must be melted, the resulting water must be raised to 100°C, and then the hot water must be fully converted into vapor: 334 kJ + 419 kJ + 2,260 kJ = <u>3,013 kJ</u>.

31. **A**   Vapor → liquid releases heat; the latent heat of vaporization is 2,260 kJ. Choice B is incorrect because heat is not removed from the environment. Choices C and D give incorrect kJ quantities of heat. The passage clearly states that 2,260 kJ/kg of energy is associated with the heat of vaporization of water.

32. **B**   You should expect that electrons are pulled over toward O because O is highly electronegative. Knowing that the dipole moment vector points from the negative charge to the positive charge, the structure in choice B the best answer.

33. **A**   Melting 1 kg of snow requires 334 kJ; heating 1 kg of water from 0°C to 100°C requires 429 kJ; therefore, it is wiser to melt snow.

PASSAGE V

34. **D**   The potential energy of a system = mgh. In this problem, the masses pass each other at h = d/2. The mass of the pulley does not affect the gravitational potential energy of the system. Thus, the potential energy of the system will be the product of the sum of the masses, g, and (d/2).

35. **D**   This question is difficult. This problem involves KE components because of the masses and the pulley. Recall that the KE = 1/2 mv^2 for the masses and KE = Iω^2/2 for the pulley. Thus, the KE of masses is (m_1 + m_2)v^2/2; KE of the pulley is Iω^2/2 and ω = v/r; I = Mr^2/2. Choice D shows the substituted values in one expression for KE.

36. **B**   Statement I is incorrect. Gravitational potential energy can be converted to kinetic energy, but the reverse is not always true. Statements II and III accurately describe this system, recalling the principle of conservation of energy. The best choice is B.

37. **C**   The force acting on the system is proportional to (m_1 − m_2). Increasing the mass of the pulley increases the inertial mass of the system, but does not change the force acting on the system. Consider what the effect of a pulley with a greater mass will have on the system. A pulley of greater mass has a greater moment of inertia and is more resistant to rotation. You might expect this resistance of rotation to affect a_2 and perhaps make it less than a_1.

38. **A**   You can arrive at the correct answer by just being clever. Recall that tension has units of force. Choices answers B and D have units of energy and can be eliminated for this reason alone. Pulley mass does not affect tension, and so choice C can be eliminated. The best answer, therefore, is choice A.

39. **B**   Because **r** points radially out from the center, **F** points tangentially counterclockwise. Therefore, **rxF/rF** = −**y.**

40. **A**   This is an easy question that is easily missed. Both r and F are unchanged by the increased mass of the pulley. Thus, the torque is unchanged, and the answer is A.

PHYSICS PRACTICE TEST 3

Time: 50 minutes

Directions: This test contains as many physics passages as you may encounter on the MCAT. The time allotted approximates the time allowed to solve the given number of questions. Choose one best answer for each question.

Passage I (Questions 1-8)

Newton's third law says that for every force, there is an equal and opposite reaction force. A good example of this and other basic laws of motion is the rocket.

Rockets propel themselves forward by throwing pieces of themselves behind them (Figure 1). Consider a rocket-powered spaceship in deep space where the net gravitational force is zero. As fuel is burned in the engine, exhaust gases are forced out the rocket nozzle. The rocket is propelled forward by the reaction force of the escaping gas. No external forces are acting on the system (the forces generated by the rocket motor are internal forces), and thus the system cannot accelerate. In fact, the center of mass of the system does not accelerate; the ship accelerates relative to the exhaust gas, but the system as a whole, the ship plus the exhaust gas, does not accelerate.

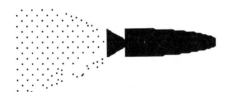

Figure 1.   Rocket-powered spaceship.

Now consider a rocket launched from Earth. The external force is gravity, and the center of mass of the rocket/exhaust gas system is accelerated toward Earth. For a rocket payload to escape the earth's gravitational pull, the rocket must throw most of itself back toward Earth. Therefore, launch vehicles are designed to consist mostly of fuel; the payload represents a tiny fraction of the mass.

A rocket achieves its maximum velocity at burnout—the point at which all of the fuel is consumed. In the absence of external forces, i.e., in deep space, v_{max} is expressed by:

$$v_{max} = V\{\ln[1+(m_f/m_o)]\}$$

V = exit speed of the exhaust gas
m_f = mass of fuel (total fuel mass before ignition)
m_o = mass of rocket without fuel

v_{max} is a logarithmic function of m_f/m_o, because the mass of the rocket **decreases** as the fuel is consumed.

1. A spaceship in deep space fires its main rocket. At constant thrust, which of the following curves best represents the velocity of the ship as a function of time, $v(t)$, relative to the center of mass of the ship-plus-exhaust system?

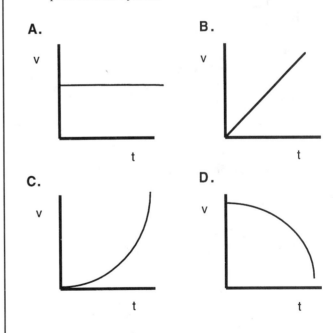

2. The rocket engines are turned off. Which of the following curves best represents the velocity of the ship relative to the center of mass of the ship-plus-exhaust system?

195

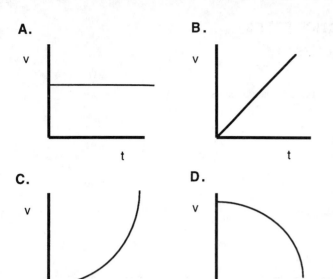

A.

v | t

B.

v | t

C.

v | t

D.

v | t

3. Which of the following statements are true?

   I. Decreasing the payload weight increases v_{max}.
   II. Increasing the exit speed of exhaust gas.
   III. In the absence of external forces, the center of mass of the rocket plus exhaust gas system does not accelerate.

   A. I and III only
   B. II and III only
   C. I only
   D. I, II, and III

4. A ship in deep space has fired its rockets and expended its fuel. The moment of inertia of the ship plus exhaust gas system for rotation about its center of mass is given by:

$$I = \sum_j m_j r_j^2$$

in which r_j is the distance from the rotation axis to the jth mass element as shown. Which of the following statements are true?

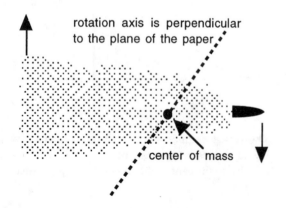

rotation axis is perpendicular to the plane of the paper

center of mass

I. I increases with time
II. I remains constant with time
III. I is greater for larger payloads

   A. I and III only
   B. II and III only
   C. II only
   D. III only

5. If I′ is the moment of inertia of the system about the rotation axis as shown, which of the following are true?

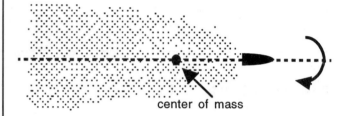

center of mass

   A. I′ > I
   B. I′ < I
   C. I′ decreases with time
   D. None are true

6. An astronaut of mass M is aboard a NASA shuttle being launched into orbit from Earth with an acceleration of 5 g (g = 9.8 m/sec²). What is the magnitude of the force the shuttle seat exerts on the astronaut?

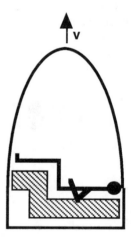

v

   A. 5 Mg
   B. 6 Mg
   C. 4 Mg
   D. 5 M/g

7. Once the shuttle is in orbit at a radius R from Earth's center, what force does the seat exert on the astronaut?

A. Mg
B. zero Newtons
C. M/g
D. Mg/R²

8. If the shuttle completes one orbit every 10^4 s and has a total mass of M_s, what is the angular momentum of the shuttle about the center of the earth?

A. $10^4 M_s R^2 / 2\pi s$
B. $10^4 M_s g R^2 / 2\pi s$
C. $2\pi \times 10^{-4} M_s R^2 / s$
D. $2p \times 10^{+4} M_s g R^2 / s$

Passage II (Questions 9-16)

Light enters the mammalian eye in Figure 2 through a variable aperture called the pupil, and is focused by the cornea-lens system on the retina, a film of nerve fibers coating the back surface of the eye. The cornea has the highest index of refraction of any of the transparent constituents of the eye and thus is responsible for most of the focusing. This structure, however, does not move or change shape and, therefore, cannot accommodate objects at variable distances from the observer.

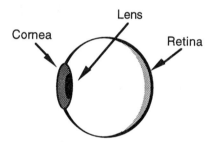

Figure 2. Mammalian eye.

Variable focusing is accomplished by a lens, the shape of which may be altered by the ciliary muscle that anchors the lens to the body of the eye. When the eye is focused on a distant object, the ciliary muscle is relaxed and the cornea-lens system has its maximum focal length, about 2.5 cm, the distance from the cornea to the retina. When an object is closer to the eye, the ciliary muscle contracts, increasing the curvature of the lens (i.e., decreasing the radius of curvature of the lens surface) slightly and thereby decreasing the focal length of cornea-lens system such that the image still falls on the retina. The cornea-lens system acts like a converging thin lens and can be described with the thin-lens equation:

$$1/s + 1/s' = 1/f$$

in which s is the distance to the object, s′ is the distance to the image, and f is the focal length.

Most common vision problems result from small deviations in the radius of curvature of the corneal surface. Because the cornea has the highest refractive index, its shape has the greatest influence on the proper functioning of the eye.

The cornea-lens system is responsible for the focusing of light on the retina (Figure 3). Normally, light focuses on the retina. In nearsightedness and farsightedness, light does not focus on the retina, and visual disturbances occur.

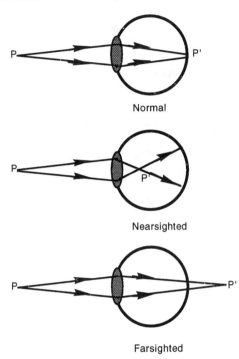

Figure 3. Focusing of light on the retina in the cornea-lens system.

9. Which of the following would cause nearsightedness?

I. The ciliary muscle fails to relax.
II. The radius of curvature of the corneal surface is larger than normal.
III. The radius of curvature of the corneal surface is smaller than normal.

A. I and III only
B. II and III only
C. I only
D. II only

10. Which type of lens would be used to correct farsightedness?

A. Converging
B. Diverging
C. Planar
D. None of the above

197

11. The index of refraction of water is greater than that of air. If a person has normal vision, what is their vision like under water?

    A.   They become effectively nearsighted.
    B.   They become effectively farsighted.
    C.   Their vision remains normal.
    D.   Not enough information to determine.

12. When focusing on a distant object, the focal length of the cornea-lens system is about 2.5 cm. When focusing on objects that are relatively close, the ciliary muscle contracts and:

    A.   the focal length increases.
    B.   the focal length decreases.
    C.   the focal length remains the same, but the magnifying power of the eye increases.
    D.   the radius of curvature of the cornea increases.

13. The cornea-lens system can be modeled as a single, thin, converging lens. The image that falls on the retina is:

    A.   virtual and erect.
    B.   real and erect.
    C.   virtual and inverted.
    D.   real and inverted.

14. Except for the fact that the lens is slightly yellow in order to filter ultraviolet light, the eye is not designed to correct for chromatic aberration—the distortion that occurs because the index of refraction is frequency dependent. Given that higher frequencies of light have a higher effective refractive index, and the eye has evolved to image objects illuminated by sunlight, which is broadly peaked in the yellow portion of the visible spectrum, where would you expect a normal eye to focus rays of red light when viewing a typical outdoor scene on a sunny day?

    A.   In front of the retina
    B.   Behind the retina
    C.   On the retina along with the rest of the image
    D.   Not enough information is provided to determine

15. The index of refraction of the cornea-lens system for blue light is slightly higher than that for red light. Therefore:

    A.   red light is refracted by the eye to a greater degree than is blue light.
    B.   red light propagates more slowly than blue light within the eye.
    C.   red light is absorbed more easily than blue light by the components of the eye.
    D.   red light has a shorter wavelength than blue light.

16. Electromagnetic waves are scattered by small dielectric spheres. The intensity of the scattered radiation relative to the primary beam is expressed by:

$$I_s/I_o = Kf^4$$

in which I_s is the intensity of the scattered light, I_o is the intensity of the incident light, f is the frequency of the incident light, and K is a constant.

    Atmospheric dust as well as N_2, O_2, and CO_2 molecules can be modeled as small dielectric spheres. The strong frequency dependence of light scattering off of these molecules and particles explains both the blue sky and red sunsets. When we look at the sky, we see blue light that has been scattered out of the primary rays emanating from the sun. Without such scattering, the sky would appear black.

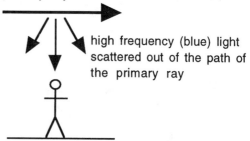

primary ray from the sun

high frequency (blue) light scattered out of the path of the primary ray

    At sunset, we look at the rays from the sun head on. Much of the blue light has been scattered out of the beam and the remaining light is shifted toward the red end of the visible spectrum.

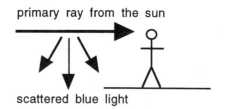

primary ray from the sun

scattered blue light

    Given that violet light has a wavelength of about 400 nm (1 nm = 10^{-9} m), and near infrared light has a wavelength of about 800 nm, what is the intensity ratio of scattered violet light to scattered near infrared light, assuming their incident intensities are the same?

    A. $I_{s(violet)}/I_{s(infrared)} = 1/8$
    B. $I_{s(violet)}/I_{s(infrared)} = 8$
    C. $I_{s(violet)}/I_{s(infrared)} = 1/16$
    D. $I_{s(violet)}/I_{s(infrared)} = 16$

Passage III (Questions 17-24)

To span the enormous dynamic range of sensory input, biologic sensors (e.g., eyes and ears) are typically logarithmic devices. A doubling of sound intensity, for example, results in a relatively small increase in the sound level perceived by the listener. It makes sense, therefore, to define a logarithmic scale to describe sound intensity. The intensity level β measured in decibels (dB) is defined by:

$$\beta = 10 \log(I/I_o)$$

in which I is the intensity of the sound and I_o is a reference level taken to be the threshold of human hearing:

$$I_o = 10^{-12} \text{ W/m}^2$$

This compressed scale actually works against us when we try to muffle sound; we have to effect a large diminution in the ambient noise to achieve a sense of quiet on the part of the listener.

One promising new method of noise reduction is anti-noise. Ambient noise is monitored by a microphone (e.g., in the tailpipe of an automobile), and sound of the same frequency and intensity is generated π out of phase with the sound that is to be muffled. The sound waves cancel each other, resulting in a degree of noise reduction unobtainable with mechanical dampening devices. This technique only works for frequencies below 1 kHz. Below this frequency, the wavelength (λ) of sound is as long or longer than commonly occurring apertures (e.g. doorways) and protrusions. The sound waves are diffracted by these physical objects, and one can then ignore the different physical paths between the listener and the noise and anti-noise sources.

17. If the speed of sound in air is 340 m/sec, what is the wavelength of a 1-kHz sound wave?

   A.   3.40 m
   B.   2.94 m
   C.   0.340 m
   D.   0.294 m

18. For noise composed of sine waves:

$$\psi_{noise} = A\sin(kx - \omega t)$$
$$\psi_{anti\text{-}noise} = A\sin(kx - \omega t + \phi)$$

For destructive interference (i.e., noise cancellation) to occur:

   A. $\phi = 0$.
   B. $\phi = \pi/2$.
   C. $\phi = \pi$.
   D. $\phi = 2\pi$.

19. A person speaking at 30 dB approaches a stationary listener while speaking. The perceived frequency heard by the listener is:

   A.   less than 30 dB.
   B.   greater than 30 dB.
   C.   equal to 30 dB.
   D.   unknown because not enough information is provided.

20. Which of the following statements are true?

Increasing ω:

   I.   decreases λ.
   II.   increases the pitch of the noise.
   III. has no effect on the intensity.

   A.   I only
   B.   II and III only
   C.   I and II only
   D.   I, II, and III

21. Normal conversation results in a sound level intensity of about 10^{-6} W/m², which corresponds to 60 dB. The threshold of pain occurs at about 1 W/m². This intensity is what you might experience standing next to a large jet taking off or directly in front of the speakers at a concert. The energy density is a million times that of normal conversation. What would be the corresponding value on the decibel scale?

   A.   180 dB
   B.   90 dB
   C.   10 dB
   D.   120 dB

22. When no definite phase relationship exists between two different sources of sound, there is no interference, either constructive or destructive, and sound intensities are additive. Such is the case with most commonly occurring sounds. At a party, you do not hear interference effects (interference would give rise, for example, to beats, dropouts, or locations in the room where the sound is amplified).

If 100 people are conversing in a room, and each pair of individuals generates 60 dB of sound, what is the sound level in the room in decibels?

   A.   80 dB
   B.   60 dB
   C.   10 dB
   D.   120 dB

23. When a stereo is playing in the next room, a person around the corner generally cannot hear the high

frequency portion of the sound very well. What is the reason for this difficulty?

A. High frequency sound is absorbed more easily.
B. High frequency sound attenuates more rapidly than $1/r^2$.
C. High frequency sound waves are not readily diffracted.
D. None of the above provide an explanation.

24. In the figure below, waves of wavelength λ impinge on an aperture of width d. Do not assume that λ and d are drawn to scale. From the behavior of the waves in the vicinity of the aperture, we can conclude that:

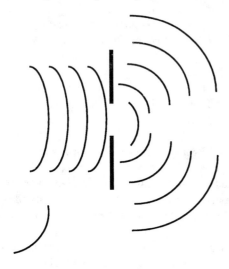

A. $\lambda \geq d$.
B. $\lambda << d$.
C. $\lambda = 1/d$.
D. None of the above

Passage IV (Questions 25-32)

Rubber bands consist of long chain polymers tangled together. Van der Waals attractive forces between functional groups on the chains tend to cause the polymers to tangle, thus increasing cross-linking between the chemically active groups. The Van der Waals interactions result in a restoring force that opposes stretching:

$$F = k[f(x)]$$

Van der Waals forces are temperature independent; however, with a change in temperature, a substantial change in the elastic properties of rubber bands can be observed. As temperature is increased, a rubber band will contract, and the value of k in the restoring force will increase. This response is an entropy-driven effect. Stretching a rubber band causes the polymer chains to straighten

out and align with one another. A stretched rubber band with polymer chains aligned roughly parallel to each other is in a more highly ordered state (therefore lower entropy) than an unstretched rubber band. At equilibrium, the free energy of a system is minimized:

$$F = E - TS$$

in which E is the internal energy (e.g., energy from the Van der Waals interactions) and S is the entropy. Clearly, entropy becomes increasingly important as temperature is raised, and increasing the entropy lowers the free energy of the system.

Consider a 1-kg weight suspended by a rubber band at two different temperatures (Figure 4). Assume that the restoring force is linear, i.e., F = kx. (**Note:** this is never true for rubber bands, which is why it is not possible to set up a simple harmonic oscillator with a rubber band. For these questions, however, assume the rubber bands act like springs.)

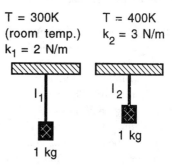

Figure 4. One-kilograms weights suspended by rubber bands at different temperature.

25. What is the length difference ($\Delta l = l_1 - l_2$) between the weighted rubber band at T = 300 K and T = 400 K?

A. $\Delta l = l_2(k_1 + k_2)$
B. $\Delta l = mg[(k_2 - k_1)/(k_2 k_1)]$
C. $\Delta l = l_2/(k_1 + k_2)$
D. $\Delta l = l_2/3$

26. Because the restoring force is a linear function of the displacement, displacing the weight from its equilibrium position will cause the system to execute simple harmonic oscillations. If the weight is pulled down by a fixed amount x_o and then released, what is the ratio of the oscillation frequency at T = 300 K relative to the frequency at T = 400 K?

A. $\omega_1/w_2 = k_1/k_2$
B. $\omega_1/w_2 = (k_1/k_2)^2$
C. $\omega_1/w_2 = \sqrt{k_1/k_2}$
D. $\omega_1/w_2 = [(k_1 + k_2)/(k_1 - k_2)]$

27. At T = 300 K, the weight is pulled down by x_o and then released. A heater is turned on until the temperature reaches 400 K. The energy associated with the oscillation is **conserved.** How does the oscillation change when the temperature is elevated?

   I.   The frequency increases
  II. The amplitude increases
 III. The period increases

  A.   I only
  B.   I and III only
  C.   II and III only
  D.   I, II, and III

28. If the weight at the end is a magnet, and an external magnetic field creates an additional downward force on the weight, how is the oscillation affected? (The system is still at T = 400 K.)

   I.   The frequency increases
  II. The amplitude increases
 III. The period increases

  A.   I only
  B.   I and III only
  C.   II and III only
  D.   None of the above

29. The weighted rubber band is immersed in a viscous liquid, like glycerine. T = 400 K and B = 0 (i.e., no magnetic field). You displace the weight by x_o and release it. What can you say about the system now?

   I.   The energy of the oscillator is no longer conserved.
  II. The amplitude of the oscillations decreases with time.
 III. The oscillation frequency remains unchanged (until the oscillations are damped out).

  A.   I only
  B.   I and II only
  C.   II and III only
  D.   I, II, and III

30. Which of the following curves best represents the elastic potential energy (potential energy associated with the harmonic oscillations), U, as a function of displacement, x, for the weighted rubber band oscillator?

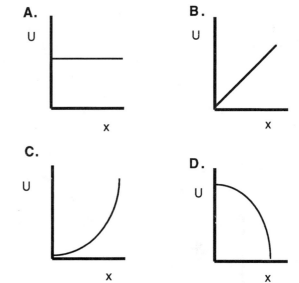

31. Consider the rubber band oscillator. When U has its maximum value, the kinetic energy is:

  A. $kx^2/2$
  B. $\sqrt{k/m}$
  C.   0
  D. $U^2/2$

32. The weighted rubber band oscillator hangs from an arm. The up-and-down motion of the arm provides a driving force for the oscillator. The response of the system is the greatest when the driving frequency is equal to:

  A. $(k/m)^2$
  B. $2\pi x/k^2$
  C. $2\pi x^2/k$
  D. $\sqrt{k/m}$

Passage V (Questions 33-40)

The sensors at intersections that control traffic lights are essentially magnetometers (devices that measure magnetic fields). A loop of wire is buried in the road bed and is connected to an ammeter (Figure 5). The iron in the body and frame of an automobile will have some randomly oriented net magnetic moment. As the car passes over the loop, a current is generated in the loop according to Faraday's law:

$$\epsilon = \Delta\phi/\Delta t$$

Electromagnetic frequency, ϵ, is equal to IR (current × resistance of the loop) and the magnetic flux, ϕ, is equal to $\mathbf{B} \cdot \mathbf{A}$ (dot product of magnetic field and area of the loop).

A = n**A,** in which **n** is a unit vector perpendicular to the plane of the loop (i.e., **n** points straight up out of the road bed). If a sufficient voltage is generated across the loop leads, the sensor control unit sends a signal to the traffic light controller, which indicates that a car is at the intersection.

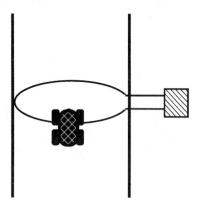

Figure 5. Sensors at an intersection connected to an ammeter signal approaching traffic.

33. Motorcycles often fail to trip the sensors at traffic intersections because their total mass (and thus the amount of iron) is low. How can a cyclist improve his or her chances of tripping the sensor?

   I Approach the intersection as slowly as possible
   II. Approach the intersection as quickly as possible
   III. Attach a high-field permanent magnet to the bottom of the cycle frame

   A. I and/or III
   B. II and/or III
   C. III only
   D. None of the above

34. You have magnetized your car in such a way that the external field it produces is large and oriented parallel to the surface of the road. Will your car trip the sensor at an intersection?

   A. Yes
   B. No
   C. Only if you approach the intersection slowly
   D. Not enough information is provided to determine

35. You have just stopped at a red light. Which of the following curves best represents the current in the loop as a function of time, I(t), while you remain stopped at the intersection?

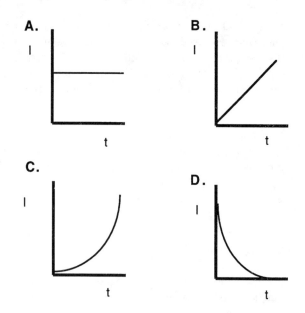

36. How does the magnetic field of the Earth affect traffic light sensors? (**Note:** The Earth's field is large relative to that produced by automobiles, and it points up from the ground at a slight angle.)

   A. Earth's field adds to the field produced by a car and effectively increases the sensitivity of traffic light sensors
   B. Earth's field has no effect on traffic light sensors because $\mathbf{B} \cdot \mathbf{A} = 0$ (here, $\mathbf{B} = \mathbf{B_{earth}}$)
   C. Earth's field has no effect on traffic light sensors because it is constant in time
   D. None of the above

37. Which of the following would increase the sensitivity of traffic light sensors?

   I. Increase the area of the loop
   II. Decrease the resistance of the loop
   III. Shield the loop from the earth's magnetic field

   A. I only
   B. I and II only
   C. I, II, and III
   D. None of the above

38. A magnetic force is created if several conditions are met. Which is NOT a condition for giving rise to a magnetic force?

   A. An electrically charged object
   B. A stationary charge
   C. An object in the vicinity of a magnetic field
   D. An object with v perpendicular to B or with a component of v perpendicular to B

39. If the sensor loop is a simple wire, which of the following would be inversely proportional to the magnitude of the B-field at a reference point X?

    A. Current
    B. Distance to point X
    C. Both current and distance to point X
    D. Neither current nor distance to point X

40. Which of the following statements are true?

    I. ϕ is not a vector.
    II. B is a vector.
    III. E is a vector.

    A. I only
    B. I and II only
    C. II and III only
    D. I, II, and III

Answers and Explanations to Physics Practice Test 3

PASSAGE I

1. **B** Recall that constant acceleration (thrust) means v is proportional to t. You are looking for a graph that shows a constant rate of change of velocity versus time. Choice A shows constant velocity (zero acceleration). Choice C demonstrates increasing acceleration. Choice D shows deceleration changing with time. Choice B is the best answer.

2. **A** In this situation, you should expect zero acceleration, i.e., v is constant.

3. **D** In the formula, v_{max} is increased by decreasing m_o and increasing V. Thus, statements I and II are true. By elimination, choice D is best.

4. **A** Evaluating each of the statements carefully, look at the value of I. The moment of inertia (I) increases when the radius increases and/or the mass increases. The ship continues to move at constant velocity to the right, and the fuel and payload continue to move in opposite directions with constant velocity, which all act to increase the r_j term of the moment of inertia equation. This change increases I over time. Statement I is correct. Statement II is incorrect. Statement III is correct, because a heavier payload means larger m_j values. The best answer is A.

5. **B** Comparing the figure in Question 5 to the figure in Question 4, the mass is closer to the rotation axis, which means the moment of inertia is less in the figure from Question 5 than in the preceding figure.

6. **B** The astronaut will feel 5 g from shuttle acceleration and 1 g acceleration from Earth's gravity for a total of 6 Mg force exerted by the seat. Choice A is incorrect because it does not take into account the baseline acceleration of gravity at rest. Choice C is incorrect because it subtracts the baseline acceleration of gravity at rest from the acceleration of the shuttle. The best answer is choice B.

7. **B** Space travel and being in orbit in space is similar to a free fall situation; i.e., there is no force. Choices A, C, and D are included to confuse you and to draw you into thinking this simple conceptual question requires some type of calculation.

8. **C** A simple calculation is all that is required. Recall that the angular momentum $= L = I\omega$. Because $I = mr^2$, $I = M_sR^2$. The angular velocity equals the change in ω (angle rotated through) divided by change in time. When one rotation equals 2π, $2\pi/10^4$ s. Therefore, $L = M_sR^2 2\pi/10^4$ s.

PASSAGE II

9. **A** The passage states that the ciliary muscle anchors the lens to the body of the eye. When focusing on a distant object, the ciliary muscle relaxes, which gives the cornea-lens complex its maximum focal length. You should predict that this change will allow the lens to become more concave. Thus, contracted ciliary muscle means <u>more</u> curvature of lens; relaxed ciliary muscle means <u>less</u> curvature of the lens.

    Failure of the ciliary muscle to relax (statement I) would mean more curvature of the lens and focusing of the image before reaching the retina (nearsighted diagram). A decreased radius of curvature of the cornea (statement III) means that the curvature of cornea has increased, also leading to nearsightedness. Thus, statement III is correct and statement II is incorrect. The best answer is choice A.

10. **A** Figure 3 (farsighted image) shows you that you need more convergence to focus an image on the retina. A diverging lens is useful for nearsightedness to focus the image farther toward the back of the eye toward the retina. A planar lens does not move the image.

11. **B** Review the concept of index of refraction. Water lowers the difference in refractive index between the propagation medium and the eye. This change lowers the degree of refraction that occurs at the eye, and the person becomes effectively farsighted.

12. **B** You can infer from the discussion of the action of the ciliary muscle that when focusing on a near object, the muscle contracts and the cornea-lens system has decreased focal length. For this question, you can expect that the lens becomes more curved, more refraction occurs, and the focal length decreases. Choice A is incorrect because it describes a state of ciliary muscle relaxation. Choice C is incorrect because the focal length changes. Choice D is incorrect because no data support statements about the radius of curvature of the cornea.

13. **D** By either drawing a ray diagram (see the optics chapter of the physics review notes) or looking at the thin lens equation, you see that a single converging lens produces a real and inverted image.

14. **B** Red light has a low frequency compared to other colors in the visible spectrum (see Physics Review Notes). The question implies that frequency tends to relate to refractive index, i.e., the low frequency of red light equates to a low index of refraction. A low index of refraction means less refraction and imaging behind the retina.

15. **B** The index of refraction $= n = c/v =$ (sp. of light in vacuum)/(sp. of light in medium); thus, red light (lower n) must travel slower than blue light within the human eye. Choice A is incorrect because greater n means greater refraction. Choice D is incorrect because red light has lower energy, thus a greater wavelength than blue light (higher energy, lower wavelength). No information is given to allow you to support choice C.

16. **D** The introductory section of this question includes much new material, diagrams, a new formula, and a great deal of verbiage. You are told that the intensity is proportional to the frequency to the power of four. The important information is that the ratio of the frequencies $f'/f = 2$, which can be derived from the wavelength values given (400 nm and 800 nm). Recall that the velocity equals the product of frequency and wavelength, so a ratio of wavelength of 1:2 gives a frequency ratio of 2:1. If the ratio of the frequencies of violet to infrared is 2, the intensity ratio should be $2^4 = 16$.

---

17. **C** A simple calculation is needed: wavelength $= v_s/f = $ (340 m/sec)/(1000/sec) $=$ 0.34 m.

18. **C** Recall the concept of interference. Destructive interference occurs when coherent waves of the same amplitude are π (or 180°) out of phase with one another. Thus, choice C is the best answer.

19. **B** The Doppler effect allows the measurement of compression and stretching of waves as changes in frequency. Consider how you perceive different frequencies of engine sounds at a race track depending on if the car is coming toward you or if it is passing you. A sound source moving away from a stationary listener is heard at a lower perceived frequency compared to a stationary source. Similarly, a sound source approaching a stationary listener is heard at a higher perceived frequency than if the source were stationary.

20. **D** Pitch is the perceived predominant frequency of a sound source. Recall that angular velocity $= 2\pi f$. Thus, an increase in angular velocity leads to an increase in frequency and a decrease in wavelength, supporting all three statements. Intensity is not effected by changes in ω or f.

21. **D**   Use the formula provided to measure intensity level in decibels. The intensity level you are looking for is 1 W/m², which can be written as 10^0 W/m². Thus, the intensity level in decibels = 10 log($10^0/10^{-12}$)ç = 10 log(10^{12}) = 120 dB.

22. **A**   Solving this problem requires an understanding of the intensity formula provided and of the basic concepts of sound intensity. Some of the answer choices do not make sense and can be eliminated before calculating an answer. Choice C is incorrect because sound intensity is certainly greater than 60 dB if many persons are speaking simultaneously. By the same reasoning, choice B can be eliminated. To choose between choices A and D, perform this simple calculation: 60 dB = 10^{-6} times 100 people = 10^{-4} and $\beta = 10_{\log}(10^{-4}/10^{-12}) = 10_{\log}(10^8) = 80$ dB.

23. **C**   High frequencies are not diffracted because their wavelengths are short relative to common obstructions. You only hear high frequencies well when the path between you and the source is unobstructed. Answer this question by the process of elimination. No information is provided in the passage or no basic conceptual principles support choices A and B. Choice C is the best answer.

24. **A**   Look carefully at the diagram and reason carefully. What can you say about this figure, and why is it provided? You are told that the wavelengths and aperture may not be drawn to scale. Note, however, that diffraction of waves is occurring at the aperture. Therefore, wavelength must be equal to or larger than the width of the aperture (choice A).

PASSAGE IV

25. **B**   A calculation is required: $l_1 = l_o + mg/k_1$; $l_2 = l_o + mg/k_2$. To find the answer, subtract one from the other: $\Delta l = mg(1/k_1 - 1/k_2) = mg[(k_2 - k_1)/k_2k_1]$.

26. **C**   This question appears difficult until you recall that the oscillation frequency = $\omega = \sqrt{k/m}$. Thus, the ratio of the oscillation frequencies equals the square root of the ratio of the k values at the different temperatures.

27. **A**   Raising the temperature increases k, which increases ω (because $\omega = \sqrt{k/m}$). Thus, frequency also increases (statement I is true). A is proportional to the square root of E, but the passage stated that E is conserved (statement II is false). The period is proportional to $1/\omega$, so when ω increases, the period decreases (statement III is false). Choice A is the best answer.

28. **D**   A magnet and a magnetic field are added to confuse you. The magnet does increase the mass of the oscillating system, which makes the equilibrium position of the weight change, but everything else remains the same. The items of concern in an oscillating system are the value of k and the distance of the system from the equilibrium position. Thus, statements I, II, and III are all incorrect.

29. **D**   When the weight is displaced and released, the E is lost to glycerine. Thus, statement I is true. Statements II and III are true because A decreases and ω remains unchanged until motion stops.

30. **C**   Recall that the potential energy of a mass-spring oscillator = $U = kx^2/2$. You are looking for the graph that shows an exponential function that increases as the value of x increases—choice C. Choice D is incorrect because it suggests that as x increases, U decreases.

31. **C**   Consider the concept of conservation of energy. KE and U trade off against one another, but the sum of the two (total energy) is conserved. When U is maximum, KE is zero and when KE is maximum U is zero. The other choices are included to confuse you and to infer that some complex calculation is required.

32. **D**   The maximal response of the system (resonance) occurs when the system is driven at the natural frequency $\omega = \sqrt{k/m}$.

PASSAGE V

33. **B**   Look at the statements carefully to determine whether a slow or a fast approach gives a better chance of tripping the sensor. Use the formula provided to decide if the chance of sensor activation increases. A quick approach makes Δt small, thus making $\Delta flux/\Delta t$ larger. The chance of tripping the sensor is then in-

creased. Attaching a permanent magnet makes B larger, and should increase Δflux, which also increases the chance of tripping the sensor. Statements II and/or III are correct, making choice B the best answer.

34. **B** $\mathbf{B} \cdot \mathbf{A} = 0$, since $\mathbf{B}$ is perpendicular to $\mathbf{A}$. Thus, there is no magnetic flux, and the sensor is not activated.

35. **D** Approaching the intersection generates current in the loop, but Δflux = 0 once the car is stopped. The current decays because of resistance, R, of the loop. Choice D is the best answer because it shows the current was maximal at the instant the car stopped. It then shows that the current decays as a function of time. The other choices are incorrect because they show either a constant current or a current that is increasing.

36. **C** Evaluate each choice carefully to determine whether or not the Earth's field is constant. B_{earth} is constant, which mean Δflux/Δt because of the Earth's field is zero. Choice A is not the best answer because it fails to address the change in the Earth's field (Δflux). In addition, the sensitivity of the sensors are not increased by the Earth's field. Choice B is incorrect because the magnetic flux of the Earth is not zero (B and A would be parallel). Choice C is the best answer because is addresses the constant nature of the Earth's field.

37. **A** Statement I is correct because increasing area does increase flux. Statement II is incorrect because decreasing R decreases V (V = IR) and V is what you measure. Statement III is incorrect because the Earth's field has no effect on sensitivity of the sensors. Thus, the best answer is choice A.

38. **B** This conceptual question does not appear directly related to the passage. A magnetic force is created and can act on an object if and only if the object of interest is electrically charged, moves with a speed v, is in the vicinity of a B-field, and moves so that the v vector is perpendicular to the B vector or a component of v is perpendicular to B. Choice B is not correct because the charge must be moving to generate a magnetic force.

39. **B** Review your conceptual understanding of B-fields. The magnitude of a B-field or B is proportional to the current running through the wire and inversely proportional to the distance from the wire to the point of interest. Because choice A is incorrect, choice C must also be incorrect. Therefore, choice B is the correct answer.

40. **D** Flux is a scalar quantity (magnitude only) because it is the result of a dot product. B-fields and E-fields are both vector quantities. Thus, all the statements are true.

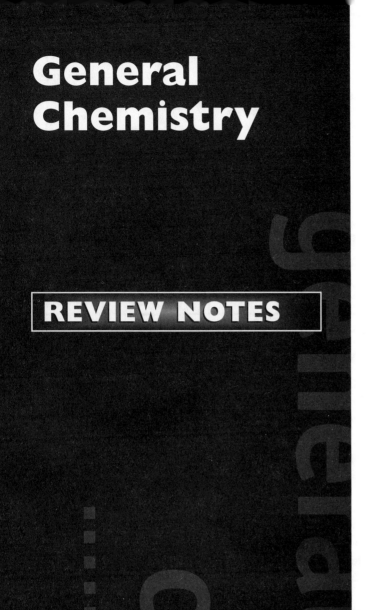

General Chemistry

REVIEW NOTES

SECT. 11
GENERAL
CHEMISTRY
REVIEW
NOTES

209

Introductory Concepts

**I. Basic Definitions and Relationships
Used in Chemistry**

II. Describing Reactions by Chemical Equations

I. Basic Definitions and Relationships Used in Chemistry

Most students learn college chemistry with a quantitative emphasis. Although being able to calculate unknown quantities is important, almost two-thirds of the general chemistry questions on the MCAT are conceptual. The review notes in this section focus on both the concepts and important calculation techniques you will need to answer these questions. The first chapter gives you an overview of the basics of stoichiometry, oxidation-reduction, and the balancing of chemical equations. An understanding of these topics is important for both conceptual understanding of the chapters that follow and success on the MCAT.

An **atom** is the smallest neutral component of an element that has all the chemical properties of the element. As is reviewed in Chapter 2 of the General Chemistry Review Notes, atoms are composed of subatomic particles: **protons, neutrons,** and **electrons.** For all practical purposes, you can think of the atom as having a very small core, the **nucleus,** which contains both protons and neutrons. Electrons form a cloud around the nucleus. The space occupied by electrons (electron cloud) is massive compared to the nucleus. The **atomic number** of an atom is the number of protons that the atom contains.

In many substances, groups of atoms are joined together by chemical bonds to form **molecules.** You can express the composition of a molecule using its **molecular formula,** by writing the symbols of the atoms it contains, with numeric subscripts showing how many of that kind of atom are present in the molecule.

A **mole** is the amount of a substance that contains **Avogadro's number** of particles of that substance. Avogadro's number is about 6.02×10^{23}. Thus, a mole of atoms contains 6.02×10^{23} atoms.

The **atomic weight** of an element is an average of the weights of all the isotopes of the element. **Isotopes** are atoms of the same element that differ in mass but not in atomic number (atoms with the same number of protons but different number of neutrons). **Stoichiometry** is the study of the molar relationships between atoms and compounds.

A. Atomic and Molecular Weight

In chemical calculations, you often need to know the mass of an element. This is accomplished by finding the **atomic weight** of the element on the periodic table. The atomic weight is the larger of the two numbers given for each element. The smaller number is usually the atomic number. To calculate **molecular weight,** you add the individual atomic weights of the elements comprising the compound. Example 1-1 illustrates the calculation of molecular weight.

Example 1-1: What is the molecular weight of C_6H_6?

Solution: Look up the atomic weights of both carbon and hydrogen (C = 12 and H = 1). Multiply each by the number of that type of atom, then add the result. Molecular weight = $(12 \times 6) + (1 \times 6) = 78$ g/mol.

One common mistake in the calculation of molecular weight is not multiplying through by the subscripts in a molecular formula. For example, a molecule with a formula of $Al_2(SO_4)_3$ would actually be thought of as $Al_2S_3O_{12}$ for calculating molecular weight.

B. Empiric Formula Versus Molecular Formula

Chemical formulas are derived empirically, which means that experiments must be done to determine the actual mass of the elements in a compound or their percentage by weight. The **empiric formula** (E.F.) of a compound is the smallest possible integer ratio of the different kinds of atoms present in a compound.

The **molecular formula** (M.F.) is an integral multiple of the empiric formula. It expresses the actual number of atoms joined by chemical bonds to form a molecule. For example, the molecular formula for benzene is C_6H_6. Notice the 1:1 ratio of carbon and hydrogen, making the empiric formula CH.

The molecular formula can be determined if the molecular weight and the empiric formula of a compound are known. The ratio of the molecular weight of the compound to the molecular weight of the empiric formula provides the integral multiple from which the molecular formula can be determined. Example 1-2 shows how a molecular formula is determined from the molecular weight and empiric formula.

Example 1-2: Glucose has an empiric formula CH_2O and a molecular weight of 180 g/mol. What is its molecular formula?

Solution: The empiric weight of glucose is 12 + 1 + 1 + 16 = 30. 180/30 = 6 of the empiric unit in the molecule. The molecular formula is $C_6H_{12}O_6$.

How do you experimentally determine the molecular weight of a compound? Usually from studies of the compound in its gaseous state. If a compound is weighed and then vaporized at constant temperature and volume, the gaseous molecular weight can be determined.

SECT. II
GENERAL
CHEMISTRY
REVIEW
NOTES

211

C. Description of Composition by Percent Mass

Many analytic methods do not give an empiric formula directly. Instead, a **percent mass** is provided for each of the elements in the sample. The empiric formula can then be determined from the composition by percent mass (Example 1-3). To determine the empiric formula from percent composition, follow the following steps:

1.   Assume 100 g of the compound. (This amount makes the calculation easier.)

2.   Find the number of moles of each element in the compound.

3.   Divide each of these numbers of moles by the smallest value arrived at in step 2.

4.   Finally, multiply all by the smallest factor that provides whole numbers. These numbers are the subscripts in the empiric formula.

Example 1-3: A hydrocarbon was determined to contain 20% hydrogen by mass. Determine its empiric formula.

Solution: First, realize that a hydrocarbon contains only carbon and hydrogen, so the actual percent composition is 20% hydrogen and 80% carbon. Then, follow these steps:

1. **Assume** 100 g of the hydrocarbon: Because 20% of 100 g is 20 g, and 80% of 100 g is 80 g, there are 20 g of hydrogen and 80 g of carbon.
2. **Convert** each of these masses to moles:
   $(80 \text{ g}) (1 \text{mol}/12 \text{ g C}) = 6.67 \text{ mol}$
   $(20 \text{ g}) (1 \text{mol}/1 \text{ g H}) = 20 \text{ mol}$
3. **Divide** each of these by the smallest number:
   $6.67 / 6.67 = 1$
   $20 / 6.67 = 3$
4. **Multiply** by the smallest factor that makes these whole numbers (1 in this case). Thus, the empiric formula is CH_3.

D.   Mole Concept and Avogadro's Number

Although we have already defined some of these terms, we should talk about them in more detail because an understanding of the mole concept is critical to success on the MCAT.

Elements react in certain ratios by weight. This observation led to the modern understanding of moles and stoichiometry. Because molecules and atoms are extremely small, it is not convenient to use quantities such as dozens or scores to define a quantity of atoms or molecules. The number of dozens of atoms needed to add up to 1 gram is an extremely large number. The mole is a quantity that makes dealing with huge numbers of molecules much easier. **A mole of atoms is the number of atoms of C-12 that weigh exactly 12.0 g.** Also, as defined previously, a mole of atoms is equivalent to 6.02×10^{23} atoms.

Conveniently, a mole of any type of atom or compound is the number of atoms the weight of which is equal to the atomic or molecular weight. Therefore, an appropriate unit for the atomic weights on the periodic table is grams per mole (g/mol).

Examples 1-4 and 1-5 show that the number of moles of a substance equals the gram quantity times the molecular weight of the substance.

Example 1-4: How many moles of O_2 are in 48 g of O_2?

Solution: Moles O_2 = (48 g) (1mol/32 g) = 1.5 mol

Example 1-5: How many moles is 50.0 g CH_4?

Solution: Moles CH_4 = (50.0 g)(1 mol/16.04 g) = 3.12 moles

Because you know that a mole of a substance contains Avogadro's number of particles of that substance, it is easy to calculate how many atoms are in a mass quantity of a compound. A good example of this calculation is given in Example 1-6.

Example 1-6: How many carbon and hydrogen atoms are in 25 g of CH_4?

Solution: $[25$ g $CH_4/$ (mol $CH_4/16$g$)](1$ mol C/1 mol $CH)(6.02 \times 10^{23})$
= 9.41×10^{23} C atoms

25 g $CH_4/$ (mol $CH_4/16$g$)(4$ mol H/1 mol $CH_4)(6.02 \times 10^{23})$
= 3.76×10^{24} H atoms

E. Density

Matter is something that possesses mass and occupies space or volume. Density is a relationship that describes how mass is related to volume and is given by the relationship:

$$\textbf{density} = \textbf{m/v}$$

in which m is the mass (unit: usually grams) and v is the volume (unit: liters, milliliters, or cm³).

Density is an **intrinsic property** of a substance, meaning that it is not dependent on the amount of matter. The volume of a substance does change with temperature, however, so density is dependent on temperature and therefore is usually reported at a given temperature.

You are probably aware of density differences in things around you. For example, you know that a block of iron weighs more than a block of wood of equal volume and that oil floats above water. You have also seen examples of density differences in the organic laboratory, when a liquid such as chloroform ($CHCl_3$) tends to form a layer beneath a less dense aqueous layer.

SECT. II
GENERAL
CHEMISTRY
REVIEW
NOTES

213

F. Oxidation Number

Before beginning a review of oxidation numbers, you should review the meaning of oxidation and reduction.

Oxidation: a loss of electrons or an increase in oxidation number

Reduction: a gain of electrons or a decrease in oxidation number

The **oxidation number or oxidation state of an atom in a compound is an assigned numeric representation of the positive or negative character of the atom.** In other words, it is the number of electrons that an atom appears to have gained over or lost from its normal complement when it is combined with other atoms.

You should become familiar with some of the **basic rules for assigning oxidation numbers,** which are summarized as follows:

a. The sum of the oxidation numbers of atoms in a molecule or ion must equal the overall charge on the species (e.g., for O_2, the sum of the oxidation states of the two oxygen atoms must be zero; for SO_4^{2-}, the oxidation states on the sulfur and four oxygen atoms must sum to -2).

b. The oxidation number of a free, uncharged element is zero (e.g., O_2, H_2, Na, Cl_2).

c. Alkali metals, found in the first column of the periodic table (group I), have an oxidation number of $+1$ in compounds (e.g., Na^+, K^+).

d. Alkaline earth metals, found in the second column of the periodic table (group II), have an oxidation number of $+2$ (e.g., Ca^{2+}, Mg^{2+}).

e. Halogens, found in the column of the periodic table second from the right (group VII), usually have an oxidation number of -1 (e.g., Cl^-, Br^-).

f. Oxygen has an oxidation number of -2, except in peroxides (e.g., H_2O_2) in which it is -1, or in compounds with fluorine (e.g., OF_2), in which it is $+2$.

g. Hydrogen has an oxidation number of $+1$ when bonded to a nonmetal and -1 when bonded to a metal (e.g., in H_2O, the hydrogen is bonded to oxygen, a nonmetal, so its oxidation state is $+1$; in LiH, hydrogen is bonded to a metal, so its oxidation state is -1).

1. **Common oxidizing and reducing agents**

    Oxidizing agent: The species in a redox reaction that accepts electrons. The result of this action is that the oxidizing agent is reduced and the other species is oxidized. Usually nonmetal elements such as groups VI (e.g., oxygen) and VII (e.g., chlorine) gain electrons to obtain a noble gas configuration.

    Reducing agent: The species in a redox reaction that donates electrons. The result of this action is that the reducing agent is oxidized and the other species is reduced. Usually metallic elements from groups I or II (e.g., sodium and magnesium) or transition metals (e.g., silver and titanium) lose electrons to obtain a more stable electron configuration.

2. **Redox titration**

    As in other titrations, a redox titration uses a known concentration of one reactant in a quantitative reaction with a known stoichiometry to determine the unknown concentration of a different reactant. The distinguishing feature of a redox reaction is that it involves oxidation and reduction of the reacting species. Example 1-7 is a redox titration used in the quantitative analysis of iron ore.

Example 1-7: Given the following reaction in which 34.6 ml of 0.11 M $KMnO_4$ was required to oxidize all the Fe^{+2} in a 3.52-g sample of iron ore, determine the mass percent of iron in the sample.

$$5\ Fe^{2+}(aq) + MnO_4^-(aq) + 8\ H^+ \longrightarrow 5\ Fe^{3+}(aq) + Mn^{2+}(aq) + 4\ H_2O(l)$$

Solution:

Calculate the number of moles oxidizing agent:
mol $KMnO_4$ = (0.11 mol/L)(0.0346 L) = .00381 mol
Use the stoichiometry of the reaction to calculate the number of moles of the unknown reagent:
mol Fe^{2+} = (.00381 mol $KMnO_4$)(5 mol Fe^{2+}/1 mol $KMnO_4$)
= 0.01905 mol Fe^{2+}
Convert this value to grams:
g Fe^{2+} = (0.01905 mol Fe^{2+})(55.85 g/mol Fe^{2+}) = 1.064 g Fe^{2+}
Calculate the percentage by mass:
mass % Fe^{2+} = (1.064 g Fe^{2+}/3.52 g ore)(100%) = 30.2%

II. Describing Reactions by Chemical Equations

Chemical reactions can be described in words, but chemists use chemical equations as a "shorthand" to describe these reactions.

A. Conventions for Writing Chemical Equations

The reactants are the substances that react with each other; they are shown on the left-hand side of the equation. The products are the substances formed in the reaction; they are shown on the right-hand side of the equation. A left-to-right arrow indicates that the reactants are converted to products (Example 1-8).

Example 1-8:

$$Na(s) + \frac{1}{2}Cl_2(g) \longrightarrow NaCl(s)$$

Reactants   form   Products

The symbols after the chemical formulas represent the physical state of the substances:

(s) = solid

(g) = gas

(l) = liquid

(aq) = aqueous solution

B. Balancing Equations, Including Oxidation–Reduction Equations

Two basic rules for balancing an equation follow:

Mass balance: The number of each type of atom on both sides of the equation must be equal.

Charge balance: The net charge on both sides of the equation must be equal.

SECT. II
GENERAL
CHEMISTRY
REVIEW
NOTES

215

For most equations, you should balance by inspection (trial and error). Example 1-9 shows the mass balance concept. Note that balancing is done by trial and error.

Example 1-9:

$$Na(s) + Cl_2(g) \longrightarrow NaCl(s)$$

This equation does not obey the mass balance condition. To balance it, make sure you have 2 chlorine atoms on both sides:

$$Na(s) + Cl_2(g) \longrightarrow 2\ NaCl(s)$$

This change disrupts the mass balance of the sodium atoms, so put a 2 in front of the sodium on the left.

$$2\ Na(s) + Cl_2(g) \longrightarrow 2\ NaCl(s)$$

In redox reactions, balancing by trial and error is difficult and inefficient. These equations are hard to balance because of the different numbers of different kinds of atoms on the two sides of the equations. In addition, the charges often do not balance. Although the techniques outlined subsequently seem advanced for this first chapter of the review notes, the principles involved are simply an application of the mass and charge balancing rules.

The two systematic approaches used to balance redox equations are outlined side-by-side in Table 1-1, followed by examples showing both methods. Method 1 is commonly used in textbooks to emphasize that redox reactions involve transfers of electrons. **Most students seem to find method 2 a little easier and faster.** Do not get frustrated by redox equation balancing. It gets easier with practice.

TABLE 1-1. Rules for balancing oxidation–reduction reactions

Method 1	Method 2
i. Identify species being oxidized and reduced	**i.** Identify species being oxidized and reduced
ii. Separate into half reactions	**ii.** Determine oxidation states
iii. Balance all elements except O and H	**iii.** Balance all elements except O and H
iv. Balance with respect to O	**iv.** Make changes in oxidation state opposite
a. In acid, add H_2O to the side with less O	**v.** Balance charge; use H^+ in acid or OH^- in base
b. In base, add H_2O to the side with more O to equal amount necessary on other side	**vi.** Balance hydrogen and oxygen with H_2O
v. Balance each half reaction with respect to H	
a. In acid, add H^+ to the side deficient in H	
b. In base, add OH^- to the side deficient in H	
vi. Balance charge with electrons	
vii. Make the electrons in each half reaction equal by multiplying by the appropriate factor	
viii. Add the half reactions and cancel or combine like terms	

Examples 1-10 and 1-11 show use of both of the methods just described to balance oxidation-reduction reactions. Try to follow the examples carefully. For the MCAT, you only need to know one technique for balancing redox equations. Typically, if you are asked to balance a redox equation, it is a fairly easy equation to balance. Remember to use whichever technique you find easier! Example 1-10 shows a redox equation being balanced in **acidic solution,** and Example 1-11 shows the same steps for a reaction in a **basic solution.**

Example 1-10:

Balance this chemical reaction in acid: $Fe^{+2} + O_2 \longrightarrow Fe^{+3} + H_2O$

Method 1

i and ii. Oxidation: $Fe^{+2} \longrightarrow Fe^{+3}$
Reduction: $O_2 \longrightarrow H_2O$

iii. All elements except O and H balanced

iv. $O_2 \longrightarrow 2\,H_2O$

v. $4\,H^+ + O_2 \longrightarrow 2\,H_2O$

vi. $Fe^{+2} \longrightarrow Fe^{+3} + e^-$
$4\,H^+ + O_2 + 4\,e^- \longrightarrow 2\,H_2O$

vii. $4\,Fe^{+2} \longrightarrow 4\,Fe^{+3} + 4\,e^-$
$4\,H^+ + O_2 + 4\,e^- \longrightarrow 2\,H_2O$

viii. $4\,H^+ + 4\,Fe^{+2} + O_2 \longrightarrow 4\,Fe^{+3} + 2\,H_2O$

Method 2

i and ii.

Species	Oxidation state on left	Oxidation state on right
Fe	+2	+3
O	0	-2

iii. All elements except O and H balanced

iv. Change in oxidation state of Fe = (3-2) = 1
Change in oxidation state of O = $2 \times (-2-0)$ = -4
Therefore: $4\,Fe^{+2} + O_2 \longrightarrow 4\,Fe^{+3} + H_2O$

v. Charge = 8 on left, 12 on right
$4\,H^+ + 4\,Fe^{+2} + O_2 \longrightarrow 4\,Fe^{+3} + H_2O$

vi. $4\,H^+ + 4\,Fe^{+2} + O_2 \longrightarrow 4\,Fe^{+3} + 2\,H_2O$

SECT. II
GENERAL
CHEMISTRY
REVIEW
NOTES

217

Example 1-11: Balance this chemical reaction in base:

$$BrO_3^- + F_2 \longrightarrow BrO_4^- + F^-$$

Method 1

i. and ii. Oxidation: $BrO_3^- \longrightarrow BrO_4^-$

Reduction: $F_2 \longrightarrow F^-$

iii. $F_2 \longrightarrow 2\ F^-$

iv. $BrO_3^- \longrightarrow BrO_4^- + H_2O$

$F_2 \longrightarrow 2\ F^-$

v. $2\ OH^- + BrO_3^- \longrightarrow BrO_4^- + H_2O$

$F_2 \longrightarrow 2\ F^-$

vi. $2\ OH^- + BrO_3^- \longrightarrow BrO_4^- + H_2O + 2e^-$

$F_2 + 2e^- \longrightarrow 2\ F^-$

vii. Not needed

viii. $2\ OH^- + BrO_3^- + F_2 \longrightarrow BrO_4^- + 2\ F^- + H_2O$

Method 2

i. and ii.

Species	Oxidation state on left	Oxidation state on right
Br	+5	+7
F	0	-1

iii. $BrO_3^- + F_2 \longrightarrow BrO_4^- + 2\ F^-$

iv. Change in oxidation state of Br = (7-5) = 2

Change in oxidation state of F = $2 \times (-1-0) = -2$

Therefore: $BrO_3^- + F_2 \longrightarrow BrO_4^- + 2\ F^-$

v. Charge = -1 on left, -3 on right

$2\ OH^- + BrO_3^- + F_2 \longrightarrow BrO_4^- + 2\ F^-$

vi. $2\ OH^- + BrO_3^- + F_2 \longrightarrow BrO_4^- + 2\ F^- + H_2O$

Electronic and Atomic Structure

I. Orbitals and Simple Quantum Mechanics   **HIGH-YIELD TOPICS**

Questions on the MCAT require a working knowledge of simple quantum mechanics. This chapter provides a review of the basics of this topic at the level that you need to know for the test.

An understanding of electronic and atomic structure allows you to predict and understand the chemical and physical properties of chemical compounds. Our review of this material begins by examining the atomic structure of hydrogen, which is the simplest atom with which to work.

I. Orbitals and Simple Quantum Mechanics

A. Orbital Structure of the Hydrogen Atom as a Model

The basic unit of matter is the atom, which is the smallest particle of an element that has the same properties as that element. An atom consists of smaller particles that are common to all elements but are present in different amounts in different elements.

The mass of an atom is very small. A special unit for atomic mass is the **atomic mass unit** (amu) or **dalton.** The amu or dalton is defined as $\frac{1}{12}$ of the mass of one atom of the carbon-12 isotope (^{12}C).

TABLE 2-1. Properties of subatomic particles.

Particle	Location	Charge	amu
Proton	Nucleus	+1	1.0073
Neutron	Nucleus	0	1.0087
Electron	Orbital	−1	0.00055

As shown in Table 2-1, the mass (as indicated by entries in the amu column) of an atom depends on how many protons and neutrons are present. Electrons have such a small mass compared to the nucleus that their mass can be ignored. Many physical properties are related to the mass of an element. This statement implies that the **physical properties are primarily dependent on the number of protons and neutrons.** The size of an atom, however, is determined by the electrons that are outside of the nucleus. Therefore, when atoms interact, it is primarily their **electrons that determine their chemical reactivity.**

SECT. II
GENERAL
CHEMISTRY
REVIEW
NOTES

219

The hydrogen atom is the simplest element. It has one proton, one electron, and no neutrons. Figure 2-1 shows a simplified diagram of the hydrogen atom and the atomic symbol for hydrogen.

FIGURE 2-1.

Diagram of the hydrogen atom (left) and the atomic symbol for hydrogen (right).

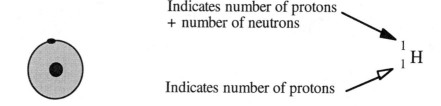

Indicates number of protons
+ number of neutrons

Indicates number of protons

$$_1^1 H$$

The simplified picture of the hydrogen atom implies that hydrogen has only one orbital for its single electron. Actually, hydrogen has only one **occupied** orbital. The single electron is not constrained to remain in only one orbital. It tends to remain in the orbital closest to the nucleus (the most stable orbital) unless electromagnetic energy of an appropriate wavelength is provided. This energy can stimulate the electron to move to a higher energy state farther from the nucleus. Energy must then be given off (frequently as electromagnetic energy) before the electron can return to the most stable position.

B.   Quantum Numbers and Simple Quantum Mechanics

The electronic structure of elements is described by several quantum numbers. **Each quantum number describes one aspect of the position of an electron within the overall electronic structure of an atom.** Each electron in an atom has a unique combination of four quantum numbers: **n,** l**, m,** and **s.**

An atomic orbital describes the probability distribution of finding an electron with a specific energy, defined by three specific values of the quantum numbers n, l, and m. The details of orbitals are described subsequent to a review of the quantum numbers.

1.   **n: the principal quantum number**

This quantum number indicates the ***principal energy level of an electron.*** The principal quantum number can assume any positive integer: $n = 1, 2, 3 \ldots$ and n is proportional to the energy and the distance of the electron from the nucleus. As **n** increases, the energy of the electrons with that **n** increases and their distance from the nucleus increases. The value of **n** for any valence (outer) electron corresponds to the row of the periodic table in which the element is located.

2. l**: the azimuthal, orbital, or angular momentum quantum number**

This quantum number, which can have any integral value from **(0 to n-1)** inclusive, describes the ***shape of the orbital*** in which the electron is found. The values for l correspond to different orbitals:

l	0	1	2	3	. . .
designation	s	p	d	f	. . .

Note the shapes of the s and p orbitals in Figure 2-2. The **s orbitals are spherical** and the **p orbitals** (p_x, p_y, and p_z orbitals) are dumbbell-shaped with the electron density located on the appropriate axis. A **node,** defined as a point with a very low probability of finding an electron, is located at the origin for the p orbitals.

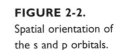

FIGURE 2-2.
Spatial orientation of
the s and p orbitals.

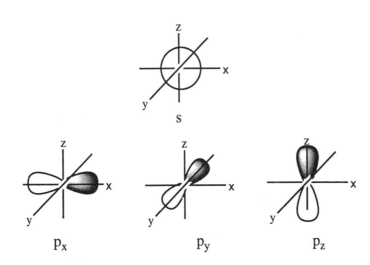

An orbital is described by stating the value of **n** with the letter designation of *l*. For example, if **n** = 1, then *l* = 0, and the result is a spherically symmetric 1s orbital. On the basis of the equations just reviewed, if you are given **n** = 2, then *l* = 0 and 1. When *l* = 0, the result is a 2s orbital in which the electron, on average, will be further from the nucleus than an electron in a 1s orbital. There are three **m** values for *l* = 1, so there are three 2p orbitals. You should be able to figure out how many orbitals are in the third energy level (**n** = 3). This level has nine orbitals: one 3s orbital, three 3p orbitals, and five 3d orbitals. If you are having trouble picturing what is going on, the table in the next section will help because it displays several common quantum numbers and orbitals.

3. **m (Sometimes referred to as m$_l$): The magnetic quantum number**

    This quantum number can have any integral value from $-l$ to $+l$. Remember that *l* tells you the shape of an orbital and **m$_l$ tells you the spatial orientation of the orbital.** There is a different value of **m** for each orbital of a particular type.
    For an s orbital *l* = 0, so the only possible value of **m** is 0. Thus, there is only one possible spatial orientation for an s orbital. This concept should make sense because it is difficult to think of two ways to orient a sphere. For a p orbital *l* = 1, and the possible values of **m** are -1, 0, and 1. Thus, there are 3 different orientations of the p orbitals (p$_x$, p$_y$, and p$_z$).

4. **s (sometimes referred to as m$_s$): The spin quantum number**

    This number **differentiates between the two electrons that can occupy the same orbital** (having the same values for **n, l,** and **m**). The spin quantum number can have only two possible values, $+\frac{1}{2}$ or $-\frac{1}{2}$, corresponding to spin up or spin down for each electron. When an atom is placed in a magnetic field, two electrons in an orbital will line up so one has a spin aligned with the magnetic field $(+\frac{1}{2})$ and one has a spin against the magnetic field $(-\frac{1}{2})$.

C. Orbitals and Number of Electrons per Orbital in More Complex Atoms

Table 2-2 shows that electrons are associated with four quantum numbers: a principal quantum number, an angular momentum quantum number, and both magnetic and spin quantum numbers. These four quantum numbers completely specify the state of the electron. Note also that the quantum numbers have orbitals associated with them.

SECT. II
GENERAL
CHEMISTRY
REVIEW
NOTES

221

TABLE 2-2. The four quantum numbers and their associated orbitals.

n	l (0 to n-1)	m (−l to l)	$s \left(\pm \frac{1}{2}\right)$	Orbital	Total Number of Electrons
1	0	0	$+\frac{1}{2}, -\frac{1}{2}$	1s	2
2	0	0	$+\frac{1}{2}, -\frac{1}{2}$	2s	2
	1	−1,0,1	$+\frac{1}{2}, -\frac{1}{2}$	$2p_x, 2p_y, 2p_z$	6
3	0	0	$+\frac{1}{2}, -\frac{1}{2}$	3s	2
	1	−1,0,1	$+\frac{1}{2}, -\frac{1}{2}$	$3p_x, 3p_y, 3p_z$	6
	2	−2−1,0,1,2	$+\frac{1}{2}, -\frac{1}{2}$	five 3d	10

PAULI EXCLUSION PRINCIPLE

No two electrons in the same atom can have the same values of all four quantum numbers.

In complex polyelectronic atoms, electrons usually fill orbitals in a predictable order. The **ground state** for an atom is the lowest energy state for that atom based on electron orbital filling. The electron configuration for an atom, filling its ground state, is illustrated in Figure 2-3. In general, electrons occupy the lowest energy orbitals available before entering the higher energy orbitals. Note also that the maximum number of electrons that can fill each listed orbital or group of orbitals is shown.

FIGURE 2-3.
Order of orbital filling by electrons.

$$1s^{2e \; max}, \; 2s^{2e \; max}, \; 2p^{6e \; max}, \; 3s^{2e \; max}, \; 3p^{6e \; max}, \; 4s^{2e \; max}, \; 3d^{10e \; max},$$
$$4p^{6e \; max}, \; 5s^{2e \; max}, \; 4d^{10e \; max}, \; 5p^{6e \; max}, \; 6s^{2e \; max}, \; \text{etc.}$$

A great way to help you remember the order of orbital filling is illustrated in Figure 2-4. Write out the orbitals as shown and follow the arrows from head to tail. By filling the orbitals in the proper order, you can write a ground electronic state (Example 2-1).

FIGURE 2-4.
Head-to-tail method of remembering order of orbital filling.

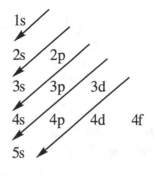

Example 2-1:

Sulfur = 16e⁻. Ground electronic state = $1s^2 \; 2s^2 \; 2p^6 \; 3s^2 \; 3p^4$

The sum of superscripts should add up to the number of electrons in a given atom or ion. If the atom is neutral, then this number represents the atomic number of the atom. If an ion is positively charged, then this number will be less than the atomic number. This idea makes sense because a positively charged ion has fewer electrons than the neutral atom. If an ion is negatively charged, then the sum of the superscripts will be greater than the atomic number.

An atom is said to be isoelectronic with another atom when they have the same number of electrons.

HUND'S RULE

Another important rule in quantum mechanics is **Hund's rule,** which states that **equal energy orbitals are each occupied by a single electron before the second electron of opposite spin(s) enters the orbital.** Thus, in orbitals of the same energy level, electrons remain unpaired and parallel in spin when possible to minimize electron–electron repulsion. For example, each of the three 2p orbitals ($2p_x$, $2p_y$, $2p_z$) will hold a single electron before any receives a second electron. Example 2-2 demonstrates Hund's rule:

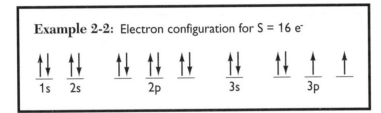

Example 2-2: Electron configuration for S = 16 e⁻

Note that in the filled orbitals (1s, 2s, 2p, 3s), all of the electrons are paired. In the case of the unfilled 3p orbital, you should put a single electron with the same spin (Hund's rule) into each orbital before pairing the electrons in the first 3p orbital.

Electronic configurations allow you to determine the number of unpaired electrons. As shown in Example 2-2, sulfur has two unpaired electrons. The presence of these unpaired electrons is important because they affect properties of the elements, such as chemical reactivity and attraction to a magnetic field. Substances with unpaired electrons tend to be attracted to magnetic fields and are said to be **paramagnetic.** Substances in which all of the electrons are paired are slightly repelled by magnetic fields and are termed **diamagnetic.**

SECT. II
GENERAL
CHEMISTRY
REVIEW
NOTES

223

Periodic Table

HIGH-YIELD TOPICS

I. Basic Principles

II. Important Periodic Trends

In the general chemistry section of the MCAT, you frequently are asked to answer questions based on the principles and trends of the periodic table. You are also given a copy of the table at the beginning of both the physical and the biologic sciences sections of the test. Therefore, it is critical that you understand the periodic table.

The name "periodic table" derives from the observation that many properties of the elements are periodic (repeating) as the atomic numbers of the elements increase. The periodic table is just an array of the elements arranged in order of increasing atomic number, with elements having similar chemical properties arranged in vertical columns called **groups.** A **period** is a horizontal row, where the period number (1 through 7) corresponds to the principal energy level.

I. Basic Principles

A. Structure

Properties such as the tendency to form ions of a particular charge, heat and electrical conduction, electronegativity, and ionization energy tend to repeat themselves as the atomic numbers of the elements increase. This repetition is related to the

FIGURE 3-1.
The periodic table. A copy is provided on the MCAT.

IA																	VIIIA
1 H	IIA											IIIA	IVA	VA	VIA	VII A	2 He
3 Li	4 Be											5 B	6 C	7 N	8 O	9 F	10 Ne
11 Na	12 Mg											13 Al	14 Si	15 P	16 S	17 Cl	18 Ar
19 K	20 Ca	21 Sc	22 Ti	23 V	24 Cr	25 Mn	26 Fe	27 Co	28 Ni	29 Cu	30 Zn	31 Ga	32 Ge	33 As	34 Se	35 Br	36 Kr
37 Rb	38 Sr	39 Y	40 Zr	41 Nb	42 Mo	43 Tc	44 Ru	45 Rh	46 Pd	47 Ag	48 Cd	49 In	50 Sn	51 Sb	52 Te	53 I	54 Xe
55 Cs	56 Ba	57 La	72 Hf	73 Ta	74 W	75 Re	76 Os	77 Ir	78 Pt	79 Au	80 Hg	81 Tl	82 Pb	83 Bi	84 Po	85 At	86 Rn
87 Fr	88 Ra	89 Ac															

number of valence electrons of an atom. For example, if you look at the chemical properties of the elements in group IA on the periodic table in Figure 3-1 (e.g., Li, Na, K), you will note that they are all soft metals, the color of silver, with a low melting point.

The periodic table can be used to estimate relative properties of elements. This application prevents a great deal of unnecessary memorization and is of great value for the MCAT.

B. Terms and Definitions

The following definitions apply to the periodic table. You should become familiar with these terms.

1. **Periods:** Horizontal rows

2. **Groups or families:** Vertical columns

3. **Group designations:**
   IA = Alkali metals
   IIA = Alkaline earth metals
   VIA = Chalcogens
   VIIA = Halogens
   VIIIA = Noble, "inert," or "rare" gases

4. **Representative elements:** Elements that fill the s and p blocks (groups IA to VIIA)

5. **Transition elements:** Elements that fill the d block (IB-VIIB, and VIIIB, which consists of three families)

6. **Inner transition elements:** Elements that fill the f block. These include the Lanthanides (top period elements 58-71) and the Actinides (bottom period elements 90-103).

C. Organization Based on Valence Electrons

Valence electrons occupy the outermost set of orbitals of an atom. They are responsible for bonding. The outermost orbitals have the largest principal quantum number (e.g., for carbon, the 2s and 2p orbitals). In the periodic table, all elements of any given group have the same number of valence electrons. For example, all of the alkali metals have one valence electron (Example 3-1).

Example 3-1: $Na = 1s^2 \, 2s^2 \, 2p^6 \, 3s^1$ (1 valence electron)

$K = 1s^2 \, 2s^2 \, 2p^6 \, 3s^2 \, 3p^6 \, 4s^1$ (1 valence electron)

As expected, Na and K have similar reactivity, because they have the same number of valence electrons. They both tend to form cations in the +1 oxidation state. This tendency to donate an electron makes them reducing agents. They also are highly reactive metals. Again, because elements with the same number of valence electrons are placed in the same group, you can predict similar chemistry of the elements within that group.

SECT. II
GENERAL
CHEMISTRY
REVIEW
NOTES

225

II. Important Periodic Trends

A. First and Second Ionization Energies

Ionization energy (IE) is that **amount of energy required to remove an electron** from a gaseous atom. Atoms can be stripped of all their electrons, one by one, giving ions with one, two, or more positive charges. Generally, more and more energy is required to remove successive electrons from an atom.

The species losing the electron is said to have become oxidized. The IE is always positive and hence appears on the reactants side of an equation showing the ionization:

1st Ionization energy $X_{(g)} + \text{1st IE} = X^+_{(g)} + e^-$ (Energy required to remove the first electron from a neutral atom in the gas phase)

Figure 3-2 shows the first ionization energies for different elements with increasing atomic number. Note that the IA atom, Li, has the lowest ionization energy. It has only one valence electron. On the other hand, note the high ionization energy of Ne. This element is in the VIIIA group and is a noble gas. It has eight valence electrons and is unreactive. Its valence electrons are stable, and a great deal of energy is required to remove one.

FIGURE 3-2.
The first ionization energies of various elements. Appreciate that the number of valence electrons of these elements is increasing: Li$^+$ has one valence electron; Ne has eight valence electrons.

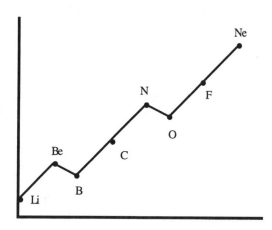

Generally, it is easier to ionize an element when that process results in a stable configuration.

2nd Ionization energy: $X^+_{(g)} + \text{2nd IE} = X^{+2}_{(g)} + e^-$ (Energy required to remove the second electron from a +1 charged ion in the gas phase)

The same considerations apply to the second ionization energy as to the first. It is easier to ionize an element when the ionization results in a noble gas configuration, as shown in Example 3-2.

Example 3-2: Calcium has a low second ionization energy because the calcium +2 ion has the neon electron configuration:

$$Ca^+ \longrightarrow Ca^{+2} \text{ (Ne configuration)}$$

General trends are as follows:

1. **Ionization energy increases from left to right and bottom to top on the periodic table.**

2. **The lower the ionization energy, the more metallic the element.**

B. Electron Affinity

Electron affinity (EA) is a measure of the amount of energy associated with a gaseous atom gaining an electron. When an atom gains electrons, energy is released. The greater the amount of energy released, the higher the electron affinity. The more stable the ion that results from this gain of electrons, the greater the amount of energy released. Stability follows the same guidelines described for ionization energy. An ion is more stable if it has a noble gas configuration.

General trends are as follows:

1. **Within a period, the halogens have the highest EA** (the gain of one electron gives them a noble gas configuration) and **the noble gases have the lowest EA.**

2. **EA generally increases from left to right along a row,** and from **bottom to top along any column.**

C. Electronegativity

Electronegativity is a measure of the attraction an atom has for shared electrons (i.e., the electrons in bonds). If there is a covalent bond between two atoms that have different electronegativities, the electrons in the bond will spend more time around the more electronegative atom.

General trends are as follows:

1. **Metals have extremely low electronegativity values,** whereas nonmetals may have high electronegativity values.

2. **Electronegativity increases from left to right along any row.**

3. **Electronegativity increases from bottom to top in any column.**

D. Variation of Properties within Groups and Rows

1. **Within a period, increasing atomic number leads to:**

   a. **Decreasing atomic radius.** This result is the opposite of what you would expect to happen when the atomic weight increases. The atomic radius actually decreases across a period because all orbitals at the same principal quantum number are at about the same distance from the nucleus. When the atomic weight increases, there are more protons, which increases the positive charge in the nucleus. This change exerts a greater pull on the electrons and decreases the radius of the electron cloud. Thus, the atoms actually get smaller as you move across a period.

   b. **Decreasing metallic properties**

   c. **Increasing ionization energy.** Elements closer to the right side of the periodic table more easily achieve the noble gas configuration by gaining electrons. Thus, removing an electron from them is difficult.

2. **Within a group, increasing atomic number leads to:**

   a. **Increasing atomic radius.** The occupation of orbitals with a larger principal quantum number causes a significant jump in the size of the atom.

SECT. II
GENERAL
CHEMISTRY
REVIEW
NOTES

227

b. Increasing metallic properties

c. Decreasing ionization energy. The farther away an electron is from the nucleus, the more shielded it is from the attraction of the nucleus. Thus, electrons with higher principal quantum numbers require less energy to remove.

d. Decreasing electronegativity. This effect is also related to the shielding of the valence electrons from the nuclear charge by all of the electrons in the lower-lying orbitals.

3. **Alkali and alkaline earth metals become more reactive as the atomic weight increases because of shielding of the nucleus by inner electrons.**

E. Trends for Covalent Radii for Atoms and Ions Based on Atomic Number

As described previously, **atomic radii tend to decrease across periods and increase down groups in the periodic table.**

The size of a cation is smaller than the size of its parent atom because of the greater concentration of positive charge in the nucleus relative to the number of electrons. The result is a greater "pull" on the electrons by the nucleus, and a smaller ion. **The size of an anion is larger than the original atom** because of the greater concentration of negative charge in the orbitals. The result is less attraction to the nucleus per electron, and the radius increases.

The only comparison that can be made between anions, cations, and atoms that are not from the same element is when they are isoelectronic (same number of electrons). **In an isoelectronic series, the cation with the largest positive charge will be the smallest, and the anion with the greatest negative charge will be the largest.** This phenomenon occurs because of the differing number of protons in the nucleus. The more protons, the more "pull" on the electrons and the smaller the size. Example 3-3 shows an isoelectronic series. Each ion or atom has 18 electrons. Note, however, that each ion or atom has a different number of protons; e.g., calcium has 20 protons, whereas sulfur has 16. Example 3-3 shows that calcium ion has the smallest radius because it has the most protons for the same number of electrons. The greater number of protons "pulls" on the electron cloud and decreases the radius of the ion relative to the other species.

Example 3-3: Rank the following isoelectronic species from smallest to largest: S^{-2}, Cl^-, Ar, K^+, Ca^{+2}

Solution: Note the decreasing order of atomic/ionic radii. Calcium has the greatest radius because it has the greatest number of protons for the same number of electrons:

$$Ca^{+2} < K^+ < Ar < Cl^- < S^{-2}$$

Bonding $\left(4 \right)$

Bonding

I. **Ionic and Covalent Bonds**	
II. **Lewis Dot Structures**	**HIGH-YIELD**
III. **Molecular Geometry**	**TOPICS**

I. Ionic and Covalent Bonds

A. Ionic Bond

Ionic bonds are formed by the electrostatic attraction between ions. Ionic bonds result from the transfer of electrons from one species to another. When an electron is transferred from one atom to another, a positive ion and a negative ion are formed. The subsequent attraction between the ions is the bond.

Ionic bonds are formed between an electropositive metal (usually group IA or IIA metals) and a nonmetal (usually group VIA or VIIA). The metal gives an electron to the nonmetal, forming a cation (metal) and an anion (nonmetal), both gaining noble gas configurations. The resulting ions have a powerful electrostatic attraction for one another.

Look at Figure 4-1. Sodium has one valence electron and low ionization energy. Thus, it does not take much energy to remove one electron from sodium. Sodium gives up its $3s^1$ electron and becomes a sodium ion. It now has a noble gas configuration of its electrons (configuration of Ne) and is stable. Therefore, sodium is a good *electron donor.* Chlorine has a high electron affinity and is a good *electron acceptor.* It has seven valence electrons and would like one additional electron to produce the noble gas configuration (configuration of Ar). When Na and Cl atoms combine, an electron is transferred from Na to Cl, resulting in stable Na^+ and Cl^- ions, which attract each other.

FIGURE 4-1.

Formation of ions by electron transfer. The resulting ions form an ionic bond by electrostatic attraction.

$$Na(3s^1) + Cl\ (3s^23p^5) \rightarrow Na^+[Ne] + Cl^-[Ar]$$

Ionic compounds tend to form ionic crystals, which are held together by electrostatic attraction. Ionic compounds usually have high melting points (800°C for NaCl), which is indicative of **strong bonds.**

229

B. Covalent Bond

When two atoms **"share" a pair of electrons,** they form what is commonly known as a covalent bond. A simple way of indicating covalent bonding in molecules is through the use of the Lewis electron dot diagram. Only valence (outer shell) electrons are depicted in these diagrams, which are represented by a dot or dots placed beside the chemical symbol.

How do you know the number of valence electrons for any given element? Simple. It is the same number as the family or group number (vertical column) in the periodic table. There are eight groups among the main elements. You reviewed this concept in Chapter 3 of the General Chemistry Review Notes, but the periodic table is shown in Figure 4-2 for convenience. Note that H, Li, Na, K, Rb, Cs, and Fr (group IA elements) have only one valence electron, which is represented by a single dot. Group IIA elements (Be, Mg, Ca, Sr, Ba, and Ra) have two valence electrons; group IIIA (B, Al, Ga, In, Tl), three valence electrons; group IVA (C, Si, Ge, Sn, Pb), four valence electrons, and so on. **A stable molecule results whenever the noble gas configuration has been achieved** (called an **octet**).

FIGURE 4-2.
Periodic table. Note that the table is organized so it is easy to see the number of valence electrons for any given element. Know that the valence electrons of the elements participate in bonds.

IA																	VIIIA
1 H	IIA											IIIA	IVA	VA	VIA	VIIA	2 He
3 Li	4 Be											5 B	6 C	7 N	8 O	9 F	10 Ne
11 Na	12 Mg											13 Al	14 Si	15 P	16 S	17 Cl	18 Ar
19 K	20 Ca	21 Sc	22 Ti	23 V	24 Cr	25 Mn	26 Fe	27 Co	28 Ni	29 Cu	30 Zn	31 Ga	32 Ge	33 As	34 Se	35 Br	36 Kr
37 Rb	38 Sr	39 Y	40 Zr	41 Nb	42 Mo	43 Tc	44 Ru	45 Rh	46 Pd	47 Ag	48 Cd	49 In	50 Sn	51 Sb	52 Te	53 I	54 Xe
55 Cs	56 Ba	57 La	72 Hf	73 Ta	74 W	75 Re	76 Os	77 Ir	78 Pt	79 Au	80 Hg	81 Tl	82 Pb	83 Bi	84 Po	85 At	86 Rn
87 Fr	88 Ra	89 Ac															

Sulfur has six valence electrons. In the molecule disulfide (S_2), each sulfur atom wants to obtain an octet. Sulfur can obtain an octet by sharing electrons, as shown in Example 4-1.

Example 4-1: S_2

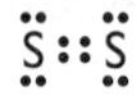

S̈ :: S̈

The unshared electron pairs in the Lewis dot diagram are known as lone pairs, and make no contribution to the bond between the atoms. Elements at the right of the periodic table (N, O, S, and the halogens) frequently have lone pairs. One final note: hydrogen always forms a duet (not an octet) because it needs only two electrons to attain the noble gas configuration.

II. Lewis Dot Structures

A. Drawing a Lewis Dot Diagram

Lewis dot diagrams show how atoms are connected to one another to form a molecule. It gives no information, however, regarding molecular geometry (i.e., how the atoms are arranged in three dimensions).

The first step in drawing a Lewis diagram is to decide what atoms are directly attached to each other. The hardest part may be in deciding which is the **central atom.** In many cases, the arrangement of atoms can be inferred directly from the molecular formula, because it is common practice to write the central atom of a molecule first in the molecular formula, followed by the atoms that surround the central atom. For example, in CO_2, carbon is the central atom surrounded by two oxygen atoms, as shown in Example 4-2.

Example 4-2: CO_2

$\ddot{O}::C::\ddot{O}$

This same principle applies to molecules such as NH_3, NO_2, SO_3, and many others. You cannot, however, always count on this rule. For example, molecules such as H_2O and H_2S have O and S as the central atoms. Thus, the Lewis electron dot diagram is not always obvious. If you must guess, **the most symmetric arrangement of atoms has the greatest chance of being correct.**

Once the arrangement of atoms has been chosen, one bond is made between each pair of attached atoms. The octet rule must then be satisfied for each atom (except H). The remaining electrons can be placed as lone pairs or multiple bonds. The Lewis structure **must** have the correct total number of valence electrons.

Drawing a diagram involves the following steps:

Step 1.

Remember to count all the valence electrons for each atom in the molecule. You will then know how many dots to put in the diagram. Also, if the molecule is an ion, add an additional electron for each negative charge or subtract an electron for each positive charge. See Examples 4-3 and 4-4.

Example 4-3: SO_4^{-2}

S: 6 valence e⁻ = 6 dots
O: 6 valence e⁻ × 4 atoms = 24 dots
Charge: add 2 valence e⁻ = +2 dots
_____
TOTAL = 32 dots

Example 4-4: NO^+

N: 5 valence e⁻ = 5 dots
O: 6 valence e⁻ = 6 dots
Charge: subtract 1 valence e⁻ = -1 dot
_____
TOTAL = 10 dots

Step 2.

Draw the molecular skeleton. Remember that the **most symmetric arrangement of atoms has the greatest chance of being correct.** See Example 4-5.

SECT. II
GENERAL
CHEMISTRY
REVIEW
NOTES

231

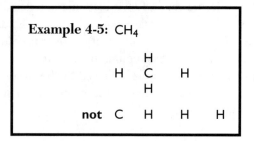

Example 4-5: CH_4

$$
\begin{array}{ccc}
 & H & \\
H & C & H \\
 & H & \\
\end{array}
$$

not C   H   H   H

Step 3.

Place one pair of electrons in each bond to the central atom. See Example 4-6.

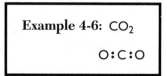

Example 4-6: CO_2

O:C:O

Step 4.

Remember that this step is the octet rule. Complete the octets of the atoms bonded to the central atom with remaining electrons. See Example 4-7.

Example 4-7: CO_2

:Ö:C:Ö:

Step 5.

Subtract the number of electrons so far distributed from the total determined in **step 1,** and place any (if any) additional electrons on the central atom **in pairs.** See Example 4-8.

Example 4-8: CO_2

C: 4 valence e⁻   = 4 dots
O: 6 valence e⁻ × 2 atoms = 12 dots
                      TOTAL = 16 dots

Structure in step 4 (see Example 4-7) has 16e⁻, so add none

Step 6.

If the central atom still has less than an octet, you must form multiple bonds so that each atom has its own octet. See Example 4-9.

> **Example 4-9:** CO_2
>
> Structure from step 4, (see Example 4-7) has only 4 electrons around carbon. Move in lone pairs from oxygen to make double bonds:
>
> $\ddot{O}::C::\ddot{O}$

Step 7.

Make sure that the electrons you counted in **step 1** are all accounted for with dots.

Step 8.

Calculate any formal charges. The formal charge for each atom equals the number of valence electrons minus the number of bonds and number of lone electrons. The formal charge can be used to determine several things and is described later in this chapter. Example 4-10 shows how to find the formal charge of atoms in a molecule.

> **Example 4-10:** NO^+
>
> $:N::O:$
>
> $FC_N = 5$ valence e^- - 3 bonds - 2 lone e^- = 0
> $FC_O = 6$ valence e^- - 3 bonds - 2 lone e^- = +1

B. Multiple Bonds

Some molecules have more than one pair of electrons shared by two atoms. To determine whether or not a molecule has multiple bonds, follow steps 1 through 5 as described and then proceed to step 6. **If the central atom still has less than an octet, you must form multiple bonds so that each atom has its own octet.** In other words, you may have double bonds or triple bonds in the molecule (Figure 4-3).

Double bonds in a Lewis diagram.

$$
\begin{matrix}
H & & H \\
.. & & .. \\
C & :: & C \\
.. & & .. \\
H & & H
\end{matrix}
$$

FIGURE 4-3.
Double and triple bonds in Lewis dot diagrams.

Triple bonds in a Lewis diagram. $H:C:::C:H$

C. Exceptions to the Octet Rule

Although most molecules satisfy the octet rule with a maximum of octets drawn for each atom in the Lewis dot diagram, there are exceptions. Some molecules have in-

SECT. II
GENERAL
CHEMISTRY
REVIEW
NOTES

233

complete octets. Look at the diagram for beryllium dichloride in Example 4-11. Beryllium, the central atom, has four electrons around it and not the conventional eight. Don't get upset! You should know that incom-plete octets are rare and are formed mostly by atoms on the left side of the periodic table.

Example 4-11: $BeCl_2$

$$:\overset{..}{\underset{..}{Cl}}:Be:\overset{.}{\underset{..}{Cl}}:$$

Another exception includes those rare cases in which the central atom has more than eight electrons in its valence shell, called an **expanded octet or valence expansion.** Some typical examples of expanded octets are PCl_5 and SF_6. In fact, expanded octets are common for phosphorus and sulfur because these elements have a valence shell that can accommodate more than eight electrons (both P and S are in the third period and the third shell can contain as many as 18 electrons because of the availability of the third orbitals). Only elements in the third period or below can have a valence expansion.

D. Resonance Structures

Often more than one Lewis electron dot diagram can be drawn for a molecule. When this occurs, don't panic! Look at the possible Lewis electron dot diagrams for CO_3^{2-} in Example 4-12.

Example 4-12: CO_3^{2-}

A   B   C

These diagrams represent the resonance structures for the carbonate ion. In fact, the actual electronic structure of CO_3^{2-} does not correspond to A, B, or C, but instead to a structure somewhere in between that has properties of A, B, and C (i.e., a **"resonance hybrid"** of structures A and B and C). The negative charge is evenly distributed or **"delocalized"** over all three oxygen atoms. In other words, none of the Lewis structures shown for this ion are structurally correct. We arrive at a correct description of carbonate if we take A, B, and C and conceptually create an **average structure** out of all three—the resonance hybrid. Therefore, CO_3^{2-} is a resonance hybrid of all three resonance structures.

Resonance structures are purely hypothetical; they exist only on paper and cannot be isolated or even observed. Just as a mule is a hybrid of a donkey and a horse, CO_3^{2-} is the hybrid offspring of its three "parents"—resonance structures A, B, and C.

E. Formal Charge

Formal charges added together give the overall total charge on the molecule or ion. Formal charges can also tell you where charges are likely found in a molecule. Remember that the formal charge is equal to:

Formal Charge = (# valence electrons) − (# bonds) − (# lone electrons)

As an example, consider the nitrite ion (NO_2^-). The main question concerns where exactly the −1 charge formally resides. The whole ion carries a −1 charge, but on which atom(s) is this charge "formally" located? To find the answer, begin by drawing the correct Lewis dot diagram for NO_2^-.

Example 4-13: Draw the correct Lewis electron dot diagram for NO_2^-.

Step 1. How many valence electrons?

> N: 5 valence e⁻ = 5 dots
> O: 6 valence e⁻ × 2 atoms = 12 dots
> Charge: add 1 valence e⁻ = +1 dot
> _____
> TOTAL = 18 dots

Step 2. Molecular skeleton:

> O   N   O

Step 3. Place a pair of electrons in each bond to the central atom.

> O:N:O

Step 4. Complete the octets of the atoms bonded to the central atom.

> :Ö:N:Ö:

Step 5. Place any additional electrons (18-16 = 2) on the central atom in pairs.

> :Ö:N̈:Ö:

Step 6. Form multiple bonds if the central atom does not have a complete octet.

> :Ö:N̈::Ö

Step 7. 18 total dots used in the diagram. This confirms step 1.

Step 8. Calculate formal charge (FC). For each atom, count the number of valence electrons and subtract from this the number of bonds and lone electrons:

> O (left)   FC = 6 - 1 bond - 6 lone electrons = -1
> N   FC = 5 - 3 bonds - 2 lone electrons = 0
> O (right) FC = 6 - 2 bonds - 4 lone electrons = 0

SECT. II
GENERAL
CHEMISTRY
REVIEW
NOTES

235

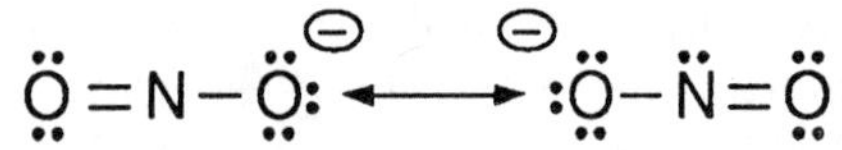

FIGURE 4-4.
Structure of nitrite and its
resonance structure. The arrow indicates resonance structures, not equilibrium.

Notice that the sum of the formal charges on the atoms equals the overall charge of the
molecule (-1). The diagram also reveals that the -1 charge is localized on the oxygen
with one bond. Nitrite actually has another equivalent Lewis dot diagram (resonance
structure) in which the (-1) charge is localized on the other oxygen atom. The structure of nitrite and its resonance structure are shown in Figure 4-4. Notice that the sum
of the formal charges on the atoms equals the overall charge of the molecule (-1).

$$\ddot{O}=N-\ddot{\underset{..}{O}}: \longleftrightarrow :\ddot{\underset{..}{O}}-\ddot{N}=\ddot{O}$$

III. Molecular Geometry

A. VSEPR Geometry

The number of valence electron pairs in a covalently bonded molecule is the most important factor in determining the geometric arrangement of the atoms, because each
electron pair stays as far away from other pairs as possible. Thus, the angle of separation between atoms in a molecule depends on the number of electron pairs.

   VSEPR stands for valence shell electron-pair repulsion. VSEPR predicts
molecular geometry based on the principle of maximum electron pair separation on
the assumption that electron pairs, both bonding and lone pairs, want to be as far
apart as possible. Figure 4-5 shows common shapes resulting from different numbers
of electron pairs. You should become familiar with these basic shapes as you prepare
for the MCAT.

FIGURE 4-5.
VSEPR geometry. Basic shapes,
structures, and examples of
some common compounds
that are important to review
and remember.

e⁻ pairs	Shape	Structure	Example
2	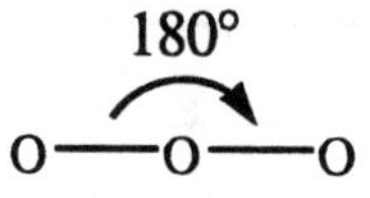 180° linear	linear	$BeCl_2$, $MgBr_2$
3	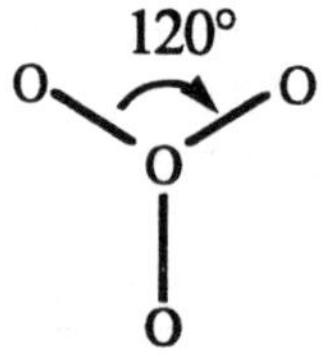 120°	trigonal planar	BCl_3, $AlCl_3$
4	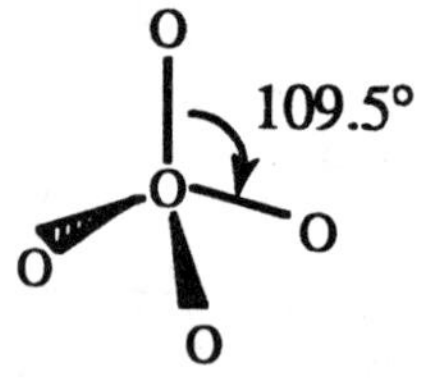 109.5°	tetrahedral	CH_4, CCl_4
5	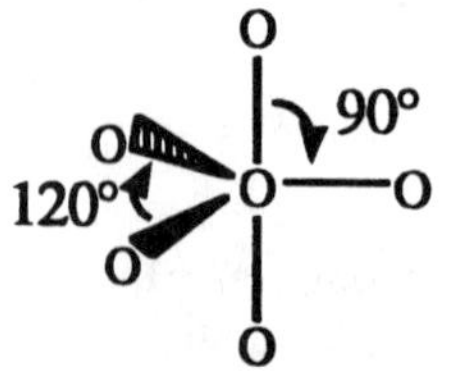 90° 120°	trigonal bipyramidal	PCl_5, $SbCl_5$
6	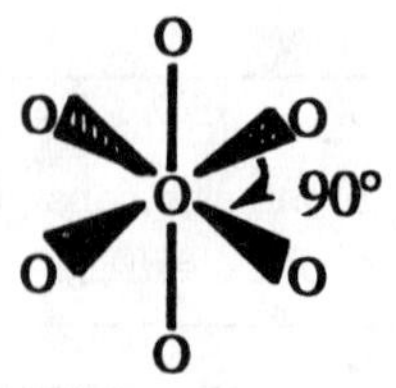 90°	octahedral	PCl_6, SF_6

B. Polar Covalent Bonds

The next concept that you must understand is the role of electronegativity in determining charge distribution. **It is the difference in electronegativity of two atoms in a covalent bond that determines how the electrons in a bond are shared.** If the electronegativity of the two atoms differs, electrons in the bond are not shared equally and the bond is said to be a **polar bond.** The electrons are shifted toward the more electronegative atom, resulting in a partial negative charge (δ^-) on the electronegative atom and a partial positive charge (δ^+) on the less electronegative atom.

Look at Example 4-14. The Cl atom is more electronegative than the H atom. Thus, the electrons are shifted toward the Cl and it takes on a partial negative charge (δ^-), creating a polar bond.

Example 4-14: HCl

$$\delta^{v+}\delta^-$$
$$H - Cl$$
$$\longmapsto$$

C. Dipole Moment

Now that you understand how the molecular geometry of molecules can be determined, you can appreciate that the polarity of entire molecules depends in part on their geometry. One measure of polarity of a molecule is its dipole moment. **The dipole moment of a molecule is the vector sum of the bond moments** in a molecule. **The bond moments are a measure of the polarity of a diatomic covalent bond.** Thus, the dipole moment gives you a measure of the polarity of molecules, which is dependent on molecular geometry.

The dipole moment is represented as an arrow pointing along the bond from δ^+ to δ^-. As shown in Example 4-15, drawing the water molecule with the correct geometry is important to see if the bond moments cancel. You can see that the two bond dipoles add vectorially to give a net dipole moment.

Example 4-15: H_2O

Net dipole

Bond dipole

Bond dipole

Drawing correct molecular geometry is important because sometimes the bond dipoles can cancel. In this case, there may be a dipole moment of zero. In Example 4-16, notice the polar bonds. Oxygen is more electronegative than carbon. Because of the symmetry of the molecule, however, the vector sum of these polar dipoles is zero. Thus, the dipole moment of carbon dioxide is zero. In some symmetric

SECT. II
GENERAL
CHEMISTRY
REVIEW
NOTES

237

molecules, the dipoles cancel even though there are polar bonds. Other symmetric molecules, such as CH_4 and C_2H_4, have a zero dipole moment.

Example 4-16: CO_2

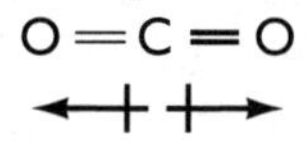

$$O = C = O$$

$\longleftarrow + \longmapsto$

No net dipole

5

Gases and Liquids

iquids

| **I.** Gas Phase: Key Ideas and Equations | **HIGH-YIELD** |
| **II.** Liquid Phase: Intermolecular Forces | **TOPICS** |

Compounds can exist in several different physical states, including gases and liquids. In Chapter 6 of the General Chemistry Review Notes, you will review phase equilibria. This chapter provides an overview of the basic gas laws needed to answer MCAT questions. In addition, the intermolecular forces affecting liquids are discussed.

Because of the great distance between molecules in the gas phase, gases are sometimes called the **expanded phase.** In the liquid or solid phase, molecules are closer together, and these phases are called **condensed phases.**

I. Gas Phase: Key Ideas and Equations

A. Definitions

A **gas** is a particular state of matter in which the molecules or atoms that make up the sample of matter are small compared to the distances between them. In a gas, the particles are in **constant motion,** bumping into the walls of the container. The collision of these gas particles with the container walls creates the pressure of a gas.

The **state** of a gas is given by its **volume, temperature, pressure, and composition.** You need to understand each of these terms.

The **volume** of a gas equals the volume of its container.

The **pressure** of a gas is the force exerted by the gas molecules on each unit area of a surface. Usually, this surface is the wall(s) of the container. Pressure is measured in atmospheres, torr, or millimeters of mercury (mm Hg). Know that 1 atmosphere = 760 torr = 760 mm Hg.

Temperature is a measure of kinetic energy. The unit used to describe temperature when working with gases is the kelvin degree (K). Remember that K = °C + 273.

The **composition** of a gas is given by the relative amounts of each gas present in a mixture. If you are given a mixture of gases, and are asked for the partial pressure of one particular gas, start by determining the mole fraction of the gas in which you are interested. The **mole fraction** is the number of moles of the desired gas divided by the total number of moles of all gases in the mixture. The **partial pressure** of a gas is the mole fraction of that gas multiplied by the total pressure of the gas mixture.

SECT. II
GENERAL
CHEMISTRY
REVIEW
NOTES

239

You should also be familiar with the term **STP,** which stands for **S**tandard **T**emperature and **P**ressure. The conditions of STP are **P = 1 atm, T = 0°C (273 K).** Also know that for an ideal gas, 1 mole of gas at STP occupies 22.4 liters.

B. Kinetic Molecular Theory of Ideal Gases

An ideal gas satisfies several postulates.

1. Ideal gases have no volume (e.g., they are volumeless points of mass or small hard spheres).
2. They are in a constant state of random molecular motion.
3. They exert no forces on one another other than through the impact of collisions.
4. No loss of energy occurs because of friction (all collisions are elastic).

C. Important Gas Equations

Before you review the key equations of gases, look over the meaning of each of the variables used in the equations:

P   = the pressure in atm

T   = the temperature in K (absolute temperature)

V   = the volume in liters (l)

n   = the number of moles of an ideal gas

k   = the appropriate gas constant

R   = the universal gas constant (0.0821 L atm/mol K or 8.3 J/mol K)

MW = molecular weight (g/mol)

N_A = Avogadro's number

A key equation to know for the MCAT is the ideal gas law. Most of the other equations discussed in this section can be derived from this equation.

1. **The Ideal Gas Law and The Combined Gas Law**

    The **ideal gas law** describes the behavior of all gases under any combination of amount, temperature, pressure, and volume:

    $$PV = nRT \qquad \text{(R = Universal Gas Constant)}$$

    Notice that this equation has four variables. This law is useful in calculations when you have three known quantities and one unknown quantity.

    The **combined gas law** is also useful on the MCAT. If you are given a problem with a single sample of gas (constant number of moles) or two samples of gas containing the same number of moles, you can rapidly solve for unknown variables. For example, if you know the pressure, temperature, and volume of a gas, it is easy to find the volume of the gas if the temperature and pressure are changed and this change is known. All you have to do is plug the numeric values into the combined gas law equation (remember to use kelvin for the temperature units):

    $$P_1 V_1 / T_1 = P_2 V_2 / T_2$$

    Note that the subscripts 1 and 2 refer to the initial and final states of the gas, respectively.

2. **Avogadro's Law**

    Avogadro's law shows that at constant temperature and pressure, equal volumes of gases contain equal numbers of moles or molecules. The volume of an ideal gas is directly proportional to its amount in moles. Thus, $V = n \times$ constant. This relationship can be rearranged to give a more useful equation.

    $$V_1/n_1 = V_2/n_2$$

    Note that the subscripts 1 and 2 refer to the volumes and numbers of moles of two gases.

3. **Boyle's Law**

    Boyle's law states that the volume of a fixed amount of an ideal gas is inversely proportional to its pressure at constant temperature. Thus, $V = 1/p \times$ constant, or $PV =$ constant. A more useful form of this law is as follows:

    $$P_1V_1 = P_2V_2$$

    Note that the subscripts 1 and 2 refer to initial and final states of a gas. The number of moles of gas and temperature remain constant.

4. **Charles' Law**

    Charles' law shows that the volume of a fixed amount of an ideal gas is directly proportional to its absolute temperature at constant pressure. Thus, $V = T \times$ constant, or $V/T =$ constant. A more useful form of this law is as follows:

    $$V_1/T_1 = V_2/T_2$$

5. **Equations Relating to the Kinetic Theory of Gases**

    Remember that the kinetic theory of gases reviewed previously in this chapter states that an ideal gas is in continuous random motion in a straight line, occupies negligible volume, and has point mass. In addition, the ideal gas undergoes elastic collisions and has an average kinetic energy proportional to temperature in kelvins.

    a. **Kinetic Energy**

        Understanding the principle assumptions of ideal gas behavior at the molecular level, you should not be surprised that the kinetic energy of an ideal gas is related to the following equations:

        $$^*\text{K.E.} = 1/2\ mv^2 = (3/2)nkT \quad \{\text{J/molecule}\}$$

        $$\text{K.E.} = (3/2)nRT \quad \{\text{J/mole}\}$$

        in which m = mass; v = average velocity; k = Boltzmann's constant = R/N_A; $R = 8.3$ J/mole-K (in this formula); and N_A = Avogadro's number. Notice that these two equations are similar and just give you different units. You do not need to memorize these equations for the MCAT; just know the variables that relate to KE.

    b. **Velocity**

        The next important concept relates the velocity to absolute temperature and molecular weight. Recalling that $PV = nRT$, then $\text{K.E.} = 3/2\ PV = 3/2\ nRT$.

SECT. II
GENERAL
CHEMISTRY
REVIEW
NOTES

241

Solving for velocity, you find that:

$$v = [3RT/MW]^{1/2} \text{ (MW in kg/mol)}$$

This equation gives "root mean square" velocity, which is not quite the same as average velocity, although it does give you a good approximation. This concept is discussed in more detail in the physics section. Just be familiar with this relationship.

From analyzing the preceding concepts of velocity, and realizing that diffusion rate (R) is directly proportional to the average velocity of an ideal gas, you can define **Graham's law of effusion.**

c. **Graham's Law of Effusion**

The ratio of effusion rates of two gases is inversely proportional to the square root of the ratio of the molecular weights:

$$R_1/R_2 = [M_2/M_1]^{1/2}$$

The best example of this law is how quickly a helium balloon goes flat compared to an air-filled balloon. A helium balloon contains a gas with a molecular weight of 4 g/mol. An air-filled balloon contains a mixture of gases, but for the sake of simplicity, assume that only nitrogen is present. The molecular weight of nitrogen (N_2) is 28 g/mol. $R_{He}/R_{N2} = [28/4]^{1/2} \sim 2.5$. This calculation shows that a helium balloon will deflate about two and one-half times as fast as a balloon filled with air.

6. **Deviation of Real Gases From Ideal Gas Laws**

An ideal gas is a hypothetical concept; in nature, gases tend to behave as **real gases.** Real gases occupy some volume of the container that holds them, and their particles exert forces on one another. Some of these forces are attractive and others are repulsive. The **van der Waals gas equation** explains these deviations from ideality:

$$\{P + an^2/V^2\} \{V - nb\} = nRT$$

For purposes of the MCAT, **you need to understand this equation.** Basically, the "a/V^2" term accounts for the intermolecular attractions that a real gas feels. The "b" term accounts for the volume actually occupied by the real gas molecules. Because the volume of an ideal gas does not include any contribution from the intrinsic volume of the molecules, the "b" term must be subtracted from the measured volume of a real gas.

This equation is a simple modification of the ideal gas law. The van der Waals equation gives results that match experimental results of real gases better than does the ideal gas equation.

7. **Dalton's Law of Partial Pressures**

You briefly reviewed some of these concepts in the beginning of this chapter, but this important topic warrants a more detailed discussion.

Partial pressure is the pressure that one component of a gas mixture exerts independent of the other components in the mixture. As shown in the subsequent equations, the partial pressure of component (i) in a gas mixture is equal to the mole fraction of component (i) times the total pressure (equation #2). The sum of the partial pressures in a mixture must equal the total pressure (equation #3).

1. X_i = mole fraction = $\dfrac{mole_i}{total\ moles}$

2. $P_i = X_i(P_T)$

3. $P_T = P_A + P_B + P_C + \ldots =$ {Sum of partial pressures}

For practice, look at the partial pressure calculation using Dalton's law provided in Example 5-1.

Example 5-1: A mixture of 2.4×10^{-3} moles $N_2(g)$, 4.5×10^{-3} moles $N_2O(g)$, and 3.7×10^{-3} moles $CO_2(g)$ in a flask had a total pressure of 1.75 atm. What is the partial pressure of each gas in the mixture?

Solution:

Step 1. To use Dalton's $P_i = X_iP_T$, you need to find the mole fraction of each gas. First, add the moles of each gas to find the total moles. Then, divide total moles by the moles of each gas:

$$X_{N_2} = \frac{2.4 \times 10^{-3}\ mol}{10.6 \times 10^{-3}\ mol} = 0.23$$

$$X_{N_2O} = \frac{4.5 \times 10^{-3}\ mol}{10.6 \times 10^{-3}\ mol} = 0.42$$

$$X_{CO_2} = \frac{3.7 \times 10^{-3}\ mol}{10.6 \times 10^{-3}\ mol} = 0.35$$

Step 2. Apply Dalton's law to each gas:

$$P_{N_2} = X_{N_2}P_T = (0.23)(1.75\ atm) = 0.40\ atm$$

$$P_{N_2O} = X_{N_2O}P_T = (0.42)(1.75\ atm) = 0.74\ atm$$

$$P_{CO_2} = X_{CO_2}P_T = (0.35)(1.75\ atm) = 0.61\ atm$$

II. Liquid Phase: Intermolecular Forces

Liquids have no fixed or definite shape because their molecules move about at random and are not ordered. Liquids are in a fluid state. In Chapter 6, you will review some of the properties of fluids, including boiling point, freezing point, osmotic pressure, and vapor pressure. The focus of this section is on the forces that act between molecules of a liquid. These **intermolecular forces** play an important role in the properties of fluids.

The three important intermolecular forces that you should know for the MCAT are **hydrogen bonding, dipole interactions,** and **London dispersion forces.** Dipole interactions and London dispersion forces are two types of **van der Waals forces.**

A. Hydrogen Bonding (Strength ≈ 7 − 10 kcal/mol)

A hydrogen bond is an intermolecular force that occurs between molecules in which a hydrogen covalently bound to an O, N, or F is attracted to another O, N, or F atom in another molecule. **These bonds depend on the electronegativity of O, N, or F.** You should understand that hydrogen bonds form between molecules as a result of the electronegative atom attaining a partial negative charge by attracting electrons

SECT. II
GENERAL
CHEMISTRY
REVIEW
NOTES

243

from neighboring atoms (hydrogens). The hydrogen atoms acquire a partial positive charge as their electrons are "pulled" toward the electronegative O, N, or F. As a result, an attraction is created between the hydrogen (partial positive charge) and the O, N, or F of a neighboring molecule (partial negative charge).

A great example of a hydrogen bond is shown in Figure 5-1. Notice the importance of the partial charges in creating the bond. You can see that two water molecules are participating in a hydrogen bond. Hydrogen bonds play a key role in the properties of water. Water would undoubtedly not have a boiling point as high as 100°C if hydrogen bonding did not occur. You will see in the organic chemistry section that hydrogen bonding is an important intermolecular force.

Hydrogen bond

B. Dipole Interactions (Strength ≈ 5 kcal/mol)

This type of intermolecular attraction takes place between **polar molecules.** These molecules do not have to possess an O, N, or F atom as long as the molecules have a dipole. The positive end of the dipole on one molecule is attracted to the negative end of another molecule. Figure 5-2 shows two examples of dipole interactions.

dipole interation

C. London Dispersion Forces (Strength ≈ 2 kcal/mol)

Attractive forces exist between molecules that do not appear to have an obvious dipole. Because electrons are in constant motion, the charge distribution of a neutral molecule fluctuates. At any instant of time, a molecule may generate a temporary dipole based on the distribution of its electrons. This dipole may set up a dipole in a neighboring molecule. **These temporary or instantaneous dipoles lead to attractive forces termed London forces, or van der Waals forces.**

Van der Waals forces tend to increase with the increasing molecular weight of a molecule because the number of electrons is proportional to molecular weight. You also find that these forces increase with symmetry and decrease with molecular branching. Also, note that all types of molecules have London forces, even if they are polar, are able to hydrogen bond, or both.

Although in some textbooks van der Waals forces include both London forces and dipole–dipole interactions, the terms van der Waals forces and London forces have been used interchangeably on the MCAT.

6

Phase Equilibria

I. Phase Changes and Phase Diagrams

This short chapter is a review of phases and phase diagrams. The MCAT frequently tests your understanding of these concepts. In the physics section, you will review the energy associated with phase changes.

The physical state of a compound depends on temperature and pressure. Changes in temperature and pressure lead to changes of phase. Phase changes are always **reversible** and are therefore in **equilibria.** The different phase changes of a compound are shown through the use of a phase diagram.

I. Phase Changes and Phase Diagrams

A. Solids

Before moving into the phase change material, you should understand something about solids (see Chapter 5 of the General Chemistry Review Notes for a discussion of gases and liquids). **A solid has a definite shape that is resistant to change. At a given temperature, a solid has a fixed volume and density.** The two major types of solids are **amorphous and crystalline solids.**

1. **Amorphous Solids**

   The atoms, molecules, or ions that make up an amorphous solid occur at random positions. The arrangement of particles in the solid follows no ordered pattern. A great example of an amorphous solid is glass.

2. **Crystalline Solids**

   The atoms, molecules, or ions that make up a crystalline solid have a characteristic repetitive pattern. Four important examples of crystalline solids include: **metallic solids** (e.g., iron, aluminum), **molecular solids** (e.g., sugar), **covalent network solids** (e.g., diamond), and **ionic solids** (e.g., NaCl).

B. Phase Changes

Looking at Table 6-1 is the easiest way to review this topic. This simple relationship shows the transition that occurs between the various states of matter. Starting with the lowest energy phase (solid) and adding energy, the entropy (randomness)

SECT. II
GENERAL
CHEMISTRY
REVIEW
NOTES

245

increases, heat is absorbed, and, generally, molar volume increases. This process brings you to the liquid phase. As more energy is added, the liquid phase can undergo a phase change to the gas phase. This change is also associated with an entropy increase and a volume expansion.

TABLE 6-1. Phase changes and associated trends: solid → liquid → gas.

Trends in → direction
Entropy increases
Heat is absorbed
Molar volume increases (exception: ice melting results in a decrease in molar volume)
Boiling occurs when the vapor pressure equals the atmospheric pressure

C. Phase Diagrams

The phase diagram is important because it allows you to predict the phase of a substance based on its temperature and pressure. This diagram is unique for a given substance and shows three phases of the substance plotted as a function of temperature and pressure. A classic phase diagram is shown in Figure 6-1. **The liquid is shown in region A, gas in B, and solid in C.**

FIGURE 6-1.
A phase diagram.

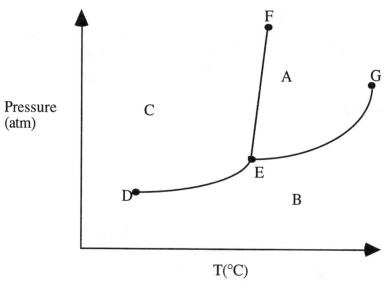

Several terms are important to learn for the MCAT. The line separating solid and gas (line D-E) is the **sublimation line,** which represents where solid and gas are in equilibrium. The line separating solid and liquid (line E-F) is **the freezing or melting line,** which represents where solid and liquid are in equilibrium. The line separating liquid and gas (line E-G) is the **vaporization line,** which represents the equilibrium between vapor and liquid. Finally, point E is the **triple point,** where solid, liquid, and vapor are in equilibrium.

D. Freezing Point, Melting Point, Boiling Point, and Sublimation Point

The definitions of the following terms are important to know. Understand that a compound can change phase at many combinations of temperature and pressure, but the normal values are tabulated at atmospheric pressure.

Freezing point: the temperature at atmospheric pressure at which a liquid changes to the solid phase.

Melting point: the temperature at atmospheric pressure at which a solid changes to the liquid phase.

Boiling point: the temperature at atmospheric pressure at which the liquid changes to a gas. At this point, the vapor pressure is equal to the ambient pressure.

Sublimation point: the temperature at atmospheric pressure at which the solid changes to a gas.

SECT. II
GENERAL
CHEMISTRY
REVIEW
NOTES

247

7

Solution Chemistry

Solution
Chemistry

HIGH-YIELD TOPICS	**I. Definitions and Concepts** **II. Colligative Properties** **III. Solubility and Ksp**

Much of the study of chemistry involves compounds in solution. This topic is critical to your future studies in medical school. Just think . . . the human body is bathed in fluids that represent complex solutions! Understanding solution chemistry is also important in environmental studies, many types of quantitative and qualitative analysis, and many biologic systems.

I. Definitions and Concepts

A. Some Important Definitions

A solution is a homogeneous mixture of two or more substances. Usually, gases or solids are dissolved in liquids. The liquid in which a substance is dissolved is the solvent. The substance that dissolves in the liquid is the solute. Consider the solution made by dissolving salt in water. Salt is the solute and water is the solvent.

Molality is defined as the moles of solute dissolved per kilogram of solvent. If 2 moles of sugar (solute) is dissolved in 1 kilogram of water, the molality is **2 molal.** Molality is an important unit of concentration for the determination of properties that depend on the number of particles in solution. These **colligative properties** are discussed in the next section.

$$\text{Molality (m)} = \frac{\text{moles solute}}{\text{kg solvent}}$$

Ionic compounds dissolve to form more than one particle per solute molecule. In these situations, use the **colligative molality** (m_c):

$$\text{Colligative molality} = m_c = im$$

in which **i** is the number of particles that the ionic compound dissolves into (i.e., $NaCl = 2$, $Mg(OH)_2 = 3$) and **m** is molality.

Miscible solutions are mixtures of two polar solutions (e.g., water and alcohol) or two nonpolar solutions (e.g., carbon tetrachloride and benzene) forming homogeneous, one-phase solutions.

Immiscible solutions are mixtures of a polar with a nonpolar liquid (e.g., water and carbon tetrachloride) forming a two-phase solution.

Ideal solutions are solutions that follow Raoult's law ($P = P_A°X_A + P_B°X_B$). In these solutions, the solute and solvent are chemically similar so that solvent–solute intermolecular forces are equally strong as solvent–solvent or solute–solute intermolecular forces. **Non-ideal solutions** do not follow Raoult's law.

B. Some Important Concepts: Ions in Solution

To understand solutions, you need to picture what is going on at the molecular level. Consider an ionic compound that dissociates to give anions and cations. When ionic compounds are dissolved in water, the species produced are usually individual ions (from the crystalline solid) surrounded by water molecules. Notice in Figure 7-1 that the water molecules are organized so that the negative end of the net dipole (the oxygen atom) is pointed toward the cations (Na^+) and the positive end of the net dipole (the hydrogen atoms) is pointed toward the anions (Cl^-). This positioning helps to dissolve the ionic solid and accounts for the water solubility of many ionic substances.

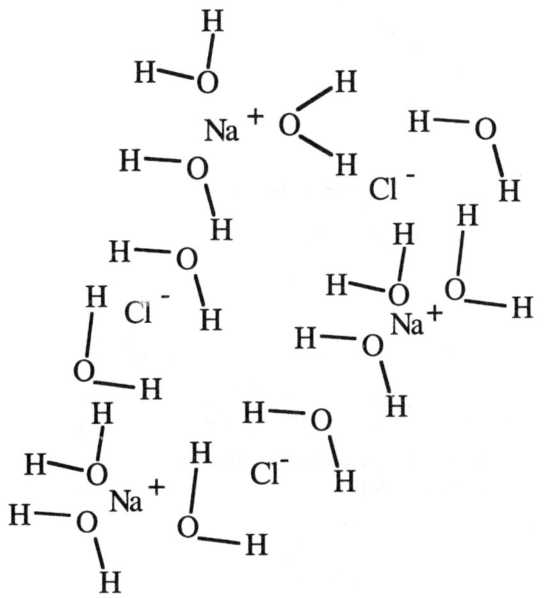

FIGURE 7-1.
An ionic compound dissolving in water.

If ionic compounds can dissolve in a way similar to that shown in Figure 7-1, what about covalent compounds? Unlike ionic compounds, covalent compounds generally do not dissolve by dissociating. Covalent bonds, being less polarized, do not attract water molecules to the extent that the water molecules replace the covalent bonds. On the other hand, ionic compounds dissociate because the strong interaction between the cations and anions can be replaced by many weaker interactions between the ions and the dipoles of the water molecules.

II. Colligative Properties

This topic is frequently tested on the MCAT!

A **colligative property of a solution is any property that varies in proportion to the number of solute particles present** in a given volume of solution. **The identity of the solute is not important.**

This section reviews four specific colligative properties.

A. Solution Vapor Pressure (Raoult's Law)

When you dissolve a solute (nonvolatile) in a solvent (volatile), the vapor pressure of the solution is **lower** than the vapor pressure of the pure solvent.

SECT. II
GENERAL
CHEMISTRY
REVIEW
NOTES

249

The extent of the lowering of the vapor pressure ΔP is the product of the mole fraction of the nonvolatile solute (X_B) and the vapor pressure of the pure solvent (P_A°):

Lowering of vapor pressure of pure solvent: $\Delta P = X_B P_A^\circ$

Figure 7-2 shows what happens as the mole fraction of solvent decreases (right to left). You would expect that pure solvent would have the greatest vapor pressure. As you add solute and the mole fraction of solvent decreases, the vapor pressure decreases.

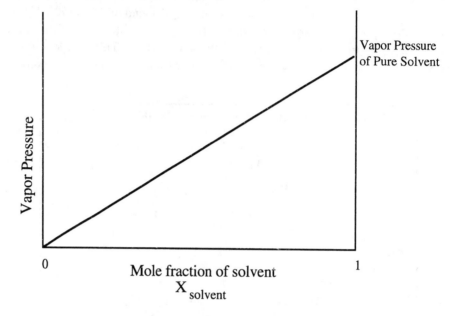

Remember that the sum of the mole fractions is 1, and that the vapor pressure lowering is equal to the pure pressure minus the vapor pressure of the solvent above the solution (P_A). It makes sense that the vapor pressure over the solution, P_A, will be the product of the mole fraction of solvent (X_A) and the vapor pressure of pure solvent (P_A°). This important relationship is known as **Raoult's law.**

$$P_A = X_A\ P_A^\circ$$

P_A = vapor pressure of solvent above solution
X_A = mole fraction of solvent
P_A° = vapor pressure of pure solvent

Example 7-1 shows how you can use Raoult's law to solve problems.

Example 7-1: The vapor pressure of pure water is 350 torr at 78°C. If 0.1 mol of sucrose is dissolved in 50 g of pure water at 78°C, what is the vapor pressure of the solution?

Solution: We use Raoult's law, $P_A = X_A P^\circ_A$:

$$X_A = \frac{\text{mol } H_2O}{\text{mol } H_2O + \text{mol sucrose}}$$

$$\text{mol } H_2O = (50 \text{ g})[(1 \text{ mol } H_2O)/(18 \text{ g } H_2O)] = 2.8 \text{ mol } H_2O$$

$$X_A = \frac{2.8 \text{ mol } H_2O}{2.8 \text{ mol } H_2O + 0.1 \text{ mol sucrose}} = 0.97$$

$$P_A = (0.97)(350 \text{ torr}) = 340 \text{ torr}$$

B. Boiling Point Elevation

When you add a nonvolatile solute to a solution, you **raise** the boiling point of the solution. The boiling point elevation (ΔT_b) of a solution is directly proportional to the **molality** (not molarity) of the solute.

$$\Delta T_b = ik_b m$$

ΔT_b = boiling point elevation

i = number of particles into which the solute dissociates when dissolved in solvent

k_b = constant characteristic for the solvent − units: {(°C)(kg)/(mol)}

m = molality

The higher the concentration of solute added to a pure solvent, the higher the boiling point of the solution. Adding salt to pure water raises the boiling point of the water. The more salt you dissolve in water, the higher the boiling point.

When you add a solute that dissociates in solution, you must take into account each dissociated particle. If you add glucose to water, glucose does not dissociate. You would use an "i" value of 1 for glucose in the equation. If the solute was NaCl, it dissolves in water to give two particles, and you would use an "i" value of 2 in the equation.

As mentioned previously, k_b is a constant of the solvent. For water, the numeric value of the constant is 0.52. Do not worry about memorizing these constants. In any calculation question on the MCAT, the value of k_b will be given. Example 7-2 shows a typical calculation for boiling point elevation:

Example 7-2: 2.0 g NaCl was dissolved in 100 g of water. What was the boiling point of the solution produced?

Solution: We use the boiling point elevation equation, $\Delta T_b = ik_b m$. Note that NaCl dissociates into **2** particles. We will take into account the "i" term in the first equation:

$$m = \frac{\text{mol NaCl}}{\text{kg } H_2O} \times 2 = \frac{2.0 \text{ g NaCl} \times \dfrac{1 \text{ mol NaCl}}{58.5 \text{ g NaCl}}}{0.100 \text{ kg } H_2O} \times 2 = 0.684$$

$$\Delta T_b^\circ = (0.684 \text{ mol/kg})(0.52 \text{ kg}^\circ\text{C/mol}) = 0.36\,^\circ\text{C}$$

$$T_b = 0.36^\circ\text{C} + 100.00^\circ\text{C} = 100.36^\circ\text{C}$$

C. Freezing Point Depression

The freezing point depression is similar in concept to boiling point elevation. **Solutions have lower freezing points than pure solvents.** The change in freezing point of the solution is directly proportional to the molality of the solute.

$$\Delta T_m = -ik_f m$$

ΔT_m = Freezing point depression

i = number of particles into which solute dissolves when dissolved in solvent

k_f = freezing point constant

m = molality of the solution

SECT. II
GENERAL
CHEMISTRY
REVIEW
NOTES

251

The higher the concentration of solute, the lower the freezing point of the solution. The freezing point depression constant for water is 1.86°C kg/mol, which means that each mole of solute per kilogram of water lowers the freezing point of water by 1.86° C. A practical application for freezing point depression is the use of salt on roads and sidewalks during the winter months. Salting lowers the freezing point of collected water and minimizes ice formation. Another good example is the addition of antifreeze to the radiator of a car to lower the freezing point of water in the radiator.

D. Osmotic Pressure

This term describes **the pressure that would have to be applied to a solution to stop the passage of molecules from the pure solvent through a semipermeable membrane into the solution.**

$$\text{Osmotic pressure} = (n/V)RT = MRT$$

n = number of moles of solute

V = solution volume

R = gas constant

T = Kelvin temperature

M = n/V or molar concentration of solute

To see if you understand osmotic pressure, look at Example 7-3:

Example 7-3: You are given two solutions of particles A and B separated by a semipermeable membrane through which A may pass but B may not. What will happen?

Solution: Particles from solution A will diffuse toward the side with the greater concentration of B particles until the pressure of this diffusion ("osmotic pressure") is balanced by increasing hydrostatic resistance. The osmotic pressure is directly proportional to the concentration difference of B particles across the membrane.

III. Solubility and Ksp

Solubility is the amount of solute that dissolves in a fixed amount of solvent so as to produce a saturated (equilibrium) solution. Solubility varies with temperature. Polar or charged compounds (ions) are usually soluble in polar solvents (e.g., water).

A. Units of Concentration

Stoichiometric calculations can also be made for species in solution. The following concentration units help to establish the stoichiometric link. **Molarity** is moles of solute per liter of solution. **Molality** is moles of solute per kilogram of solvent. **Normality** is moles of equivalents per liter of solution. An equivalent of acid is 1 mole of H^+ ions and an equivalent of base is 1 mole of OH^- ions.

Equivalents are determined according to the following guidelines:

1. H^+ if the species involved is an acid (e.g., H_2SO_4 has 2 equivalents of H^+, and H_3PO_4 has 3 equivalents of H^+)
2. OH^- if the species involved is a base (e.g., NaOH has 1 equivalent of OH^-, whereas $Ba(OH)_2$ has 2 equivalents of OH^-)

B. Solubility Product Constant (K_{sp}), and the Equilibrium Expression

On the MCAT, you may be asked to predict whether or not a solution will precipitate or whether or not a solution is saturated. A useful relationship to know about is the solubility product constant, or K_{sp}. The symbol [ ] represents the concentration in moles per liter.

Given an equation for an ionic solid dissolving in water:

$$A_xB_y(s) \rightarrow xA^+(aq) + yB^-(aq)$$

K_{sp} is defined as follows:

$$\mathbf{K_{sp} = [A^+]^x[B^-]^y}$$

The K_{sp} can be used to predict when precipitation will occur. Because the K_{sp} represents the maximum value of the ion product, **any calculated ion product that is greater than K_{sp} means that precipitation will occur.**

Consider an ionic solid, like NaCl, that dissociates in water. The concentration of the sodium ion multiplied by the chloride ion is the equilibrium expression for this dissociation. If the product of the concentration of sodium and chloride ion exceeds the given K_{sp} for this reaction, NaCl will precipitate. If the equilibrium expression is less than K_{sp}, precipitation will not occur. Another useful piece of information: **the higher the K_{sp}, the more soluble the compound.**

C. Quantitation of Solubility

You may be asked to solve simple solubility problems. These problems involve a solid that is dissolved in water to saturation. You may be asked to calculate the concentration of ions in this system. Always make sure that the solution is at *equilibrium*. Words like "saturated" and "solubility" imply equilibrium (Examples 7-4 and 7-5).

Example 7-4: Calculate the solubility of AgCl and estimate the concentrations of ions in the saturated solution. The K_{sp} of AgCl = 10^{-10}.

Solution: Define x as the amount of solid that dissolves in moles per liter:

1. Write the dissolution reaction:

     $AgCl(s) \longrightarrow Ag^+(aq) + Cl^-(aq)$

2. Set up an inventory in which I = **initial** concentrations of ions before any solid dissolves, C = change in amounts **during the reaction**, and E = **equilibrium** concentrations. The initial amount of solid is irrelevant because the solution is saturated with it and therefore it had unit activity:

	AgCl(s) $\longrightarrow$	Ag$^+$	+	Cl$^-$
I		0		0
C	-x	+x		+x
E	-----	x		x

3. Plug into the K_{sp} expression and solve for x:

     $K_{sp} = [Ag^+][Cl^-] = [x][x] = x^2 = 10^{-10}$
     $x = 10^{-5}$, therefore the solubility = 10^{-5} M and $[Ag^+] = [Cl^-] = 10^{-5}$ M

SECT. II
GENERAL
CHEMISTRY
REVIEW
NOTES

253

Example 7-5: Consider that we added enough of the hypothetic solid A_2B to form a saturated solution. Electrolysis studies demonstrate 0.0002 mol of A^+ per liter of solution. Calculate the solubility product for the hypothetical solid.

Solution:

1. Write the dissolution reaction:
$$A_2B(s) \longrightarrow 2A^+(aq) + B^{2-}(aq)$$

2. Set up an appropriate inventory table:

	$A_2B(s)$	=	$2A^+$	+	B^{2-}
I			0		0
C	-x		+2x		+x
E			2x		x

3. Write the K_{sp} expression:
$$K_{sp} = [A^+]^2[B^{2-}] = (2x)^2(x) = 4x^3$$

4. Now the hard part: realize that because the concentration of A is known, you know the value of 2x. 2x = 0.0002 M, hence x = 0.0001 M. Now you can plug into the equilibrium expression above and solve for the K_{sp}:
$$K_{sp} = 4(0.0001)^3 = 4(10^{-4})^3 = 4 \times 10^{-12}$$

D. Common Ion Effect

The solubility of a salt is decreased if an ion of this salt is already present in a solution. This principle is known as the **common ion effect.** Take for example the addition of KCl to a solution containing NaCl. The solubility of KCl is less than it would otherwise be because the solution contains a source of Cl^- ions. The Cl^- ion in this case is called the **"common ion."** The presence of a common ion decreases the solubility of KCl.

In general, the addition of an ion A^+ or B^- (as part of another component) to the same solution decreases the solubility of A and/or B and leads to more AB "precipitating out." These changes can be predicted by applying Le Chatelier's principle (see Chapter 12 of the General Chemistry Review Notes). To better understand the common ion effect, consider Example 7-6.

Example 7-6: What would be the solubility of AgCl in 1.0 M NaCl? How does this value compare to the results obtained in Example 7-4?

Solution:

1. Write the dissolution reaction:
$$AgCl(s) \longrightarrow Ag^+(aq) + Cl^-(aq)$$

2. Set up the appropriate inventory chart **(note the difference!)** 1.0 M NaCl dissolves to give 1 mole Cl^- ions.

	$AgCl(s)$	=	Ag^+	+	Cl^-
I			0		1.0
C	-x		+x		+x
E			x		1.0 + x

3. Write the equilibrium constant, K_{sp}, expression:

$$K_{sp} = [Ag^+][Cl^-] = (x)(1.0 + x) = 10^{-10}$$

4. Solve for x: You can assume that x is small in comparison to 1.0 M so the Cl⁻ concentration can be assumed to be 1.0 M.

$$K_{sp} = x = 10^{-10} M = [Ag^+]$$

Without added chloride, the concentration of Ag^+ is 10^{-5}, which is 10^5 times more concentrated. You can see that the common ion effect **greatly decreases the solubility of a compound.**

E. Nomenclature, Formulas, and Charges of Some Common Ions

Table 7-1 summarizes some common ions. Remember that the most frustrating type of MCAT question to miss is one that would have been easy to answer if you only knew which compound (or ion) the test writers were talking about!

TABLE 7-1. Common ions.

Name	Formula	Charge
Ammonium	NH_4	+ 1
Mercurous	Hg_2	+ 2
Carbonate	CO_3	− 2
Chlorate	ClO_3	− 1
Chromate	CrO_4	− 2
Cyanide	CN	− 1
Dichromate	Cr_2O_7	− 2
Dihydrogen phosphate	H_2PO_4	− 1
Hydrogen carbonate (bicarbonate)	HCO_3	− 1
Hydrogen phosphate	HPO_4	− 2
Hydrogen sulfate (bisulfate)	HSO_4	− 1
Hydroxide	OH	− 1
Nitrate	NO_3	− 1
Nitrite	NO_2	− 1
Permanganate	MnO_4	− 1
Peroxide	O_2	− 2
Phosphate	PO_4	− 2
Sulfate	SO_4	− 2
Sulfite	SO_3	− 2
Thiocyanate	SCN	− 1

SECT. II
GENERAL
CHEMISTRY
REVIEW
NOTES

255

Acids and Bases

and Bases

HIGH-YIELD TOPICS	**I.** Acid–Base Systems
	II. Acid–Base Strength
	III. Acid–Base Titrations

Understanding acid–base reactions is one of the most important facets of chemistry. Three systems are used to classify acids and bases, and each system has its own advantages. This chapter provides a review of each of these classification systems, as well as the major concepts that are covered on the MCAT. Try to understand both the qualitative and quantitative aspects of this material.

I. Acid–Base Systems

A. Three Acid–Base Systems

1. **Arrhenius Acids–Bases**

   The first and simplest definition of acids and bases is the Arrhenius definition. **An Arrhenius acid is a substance that dissociates to form H⁺ in water. An Arrhenius base is a substance that dissociates to form OH⁻ in water.** This definition of acids–bases has been superseded by the more useful Brønsted and Lewis definitions of acids and bases.

2. **Brønsted Acids–Bases**

   A **Brønsted-Lowry acid is a species that donates protons (H⁺). A Brønsted-Lowry base is a species that gains or accepts protons.** Look at Example 8-1. Water is acting as a Brønsted-Lowry acid and donating a proton to ammonia. The ammonia acts as a Brønsted-Lowry base and accepts the proton. Conjugate acids and bases are formed (see review in subsequent section of this chapter).

Example 8-1: NH_3 + H_2O ⟶ NH_4^+ + OH^-
(base)   (acid)   (conjugate acid)   (conjugate base)

---

3. **Lewis acids-bases**

A **Lewis acid is a species that accepts electrons. A Lewis base is a species that donates electrons.** The Lewis system is useful for classifying reactions that occur in solvents other than water or in situations in which there is no solvent. A Lewis acid–base reaction is shown in Example 8-2.

$$\text{Example 8-2: } BF_3 \; + \; F^- \longrightarrow BF_4^-$$
$$\qquad\qquad\quad \text{(acid)} \quad \text{(base)}$$

B. Ionization of Water

1. **Definition of K_w**

The dissociation constant K_w is a measure of the tendency of water to dissociate into H^+ and OH^-. Quantitatively, it is a measure of the stability of water and has a constant value at room temperature of 1.0×10^{-14}.

$$H_2O \rightarrow H^+ + OH^- \quad \mathbf{K_w = [H^+][OH^-] = 1.0 \times 10^{-14}}$$

Because water does not appear in the equilibrium constant expression, K_w is sometimes referred to as an ion-product, as is K_{sp}. By looking at the small numeric value of K_w, notice that water does not tend to dissociate and is therefore stable.

2. **Definition of pH**

The pH and pOH of pure water are as follows:

$$\mathbf{pH = -\log_{10}[H^+] \quad pOH = -\log_{10}[OH^-]}$$

The pH of pure water is 7 at room temperature. Acid solutions have pH < 7, whereas bases have pH > 7 at room temperature.

C. Conjugate Acids and Bases

Think about what happens in a Brønsted-Lowry acid–base reaction. When a Brønsted-Lowry acid donates a proton, it loses its proton to form the conjugate base of that acid. When a Brønsted-Lowry base gains the proton lost by the original acid, it is converted into the conjugate acid of that base.

Look at Figure 8-1. Notice that HA, a weak acid, has donated a proton to water. HA then becomes the conjugate base, A^-. When water accepts a proton, it acts as a Brønsted-Lowry base and forms its conjugate acid, H_3O^+. Notice that conjugate acid–base pairs differ by only one proton.

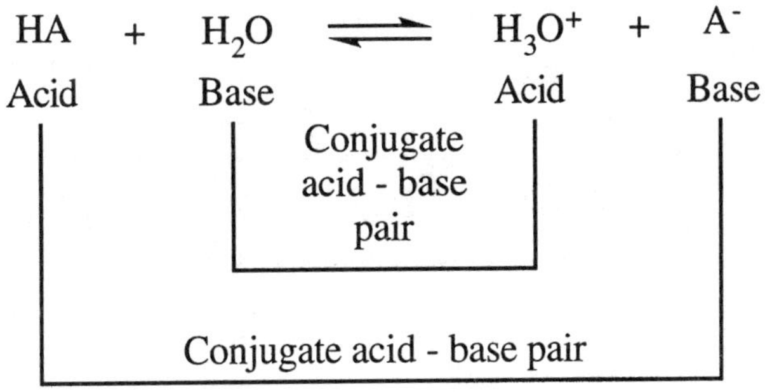

$$HA \; + \; H_2O \; \rightleftharpoons \; H_3O^+ \; + \; A^-$$

Acid   Base   Acid   Base

Conjugate
acid - base
pair

Conjugate acid - base pair

FIGURE 8-1.
Formation of conjugate acid–base pairs.

SECT. II
GENERAL
CHEMISTRY
REVIEW
NOTES

257

II. Acid–Base Strength

A. Strong Acids and Bases

Strong acids and bases **dissociate completely** in aqueous solutions.

$$\text{Strong Acid: } HX + H_2O \rightarrow H_3O^+ + X^-$$

$$\text{Strong Base: } YOH \rightarrow Y^+ + OH^-$$

When the dissociation reactions have gone to completion, there is no measurable concentration of HX or YOH; all of the acid or base has completely dissociated.

Study the important strong acids and bases listed in Table 8-1. This knowledge will help you decide whether or not the acid or base is completely dissociated. Knowing about the dissociation helps you solve both conceptual and calculation-based problems.

TABLE 8-1. Important strong acids and bases.

Strong Acids		Strong Bases	
$HClO_4$	Perchloric acid	Most Group I and II hydroxides, including:	
HNO_3	Nitric acid	LiOH	Lithium hydroxide
H_2SO_4	Sulfuric acid (first proton)	NaOH	Sodium hydroxide
HCl	Hydrochloric acid	KOH	Potassium hydroxide
HBr	Hydrobromic acid	$Ca(OH)_2$	Calcium hydroxide
HI	Hydroiodic acid		

B. Weak Acids

Unlike strong acids, **weak acids are only partially dissociated in water.** A weak acid, such as acetic acid, is less than 2% dissociated in water. You can write the following acid dissociation (ionization) reaction for weak acids in water:

$$HA + H_2O \rightleftharpoons H_3O^+ + A^-$$

1. Acid Ionization Constant

Like other equilibrium reactions, you can write an equilibrium expression, called an acid ionization expression, with the corresponding acid ionization constant (K_a).

$$K_a = \frac{[H_3O^+][A^-]}{[HA]}$$

An "a" is added to the equilibrium constant to remind you that K_a is an acid-dissociation constant. Notice that the $H_2O_{(1)}$ does not appear in the expression for K_a and can be ignored. Example 8-3 shows you how to calculate the K_a:

Example 8-3: At equilibrium, a 0.050 M aqueous solution of chloroacetic acid, $ClCH_2COOH(aq)$, was found to contain 7.57×10^{-3} M H_3O^+. What is the K_a for this reaction?

Solution:

    1. Write the reaction:

$$ClCH_2COOH + H_2O \rightleftharpoons H_3O^+ + ClCH_2COO^-$$

    2. Write the K_a expression:

$$K_a = \frac{[H_3O^+][ClCH_2COO^-]}{[ClCH_2COOH]}$$

    3. Determine equilibrium concentrations:

$$[H_3O^+] = [ClCH_2COO^-] = 7.57 \times 10^{-3} \text{ M}$$

$$[ClCH_2COOH] = 0.050 \text{ M} - 7.57 \times 10^{-3} \text{ M} = 0.042 \text{ M}$$

$$K_a = \frac{(7.57 \times 10^{-3} \text{ M})^2}{0.042 \text{ M}} = 1.4 \times 10^{-3} \text{ M}$$

Acids with large K_a values are stronger than those with small K_a values. Consider chloroacetic acid ($K_a = 1.36 \times 10^{-3}$ M). You would expect chloroacetic acid to be stronger than acetic acid ($K_a = 1.74 \times 10^{-5}$ M) because chloroacetic acid has a larger K_a value.

Strong acids have K_a values greater than 1. Weak acids have K_a values considerably less than 1.

Many times it is more convenient to compare the pK_a of an acid, which is defined by the following equation:

$$\mathbf{pK_a = -\log K_a}$$

The smaller the pK_a, the stronger the acid. Considering the preceding example of chloroacetic acid and acetic acid, you would expect the chloroacetic acid to have the smaller pK_a because it is the stronger acid (pK_a of chloroacetic acid is 2.87 and the pK_a of acetic acid is 4.76).

2. **Calculating the pH of Weak Acid Solutions**

When calculating the pH of a weak acid solution, you may want to set up a concentration table similar to the one you use for solubility problems. For the general reaction below, you can make the following table:

Concentration	HA	+	H_2O	$\rightleftharpoons$	H_3O^+	+	A^-
Initial	Y		——		O		O
Change	$-X$		——		$+X$		$+X$
Equilibrium	$Y - X$		——		X		X

Now you can plug the values that you listed in the table back into the equilibrium expression:

$$K_a = \frac{[H_3O^+][A^-]}{[HA]} = \frac{X^2}{Y - X}$$

In the next step, solve for X. You can either use the quadratic equation, or simplify the equation by making an assumption. Do not expect to have to solve the quadratic equation on the MCAT. The assumption that must be made is that X is small compared with Y. When X is small compared with Y, $Y - X$ is approx-

SECT. II
GENERAL
CHEMISTRY
REVIEW
NOTES

259

imately equal to Y:

$$K_a \approx \frac{X^2}{Y}$$

Example 8-4 shows a typical weak acid problem:

Example 8-4: The value of K_a for an aqueous solution of hypochlorous acid, $HClO$ (aq), is 3.0×10^{-8} M. What is the pH of a 0.1 M solution?

Solution:

Step 1. Set up a table:

Reaction	$HClO + H_2O$	$\rightleftharpoons$	H_3O^+	$+$	ClO^-
[Initial]	0.1 M		0		0
[Change]	-X		+X		+X
[Equilibrium]	0.1 M - X		X		X

Step 2. Make the assumption that X is less than 0.1 M, and write the K_a expression:

$$K_a = \frac{X^2}{0.1\ M} = 3.0 \times 10^{-8}\ M$$

Step 3. Solve for X:

$$X = 5.4 \times 10^{-5}\ M$$

Step 4. Calculate the pH:

$$pH = -\log 5.4 \times 10^{-5}\ M = 4.26$$

C. Weak Bases

Weak bases, unlike strong bases, do not usually dissociate to produce hydroxide. Weak bases act as **proton acceptors,** according to the Brønsted definition of bases.

Water acts as the proton donor, producing hydroxide. You can write a base protonation equation using either of two forms:

1. $B + H_2O \rightleftharpoons BH^+ + OH^-$

2. $B^- + H_2O \rightleftharpoons BH + OH^-$

Like weak acids, the equilibrium lies well to the left, and you describe it with a base ionization equilibrium expression.

1. Base Ionization Constant

The base ionization constant K_b is analogous to the K_a, although the "b" is added to designate that the ionization constant is for the base. Considering equations 1 and 2, the K_b expressions would take the following form:

$$K_b = \frac{[BH^+][OH^-]}{[B]} \quad \text{equation 1}$$

$$K_b = \frac{[BH][OH^-]}{[B^-]} \quad \text{equation 2}$$

Just as for K_a, **the larger the K_b, the stronger the base.** You can also use pK_b for ease of comparison.

$$pK_b = -\log K_b$$

The smaller the pK_b, the stronger the base. For example, ammonia has a pK_b of 4.74, whereas water has a pK_b of 7. Thus, ammonia is a stronger base than water.

In aqueous solutions, two important relationships are true at 25°C and are useful in MCAT calculation questions:

1. **pH + pOH = 14.** This relationship is derived from the K_w expression.

2. **$K_a K_b = K_w$.** This relationship is true for any acid-conjugate base pair, and can be proven by simply substituting $[A^-][H^+]/[HA]$ for the K_a and $[HA][OH^-]/[A^-]$ for the K_b.

2. **Calculating the pH of an Aqueous Solution of a Weak Base**

This calculation is similar to that for a weak acid. Assume that the amount of OH^- formed at equilibrium is small. For a general base reaction, you can make the following table:

Reaction	B	+	H_2O	$\rightleftharpoons$	BH^+	+ OH^-
Initial	Y		——-		0	0
Change	−X		——-		+X	+X
Equilibrium	Y − X		——-		X	X

Now, set up the K_b expression and plug in the values from the table. Assume that because you are dealing with a weak base, X will be small and thus, Y − X = Y. Your value for K_b should be:

$$K_b = \frac{X^2}{Y}$$

Example 8-5 shows how to work with weak base problems.

Example 8-5: Calculate the pH of a 0.1 M aqueous solution of ammonia if ammonia has a K_b of 1.8×10^{-5}.

Solution:

Step 1. Set up a table:

Reaction	$NH_3 + H_2O$	$\rightleftharpoons$	NH_4^+	+ OH^-
[Initial]	0.1		0	0
[Change]	-X		+X	+X
[Equilibrium]	0.1 - X		X	X

Step 2. Make the assumption that X is less than 0.1 M, and write the K_b expression:

$$K_b = \frac{X^2}{0.1\ M} = 1.8 \times 10^{-5}$$

SECT. II
GENERAL
CHEMISTRY
REVIEW
NOTES

261

Step 3. Solve for X:

$$X = 1.3 \times 10^{-3} \text{ M}$$

Step 4. Calculate the pH (a short cut for solving for the pH of a basic solution uses the following relationship presented previously):

$$pOH + pH = 14 \text{ and } pH = 14 - pOH$$
$$pOH = -\log OH^- = -\log(1.3 \times 10^{-3})M = 2.87$$
$$pH = 14.00 - 2.87 = 11.13$$

D. Acidity or Basicity of Aqueous Salt Solutions

Hydrolysis is the reaction of a salt (from the conjugate acid or base of a weak acid or base, respectively) with water to produce an acidic or a basic solution. Recall that the conjugate base of the weak acid HA is A^-, and the conjugate acid of the base NH_3 is NH_4^+.

1. Hydrolysis Constant

This concept is similar to the base association concept. Hydrolysis has a characteristic constant called **K_h,** which is the same as the K_a if the salt contains the conjugate acid of a weak base, or the same as the K_b if the salt contains the conjugate base of a weak acid. **This constant measures the tendency of a conjugate acid or conjugate base to associate with water.** Examples of this concept follow:

Acidic Solution: $NH_4^+ + H_2O \rightleftharpoons H_3O^+ + NH_3$ (The ammonium ion acts as an acid)

$$K_h = K_a = [NH_3][H_3O^+]/[NH_4^+] = K_w/K_b$$

Basic Solution: $CN^- + H_2O \rightleftharpoons HCN + OH^-$ (The cyanide ion acts as a base)

$$K_h = K_b = [OH^-][HCN]/[CN^-] = K_w/K_a$$

Negatively charged ions usually act as bases, and positively charged ions usually act as acids (Example 8-6).

Example 8-6: Solve for the pH of a 1.0 M NaA solution.
K_a for HA $= 1.0 \times 10^{-6}$.

1. Write the hydrolysis reaction for a base in water:
$$A^- + H_2O \rightleftharpoons HA + OH^-$$

2. Set up an inventory and solve the problem:

	A^-	+	H_2O	$\rightleftharpoons$	HA	+	OH^-
I	1.0				0		0
C	-X				+X		+X
E	1.0 - X				X		X

$$K_b = K_w/K_a = [HA][OH^-]/[A^-] = (X)(X)/(1-X) = 1.0 \times 10^{-8}$$

Thus, $X = 1.0 \times 10^{-4}$ M, pOH = 4 and pH = 10

---

2. **Calculation of pH of Solutions of Weak Acids or Bases and their Salts**

The calculation of the pH of solutions containing either an acid and its conjugate base from different sources or a base and its conjugate acid from different sources is not any more difficult than any other calculation. The main difference is that initial concentrations for two species are now a value other than zero (Example 8-7).

Example 8-7: Calculate the pH of a 1.0 M NH_3 solution in 0.1 M NH_4^+. K_b of ammonia is 1.8×10^{-5}.

1. Write the base hydrolysis reaction:
$$NH_3 + H_2O \rightleftharpoons NH_4^+ + OH^-$$

2. Set up an the appropriate inventory chart:

	NH_3	$+ H_2O \rightleftharpoons$	NH_4^+	$+ OH^-$
i	1.0		0.1	0
C	-X		+X	+X
E	1 - X		0.1 + X	X

3. Solve for X, and answer the question asked:

$K_b = [OH^-][NH_4^+]/[NH_3] = (0.1 + X)(X)/(1-X) = 10^{-5}$ M

Neglecting X in comparison to 1 and to 0.1, the equation reduces to $(0.1)(X)/(1) = 1.8 \times 10^{-5}$

Solving for X yields: $X = 1.8 \times 10^{-4}$ M = $[OH^-]$. By estimation, pOH = 3.74, and pH = 10.26

III. Acid–Base Titrations

A. Titration Curves

When strong acids or bases react with each other or with weak acids or bases, an essentially irreversible quantitative reaction takes place. **Titration is the measurement of the solution volume of one reactant that is required to react completely with a specified amount of another reactant.** If you titrate a known volume of an unknown acid or base (weak or strong) with a known amount of a strong acid or base, you can use the following relationship to calculate the concentration of the unknown:

$$N_1V_1 = N_2V_2$$

N_1 = Normality of known acid or base

V_1 = Volume of known acid or base

N_2 = Normality of unknown acid or base

V_2 = Volume of unknown acid or base

Remember that **normality** refers to the equivalents of acid (H^+) or base (OH^-) per liter of solution. You can convert molarity to normality by taking into account the number of moles of H^+ or OH^- that an acid or base produces when dissociated. A 1

SECT. II
GENERAL
CHEMISTRY
REVIEW
NOTES

263

M solution of the monoprotic acid HCl would give a 1 N solution, because HCl only produces 1 mole of H^+ when completely dissociated. On the other hand, a 1 M solution of the strong diprotic acid H_2SO_4 would give a 2 N solution, because each mole of this acid produces 2 moles of H^+ ions when completely dissociated.

In the titration of an acid with a base, a plot of the pH of the resulting solution as a function of the added base is a **titration curve.** Figure 8-2 shows the titration of strong acid by strong base.

FIGURE 8-2.

Titration of strong acid with strong base.

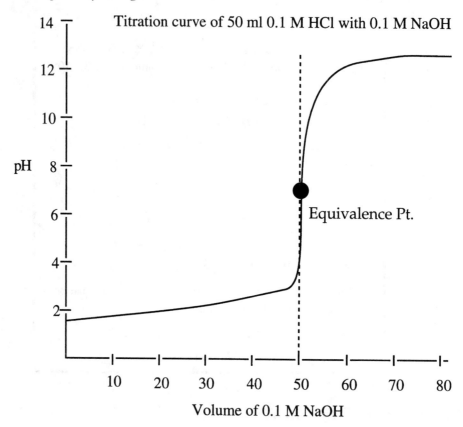

Note that the **equivalence point** is the point in the titration where a chemically equivalent amount of base and acid have been mixed. The titration of a strong acid with strong base is shown in Figure 8-2 with the equivalence point for that titration.

The shapes of the titration curves obtained from titrating acids and bases are important to know. The titration of a strong acid (e.g., HCl) with strong base (e.g., NaOH) produces the classic curve shown at left in Figure 8-3. If titration of a weak acid (e.g., acetic acid) with a strong base (e.g., NaOH) is performed, a slightly different shaped curve is obtained (at right in Figure 8-3). For the titration of a weak acid with a strong

FIGURE 8-3.

Titration curves of strong acid with strong base (left) and weak acid with strong base (right). Note the equivalence point for each titration.

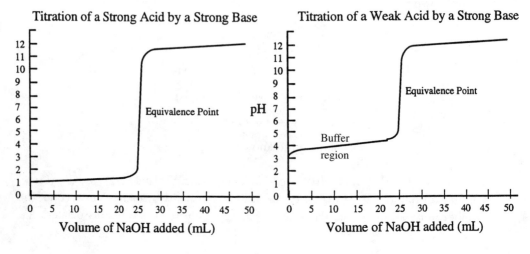

base, there is a relatively flat portion of the curve, which is called the **buffer region.** In this region, there are significant concentrations of both the weak acid and its conjugate base (thus the solution is a **buffer**). Note that the pH changes very slowly in the buffer region. Note that the titration of the weak acid starts at a higher pH because the acid is weak (not fully dissociated). For both curves, the pH changes slowly at first, then rises rapidly. For the titration of weak acid with strong base, however, notice that the pH rise is not as great as titration of strong acid by strong base.

Another important point about weak acid titrations is the **halfway point** of the titration. The halfway point occurs when half of the acid or base has been reacted. The pH corresponding to this point equals the pK_a of the acid. Why? Because at this point, $[HA] = [A^-]$, and the acid is half-converted to its conjugate base. Thus,

$$K_a = [H_3O^+][A^-]/[HA] \text{ and } [HA] = [A^-]$$

This reduces to $K_a = [H_3O^+]$. Thus, $pH = pK_a$ at the halfway point.

B. Indicators

Most acid–base titrations are colorless and no physical change takes place to indicate when the reaction has gone to completion. How are you to know when the equivalence point is reached?

Indicators are conjugate acid–base pairs that are added to titration mixtures in small molar amounts to monitor pH. **The acidic and basic forms of the indicator are different colors.** Indicators tend to react with excess acid or base in titrations to form a colored product, which you can see. The pH range at which an indicator changes color depends on its pK_a. Generally, when choosing an indicator for a titration, select the indicator that has its color change at or near the equivalence point of the titration. The indicator you select should have its color change at pH values within the steep portion of the titration curve. Table 8-2 is a list of some common indicators.

TABLE 8-2. Some common indicators*.

Indicator	Color of Acidic Form	Color of Basic Form	Range of Color Change	pK_a
Methyl orange	Red	Yellow	3.1–4.4	3.7
Bromcresol green	Yellow	Blue	3.8–5.4	4.7
Chlorophenol red	Yellow	Red	5.2–6.8	6.2
Phenol Red	Yellow	Red	6.4–8.2	7.8
Phenolphthalein	Colorless	Pink	8.0–9.8	9.7

*Do not memorize these, but note that the pK_a of the indicator is in the pH range of the color change.

C. Neutralization

Neutralization is the reaction between an acid and a base. An example of a neutralization reaction is shown in Figure 8-4. The products of the reaction of a strong acid and a strong base are an ionic compound (salt) and water. The resulting solution is neutralized if equal equivalents of acid and base are used.

$$\underset{\text{Acid}}{H_2SO_{4(aq)}} + \underset{\text{Base}}{2KOH} \rightleftharpoons \underset{\text{Salt}}{K_2SO_{4(aq)}} + 2H_2O_{(1)}$$

FIGURE 8-4.
Reaction of a strong acid and a strong base producing a salt. In this example, a neutral solution is produced.

When a strong acid and a strong base neutralize each other, a neutral solution is formed (pH = 7). When a weak acid reacts with a strong base, however, the resulting solution is basic (Figure 8-5). Likewise, reacting a weak base with a strong acid yields an acidic solution (Figure 8-6).

FIGURE 8-5.
Reaction of a weak acid and strong base. A basic solution is produced.

$$CH_3COOH_{(aq)} + NaOH_{(aq)} \rightleftharpoons CH_3COO^-Na^+ + H_2O_{(l)}$$
$$\text{Acid} \qquad\qquad \text{Base} \qquad\qquad \text{Salt}$$

FIGURE 8-6.
Reaction of a weak base with a strong acid. An acidic solution is produced.

$$NH_{3(aq)} + HCl_{(aq)} \rightleftharpoons NH_4^+ Cl^-_{(aq)} + H_2O_{(l)}$$
$$\text{Base} \qquad \text{Acid} \qquad\quad \text{Salt}$$

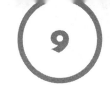
Buffers

Buffers

Buffers

| I. Major Concepts and Definitions | **HIGH-YIELD** |
| II. Effect on Titration Curves | **TOPICS** |

Buffers and their behavior are a common trouble spot for many students. For the MCAT, you need to understand what a buffer is and how buffer systems are useful in chemistry. This chapter offers a review of the meaning of buffering and how buffer solutions are important in acid–base chemistry.

As a future physician, you should know that the human body depends on buffer systems. For example, our body uses the bicarbonate/carbonic acid buffer system to resist changes in blood pH. Failure of the blood to buffer pH results in severe illness or death.

I. Major Concepts and Definitions

A buffer is a solution that contains either a weak acid and its conjugate base or a weak base and its conjugate acid. Buffer solutions resist a change in pH by neutralizing either an added acid or an added base.

The graph in Figure 9-1 differs from a titration curve because pH is plotted on the x-axis. Consider a buffer solution, which contains a weak acid and its conjugate base (salt).

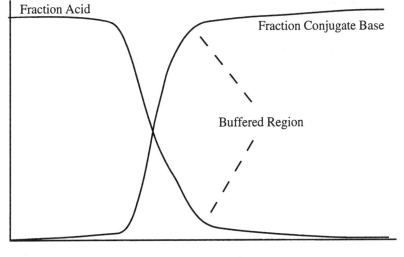

FIGURE 9-1.
pH stability within a buffered region. Note that the buffer region occurs when both the acid and its conjugate base are present.

SECT. II
GENERAL
CHEMISTRY
REVIEW
NOTES

267

Note that at very low pH, the only form present is the acid form. As the pH increases, both the acid form and its conjugate base are present. When both an acid and its conjugate base are present, the solution is buffered; added acid or base will change the proportion of acid and conjugate base without strongly affecting the pH (see the region of the graph labeled "buffered region"). Notice that this region occurs within a narrow pH range. At very high pH, only the basic form is present and the pH changes significantly with added acid and base. Thus, only when both species are present is a solution an effective buffer.

Example 9-1 shows what goes on in buffer systems.

Example 9-1: A common buffer is made from acetic acid and the salt of its conjugate base, sodium acetate. What relevant equilibria take place when an acid or base is added?

Added acid: $CH_3COO^- + H^+ \rightleftharpoons CH_3COOH$

Added base: $CH_3COOH + OH^- \rightleftharpoons CH_3COO^- + H_2O$

The **Henderson-Hasselbach equation** is used to calculate the pH of a buffer using the stoichiometric concentrations of the weak acid and conjugate base. This equation is simply a rearrangement of the K_a expression, which could also be used.

$$\text{Henderson-Hasselbach equation: } pH = pK_a + \log \frac{[\text{Base}]}{[\text{Acid}]}$$

Example 9-2 shows how to use the Henderson-Hasselbach equation.

Example 9-2: What is the pH of a buffer that is 0.1 M acetic acid and 0.1 M sodium acetate with the pK_a of acetic acid = 4.76?

Solution: Using the Henderson-Hasselbach equation:

$$pH = pK_a + \log \frac{\text{Base}}{\text{Acid}} = 4.76 + \log \frac{[0.1]}{[0.1]} = 4.76$$

This example shows that whenever the concentrations of the acid and conjugate base are equal to each other, $pH = pK_a$.

The Henderson-Hasselbach equation can also be used to calculate the pH of a buffer solution to which an acid or base has been added. Simply use an inventory table to determine the values to insert (Example 9-3).

Example 9-3: What is the pH of 100 ml of a buffer that is 0.1 M acetic acid and 0.1 M sodium acetate after the addition of 20 ml of 0.1 M HCl?

Solution:

1. Write the equation:

$CH_3COO^- + H^+ \rightleftharpoons CH_3COOH$

---

2. Calculate the moles of each species initially:

$CH_3COO^- = 0.1\ L \times 0.1\ M = 0.01$ mol

$CH_3COOH = 0.1\ L \times 0.1\ M = 0.01$ mol

$HCl\ (H^+) = 0.02\ L \times 0.1\ M = 0.002$ mol

3. Set up an inventory table:

Amount	CH_3COO^- +	H^+ $\rightleftharpoons$	CH_3COOH
Initial	0.01 mol	0.002 mol	0.01 mol
Change	-0.002 mol	?	+0.002 mol
Final	0.008 mol	?	0.012 mol

4. Solve for pH using the Henderson-Hasselbach equation:

$$pH = pK_a + \log \frac{Base}{Acid} = 4.76 + \log \frac{(0.008)}{(0.012)} = 4.58$$

Note: Be aware that you can use moles instead of concentration units in the calculation because the units divide out. Also, note the pH of the solution changed very little with the addition of acid—the importance of buffers!

The **buffer capacity** of a solution is the amount of acid or base that can be added before a drastic change in the pH of the buffer occurs. Solutions with high concentrations of acid and conjugate base have greater buffer capacity.

The **buffer region** on a titration curve is the region in which the pH does not change drastically with the addition of acid or base (see titration curves in Chapter 8 of the General Chemistry Review Notes). The buffer region is usually about 1 pH unit above and below the pK_a.

Buffers are used to control the pH of chemical and physiologic reactions. In a reaction run in a buffer, the H^+ concentration does not change as long as the buffer capacity is not exceeded. The activity of many enzymes depends greatly on pH, and numerous biochemical systems have buffer systems to control enzyme activity.

II. Effect of Buffers on Titration Curves

Buffers have a noticeable effect on the shape of a titration curve. In Chapter 8 of the General Chemistry Review Notes, two titration curves were compared: one was for strong acid titrated with strong base and the other was a weak acid titrated with a strong base. To understand what is going on at the molecular level, consider the titration of a weak acid with a strong base. This type of titration involves a buffer system. As base is added to a weak acid, some of the salt of the conjugate base forms. As more base is added, it continues to react with the weak acid rather than the H^+ in solution, and the pH changes slowly during the early part of the titration. Figure 9-2 shows the titration curve for the titration of 50 ml of 0.10 M CH_3COOH with 0.10 M NaOH.

The concentration of a species in solution at any point along the titration curve can be determined by choosing the correct equilibrium equation, and using either the K_a, K_b, or the Henderson-Hasselbach equation. The following examples use the titration curve shown in Figure 9-2 and show the calculation of the pH at points A to E. Note that the curve only shows an approximation of the location of each point. The calculated value of pH for each point is the most accurate. Rather than focusing on the details of the calculations, make sure that you understand how to arrive at the pH in each example.

SECT. II
GENERAL
CHEMISTRY
REVIEW
NOTES

269

FIGURE 9-2.
Titration of a weak acid
(acetic acid) with a strong base
(sodium hydroxide).

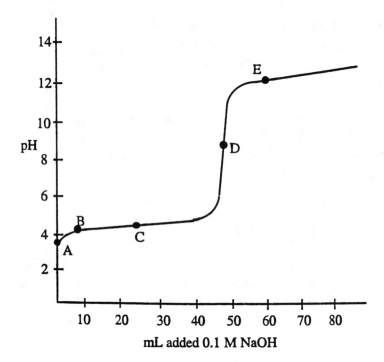

At point A in Example 9-4, only 50 ml of 0.1 M acetic acid are present.

Example 9-4: Calculate the pH at **point A** on the graph.

$$(K_a = 1.74 \times 10^{-5} \text{ M})$$

Solution:

1. Write equation:

$$CH_3COOH + H_2O \rightleftharpoons CH_3COO^- + H_3O^+$$

2. Set up an inventory table:

	$\underline{CH_3COOH}$ + H₂O $\rightleftharpoons$	$\underline{CH_3COO^-}$ +	$\underline{H_3O^+}$
Initial	0.1 M	0	0
Change	-X	+X	+X
Equilib.	0.1 M-X	X	X

3. Plug into K_a expression, assuming that 0.1-X = 0.1

$$K_a = X^2/0.1 = 1.74 \times 10^{-5} \text{ M}$$
$$X = 1.32 \times 10^{-3} \text{ M} = [H^+] \qquad pH = -\log[H^+] = 2.88$$

At point B in Example 9-5, notice that a buffer system is now present because acetic acid and acetate are in solution (weak acid and conjugate base or salt).

Example 9-5: Find the pH at **point B**.

Use the Henderson-Hasselbach equation.

Solution:

1. Write reaction:

$$CH_3COOH + OH^- \rightleftharpoons CH_3COO^- + H_2O$$

2. Because the volume is no longer 50 ml, the concentrations changed. Calculate moles of each species:

---

3. Set up an inventory table:

	CH_3COOH +	NaOH $\rightleftharpoons$	CH_3COO^- +	H_2O
Initial	0.005 mol	0.001 mol	0	-------
Change	-0.001	-0.001	0.001	-------
Equilib.	0.004	0	0.001	-------

4. Plug into Henderson-Hasselbach equation:

$$pH = pK_a + \log \frac{[base]}{[acid]} = 4.76 + \log \frac{0.001}{0.004} = 4.16$$

At point C in Example 9-6, the concentration of acetate is equal to the concentration of acetic acid. Referring back to Example 9-2, this means that $pH = pK_a$.

Example 9-6: Find the pH at **point C**

Solution:
This point is simply the half-equivalence point, and $pH = pK_a = 4.76$.

Point D in Example 9-7 is the end point of the titration. All of the acetic acid has been converted to acetate and no additional sodium hydroxide has yet been added.

Example 9-7: Calculate the pH at **point D**.

Solution:
1. Write reaction:

$$CH_3COOH + OH^- \rightleftharpoons CH_3COO^- + H_2O$$

2. Because the volume is no longer 50 ml and the concentrations changed, calculate moles of each species:

$CH_3COOH = 0.05\ L \times 0.1\ M = 0.005$ mol
$NaOH = 0.05\ L \times 0.1\ M = 0.005$ mol

These will react completely to form 0.005 moles of acetate. Thus, concentration = 0.005 mol/0.1 L = 0.05 M.

3. Set up an inventory table:

	CH_3COO^- +	H_2O $\rightleftharpoons$	CH_3COOH +	OH^-
Initial	0.05 M		0	0
Change	-X		+X	+X
Equilib.	0.05 - X		X	X

4. Plug into K_b expression. Remember K_b can be calculated from K_a because $K_a K_b = K_w$. ($K_b = 5.75 \times 10^{-10}$)

$$K_b = X^2 / 0.05 = 5.75 \times 10^{-10}\ M$$
$$X = 5.36 \times 10^{-6}\ M = [OH^-]$$
$$pOH = -\log[OH^-] = 5.27$$
$$pH = 14.00 - 5.27 = 8.73$$

SECT. II
GENERAL
CHEMISTRY
REVIEW
NOTES

271

At point E in Example 9-8, any added sodium hydroxide continues to raise the pH of the system, because the buffer capacity has been exceeded.

Example 9-8: Find the pH at **point E.**

Solution:

At this point, the excess NaOH far outweighs any contribution from the acetate. Thus, the concentration of OH⁻ is equal to the concentration of NaOH. Note that about 10 ml of NaOH has been added between points D and E.

$$M\ OH^- = (\text{excess moles } OH^-)/\text{total volume} =$$
$$(0.1\ M \times 0.01\ L)/0.110\ L = 0.0091\ M$$
$$pOH \approx 2.04$$
$$pH \approx 14 - 2 \approx 11.96$$

Acetic acid has only one proton. Examining its titration curve shows that it has a buffering region around its halfway point (where $pH = pK_a$). It is important to note that the buffer region is only within about 1 pH unit above and below the halfway point. For acetic acid, that pH is 4.76, so an acetic acid buffer system would be useful for buffering a solution in the range of 3.76 to 5.76.

When a different pH range is needed, a different buffer system must be chosen. The phosphate buffer system is useful, because it is a triprotic acid, and therefore has three buffer regions. The following three equilibria occur during the titration of phosphoric acid:

$$\text{Equilibria 1: } H_3PO_4 + H_2O \rightleftharpoons H_2PO_4^- + H_3O^+ \qquad pK_{a1} = 2.12$$

$$\text{Equilibria 2: } H_2PO_4^- + H_2O \rightleftharpoons HPO_4^{-2} + H_3O^+ \qquad pK_{a2} = 7.21$$

$$\text{Equilibria 3: } HPO_4^{-2} + H_2O \rightleftharpoons PO_4^{-3} + H_3O^+ \qquad pK_{a3} = 12.3$$

The three pK_a values are 2.12, 7.21, and 12.3, which means that phosphoric acid can buffer in the range of 1.12 to 3.12, and 6.21 to 8.21, and 11.3 to 13.3 pH units. This incredible range of buffering regions is the primary reason that phosphoric acid is such a commonly used buffer system. To discuss these equilibria more thoroughly, the titration curve of phosphoric acid by sodium hydroxide is shown in Figure 9-3. Understanding this graph is critical for the MCAT. (Similar material is presented in the amino acid section of the Organic Chemistry Notes.)

FIGURE 9-3.
Titration curve of phosphoric acid. Note that phosphoric acid is a triprotic acid. **Points A to G** are as follows. **A:** Only form of phosphoric acid present is H_3PO_4; **B:** Midpoint of equilibria 1. Concentration of H_3PO_4 and $H_2PO_4^-$ are equal, so $pH = pK_{a1} = 2.12$; **C:** End point of equilibria 1. Only form of phosphoric acid present is $H_2PO_4^-$; **D:** Midpoint of equilibria 2. Concentration of $H_2PO_4^-$ and HPO_4^{-2} are equal, so $pH = pK_{a2} = 7.21$; **E:** End point of equilibria 2. Only form of phosphoric acid present is HPO_4^{-2}; **F:** Midpoint of equilibria 3. Concentration of HPO_4^{-2} and PO_4^{-3} are equal, so $pH = pK_{a3} = 12.3$; **G:** End point of equilibria 3. Only form of phosphoric acid present is PO_4^{-3}.

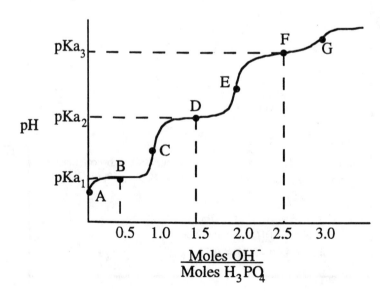

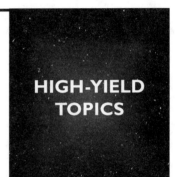

Thermochemistry

Thermochem

- **I. Major Concepts and Definitions**
- **II. Endothermic and Exothermic Reactions**
- **III. Bond Dissociation Energy/Heat of Formation**
- **IV. Calorimetry**
- **V. Entropy and Free Energy**

HIGH-YIELD TOPICS

Thermochemistry is a branch of thermodynamics. This chapter provides a review of the thermodynamic concepts you need to know for the general chemistry questions that appear on the MCAT. Other thermodynamic concepts are addressed in the physics review notes.

I. Major Concepts and Definitions

The three types of thermodynamic systems are as follows:

open: free exchange of energy and matter

closed: free exchange of energy only

isolated: no exchange of energy or matter

A state function is any function that is independent of the path. The state of a system is described by its physical parameters, which include chemical composition. The following are state functions: P = pressure, V = volume, T = temperature, E or U = internal energy, H = enthalpy, S = entropy, G = free energy.

Nonstate functions are those that do depend on the path. A good example is work. Consider doing work to fill a bucket with sand. The starting point of the process is an empty bucket and the final point is a full bucket. What would happen if the bucket of sand tips over halfway through the process of filling and you must start filling it again? As you can imagine, more total work is required for refilling. Thus, in this example, work would depend on the path from the empty bucket state to the full bucket state.

Another important concept is the **law of conservation of energy.** During any process, energy is neither created nor destroyed. This fact allows you to calculate many quantities that would otherwise be impossible if this law were not true. This concept is discussed further in the physics review notes.

SECT. II
GENERAL
CHEMISTRY
REVIEW
NOTES

273

II. Endothermic and Exothermic Reactions

A. Enthalpy and Standard Heats of Reactions

Enthalpy means heat content. The change in heat energy of a chemical system held at constant pressure is an **enthalpy change (ΔH)**. The ΔH of a system is equivalent to the difference in the final and initial enthalpies of a system:

$$\Delta H = H_2 - H_1$$

H_2 = final enthalpy of the system
H_1 = initial enthalpy of the system

The enthalpy of a system is a state function that depends only on the enthalpy of the initial and final states. Calculation of the heat of a reaction (ΔH_{rxn}) gives the heat of a unit reaction. The amount of heat produced must be handled using proper stoichiometry.

There are several kinds of enthalpy changes. **The standard enthalpy of formation ($\Delta H_f°$)** occurs when 1 mole of a substance in its most stable state at 298 K is formed from its constituent elements in their most common states at 298 K. **The standard enthalpy of a reaction ($\Delta H_r°$)** is the difference in the standard enthalpies of formation of the products less the reactants of the reaction.

A reaction that produces heat is said to be exothermic, whereas a reaction **that requires heat is endothermic.** Thus, heat is a product in exothermic reactions and a reactant in endothermic reactions. In a laboratory situation, how do you know if a reaction produces or requires heat? Try feeling the test tube that contains the reaction in progress. If the test tube is warm, the reaction is producing heat; if the test tube is cold, the reaction may be using heat.

Example 10-1 includes two examples of how the energy needed or produced by a reaction should be handled using the principles of stoichiometry. Watch out for simple math errors!

Example 10-1: The hypothetical reaction $2A + 3B \rightleftharpoons 4C + 1D$ produces 15 kcal of heat per unit reaction.

a. If 20 moles of A were reacted, what would be the maximum heat evolved assuming excess B is available?

Solution: Heat = $(20 \text{ mol A})\left(\dfrac{1 \text{ unit reaction}}{2 \text{ mol A}}\right)\left(\dfrac{15 \text{ kcal}}{\text{unit rxn}}\right) = 150 \text{ kcal}$

b. How many moles of C are produced if the reaction yields 315 kcal of heat?

Solution: Moles C = $(315 \text{ kcal})\left(\dfrac{1 \text{ unit reaction}}{15 \text{ kcal}}\right)\left(\dfrac{4 \text{ mole C}}{\text{unit}}\right) = 84 \text{ moles}$

Conceptually, enthalpy is the energy stored in the chemical bonds minus the work done by the chemical reaction:

$$\Delta H = q - w$$

ΔH = Enthalpy change
q = Heat absorbed by the system

When q < 0, heat is released. When q > 0, heat is absorbed.

$$w = \text{work}$$
$$w = -P_{ext}\Delta V \text{ (in an irreversible process at constant P)}$$

When w > 0, work is done on the system. When w < 0, work is done by the system.

Note that these statements are the **chemistry definitions** of work. Work may be defined differently in your physics textbooks. The sign definition of work should not be tested on the MCAT because of the different conventions used.

B. Hess's Law of Heat Summation

Hess's law says that for a reaction that is the result of a set of other reactions, the total enthalpy change will equal the algebraic sum of the enthalpy changes of those other reactions. More simply stated, total enthalpy change is independent of the numbers of intermediate reactions.

It is important that you know that the heats of formation can be used to determine the heat of reaction.

Important rules for Hess's law calculations involving chemical equations are as follows:

1. If you add two chemical equations with enthalpy change, ΔH_{rxn} (1) and ΔH_{rxn} (2), then the enthalpy change for the resulting equation, ΔH_{rxn} (3), is given by:

$$\Delta H_{rxn} (3) = \Delta H_{rxn} (1) + \Delta H_{rxn} (2)$$

2. If you reverse the direction of a chemical equation, the value of the enthalpy change for the resulting equation, ΔH_{rxn} (reverse), is given by:

$$\Delta H_{rxn} (\text{reverse}) = -\Delta H_{rxn} (\text{forward})$$

3. If you multiply a chemical equation with an enthalpy change of ΔH_{rxn} (1) through by n, the value of the enthalpy change for the resulting equation is:

$$\Delta H_{rxn} = n\, \Delta H_{rxn} (1)$$

The approach for using Hess's law is shown in Example 10-2.

Example 10-2: What is the ΔH_{rxn} for the following reaction given this ΔH_{rxn} data?

$$PCl_{3(l)} + Cl_{2(g)} \longrightarrow PCl_{5(s)}$$

(1) $2P_{(s)} + 3Cl_{2(g)} \longrightarrow 2PCl_{3(l)}$ $\Delta H_{rxn} = -640$ kJ/mol

(2) $2P_{(s)} + 5Cl_{2(g)} \longrightarrow 2PCl_{5(s)}$ $\Delta H_{rxn} = -886$ kJ/mol

Solution:

Step 1. Reverse equation (1) to get PCl_3 on reactant side:

(3) $2PCl_{3(l)} \longrightarrow 2P_{(s)} + 3Cl_{2(g)}$ $\Delta H_{rxn} = 640$ kJ/mol

---

SECT. II
GENERAL
CHEMISTRY
REVIEW
NOTES

275

Step 2. Add equation 2 and the new equation 3:

(2) $2P_{(s)} + 5Cl_{2(g)} \longrightarrow 2PCl_{5(s)}$ $\Delta H_{rxn} = -886$ kJ/mol

(3) $2PCl_{3(l)} \longrightarrow 2P_{(s)} + 3Cl_{2(g)}$ $\Delta H_{rxn} = 640$ kJ/mol

(4) $2PCl_{3(l)} + 2Cl_{2(g)} \cdots\!\!\longrightarrow 2PCl_{5(s)}$ $\Delta H_{rxn} = -246$ kJ/mol

Step 3. Multiply equation 4 by 1/2 to get desired equation:

$PCl_{3(s)} + Cl_{2(g)} \longrightarrow PCl_{5(s)}$ $\Delta H_{rxn} = -123$ kJ/mol

III. Bond Dissociation Energy/Heat of Formation

A. Bond Dissociation Energy

In certain reactions, it is possible to break a single chemical bond to give free atoms (e.g., a carbon–hydrogen covalent bond can be broken to give free carbon and hydrogen atoms). **The bond dissociation energy is the enthalpy per mole for breaking one and only one specific type of bond in a molecule.** Consider the molecule ammonia (NH_3), which contains three N–H bonds. Breaking the first N–H bond is associated with 435 kJ/mol of energy. Breaking the second N–H bond is associated with 377 kJ/mol of energy. The last bond is broken with only 356 kJ/mol of energy.

Similar types of bonds in the same molecule often are associated with different bond dissociation energies. To overcome this problem, the *bond energy* term was described. **The bond energy is the average amount of energy required to break one mole of bonds of the same type in a molecule.** For the example of ammonia, the bond energy can be found by adding the individual bond dissociation energies for each of the three N–H bonds, and finding the average:

$$(435 + 377 + 356)/3 = 389 \text{ kJ/mol}$$

The bond energy can be used to estimate the standard enthalpy of a reaction ($\Delta H_r°$):

$$\Delta H_r° = -(\Sigma \text{product bond energies}) + (\Sigma \text{reactant bond energies})$$

Breaking bonds requires energy, and forming bonds releases energy.

$$\Delta H_r° = (\text{bonds broken}) - (\text{bonds formed})$$

Note that the bond dissociation energies are provided for the gas phase, so they are used for estimating ΔH for gas phase reactions.

B. Heat of Formation

It is possible to calculate the $\Delta H°$ of a reaction from the *heat of formation*. **The heat of formation is the amount of heat required to form 1 mole of a compound in its standard state from its elements in their standard states.** Remember that in thermodynamics, standard refers to P = 1 atm and T = 298 K.

The heat of formation of an element is zero by definition. Example 10-3 shows some elements in their standard states.

Example 10-3: All of the following are elements in their standard state.

$$O_2(g), H_2(g), C(gr), Na(s)$$

The heat of reaction (ΔH_{rxn}) is the sum of heats of formations of each product times its stoichiometric coefficient minus the sum of the heats of formation of each reactant times its stoichiometric coefficient. This quantity is equal to the heat released or absorbed at constant pressure for a particular reaction. For our purposes, all chemical reactions occur at constant temperature and pressure. For the reaction:

$$aA + bB \rightarrow cC + dD$$

$$\Delta H_{rxn} = [c(\Delta H_f C) + d(\Delta H_f D)] - [a(\Delta H_f A) + b(\Delta H_f B)]$$

Example 10-4 shows how to use the heats of formation to calculate the ΔH of a reaction.

Example 10-4: Use the given heats of formation to calculate ΔH_{rxn} for the following reaction:

$$C_2H_5OH(l) + 3O_2(g) \longrightarrow 2CO_2(g) + 3H_2O(l)$$

$\Delta H_f [CO_2] = -393.5$ kJ/mol $\Delta H_f [H_2O] = -285.8$ kJ/mol

$\Delta H_f [O_2] = 0$ $\Delta H_f [C_2H_5OH] = -277$ kJ/mol

Solution:

$\Delta H_{rxn} = \{2 \Delta H_f [CO_2] + 3\Delta H_f [H_2O]\} - \{ 3\Delta H_f [O_2] + \Delta H_f [C_2H_2OH]\}$

$\quad = [(2 \text{ mol}) (-393.5 \text{ kJ/mol}) + (3 \text{ mol}) (-285.8 \text{ kJ/mol}) \} -$
$\quad \{(1 \text{ mol}) (-277 \text{ kJ/mol})]$

$\quad = -1367$ kJ

IV. Calorimetry

This material is presented in more detail in the review notes for physics.

The value of ΔH_{rxn} for a chemical reaction can be measured with a **calorimeter.** A simple calorimeter consists of a Dewar flask (thermos bottle) and a high precision thermometer. It works on the principle that energy is conserved by the calorimeter and none is lost to the surroundings.

Consider an exothermic reaction run in a calorimeter in which all the heat given off by the reaction is equal to the heat absorbed by the calorimeter. Using conservation of energy:

$$q_{rxn} = -(q \text{ of the calorimeter})$$

The **heat capacity** is the amount of heat required to raise the temperature of a sample by 1°C. An equation for the definition of the heat capacity at constant pressure follows:

$$\text{Heat capacity } C_p = \frac{q_p}{\Delta T}$$

Because at constant pressure, $q_p = \Delta H_{rxn}$, you can write the heat capacity as:

$$C_p = \frac{-\Delta H_{rxn}}{\Delta T}$$

SECT. II
GENERAL
CHEMISTRY
REVIEW
NOTES

277

If you know the heat capacity of the calorimeter and the temperature change, you can use the following equation to calculate ΔH_{rxn}. This equation is the one to know for the MCAT.

$$\Delta H_{rxn} = -C_p \Delta T$$

C_p = Heat capacity of the calorimeter at constant pressure

ΔT = Change in temperature

Example 10-5 shows how to use the $C_p \Delta T$ equation to calculate ΔH:

Example 10-5: A 50-ml sample of 0.2 M HCL was neutralized with 50 ml of 0.2 M NaOH in a calorimeter with a heat capacity of 3420 J/K. If $\Delta T = 0.654°C$, what was ΔH_{rxn} in kJ/mol?

Solution:

Step 1. You have the reaction:

$HCl(aq) + NaOH(aq) \longrightarrow NaCl(aq) + H_2O(l) + \Delta H_{rxn}$
Find the moles of each reactant:
Moles HCl and Moles NaOH = (0.2 mol/L)(0.05 L) = 0.01 mol
Because NaCl is in the same molar ratio as HCl and NaOH, 0.01 moles of NaCl is formed.

Step 2. Calculate: ΔH_{rxn} =
$\Delta H_{rxn} = -C_p \Delta T = (-3420 \text{ J/K})(0.652°C) = -2.2 \text{ kJ}$

Step 3. Calculate: ΔH_{rxn}/mol = -2.2 kJ/0.01 mol = -220 kJ/mol
(Note: negative sign implies an exothermic reaction)

V. Entropy and Free Energy

A. Entropy

Entropy can be thought of as a measure of randomness or disorder in a system and tends to increase as a function of the state of matter. As the temperature increases, particles in a substance move more and more vigorously. Thus, the entropy (randomness) of all pure substances increases as the temperature increases.

Relative entropy: gaseous state > liquid state > crystal state

Relative entropy, or randomness, decreases as you move from a gas to a solid state, because a gas has the highest energy state (most random) and a solid has the lowest energy state (least random, most ordered).

The entropy change (ΔS) is a measure of the increase ($\Delta S > 0$) or decrease ($\Delta S < 0$) in the disorder of a system that undergoes a change of state. The ΔS value for a reaction is determined by taking the difference of the sum of the absolute entropies of the products times their stoichiometric coefficients and the sum of the absolute entropies of the reactants times their stoichiometric coefficients.

In an **irreversible process**, the entropy of an **isolated system** always increases, thus $\Delta S > 0$. In a **reversible process**, however, the entropy of an **isolated system** is constant, thus $\Delta S = 0$.

The absolute entropy of any element is a defined quantity. The only time the absolute entropy is zero is defined by the **third law of thermodynamics:** the entropy of any perfectly ordered substance at absolute zero K is zero.

B. Free Energy

The Gibbs's free energy (G), like enthalpy, is an **intrinsic property** of a substance. Free energy (G) relates enthalpy and entropy:

$$G = H - TS$$

Even though this relationship defines G, free energy cannot be measured directly. Only changes in G are significant. Thus, **you should learn the equation for ΔG.** The free energy function (ΔG) can be thought of conceptually as the amount of energy available to do useful work.

$$\Delta G = \Delta H - T\Delta S \text{ (at constant temperature)}$$

It is interesting that all spontaneous chemical reactions are driven by the tendency to achieve maximum molecular chaos (positive ΔS) at minimum energy (negative ΔH).

Because it is a state function, you can calculate ΔG in several ways. One way is to **use the formula $\Delta G = \Delta H - T\Delta S$.** Watch out for the units because ΔH and ΔS typically have different units. Another way is to **use free energies of formation.** This process is exactly analogous to finding ΔH from enthalpies of formation. A third possibility is to **use the concept of thermodynamic equilibrium** (shown below).

The following equations allow you to calculate ΔG for a reaction at both nonequilibrium and equilibrium conditions, with a form of each equation in natural log and log base 10 form. For chemical reactions:

$$\Delta G = \Delta G° + RT \ln Q \quad \text{or} \quad \Delta G = \Delta G° + 2.3RT \log Q$$

(Notice that these equations are essentially the same)

Remember Q is the reaction quotient that allows you to use nonequilibrium values in an equilibrium-type expression.

At equilibrium, $\Delta G = O$ and $Q = K_{eq}$, therefore:

$$\Delta G° = -RT \ln K \quad \text{or} \quad \Delta G° = -2.3 \, RT \log K_{eq}$$

(Notice that these equations are essentially the same)

Recall that at equilibrium, $\Delta G = \Delta H - T\Delta S = 0$. Thus, equilibrium can be considered as the point in a system of minimum energy and maximum molecular chaos. The magnitude of the equilibrium constant is determined by these driving forces.

C. Spontaneous Reactions and DG

Criterion for spontaneity:

1. **When $\Delta G < 0$, the reaction is spontaneous in the forward direction.**

2. **When $\Delta G = 0$, the reaction is at equilibrium.**

3. **When $\Delta G > 0$, the reaction is nonspontaneous in the forward direction, but spontaneous in the reverse direction.**

SECT. II
GENERAL
CHEMISTRY
REVIEW
NOTES

279

On the MCAT, you may be given relative magnitudes for ΔH, ΔS, and ΔG. Table 10-1 provides some combinations, derived by examining the ΔG equation and evaluating the signs and magnitudes of the ΔH and $T\Delta S$ terms, that allow you to predict spontaneity.

TABLE 10-1. Relation of variables that allow prediction of spontaneity of a reaction.

$\Delta G = \Delta H - T\Delta S$		
ΔH	ΔS	ΔG
−	+	− (spontaneous)
+	−	+ (nonspontaneous)
−	−	+/− (can be +, −, or 0)*
+	+	+/− (can be +, −, or 0)*

*, ΔG varies on the actual magnitudes of ΔH and $T\Delta S$.

Kinetics

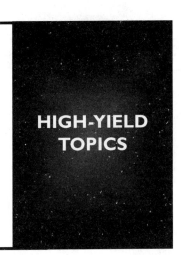

HIGH-YIELD TOPICS

Chemical kinetics is the study of reaction rates and reaction mechanisms. A reaction rate is the **velocity** with which reactants are used up and products are formed. A reaction mechanism is the **pathway** by which reactants form products. Thermodynamics (reviewed in Chapter 10 of the General Chemistry Review Notes) allows you to decide whether or not a chemical reaction is favorable, but it cannot tell you how quickly reactions may occur. A reaction can have a favorable (negative) ΔG, but occur slowly. Chemical kinetics allows you to determine how quickly a reaction occurs.

I. Reaction Rate

A. The Basics

A reaction rate is the average rate at which a product is formed or a reactant is used up (the absolute value is taken to assure a positive quantity):

$$\text{Rate} = \left| \frac{\text{Change in concentration of product or reactant}}{\text{Elapsed time}} \right|$$

For any reaction with stoichiometric coefficients other than 1, the rate of change of product formation or reactant usage must be divided by the stoichiometric coefficient. This step ensures that the same rate is obtained no matter which participant in the reaction is monitored. Example 11-1 shows a rate expression for a reaction with different coefficients of reactants and products.

SECT. 11
GENERAL
CHEMISTRY
REVIEW
NOTES

281

$$\boxed{\text{Example 11-1: } 2\,H_2O_2\,(aq) \longrightarrow 2H_2O\,(l) + O_2\,(g)}$$
$$\text{Rate} = \frac{1}{2}\left|\frac{\Delta\,[H_2O_2]}{\Delta t}\right| = \left|\frac{\Delta\,[O_2]}{\Delta t}\right|$$

B. Dependence of Reaction Rate on Concentration of Reactants

1. Rate Law

For the general reaction, $aA + bB = cC + dD$, the reaction rate can be described by the following **rate law** or **general rate equation:**

$$\text{Rate} = k_f\,[A]^x[B]^y$$

Note that the rate of the reaction depends on (1) the **concentration** of the reacting molecules (A and B in this case) raised to some power (x and y, respectively, **which are determined experimentally**); and (2) the forward **rate constant** (k_f). The rate constant is characteristic of a specific reaction but varies with temperature. The units of k also vary with reaction order.

2. Rate Constant

The reaction rate constant (k) is defined quantitatively using the Arrhenius expression:

$$k = Ae^{-E_a/RT} \text{ (A is the Arrhenius constant for a particular}$$
$$\text{reaction and } E_a \text{ is the activation energy)}$$

3. Reaction Order

The order of the reactants in a chemical reaction can be determined experimentally, or it can be deduced from the mechanism if it is known. In the preceding expression for rate, the orders are represented by the variables x and y. Thus, the reaction is said to be x-order with respect to A and y-order with respect to B. When the process is elementary (i.e., occuring in a single step), then the order of the reactant is merely its stoichiometric coefficient.

The overall order of the chemical reaction is defined as the sum of the orders for each reactant, $x + y$. When the reaction is first order, $x + y = 1$. When the reaction is second order, $x + y = 2$.

Reaction orders can be determined experimentally using the method of **initial rates.** The initial rate of a reaction is measured as one concentration is varied and the concentration of the other reactants are constant.

Table 11-1 summarizes the changes in rate as a function of concentration. The order is determined by the formula (concentration ratio)^x = (ratio of rates), in which x is the order of the reaction in the reagent varied.

TABLE 11-1. Change in rate as a function of concentration.

Concentration Change	Rate	Order
Doubled	No change	($2^0 = 1$)
Doubled	Doubled	($2^1 = 2$)
Doubled	Quadrupled	($2^2 = 4$)
Doubled	Octupled	($2^3 = 8$)

Example 11-2 is similar to a question you might see on the MCAT. A reaction was carried out and the concentration of the reactants was measured. The rate of product formation was obtained. Try to determine the overall order of the reaction and the order with respect to each reactant.

Example 11-2: The following initial-rate data was obtained
for the reaction: $2NO(g) + Br_2(l) \longrightarrow 2NOBr$
Find the reaction order with respect to NO, Br_2,
and the overall reaction:

Run	$[NO]_0$:(M)	$[Br_2]_0$:(M)	(rate)$_0$:(M/min)
1	0.50	0.50	0.65×10^{-3}
2	1.00	0.50	2.60×10^{-3}
3	0.50	1.00	1.30×10^{-3}

Solution: Comparing experiments 1 and 2, when the concentration
of NO was doubled, the rate quadrupled. Because the
concentration of Br_2 was held constant, NO must be second
order ($2^2 = 4$). Comparing experiments 1 and 3, when the
concentration of Br_2 was doubled with NO at constant
concentration, the rate doubled. Thus, Br_2 must be
first order ($2^1 = 2$).

The rate law for this reaction is therefore:
$$\text{Rate} = k\,[NO]^2[Br_2]^1$$
The overall reaction order is 3 (2+1).
The order with respect to NO is 2 and Br_2 is 1.

II. Reaction Mechanisms and Rate-Determining Step

A **mechanism** consists of a series of elementary reactions. If one step in a reaction mechanism is slower than any of the other steps, then that step effectively controls the overall reaction rate (the **rate-determining step**).

Several theories concern how reactions take place. **Collision theory** says that when particle A collides with particle B, sufficient kinetic energy must be available to allow for the rearrangement of bonds to produce products. A successful collision only occurs when the particles are in the proper orientation and when they have enough kinetic energy to overcome the bonds that hold together the reactants (either A or B).

Transition state uses the concepts of both waves and collision theory to explain reaction rates. The collision between two particles, A and B, is thought to occur in several steps. First, the bonds in A and B weaken as the particles approach each other. Next, **an activated complex or transition state** (an intermediate that is short-lived) forms. Finally, breakdown of the activated complex or transition state occurs and product is formed.

The order of the rate law is the same as the order of the rate-determining step. Consider an hourglass as an analogy. The sand in the hourglass can flow to the bottom only as fast as it can get through the constriction. Some complex reactions lack a single rate-determining step and the rate depends on the overall mechanism (Example 11-3).

SECT. 11
GENERAL
CHEMISTRY
REVIEW
NOTES

283

> **Example 11-3:** The following mechanism has been proposed for the
> reaction of hydrogen peroxide in the presence of
> iodide ion to produce water and oxygen:
>
> $$[H_2O_2(aq) \longrightarrow 2H_2O(l) + O_2(g)]$$
>
> **Step 1.** $H_2O_2 + I^- \longrightarrow H_2O + OI^-$
>
> **Step 2.** $H_2O_2 + OI^- \longrightarrow H_2O + O_2 + I^-$
>
> If step 1 is the rate-limiting step, what is the rate law?
>
> *Solution:*   The rate law must include every reactant in the rate-limiting
> step raised to their stoichiometric coefficients:
>
> Rate = $k[H_2O_2][I^-]$

III. Interpretation of Energy Profiles

A.   Some Basic Concepts

Several critical concepts and definitions are important to know for the MCAT. **The
activation energy (E_a) of a reaction is the minimum amount of energy required to make the reaction proceed.** Both forward and reverse reactions have
activation energies, which typically are different, because either the forward or reverse reaction is favored.

The overall energy change of the reaction is the activation energy of the forward reaction minus the activation energy of the reverse reaction. Numerically,
this value approximates ΔH. Conceptually, **activation energy is the amount of
energy needed to break old bonds and to create new ones in a reaction.**
When two molecules collide, they must possess a sufficient amount of energy
to weaken bonds and to form the **activated complex.** The activated complex
can then break up and form product, or can revert back to the reactants. When
new bonds are formed, heat may be released (exothermic reaction). When the new
bonds are weaker than the old bonds, the system absorbs energy and the reaction
is endothermic.

The energy diagram in Figure 11-1 illustrates the conversion of reactant A to
product B. An activated complex or transition state (AB°) is a high energy structure
formed in the reaction path (shown on a high point on the reaction energy diagram). The activation energies of both the forward and reverse reactions are also
demonstrated.

B.   An Energy Profile (curve with activation energy and ΔH)

How the energy of a reaction changes as the reaction progresses is well represented
in Figure 11-1. Note key quantities that are labeled.

In the reaction A → B, the rate at which A can be converted to B depends on
how much energy is required to make the highest energy structure on the path of the
reaction (reaction coordinate)—the transition state complex AB°. Note that the reactant (A) was a higher energy structure than the product (B), which means energy is
released by the reaction of A going to B. **The energy difference between A and
B is a good approximation of ΔH.**

Reaction Energy Diagram

FIGURE 11-1.
Reaction energy diagram.

Mechanism A $\rightleftharpoons$ AB* $\rightleftharpoons$ B

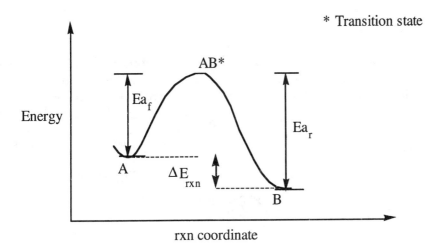

* Transition state

Ea$_f$ = Activation energy of the forward rxn.
Ea$_r$ = Activation energy of the reverse rxn
$\Delta E_{rxn} = Ea_f - Ea_r$
$\Delta E_{rxn} \approx \Delta H$

IV. Kinetic Versus Thermodynamic Control of Reactions

In many reactions, more than one product may form. In some cases, the product distribution can be strongly influenced by the reaction conditions chosen. The reaction can be **controlled** to favor the kinetic or the thermodynamic product.

The kinetic product is that which forms at the greater rate. Products form faster if they have a lower activation energy. The reaction can be influenced to yield this product **by low temperature and short reaction times.** The conditions that produce the kinetic product as the major product are the conditions of kinetic control. Figure 11-2 shows the formation of two different products, A and B, from the same reactant(s). Product A is the kinetic product. Note that it has an activated complex at a lower energy but a product with higher energy than product B.

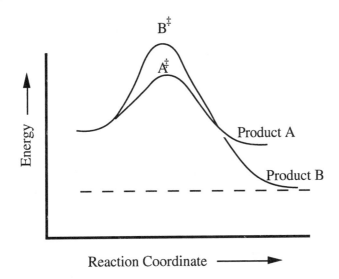

FIGURE 11-2.
Reaction energy diagram showing the kinetic product (A) and the thermodynamic product (B).

SECT. 11
GENERAL
CHEMISTRY
REVIEW
NOTES

285

The thermodynamic product is that which has the lowest energy. The formation of this product can be increased **by higher temperatures and longer reaction times.** The conditions that favor the thermodynamic product (product B in Figure 11-2) are the conditions of thermodynamic control.

V. Catalysts

A catalyst is an agent that speeds up a chemical reaction by creating a new path of lower activation energy (Figure 11-3). **Catalysts are neither produced nor consumed** in chemical reactions. Because these agents take part in the reaction, they can appear in the rate law; however, catalysts do not appear in the stoichiometric equation for a reaction.

FIGURE 11-3.

Reaction energy diagram with and without a catalyst. Note the activation energy-lowering effect of a catalyst.

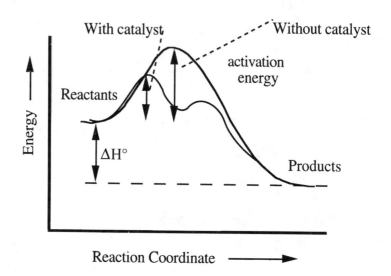

Temperature is not a catalyst because it can be produced (exothermic reactions) and consumed (endothermic reactions) in chemical reactions. Common catalysts in chemistry include metals, acids, and bases. Protein catalysts are common in biologic systems and are called **enzymes.**

Equilibrium

I. Law of Mass Action and the Equilibrium Constant

II. Le Chatelier's Principle

III. Equilibrium Constant and ΔG

HIGH-YIELD TOPICS

Chemical equilibrium is a dynamic process in which forward and reverse reactions occur at equal rates in opposite directions. When the reaction is at equilibrium, the concentration of each species remains constant at constant temperature. Many chemical reactions do not go to completion, and reach a point at which the concentrations of the reactants and products are no longer changing with time. The molecules are still changing from reactants to products and from products to reactants, but with no net change in concentrations.

Rather than complex and time-consuming equilibrium problems, MCAT questions are more likely to focus on equilibrium concepts, with particular emphasis on Le Chatelier's principle.

Many concepts of equilibrium were reviewed in Chapters 7 and 8. The following discussion addresses this topic in greater detail.

I. Law of Mass Action and the Equilibrium Constant

1. Law of Mass Action

For the reaction:

$$aA_{(g)} + bB_{(soln.)} + cC_{(s)} \rightleftharpoons xX_{(g)} + yY_{(soln.)} + zZ_{(l)}$$

the following relation is true at a given temperature:

$$\frac{[X]^x[Y]^y}{[A]^a[B]^b} = K$$

in which [ ] is equilibrium concentration and K is equilibrium constant.

Note that neither $Z_{(l)}$ nor $C_{(s)}$ appear in the expression for K because the concentration of pure liquid phases and pure solids are not included in equilibrium expressions. Example 12-1 shows how to set up an expression for K.

SECT. II
GENERAL
CHEMISTRY
REVIEW
NOTES

287

> **Example 12-1:** What is the equilibrium constant expression for this reaction?
>
> $$2\ NO_2(g) + 7\ H_2(g) \rightleftharpoons 2\ NH_3(g) + 4\ H_2O(l)$$
>
> *Solution:*
>
> $$K_{eq} = \frac{[NH_3]^2}{[NO_2]^2[H_2]^7}$$
>
> The concentration of water is not included in the equilibrium constant expression because it is a pure liquid phase.

2. Equilibrium Constant

Important points to remember follow:

a. K is a constant for any given reaction as long as the temperature does not change

b. K determines which is in greater concentration at equilibrium—the products or the reactants

c. Because K is determined by reactant and final product concentration, K is independent of the number of intermediate steps in the reaction mechanism

d. K > 1: more products than reactants at equilibrium, reaction "lies to the right"

   K < 1: more reactants than products at equilibrium, reaction "lies to the left"

II. Le Chatelier's Principle

Le Chatelier's principle states that if a stress (i.e., a change in concentration, pressure, volume, or temperature) is applied to a system at equilibrium, **the system shifts in the direction that will minimize the effects of that stress.**

When using Le Chatelier's principle, identify the applied stress. Each applied stress has a predictable effect on an equilibrium expression.

If you increase the concentration of the reactant or decrease the concentration of the product, the equilibrium will shift toward the product side. If you decrease the reactant concentration or increase the product concentration, the equilibrium will shift toward the reactant side.

An increase in pressure will shift the equilibrium toward the side with fewer moles of gas. Pressure changes only affect equilibria in gas phase reactions in which the number of moles of reactants and products differ. Determining the moles of gas in an equilibrium reaction will help you predict the effect of a pressure change. Remember that an increase in pressure can be offset by a decrease in volume, and a decrease in pressure can be offset by an increase in volume. Keep in mind that 1 mole of any gas under the same conditions occupies the same volume.

Every equilibrium system involves one endothermic and one exothermic reaction. **An increase in the temperature of a system will favor the endothermic reaction.** A decrease in the temperature of a system will favor the exothermic reaction. Remember that a change in temperature changes the value of K. Example 12-2 shows what happens to an exothermic reaction (for the forward reaction) when changes are made.

Example 12-2: Haber ammonia synthesis:

$$N_2(g) + 3H_2(g) \rightleftharpoons 2\,NH_3(g) \qquad \Delta H = -22\ \text{Kcal/mol}$$

Consider what happens with each of the following changes:

a. Concentration change: If N_2 is added, the reaction will shift to the right to relieve the stress of added reactant, and more product will be formed.

b. Pressure change: Assuming these are all ideal gases, the volume of the system depends on the number of moles of gas, regardless of which gas. This reaction has 4 moles of gas on the left and 2 on the right. Increasing the pressure on the system (usually by shrinking the volume of the container or piston) will shift the reaction in the direction that will relieve the pressure stress. You must decrease the number of moles in the system (remember pressure is proportional to moles at constant temperature); hence, the reaction shifts to the side with the least number of moles of gas. In this reaction, the shift is to the right.

c. Temperature change: This reaction is exothermic, i.e., it gives off heat when going from left to right. If the system is cooled, the reaction will tend to go to the right in an effort to heat it up again. If the system is heated, however, the reaction will go in the reverse direction. In the reverse, the heat is a reactant and the reaction can be thought of as endothermic.

III. Equilibrium Constant and ΔG

The basic relationship between ΔG and K:

$$\Delta G^\circ_{rxn} = -RT\ln K$$

can be derived from the expression for K:

$$\ln K = -\frac{\Delta G^\circ rxn}{RT}$$

in which $R = 8.314$ J/K. Example 12-3 shows how to calculate the value of K knowing the value of ΔG.

Example 12-3: Calculate the equilibrium constant for a reaction with $\Delta G^\circ = -18.7$ kJ at 25°C.

Solution:

$$\ln K = -\frac{\Delta G^\circ_{rxn}}{RT}$$

$$= \frac{(18.7 \times 10^3\ \text{J})}{(8.314\ \text{J/K})(298\ \text{K})} = +7.55$$

$$K = 1.9 \times 10^3$$

SECT. II
GENERAL
CHEMISTRY
REVIEW
NOTES

289

Understanding the qualitative relationship between ΔG°_{rxn} and K is more important than being able to calculate one from the other. Keep in mind the following **summary of the relationship between ΔG°_{rxn} and K** when dealing with equilibrium situations:

1. **When $\Delta G^\circ_{rxn} = 0$, K = 1**
   (equal amounts of products and reactants, neither side of the equation is energetically favored)

2. **When $\Delta G^\circ_{rxn} < 0$, K > 1**
   (more products than reactants, so the product side of the equation is energetically favored)

3. **When $\Delta G^\circ_{rxn} > 0$, K < 1**
   (more reactants than products, so the reactant side of the equation is energetically favored)

Electrochemistry

I. Galvanic Cells	**HIGH-YIELD TOPICS**
II. Concentration Cells	
III. Electrolytic Cells	

Chemical reactions can be used as energy sources. The oxidation-reduction reaction is particularly useful in this way. From the review in Chapter 1, remember that oxidation refers to a loss of electrons and reduction refers to a gain of electrons.

A cell that makes use of an oxidation-reduction reaction to generate electricity is a **galvanic cell.** An unusual type of galvanic cell in which the oxidation and reduction half reactions are the forward and reverse of a single reaction is a **concentration cell.** This type of cell generates electricity because of the concentration difference in the two half-cells. In the **electrolytic cell,** electricity is used to drive an unfavorable oxidation-reduction reaction.

I. Galvanic Cells

Electrons are transferred from one substance to another in oxidation-reduction (redox) reactions. As shown in Example 13-1, this electron transfer is not at all obvious, unless the overall reaction is separated into two half-reactions.

Example 13-1: $Zn(s) + Cu^{2+}(aq) \longrightarrow Zn^{2+}(aq) + Cu(s)$

This reaction can be separated into two half reactions (see Chapter 1):

$Zn(s) \longrightarrow Zn^{2+} + 2e^-$

$Cu^{2+} + 2e^- \longrightarrow Cu(s)$

If these reactions could be physically separated and connected by a wire, electrons would flow through the wire, creating an electric current. A voltmeter measures this current. Figure 13-1 illustrates a galvanic cell or electrochemical cell in which this reaction is occurring.

SECT. II
GENERAL
CHEMISTRY
REVIEW
NOTES

291

FIGURE 13-1.
A galvanic or electro-
chemical cell.

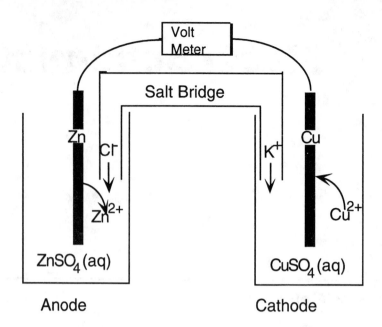

A. Half-Cell Reactions

Consider the half-cell reactions occurring in each of the containers (labeled anode and cathode) in Figure 13-1.

In the **anode half-cell,** an electrode of zinc metal has been placed in an electrolyte solution of $ZnSO_4(aq)$. As the reaction proceeds, the $Zn(s)$ of the electrode is **oxidized,** forming Zn^{2+}, which goes into solution. The anode (where oxidation occurs) is always written on the left side of the galvanic cell.

In the **cathode half-cell,** an electrode of copper metal has been placed in an electrolyte solution of $CuSO_4(aq)$. As the reaction proceeds, the Cu^{2+} of the electrolyte solution is **reduced** to $Cu(s)$ and deposited on the electrode. By convention, the cathode (where reduction occurs) is written on the right side of the galvanic cell.

Remember: oxidation occurs at the anode and reduction occurs at the cathode.

According to the half-cell reactions, you would expect that, in a short time, excess negative charge would build up in the cathode cell (SO_4^{2-}) and excess positive charge would build up in the anode (Zn^{2+}). This increase would not allow the cell to function. You can prevent this problem by adding a **salt bridge** to the cell, which usually contains a solution, such as KCl. The salt bridge completes the circuit and allows Cl^- to flow into the anode to balance the Zn^{2+} and K^+ to flow into the cathode to balance the SO_4^{2-}.

The voltmeter on a galvanic cell provides a way to measure the **electromotive force (emf or E),** which is the electrochemical potential difference between the two half-cells. The total emf for a cell is supplied by the electrode potential from each half-cell. The two half-cell reactions must occur simultaneously to generate an electrical current. The hydrogen electrode has served as a reference point for measuring electrode potentials. The potential of the hydrogen half reaction is 0 V at the standard conditions of 1 M concentration, T = 298 K (25°C), and pressure = 1 atm. The potential of a half reaction at standard conditions is known as $E°$ and is measured in volts.

B. Reduction Potentials

Table 13-1 provides the standard reduction potentials for a variety of reactions. You can predict the outcome of many redox reactions by using these values. The reduc-

TABLE 13-1. Standard reduction potentials*.

Electrode Half Reactions	$E°_{red}$ (V)
$F_2(g) + 2e^- \rightarrow 2F^-(aq)$	+2.87
$Ag^{2+}(aq) + 2e^- \rightarrow Ag(s)$	+2.07
$Cu^{2+}(aq) + 2e^- \rightarrow Cu(s)$	+0.34
$2H^+(aq) + 2e^- \rightarrow H_2(g)$	0
$Zn^{2+}(aq) + 2e^- \rightarrow Zn(s)$	−0.76
$Li^+(aq) + e^- \rightarrow Li(s)$	−3.05

*Do not memorize these reactions. Any reaction you need during the MCAT will be given to you.

tion potentials can be converted to oxidation potentials by reversing both the sign and direction of the reactions, without changing the magnitudes of the potentials.

The data in Table 13-1 are given for the half reactions at standard conditions—298 K, 1 atm pressure, and 1 M concentrations. Also, the hydrogen half reaction—$(2H^+ + 2e^- \rightarrow H_2(g)$, is taken as the standard, and therefore is set at zero volts.

Make sure you understand the meaning of E°. A positive E° indicates that the species accepting electrons is a stronger oxidizing agent than H^+. The larger the positive value of E°, the stronger the oxidizing agent. A negative E° indicates that the species donating electrons is a stronger reducing agent than H_2. The larger the negative E°, the stronger the reducing agent.

C. Cell Potentials

To combine half-cell potentials into an overall electrochemical cell potential:

1. Sum half reactions algebraically to give the overall reaction.

2. If the half reaction as tabulated is written in the opposite direction from the half reaction needed, reverse the sign on E°. Even though the half cell reaction may be multiplied by a coefficient, **do not multiply E°** by this number. E° is an intrinsic property, not dependent on the number of moles participating in the reaction.

3. Sum E° for each unit reaction to get the overall E° for the cell.

Cell potentials (E°) greater than zero are indicative of spontaneity (Example 13-2). Remember that a $-\Delta G$ is indicative of a spontaneous reaction. The relationship between ΔG and E° is as follows:

$$\Delta G° = -nFE°$$

in which $\Delta G°$ is free energy change for a reaction, n is the number of moles of electrons involved in the reaction, and F is Faraday's constant (9.65×10^4 J/Vmol).

Example 13-2: What is E° for the following cell reaction?

$$Zn(s) + Cu^{2+}(aq) \longrightarrow Cu(s) + Zn^{2+}(aq)$$

Solution: Start by finding the half-reactions in Table 13-1. Convert the zinc reaction to an oxidation and change the sign of its potential:

SECT. II
GENERAL
CHEMISTRY
REVIEW
NOTES

293

1. Relevant half reactions:

$$Cu^{2+}(aq) \longrightarrow Cu(s) \qquad E° = +0.34 \text{ V}$$

$$Zn(s) \longrightarrow Zn^{2+}(aq) \qquad E° = +0.76 \text{ V}$$

2. Sum half reactions:

$$E_{cell} = E°_{ox} + E°_{red} = 0.34 \text{ V} + 0.76 \text{ V} = +1.10 \text{ V}$$

E_{cell} is positive, so this reaction is spontaneous.

D. Direction of Electron Flow and the Nernst Equation

An electrochemical cell has polarity, meaning that one of the electrodes is positive (cathode) and one of the electrodes is negative (anode) with respect to the flow of electric current. **Electrons flow spontaneously from the negative (anode) electrode to the positive (cathode) electrode.**

Remember that our half cell reduction potentials are tabulated for half cells at 1 M concentration. If the concentrations of electrolytes are not at 1 M, use an alternate method to find the E_{rxn}.

The **Nernst equation** allows you to calculate cell potentials under nonideal conditions:

$$\mathbf{E_{rxn} = E°_{rxn} - (0.0592/n) \log \frac{[Products]}{[Reactants]}}$$

in which n is the number of moles of electrons transferred. You can also use the Nernst equation to calculate the concentration of an unknown electrolyte if you are given cell potentials (Example 13-3).

Example 13-3: Consider the following cell reaction:

$$Zn(s) + Cu^{2+}(g) \longrightarrow Cu(s) + Zn^{2+}(aq)$$

The cell voltage was measured and found to be 1.25 V with a Cu^{2+} concentration of 1 M. What is the concentration of Zn^{2+}?

$E°rxn = 1.10 V$.

Solution:

Step 1. Set up the Nernst equation:

$$E_{rxn} = E°_{rxn} - (0.0592/n) \log \frac{[Products]}{[Reactants]}$$

Note 2 moles of electrons are involved, so n = 2

$$1.25 V = 1.10 V - (0.0592/2) \log \frac{[Zn^{2+}]}{[1M]}$$

Step 2. Solve for $[Zn^{2+}]$:

$$0.15 V = -0.0296 \log \frac{[Zn^{2+}]}{[1M]}$$

$-5.07 = \log [Zn^{2+}]$. By taking inverse log of both sides:

$$[Zn^{2+}] = 8.6 \times 10^{-6} \text{ M}$$

II. Concentration Cells

Remember that in this type of cell, the oxidation reaction is the reverse of the reduction reaction (Figure 13-2). The two sides of the cell contain different concentrations of the same solution with similar electrode composition. Current flows because of the difference in concentration of the two sides. Electrons flow from the less concentrated to the more concentrated half-cell.

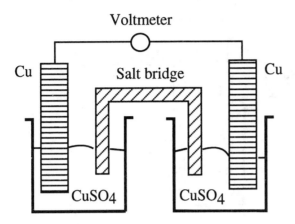

FIGURE 13-2.

A concentration cell. If different concentrations of $CuSO_4$ are in the half-cells, electrons will flow from the less concentrated to the more concentrated half-cell.

When the concentration of the two electrolyte solutions are not the same, a current will exist even though ΔE°_{rxn} is zero. Because at least one of the reactants is not at 1 M, you need to use the Nernst equation to find the E_{rxn}.

$$E_{rxn} = -(0.0592/n) \log \frac{[\text{less concentrated}]}{[\text{more concentrated}]}$$

Remember that the log of a number less than 1 is negative, so E_{rxn} will be positive under these conditions.

To understand why **electrons flow from the less concentrated to the more concentrated half-cell,** look at Example 13-4. Electron flow to the more concentrated side causes the concentrated solution on that side to gain electrons, and the ions on that side come out of solution by plating onto the electrode. This reduces the concentration on that side of the half-cell.

Example 13-4: Consider the concentration cell in Figure 13-2. If the concentration of $CuSO_4$ is 1 M on the left side and 10 M on the right side, in which direction will electrons flow?

Solution: Without memorizing any rules, think about what must occur to reach equilibrium (concentrations on both sides equal). The relevant half reaction is $Cu^{2+}(aq) \longrightarrow Cu(s)$ and the reverse. Because the concentration of Cu^{2+} is higher on the right side, Cu^{2+} must decrease during the course of the reaction, so Cu^{2+} will be consumed on the right side of the diagram. Thus, reduction will occur on the right, so electrons must flow toward the right.

SECT. II
GENERAL
CHEMISTRY
REVIEW
NOTES

295

III. Electrolytic Cells

A. The Basics

Electrolysis occurs when any oxidation–reduction reaction is induced by an electric current. A common example of an electrolytic reaction is the breakdown of water into hydrogen and oxygen gas (Figure 13-3). This reaction requires the input of electric current. Why do you need to apply the current?

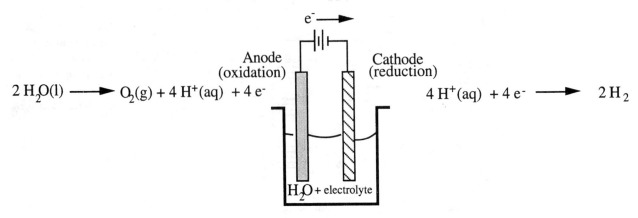

FIGURE 13-3.

An electrolytic cell. In this example of electrolysis of water, hydrogen and oxygen gas are produced at the electrodes.

Recall that if the ΔE_{rxn} for a reaction is positive, then the reaction is not spontaneous (ΔG is positive). If you pass an electric current through an electrolytic solution, the reaction can become spontaneous. The decomposition of water to form hydrogen and oxygen gas is not a favorable reaction, but electricity can be used to provide the necessary energy.

These reactions usually involve an aqueous solution of an ionic compound that dissociates into ions. It can also be a molten solution of an ionic compound, such as NaCl. The current in the electrolyte is conveyed by ions instead of electrons.

B. Anode and Cathode

As for galvanic cells, **oxidation occurs at the anode and reduction occurs at the cathode.** For example, consider the electrolysis of water. Write two half reactions:

Anode reaction: $2H_2O(l) \rightarrow O_2(g) + 4H^+(aq) + 4e^-$ *(oxidation)*

Cathode reaction: $4H^+(aq) + 4e^- \rightarrow 2H_2(g)$ *(reduction)*

Notice that oxygen is produced at the anode and hydrogen is produced at the cathode.

C. Faraday's Law and Deposition of Elements or Gas Liberated by Electrolysis (Examples 13-5 and 13-6)

Faraday's first law of electrolysis states that the extent to which an electrochemical reaction occurs depends solely on the amount of electricity passed through a solution.

Faraday's second law of electrolysis states that the mass of a substance produced by the passage of a given amount of electricity is proportional to the molar mass of the substance divided by the number of electrons transferred per formula unit.

$$\textbf{Mass of substance produced by electrolysis} = \frac{\textbf{M}}{\textbf{n}}$$

M = molar mass
n = electrons transferred per formula unit

To calculate the number of electrons in a given amount of current, use the following equation:

$$\textbf{Moles of electrons} = \frac{\textbf{Z}}{\textbf{F}} = \frac{\textbf{It}}{\textbf{F}}$$

Z = Total charge in coulombs (C)
F = Faraday's constant: 9.65 10^4 C/mol = charge on 1 mole electrons
I = Current in amperes (same as coulombs per second)
t = Time in seconds

Combine all these facts to write Faraday's law quantitatively:

$$\textbf{m} = \frac{\textbf{(It)(M)}}{\textbf{(F)(n)}}$$

Example 13-5: Consider the following two half reactions. For an electrolytic reaction, how many grams of copper metal will deposit per mole electrons? How many grams of oxygen gas will be liberated per mole electrons?

Solution: Set up a table:

Reaction	M	n	M/n
$Cu^{2+}(aq) + 2e^- \longrightarrow Cu(s)$	63.5 g/mol	2	31.78
$2H_2O(l) \longrightarrow O_2 + 4H^+ + 4e^-$	32 g/mol	4	8

Therefore, if you pass 1 mole of electrons through a Cu^{2+} solution, you can deposit 31.78 g of copper metal. Also, if you pass 1 mole of electrons through water, you can liberate 8 g oxygen gas.

Example 13-6: How much O_2 gas is liberated by the passage of 0.5 amp of current through water for 1 minute?

Solution: Two ways to solve this problem are shown. You can use Faraday's law or dimensional analysis (less memorization involved).

Faraday's law

Step 1. Write the equation and determine n:

$$2H_2O \longrightarrow O_2 + 4H^+ + 4e^-$$

n = 4   M = 32 g/mol (molar mass of O_2)

Step 2. Plug values into the equation:

$$m = \frac{(0.5 \text{ C/s})(60\text{s})(32 \text{ g/mol})}{(9.65 \times 10^4 \text{ C/mol}) (4 \text{ e}^- \text{ per formula unit})} = 0.0025 \text{ g}$$

Dimensional Analysis

$$\frac{(60\text{s}) \times (0.5\text{C}) \times (1 \text{ mol e}^-) \times (1 \text{ mol O}_2) \times (32.00 \text{ g O}_2)}{(\text{sec}) \times (9.65 \times 10^4 \text{ C}) \times (4 \text{ mol e}^-) \times (1 \text{ mol O}_2)}$$

$$= 0.0025 \text{ g}$$

SECT. II
GENERAL
CHEMISTRY
REVIEW
NOTES

297

General Chemistry

PRACTICE TESTS

SECT. II
GENERAL
CHEMISTRY
PRACTICE
TESTS

299

Time: 45 minutes

Directions: This test contains as many general chemistry passages as you may encounter on the real MCAT. There are also several independent multiple-choice questions at the end of this test. The time allotted approximates the time allowed on a real MCAT to solve the given number of questions. Choose one best answer for each question. You may refer to a periodic table as needed.

Passage I (Questions 1-8)

Although digestion begins in the mouth with the reaction between salivary amylase and carbohydrate, the stomach is the first major organ involved in the digestion of food. Between 2 L and 3 L of gastric juice is produced daily in the average adult stomach daily to facilitate digestion. Gastric juice is composed of hydrochloric acid (HCl) as well as other components, and it has a pH of 1.5.

The nonacidic components of gastric juice include the enzyme pepsin, which is activated from its inactive zymogen form, pepsinogen, in the presence of HCl. Pepsin is an important enzyme for digesting proteins. The production of gastric juice is stimulated by eating. For reasons that are not completely understood, overproduction of gastric juice can occur, which can lead to stomach ulcers.

One method of counteracting the overproduction of stomach acid is to take an antacid tablet. Antacid tablets consist of basic ingredients and possibly buffer components as well. In an effort to better understand the chemistry of antacids and to determine the comparative function of the various antacid products, a student performed a titration of 0.1000 M HCl on several commercial antacid tablets. The results are shown in Table 1.

TABLE 1. Titration results

Antacid	Initial Volume	Final Volume	Observation
Tums	24.03 ml	49.53 ml	Fizzed
Rolaids	28.09 ml	48.69 ml	Fizzed
Milk of Magnesia	14.26 ml	49.26 ml	Warm after titration
Alka-Seltzer	29.72 ml	49.62 ml	Fizzed initially

Some research into the ingredients of the various antacid products resulted in the information shown in Table 2.

TABLE 2. Antacid ingredients

Antacid	Components
Tums	Calcium carbonate
Rolaids	Dihydroxy aluminum sodium carbonate
Milk of Magnesia	Magnesium hydroxide
Alka-Seltzer	Sodium bicarbonate

1. Based on the information given in the passage, the concentration of hydrogen ion in the stomach is which one of the following values?

   A. 0.003
   B. 0.03
   C. 0.3
   D. 3

2. Based on the data given in the passage, Tums has the ability to neutralize:

   A. 0.00255 mol acid
   B. 0.0255 mol acid
   C. 2.55 mol acid
   D. 2550 mol acid

3. Which antacid is the most effective at neutralizing acid?

   A. Tums
   B. Rolaids
   C. Milk of Magnesia
   D. Alka-Seltzer

4. Milk of Magnesia was the most commonly used antacid during the nineteenth century. Based in part on the information presented in the passage, why might Milk of Magnesia no longer be as commonly used?

    A. It contains a weaker base and is therefore not as effective.
    B. It contains a stronger base and is therefore not as effective.
    C. It contains a weaker base and is therefore not as gentle on the stomach.
    D. It contains a stronger base and is therefore not as gentle on the stomach.

5. Which of the following components could be added to Tums to produce a buffered antacid?

    A. Calcium hydroxide
    B. Sodium carbonate
    C. Calcium bicarbonate
    D. Sodium hydroxide

6. Which chemical equation explains why fizzing is observed in many of the titrations?

    A. $H_2CO_3(aq) \rightleftharpoons H_2O(l) + CO_2(g)$
    B. $H_2O(l) \rightleftharpoons H_2O(g)$
    C. $H_2CO_3(aq) \rightleftharpoons H^+(aq) + HCO_3^-(aq)$
    D. $CaCO_3(aq) + HCl(aq) \rightleftharpoons H_2CO_3(aq) + CaCl_2(aq)$

7. The pH versus volume-added acid for the Milk of Magnesia titration would look like:

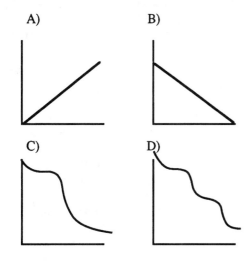

8. The pH versus volume added acid for Tums would look like:

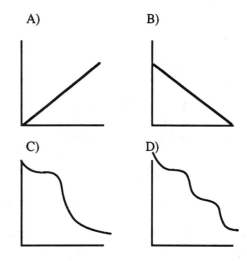

Passage II (Questions 9-15)

Almost half of the energy needs of the United States are supplied by petroleum. Petroleum is a complex mixture of alkanes, alkenes, cycloalkanes, and aromatic compounds. Petroleum deposits are widely distributed throughout the world. The actual composition of a petroleum sample varies with the location in which it was found.

Because petroleum contains thousands of compounds, separation of the compounds is necessary before petroleum can be useful. Fractional distillation is the process used to separate the compounds of petroleum into fractions based on their boiling point. A diagram of a fractional distillation column is shown below.

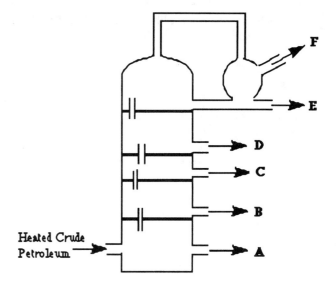

Fractional distillation of crude petroleum begins by heating the crude petroleum until vapor begins to form. This vapor moves up the column and condenses along the

301

side of the column. The liquid forms at different heights along the column based on boiling point. The lower-boiling components travel farther up the column. The major fractions of petroleum and their physical properties are shown in the following table.

TABLE 3. The major fractions of petroleum, their physical properties and uses

Fraction	Number of Carbon Atoms	Boiling Point Range (°C)	Uses
Natural gas	1–4	−161 to 20	Fuel and cooking
Petroleum ether	5–6	30 to 60	Solvent
Ligroin	7	20 to 135	Solvent
Gasoline	6–12	30 to 180	Auto fuels
Kerosene	11–16	170 to 290	Rocket and jet fuels; heating
Heating oil	14–18	260 to 350	Domestic heating
Lubricating oil	15–24	300 to 370	Machinery lubrication

9. Which of the following fractions might come off the fractionating column at the same port?

   A. Natural gas and lubricating oil
   B. Natural gas and petroleum ether
   C. Petroleum ether and ligroin
   D. Ligroin and kerosene

10. Which fraction is most likely to come off the fractionating column at port F?

    A. Natural gas
    B. Gasoline
    C. Kerosene
    D. Lubricating oil

11. Which fraction is most likely to come off the fractionating column at port A?

    A. Natural gas
    B. Gasoline
    C. Kerosene
    D. Lubricating oil

12. How could the fractionating set-up be modified to get fractions with smaller boiling point ranges?

    A. Add more ports at smaller intervals.
    B. Heat the crude petroleum to a higher temperature before introducing it to the column.
    C. Heat the crude petroleum to a lower temperature before introducing it to the column.
    D. Make the column shorter.

13. Why do the lower boiling components travel farther up the column?

    A. The top of the column is cooler than the bottom, so they travel farther before getting to their condensation temperature.
    B. The lower-boiling components are traveling more quickly up the column, so they travel farther in the same amount of time.
    C. The lower-boiling components start out at a higher temperature, so they travel farther before condensing.
    D. The lower-boiling components have a lower affinity for the walls of the column than the other components of the mixture, so they travel farther before sticking to the walls of the column.

14. What determines the composition of a sample of petroleum?

    A. The length of time it sits in storage tanks
    B. The temperature at which the sample is introduced to the fractionating column
    C. The temperature at which the sample is stored prior to fractionation
    D. The geographic location at which it is found

15. Why does the boiling point appear to increase with an increasing number of carbon atoms?

    A. Coincidence; there is no correlation between molecular weight and boiling point.
    B. A larger molecule has less energy than a smaller one, and therefore requires more energy input as heat to boil.
    C. A larger molecule has a greater capacity for intermolecular attractions, and more energy must be input as heat for a larger molecule to boil.
    D. More carbon atoms indicate more hydrogen atoms, which can bond to other molecules, and a greater energy input is required to break the hydrogen bonds.

Passage III (Questions 16-22)

Sodium carbonate (Na_2CO_3) ranks eleventh among chemicals produced in the United States. Sodium carbonate is an important material in many industrial processes, including water treatment, the glass industry, and the manufacturing of soaps, detergents, medicines, and food additives. Sulfur dioxide (SO_2) pollution in power plants can also be decreased when sodium carbonate is injected with the fuel into the furnace. The gaseous SO_2 produced during fuel combustion reacts with the added sodium carbonate to form solid sodium sulfite (Na_2SO_3).

A double exchange reaction for the formation of sodium carbonate is shown in reaction 1.

Reaction 1

$$CaCO_3(s) + NaCl(aq) \rightleftharpoons Na_2CO_3(aq) + CaCl_2(aq)$$

This reaction, however, is not industrially important because of the insolubility of the calcium carbonate and the difficulty isolating any resulting sodium carbonate from solution. The Solvay process is now used to produce sodium carbonate in large-scale operations.

The Solvay process begins with the decomposition of calcium carbonate at 1200°C, according to reaction 2. The carbon dioxide produced in reaction 2 is bubbled with ammonia through cold salt water as shown in reactions 3 and 4. The bicarbonate ion produced precipitates as the sodium salt, and it can be heated to produce sodium carbonate (reaction 5).

Reaction 2

$$CaCO_3(s) \rightarrow CaO(s) + CO_2(g)$$

Reaction 3

$$CO_2(aq) + H_2O(l) \rightleftharpoons H^+(aq) + HCO_3^-(aq)$$

Reaction 4

$$NH_3(aq) + H_2O(l) \rightleftharpoons NH_4^+(aq) + OH^-(aq)$$

Reaction 5

$$NaHCO_3(s) \rightarrow Na_2CO_3(s) + H_2O(g) + CO_2(g)$$

16. Which one of the following reactions from the passage is not balanced?

   A. Reaction 1
   B. Reaction 3
   C. Reaction 4
   D. Reaction 5

17. What reaction could be written for the precipitation that occurs during the Solvay process?

   A. $CO_3^{2-}(aq) + Ca^{2+}(aq) \rightleftharpoons CaCO_3(s)$
   B. $Na^+(aq) + HCO_3^-(aq) \rightleftharpoons NaHCO_3(s)$
   C. $Ca^{2+}(aq) + 2\ Cl^-(aq) \rightleftharpoons CaCl_2$
   D. $2\ Na^+(aq) + CO_3^{2-}(aq) \rightleftharpoons Na_2CO_3(s)$

18. How does the low solubility of calcium carbonate impact the industrial importance of reaction 1?

   A. The low concentration of calcium carbonate in solution will result in a very high equilibration constant (K_{eq}), and the right side of the reaction will be favored.
   B. The low concentration of calcium carbonate in solution will result in a very low K_{eq}, and the left side of the reaction will be favored.
   C. The low concentration of calcium carbonate in solution will result in a very low K_{eq}, and the right side of the reaction will be favored.
   D. The low concentration of calcium carbonate in solution will result in a very high K_{eq}, and the left side of the reaction will be favored.

19. Reaction 4 can be best classified as:

   A. disproportionation.
   B. acid–base.
   C. oxidation–reduction.
   D. single replacement.

20. What is the most reasonable solubility product constant (K_{sp}) for calcium carbonate based on the information inferred from the passage?

   A. 5.3×10^{-23}
   B. 6.4×10^{-1}
   C. $2.3 \times 10^{+7}$
   D. $7.8 \times 10^{+2}$

21. How would the K_{sp} expression for calcium chloride be written?

   A. $K_{sp} = [Ca^{2+}][Cl^-]^2$
   B. $K_{sp} = [Ca^{2+}][Cl^-]$
   C. $K_{sp} = [Ca^{2+}][Cl^-]^2/[CaCl_2]$
   D. $K_{sp} = [Ca^{2+}]^2[Cl^-]$

22. Why is salt water used as the solvent for reactions 3 and 4?

  A. Because the necessary ions are more soluble in salt water.
  B. Because a high chloride ion concentration is needed to promote the desired precipitation reaction.
  C. Because a high sodium ion concentration is needed to promote the desired precipitation reaction.
  D. The salt is needed as a reactant.

Passage IV (Questions 23-29)

A chemistry student studies limestone in both the chemistry laboratory and in the field. The chemistry student discovers that limestone, known chemically as ($CaCO_3$), is widespread on the Earth's surface and is in contact with the water supply in many locations. Limestone itself is insoluble but the student learns that reaction 1 can occur.

Reaction 1

$$CaCO_3(s) + CO_2(aq) + H_2O(l) \rightarrow Ca^{2+}(aq) + 2HCO_3^-(aq)$$

The student also discovers that water containing calcium or magnesium ions is called hard water. When water containing Ca^{2+} and HCO_3^- ions is boiled, reaction 1 is reversed (reaction 2).

Reaction 2

$$Ca^{2+}(aq) + 2 HCO_3^-(aq) \rightarrow CaCO_3(s) + CO_2(aq) + H_2O(l)$$

The student notes that the solid calcium carbonate formed in this way is the main component of scale deposits observed in boilers, water heaters, pipes, and tea kettles. The student also learns that often, plumbers use hydrochloric acid to remove scale deposits from water pipes.

To better understand the chemistry of limestone, the student makes some basic observations regarding solubility. These observations help explain the behavior of limestone and its associated ions. The observations are shown below:

Observation 1: All group 1A (alkali metal) hydroxides are soluble. Of the group 2A (alkaline earth metal) hydroxides, only barium hydroxide is soluble.
Observation 2: Most compounds containing chlorides, bromides, or iodides are soluble.
Observation 3: Most sulfates are soluble. Calcium and silver sulfate are only slightly soluble.

Observation 4: All compounds containing nitrate, chlorate, and perchlorate are soluble.
Observation 5: All carbonates and phosphates are insoluble, except those of ammonium and alkali metals.
Observation 6: All ammonium compounds are soluble.
Observation 7: All alkali metal compounds are soluble.

23. Which of the following factors is most important in driving reaction 2 to the right?

  A. Heat allows the reaction to proceed farther before reaching equilibrium.
  B. Heat speeds up the reaction.
  C. Solids are less soluble in boiling water.
  D. Gases are less soluble in boiling water.

24. Which of the following reactions demonstrates the net action of hydrochloric acid on scale?

  A. $CaCO_3(s) + HCl(aq) \rightarrow CaCl_2(aq) + HCO_3^-(aq)$
  B. $CaCO_3(s) + 2 HCl(aq) \rightarrow CaCl_2(aq) + HCO_3^-(aq)$
  C. $CaCO_3(s) + 2 H^+(aq) \rightarrow Ca^{2+}(aq) + H_2O(l) + CO_2(g)$
  D. $CaCO_3(s) + H^+(aq) \rightarrow Ca^{2+}(aq) + H_2O(l) + CO_2(g)$

25. What substance might be used instead of hydrochloric acid to remove scale from pipes?

  A. Hydrobromic acid
  B. Ammonium phosphate
  C. Ammonium carbonate
  D. Sodium phosphate

26. Would sulfuric acid be as effective as hydrochloric acid at removing scale from pipes?

  A. Yes, all that is required is an acid.
  B. No, sulfuric acid is not strong enough.
  C. Yes, it would work better because it is a diprotic acid.
  D. No, the calcium sulfate formed is only partially soluble.

27. Could a strong base such as sodium hydroxide be used to remove scale from pipes?

  A. No, the sodium carbonate formed is not soluble.
  B. No, the calcium hydroxide formed is not soluble.
  C. No, neither the sodium carbonate nor the calcium hydroxide formed is soluble.
  D. Yes, both sodium carbonate and calcium hydroxide are soluble.

28. If sodium bicarbonate was present in the water supply, which of the following would be true?

  A. The equilibrium position of reaction 1 would shift to the right, and the equilibrium position of reaction 2 would shift to the right.
  B. The equilibrium position of reaction 1 would shift to the right, and the equilibrium position of reaction 2 would shift to the left.
  C. The equilibrium position of reaction 1 would shift to the left, and the equilibrium position of reaction 2 would shift to the right.
  D. The equilibrium position of reaction 1 would shift to the left, and the equilibrium position of reaction 2 would shift to the left.

29. Which one of the following statements best describes hard water?

  A. It has high concentrations of ions.
  B. It has low concentrations of ions.
  C. It has a high concentration of calcium or magnesium ions.
  D. It has a low concentration of calcium and magnesium ions.

Passage V (Questions 30-36)

A colligative property is any property of a solution that varies in proportion to the concentration of the solute present in a given volume of solution. These properties can be applied to the study of solution vapor pressure, boiling point elevation, freezing point depression, and osmotic pressure. In addition, the colligative properties can be used to study the behavior of solutes in aqueous solution. The results of studies involving the colligative behavior of compounds have provided a great deal of insight into the chemistry of molecules.

In an effort to explore the basic behavior of the colligative properties, a chemist conducts experiments with several different compounds. Consider the series of freezing point experiments given below for mercury-containing compounds. Note that the $K_f = 1.9$ for water. Also recall that $\Delta T = -iKfm$, where m is the molality of particles in solution. K_f is the freezing point constant, and i is the van't Hoff factor, which equals the actual number of moles of particles formed per mole of formula units of solute when ionized.

Experiment 1

A chemist prepares a 0.01 molal solution of mercuric nitrate, $Hg(NO_3)_2$. The freezing point of the solution is measured to be $-0.060°C$.

Experiment 2

A chemist dissolves 10.8 g of mercuric chloride, $HgCl_2$, in 1000 grams of water. Trials are conducted and the freezing point of the solution is measured to be $-0.075°C$. The molecular weight of mercuric chloride is 271 g/mole.

30. Using the definition of molality and the data from experiment 2, which of the following values is the best approximation for the molality?

  A. 0.01
  B. 0.02
  C. 0.03
  D. 0.04

31. Using the measured freezing point in experiment 2, the molality of ions in the mercuric chloride solution is closest to:

  A. 0.01.
  B. 0.02.
  C. 0.03.
  D. 0.04.

32. Analysis of all data from experiment 1 allows extrapolation to which conclusion?

  I. An aqueous solution of mercuric nitrate strongly conducts electricity.
  II. Mercuric nitrate completely dissociates when placed in water.

  A. I only
  B. II only
  C. Both I and II
  D. Neither I nor II

33. Analysis of all data from experiment 2 allows extrapolation to which conclusion?

  I. An aqueous solution of mercuric chloride strongly conducts electricity.
  II. Mercuric chloride completely dissociates when placed in water.

  A. I only
  B. II only
  C. Both I and II
  D. Neither I nor II

34. Comparison of experiment 1 with experiment 2 allows for extrapolation to which of the following conclusion(s)?

   I. Mercuric chloride will elevate the boiling point of water to a greater extent than will mercuric nitrate.

   II. Preparing a 0.1 molar $HgCl_2$ solution involves a more favorable entropy change than preparing a 0.1 molar $Hg(NO_3)_2$ solution.

   III. $Hg(NO_3)_2$ dissociates more completely in water than does mercuric chloride.

   A. I only
   B. II only
   C. III only
   D. I and II only

35. If medical evidence were obtained that showed that free mercury ions were the most toxic form of mercury to humans, which of the following would be least likely to cause serious health problems if ingested?

   A. A 0.07 molal solution of $HgCl_2$
   B. A 0.05 molal solution of $Hg(NO_3)_2$
   C. A solution containing 0.07 molal $HgCl_2$ and 0.01 molal $Hg(NO_3)_2$
   D. All of the above are equally likely

36. How do the bonds to the mercury atom in the compound $HgCl_2$ compare with those in the compound $Hg(NO_3)_2$?

   A. They are more ionic in character.
   B. They are more covalent in character.
   C. They are the same type of bond.
   D. A conclusion cannot be made.

Questions 37-40 are NOT based on a descriptive passage.

37. Which of the following are state functions?

   I. S
   II. H
   III. G

   A. II only
   B. II and III only
   C. I and II only
   D. I, II, and III

38. Given the following data, calculate the heat of formation for ethanol:

   1. $C_2H_5OH + 3\ O_2 \rightarrow 2\ CO_2 + 3\ H_2O$
      $\Delta H = -327.0$ kcal/mole

   2. $H_2O \rightarrow H_2 + 1/2\ O_2$
      $\Delta H = +68.3$ kcal/mole

   3. $C + O_2 \rightarrow CO_2$
      $\Delta H = -94.1$ kcal/mole

   A. $-$ 66.1 kcal
   B. $+$ 67.2 kcal
   C. $+$ 66.1 kcal
   D. $-$ 67.2 kcal

39. Which of the following statements best explains why H_2O has an unusually high boiling point when compared with H_2S?

   A. H_2O molecules pack into a more ordered structure than H_2S.
   B. Van der Waals forces play a part.
   C. London forces play a part.
   D. Hydrogen bonding plays a part.

40. Which of the following is responsible for the changes seen in ionization energy when moving down a column in the periodic table?

   A. Increasing nuclear attraction for electrons
   B. Increased shielding of electrons and larger atomic or ionic radii.
   C. Increased shielding of electrons and increasing nuclear attraction for electrons.
   D. Increasing nuclear attraction for electrons and larger atomic or ionic radii.

answers

Answers and Explanations to General Chemistry Practice Test 1

1. **B**   To calculate hydrogen ion concentration from pH, take 10^{-pH}. There is little time for tedious calculations on the MCAT, and the multiple choice answers are often different enough that estimation will allow selection of the correct choice. Because calculators cannot be used for the MCAT, $10^{-1.5}$ can be estimated by realizing that $10^{-1} = 0.1$ and $10^{-2} = 0.01$. Thus, $10^{-1.5}$ must be between 0.1 and 0.01. Choice B, 0.03, falls within that range.

2. **A**   The number of moles of acid that Tums can neutralize will be the amount of hydrochloric acid (HCl) added during the titration. There are two values to help make this determination: the concentration of the acid (0.1000 M) and the volume added (49.53 mL − 24.03 mL = 25.50 mL). Remember that M = moles/L and that the volume units must be the same to end up with moles as the unit. The formula to use is moles = concentration × volume. Substituting values gives moles = 0.1000 M × 25.50 mL × 1 L/1000 mL = 0.00255 moles.

3. **C**   The antacid that is the most effective at neutralizing acid is the one that requires the greatest volume of acid in the titration. This is true only because the acid used with each antacid was the same concentration. Table 1 shows that the Milk of Magnesia required the greatest volume of acid.

4. **D**   The active ingredient listed for Milk of Magnesia is magnesium hydroxide. A similar and familiar compound is sodium hydroxide, which is a strong base. Another clue to the correct answer is given in Table 1, in which it is noted that Milk of Magnesia was warm after the titration. Acid–base reactions release heat, and strong acids (e.g., HCl) reacting with strong bases produce noticeably more heat than do strong acids reacting with weak bases.

5. **C**   To form a buffered solution, an acid and its conjugate base must be present. The active ingredient listed for Tums is calcium carbonate (Table 2). Calcium is neither an acid nor a base, so the answer must contain either the conjugate acid or base of the carbonate ion. Carbonate (CO_3^{2-}) does not have a conjugate base, but its conjugate acid is bicarbonate (HCO_3^-). Therefore, calcium bicarbonate would produce a buffered solution with calcium carbonate.

6. **A**   The three titrations that were observed to fizz all contained some form of carbonate. Carbonate is in equilibrium with carbonic acid (H_2CO_3), which is unstable and decomposes to form water and carbon dioxide. The observed fizzing is the result of the carbon dioxide gas being released.

7. **C**   To answer this type of question, one must know that pH versus volume means that pH is plotted on the y-axis, and volume goes on the x-axis. Recall that Milk of Magnesia is a strong base. A titration of a strong base with a strong acid starts at a high pH and ends up at a low pH. A titration of a strong base with a strong acid starts at a high pH and ends up at a low pH. Therefore, the answer, C, looks like an upside-down titration curve of a strong acid with a strong base.

SECT. 11
GENERAL
CHEMISTRY
PRACTICE
TEST

307

8. **D** The active ingredient in Tums is carbonate, which is a weak base. The titration of a weak base with a strong acid produces a sigmoidal curve. There will be one plateau for each ionization, and carbonate has two ionizations:

$$CO_3^{2-} + H^+ \rightarrow HCO_3^-$$
$$HCO_3^- + H^+ \rightarrow H_2CO_3$$

PASSAGE II

9. **C** Because fractional distillation separates substances based on boiling point, two fractions might come off at the same port if their boiling points overlap. The only two options given with overlapping boiling points are petroleum ether and ligroin, choice C.

10. **A** Port F is at the top of the fractional distillation set-up. This means that the lowest boiling fraction will be the one to reach that port. The table lists natural gas, A, as the component with the lowest boiling point.

11. **D** Port A is at the bottom of the fractional distillation set-up. This means that the highest boiling component will be the most likely substance to not go pass port A. Lubricating oil is listed in the table as the component with the highest boiling point.

12. **A** There are two ways to get better separation from a fractional distillation set-up. One is to increase the length of the column, which was not offered as a possible answer. The other is to increase the number of ports. Changing the temperature of the petroleum before introducing it to the column would either cluster the compounds closer together at the top (if petroleum is made hotter) or the bottom (if the petroleum is made cooler) of the set-up.

13. **A** The compounds that require less energy to remain in the gas phase will naturally stay in the gas phase longer. The vapor is introduced at the bottom and travels up the column, so the components with lower boiling points will travel farther before reaching their condensation temperature.

14. **D** This question requires information recall. The last sentence of the first paragraph gives the answer: The actual composition of a petroleum sample varies with the location in which it was found.

15. **C** The larger size of a molecule with more carbon atoms allows more intermolecular attractions. This tends to hold the compound in a condensed (solid or liquid) phase longer than a smaller molecule. Hydrogen bonding would also effectively hold the molecules in a condensed phase, but the components of petroleum listed in the passage do not have hydrogen atoms attached to electronegative atoms, such as oxygen, nitrogen, or fluorine.

PASSAGE III

16. **D** Reaction 5 has one sodium molecule on the left side of the equation and two sodium molecules on the right side. The hydrogen, carbon, and oxygen molecules also do not add up.

17. **B** The passage states that in the Solvay process, the bicarbonate ion produced (after reactions 3 and 4) precipitates as the sodium salt; that is, sodium bicarbonate. This eliminates choices A and C, as they do not contain sodium. Choice D contains sodium carbonate (Na_2CO_3) rather than the bicarbonate ion. That leaves choice B, which produces $NaHCO_3$, as the correct answer.

18. **D** The equilibration constant (K_{eq}) is always expressed as product concentrations over starting material concentrations. Because calcium carbonate has a very low solubility, its concentration will be low, and the denominator will be very small. Dividing by a smaller number yields a larger number (i.e., $1/1 = 1$ but $1/0.1 = 10$). When Q (which is calculated the same as K_{eq} but applies to non-equilibrium situations) is greater than K_{eq}, the reaction proceeds from right to left until $Q = K_{eq}$.

19. **B** In reaction 4, ammonia gains a proton, and water loses a proton. This is an acid–base reaction.

ANSWERS AND
EXPLANATIONS
TO GENERAL
CHEMISTRY
PRACTICE TEST I

308

20. **A** The larger the solubility product constant (K_{sp}), the greater the concentration of ions in solution. For calcium carbonate, $K_{sp} = [Ca^{2+}][CO_3]^2$. A compound with a low solubility will have a low value for K_{sp}. The most reasonable answer, therefore, is the one with the lowest K_{sp}; that is, 5.3×10^{-23}.

21. **A** The important feature of a solubility product constant (K_{sp}) compared with an equilibration constant (K_{eq}) is that only the ions from the right side of the dissociation equation appear because solids are left out of equilibrium expressions. An important feature of equilibrium expressions is that every product must appear as many times as it shows up in the balanced equation. This means that the concentration is raised to the power of the coefficient. Calcium chloride dissolves to form one calcium ion and two chloride ions. The concentration of the chloride ion must show up twice in the K_{sp}. Choice C is incorrect because it contains a term for the solid, $CaCl_2$.

22. **C** The common ion effect is extremely important in the desired precipitation reaction. Sodium bicarbonate is somewhat soluble. If a large excess of sodium is added, the product of sodium and bicarbonate ions will exceed the solubility product constant (K_{sp}), and sodium bicarbonate will precipitate. Remember that the K_{sp} includes all sodium and bicarbonate ions, regardless of their source.

---

23. **D** Although the carbon dioxide (CO_2) in reaction 2 is described as aqueous, it is still a gas. The term aqueous simply means that it is dissolved in water. In boiling water, the carbon dioxide is driven off, which pulls the equilibrium toward the right side.

24. **C** The reactions shown in choices A and B are not balanced, and they should only be considered if no other reasonable choice is offered. Choice C is more reasonable because it demonstrates that the carbonate is permanently removed as carbon dioxide. A reaction that temporarily converts calcium carbonate to a soluble species would only temporarily solve the problem.

25. **A** The solubility rules (observations) in the passage state that most compounds containing chlorides, bromides, or iodides are soluble (observation 2). Thus, hydrobromic acid would be very analogous to hydrochloric acid and could react with calcium carbonate to form calcium bromide and hydrogen carbonate, which would decompose to release carbon dioxide and water.

26. **D** Sulfuric acid would remove the scale (calcium carbonate), giving off carbon dioxide, but the calcium carbonate would simply be replaced by sulfate. Observation 3 states that calcium sulfate is only partially soluble.

27. **B** The reaction of calcium carbonate with sodium hydroxide would produce sodium carbonate and calcium hydroxide. Observation 1 indicates that of the group 2A hydroxides (which include calcium hydroxide), only barium hydroxide is soluble.

28. **C** If sodium bicarbonate was present in the water supply, the equilibria would shift away from where the added bicarbonate shows up in the reaction. In reaction 1, bicarbonate (HCO_3^-) is on the right side of the equation, so the equilibrium will shift to the left. In reaction 2, bicarbonate is on the left side, so the equilibrium will shift to the right side of the equation.

29. **C** The answer to this question is based on information recall. The first sentence after reaction 1 states that hard water contains calcium or magnesium ions.

---

30. **D** Molality (m) equals moles of solute per kilograms of solvent. For this problem, start by calculating the moles of solute. This equals 10.8 g divided by 271 g/mole, which equals 0.04 moles. The solvent is water. There is 1 kilogram of water given in this problem. Thus, the molality is (0.04 moles)/(1 kg water) = 0.04.

31. **D** $\Delta T_f = iK_f m$. K_f is the freezing point constant, and i is the van't Hoff factor, which equals the number of moles of particles formed per mole of formula units of solute when ionized. This question appears to be easy, but it is deceiving. The problem is that without knowing if the compound dissociates in solution, the

SECT. II
GENERAL
CHEMISTRY
PRACTICE
TEST

309

value of i is unknown. To figure out if the compound dissociates, the molality calculation from question 30 is used. Thus, $0.075 = -(i)(1.9)(0.04)$. When solving for i, i is found to equal 1, which means that the compound does not dissociate in water. The calculation of molality based on the freezing point depression can proceed: $0.075 = (1)(1.9)(m)$. Therefore, m = 0.04.

32. **C** A good way to solve this problem is to work backward. Using the freezing point of the mercuric nitrate solution, it is known that $-0.06 = (i)(1.9)(0.01)$. This means that i is approximately equal to 3. This should suggest that the compound dissociates into its respective ions and is soluble. In addition, ionic solutions strongly conduct electricity.

33. **D** Using the freezing point of the mercuric chloride solution to find the molality (m), it is found that m = 0.04, similar to question 31. This suggests that $HgCl_2$ does not dissociate into Hg^{2+} and $2 Cl^-$. Therefore, the solution is nonionic, and nonionic solutions do not conduct electricity.

34. **C** Because mercuric chloride does not dissociate and mercuric nitrate does dissociate, mercuric chloride will not elevate the boiling point of water to the extent that mercuric nitrate will. Thus, statement I is false. Remember that entropy is a measure of the disorder within a system. Note that the more entropic solution will have a greater number of particles, therefore, statement II is false. Statement III is true because, as stated, mercuric nitrate does dissociate and does elevate the boiling point of water.

35. **A** The data from experiments 1 and 2 demonstrate that mercuric nitrate dissociates more completely than mercuric chloride. Choice A, mercuric chloride, is the least likely of the choices to cause serious health problems if ingested. Choice B is mercuric nitrate, and choice C contains mercuric nitrate, so both could cause health problems. Choice D is wrong because choices B and C are eliminated.

36. **B** Water is excellent at dissolving ionic and polar compounds. Therefore, solubility can be used as a measure of ionic character. Because mercuric nitrate dissociates completely in solution, it must be ionic. Therefore, the bonds in mercuric chloride must be more covalent than those in mercuric nitrate.

37. **D** Entropy, enthalpy, and free energy are state functions because they depend only on the initial and final states of the system. They are independent of the path taken to reach the final state.

38. **A** This question can be answered by doing the following steps. First, reverse the first equation and change the sign of ΔH:

$$2 CO_2 + 3 H_2O \rightarrow 3 O_2 + C_2H_5OH; \Delta H = +327.0$$

Next, reverse the second equation and multiply by 3:

$$3(H_2 + 1/2 O_2 \rightarrow H_2O); \Delta H = 3(-68.3)$$

Next, multiply the third equation by 2:

$$2(C + O_2 \rightarrow CO_2); \Delta H = 2(-94.1)$$

Add all three equations above and their respective ΔH values:

$$327.0 + 3(-68.3) + 2(-94.1) = -66.1 \text{ kcal.}$$

39. **D** The order of interaction strengths from strongest to weakest in this question is: hydrogen bonding, polar forces, van der Waals forces. Oxygen is more electronegative than sulfure, and it allows the water molecule to form strong hydrogen bonds.

ANSWERS AND
EXPLANATIONS
TO GENERAL
CHEMISTRY
PRACTICE TEST 1

310

40. **B** The elements at the bottom of the periodic table have low ionization energies because they are shielded from the positive charge of the nucleus, and these elements have large atomic radii (choice B). The farther the electrons are from the nucleus, the easier it is for the outer electrons to be lost.

GENERAL CHEMISTRY PRACTICE TEST 2

Time: 45 minutes

Directions: This test contains as many general chemistry passages as you may encounter on the real MCAT. There are also several independent multiple-choice questions at the end of this test. The time allotted approximates the time allowed on a real MCAT to solve the given number of questions. Choose one best answer for each question. You may refer to a periodic table as needed.

Passage I (Questions 1–7)

Kinetic theory provides several gas laws that explain the movement of gases and allow quantification of molecular speed. The average molecular speed is proportional to the square root of the absolute temperature and is inversely proportional to the square root of the molecular mass.

Kinetic theory also allows the derivation of another gas law describing the movement of gases. This is known as Graham's law. Gases move through an open space or through a permeable barrier by a process known as diffusion. Effusion, on the other hand, refers to a process whereby a gas escapes through a small hole in a container. Graham's law of effusion states that the relative rates of gases escaping through a pinhole is inversely proportional to the square root of the molecular weight of the gas.

A student performed an experiment using balloons filled with equal volumes of gases to observe Graham's law. The experimental design and results are given below:

Experimental design

The student asked the instructor to choose two unknown gases and fill separate balloons with 1 L of each of those pure gases. The student filled balloons with 1 L each of hydrogen, helium, neon, argon, nitrogen, oxygen, and krypton.

Experimental results

At the end of 3 days, the student ranked the balloons by increasing size. The result was hydrogen, helium, neon, nitrogen, unknown 1, oxygen, unknown 2, argon, krypton.

1. If a balloon is filled with equal volumes of each of the gases below, which one will be the largest at the end of a week?

    A. Helium
    B. Hydrogen
    C. Oxygen
    D. Neon

2. If a single balloon is filled with equal volumes of hydrogen, helium, nitrogen, neon, and oxygen, which gas will be depleted first?

    A. Helium
    B. Hydrogen
    C. Nitrogen
    D. Neon

3. Unknown 1 could be which one of the following?

    A. Carbon dioxide
    B. Carbon monoxide
    C. Nitrogen monoxide
    D. Methane

4. Unknown 2 could be which one of the following?

    A. Fluorine
    B. Hydrogen sulfide
    C. Carbon monoxide
    D. More than one of the above

311

5. Which one of the following equations describes the relationship between the effusion rates of oxygen (E_o) and unknown 1 (E_u)?

   A. $E_o/E_u = MW_u/MW_o$
   B. $E_o/E_u = (MW_u/MW_o)^{1/2}$
   C. $(E_o/E_u)^2 = (MW_u/MW_o)^{1/2}$
   D. $E_o/E_u = (MW_o/MW_u)^{1/2}$

6. If a balloon filled with 1 L of a mixture of hydrogen and helium is compared to a balloon filled with 1 L of either hydrogen or helium, the relative size at the end of 3 days will be:

   A. mixture > hydrogen > helium.
   B. mixture > helium > hydrogen.
   C. hydrogen > mixture > helium.
   D. helium > mixture > hydrogen.

7. Considering a balloon filled with equal volumes of hydrogen, helium, and neon, what will be the final proportion of gases, in decreasing volume, after 3 days?

   A. Neon > helium > hydrogen
   B. Hydrogen > neon > helium
   C. Helium > hydrogen > neon
   D. Neon > hydrogen > helium

Passage II (Questions 8–13)

There are several important theories as to how chemical reactions take place. One of the prominent theories is known as collision theory. This theory postulates that when two different particles collide (reactants), sufficient kinetic energy must be available to allow for the rearrangement of bonds in the particles to occur and to lead to the formation of products. The rate at which the reaction can occur leading to product formation depends on the number of collisions between reactant particles per unit time and the fraction of collisions that possess enough energy for reaction.

Two important terms are frequently used in chemical kinetics. The activation energy is an important consideration when studying chemical kinetics. The activation energy is considered the extra energy necessary to alter the valence–electron configuration of the reactants to that of the activated complex. One can think of the activation energy as an "energy hill" that the reactants must climb to form products. The activated complex, or transition state, is an intermediate form between reactants and products.

The following plots show the thermodynamic diagrams for the reaction progress of three different reactions:

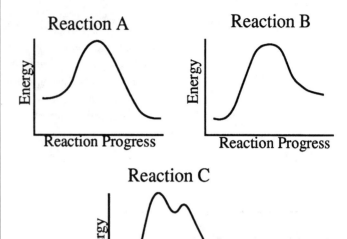

Figure 1 The reaction progress for reactions A, B, and C.

8. Which of the reactions is exothermic?

   A. Reaction A
   B. Reaction B
   C. Reaction C
   D. Reactions B and C

9. Which of the reactions would most likely absorb heat energy from the surroundings?

   A. Reaction A
   B. Reaction B
   C. Reaction C
   D. Reactions B and C

10. In reaction C, the diagram has a region where the energy is low relative to the energy "hills" on either side. This region signifies:

   A. the transition state.
   B. an isolatable product that can be reacted to form the lower energy product.
   C. a temporary intermediate that cannot be isolated.
   D. an experimental error.

11. The highest point on the curve representing reaction B signifies:

    A. the transition state.

    B. an isolatable product that can be reacted to form the lower energy product.

    C. a temporary intermediate that cannot be isolated.

    D. an experimental error.

12. A noticeable difference in the mechanism of reaction C versus reactions A and B is:

    A. it has two transition states.

    B. it requires two steps.

    C. the rate-determining step is the first step.

    D. it has two transition states and requires two steps.

13. The addition of a catalyst would have which of the following effects on the diagram for reaction B?

    A. It would raise the energy of the starting materials closer to the energy of the transition state so that the reaction can proceed faster.

    B. It would lower the energy of the transition state but not effect any other part of the diagram.

    C. It would change the mechanism of the reaction so that it could proceed along a lower energy path, which may or may not have the same general shape.

    D. Either B or C could occur.

Passage III (Questions 14–19)

Absorption spectroscopy can give valuable qualitative and quantitative information about substances that absorb light in the visible region. Absorbance is a unitless measure of the amount of light absorbed by a sample.

The details of light absorption are quite complex. When an atom absorbs a photon, the total angular momentum of the atom and photon must be constant. Thus, because the photon carries angular momentum, the electron that absorbs that photon must change its angular momentum.

The absorbance of a substance at a given wavelength is quantitatively related to the concentration of that substance in solution by Beer's law (i.e., $A = \epsilon bc$), where A is absorbance, ϵ is the molar extinction coefficient (L/mole-cm), b is the path length through which the light must travel in the solution being measured (cm), and c is the concentration (moles/L).

Qualitative information can be obtained by running a scan over a range of wavelengths for a single solution. Consider an unknown, solution A. Two figures are given below for solution A. Figure 2 demonstrates the concentration versus absorbance, and Figure 3 demonstrates the wavelength versus absorbance for this particular solution. Table 1 demonstrates the wavelength and color relations of the visible spectrum.

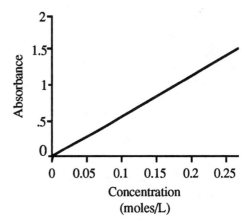

Figure 2   Concentration versus absorbance curve for solution A at 550 nm.

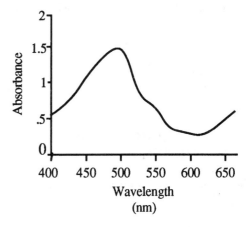

Figure 3   Wavelength versus absorbance curve for solution A.

TABLE 1. Wavelength and Color Relations of the Visible Spectrum

Color:	Red	Orange	Yellow	Green	Blue	Indigo	Violet
Nanometers:	700	650	600	550	500	450	400

14. Was the concentration-versus-absorbance curve measured at an appropriate wavelength for determining the concentrations of very dilute solutions?

    A. Yes, because it is linear down to zero concentration.
    B. No, measuring the absorbance-versus-concentration curve at the wavelength where maximum absorbance was measured would be more appropriate for very dilute solutions.
    C. Yes, because increasing the wavelength would decrease the absorbance, which would make the measurement of dilute solutions more difficult.
    D. Yes, because the choice of wavelength does not affect Beer's law.

15. If the absorbance of an unknown solution is measured at 550 nm and is found to be 0.5, what is the approximate concentration of that solution?

    A. 0.005 M
    B. 0.01 M
    C. 0.05 M
    D. 0.1 M

16. According to Figures 2 and 3, which color is solution A least likely to appear?

    A. Red
    B. Orange
    C. Yellow
    D. Blue

17. Absorption spectroscopy would be a good quantitative tool for which of the following measurements?

    A. Food dye in fruit drinks
    B. Sugar in fruit drinks
    C. Amount of alcohol in liquors
    D. Both B and C

18. How could the molar extinction coefficient be determined from Figure 2?

    A. It is equal to the y-intercept.
    B. It is equal to the slope.
    C. It is equal to the slope divided by b.
    D. It is equal to the y-intercept divided by b.

19. If the molar extinction coefficient is 100 L/mol-cm at 500 nm, and the absorbance measured for an unknown solution in a cuvette with a 1-cm path length is 0.5, what is the concentration?

    A. 0.1 M
    B. 0.5 M
    C. 0.05 M
    D. 0.005 M

Passage IV (Questions 20–27)

When an object at one temperature is placed on or near a second object at a higher temperature, energy is transferred to the cooler object. This object then experiences an increase in temperature. When a ratio is taken between the amount of energy and the temperature change, the ratio is known as the heat capacity.

Heat capacities are important properties of substances. For example, water has a high heat capacity. This property makes water useful for cooling engines and for storing heat in solar energy heating systems. Heat capacities and the heat associated with reactions are often measured by calorimeters.

The determination of ΔE is frequently performed in an apparatus called a bomb calorimeter. This piece of equipment has strong, well-insulated walls that minimize the exchange of heat with the surroundings and maintain a constant volume. The following figure shows the design of a bomb calorimeter.

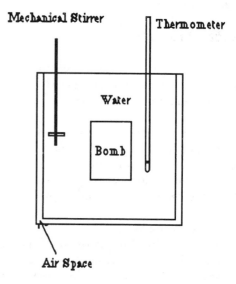

Figure 4   A bomb calorimeter.

The measurement of the ΔE for a reaction requires that the reaction occur quickly, yield definite products without side reactions, and essentially go to completion.

20. Reactions that go to completion generally have what type of value for their equilibrium constants?

   A. Zero
   B. Very small
   C. Average
   D. Very large

21. Why would a reaction have to occur quickly for measurement of the ΔE?

   A. Heat exchange with the surroundings is maximized.
   B. Reactions that take a long time probably will not go to completion.
   C. Reactions that take a long time probably produce side products.
   D. The longer a reaction takes, the more chances there are for heat exchange with the surroundings.

22. ΔE represents what kind of physical change?

   A. Heat absorbed at constant pressure
   B. Heat lost at constant pressure
   C. Heat absorbed at constant volume
   D. Heat lost at constant volume

23. Could ΔH be measured directly in a bomb calorimeter? Why or why not?

   A. It could because ΔH is the heat absorbed at constant pressure.
   B. It could not because ΔH is the heat absorbed at constant pressure.
   C. It could because ΔH is the heat absorbed at constant volume.
   D. It could not because ΔH is the heat absorbed at constant volume.

24. Which of the following types of processes would be the best candidate for determination of ΔE by bomb calorimetry?

   A. Acid–base reactions
   B. A salt dissolving in water
   C. Combustion
   D. Precipitation

25. Which of the following is the balanced combustion equation for sucrose $(C_{12}H_{22}O_{11})$?

   A. $C_{12}H_{22}O_{11} + 6\ O_2 \rightarrow 12\ CO + 11\ H_2O$
   B. $C_{12}H_{22}O_{11} + O_2 \rightarrow CO_2 + H_2O$
   C. $C_{12}H_{22}O_{11} + O_2 \rightarrow CO + H_2O$
   D. $C_{12}H_{22}O_{11} + 12\ O_2 \rightarrow 12\ CO_2 + 11\ H_2O$

26. If 3.42 g of sucrose (MW = 342 g/mole) were burned in a bomb calorimeter (assume that the heat capacity of the calorimeter is 10.00 kJ/K), and the temperature changed 5.647 K, what is the heat of combustion of sucrose at constant volume?

   A. 5.647 kJ/mole
   B. −5.647 kJ/mole
   C. 56.47 kJ/mole
   D. −5647 kJ/mole

27. The best reason why water is useful for cooling engines and storing heat in solar heating systems is that:

   A. water stores a large amount of energy for a large temperature change.
   B. water stores a small amount of energy for a large temperature change.
   C. water stores a large amount of energy for a small temperature change.
   D. water stores a small amount of energy for a small temperature change.

Passage V (Questions 28–35)

Acid–base reactions are one of the most important reaction types in chemistry. Although there are three systems for classifying acids and bases, the Brönsted-Lowry system is the most popular. In this system, an acid is any molecule or ion that can donate a proton, and a base is any molecule or ion that can accept a proton.

Acids and bases can be rated by the concentrations of their hydrogen and hydroxide ions, respectively. Because the concentrations of these species are often very small, chemists simplify concentration expressions by using a logarithmic base-ten scale for hydrogen and hydroxide ion concentrations. The terms pH and pOH are defined as the negative logarithm of the hydrogen ion and hydroxide ion concentrations, respectively.

A series of experiments were performed with reagents to explore reactions in acid–base systems. For the following experiments, consider HA to be a weak acid with an unknown pK_a (negative logarithm of the acid ionization constant). HZ is an acid (it is unknown whether HZ is weak or strong), and NaA is the salt of the weak acid HA.

Experiment 1

A premedical student prepares a 0.10M solution of HA. She measures the pH of the solution to be 5 using a pH meter.

Experiment 2

A premedical student finds by titration that 15 grams of HZ is neutralized by 100 ml of 1.0M NaOH. She performs conductivity studies on HZ and is surprised at how well an aqueous solution of HZ conducts electricity.

Experiment 3

The premedical student who performed experiment 1 now dissolves NaA in water, such that the molarity of NaA is 0.10M. She tries to measure the pH of this solution with the pH meter, but she finds that the pH meter is broken.

28. What is the concentration of H^+ in the solution prepared in experiment 1?

   A. 10^{-9}
   B. 10^{-5}
   C.   0.01
   D.   0.10

29. What is the concentration of A^- in the solution prepared in experiment 1?

   A. 10^{-9}
   B. 10^{-5}
   C.   0.01
   D.   0.10

30. The pKa of HA using the results of experiment 1 is closest to:

   A.   5
   B.   7
   C.   8
   D.   9

31. The fact that an aqueous solution of HZ strongly conducts electricity suggests that:

   A.   the HZ bond is stable in water.
   B.   the HZ molecule is really a base.
   C.   the HZ molecule dissociates completely into ions in water.
   D.   an oxidation–reduction reaction is occurring.

32. An estimation of the pH of the solution made by the premedical student in experiment 3 would be:

   A.   5
   B.   7
   C.   9
   D.   11

33. Consider the solution made by mixing equal volumes of equimolar solutions of HZ and NaA. Which of the following statements are correct?

   I.   The pH of the resulting mixture is 7.
   II.   The resulting solution is a buffer.
   III.   No net reaction occurs.

   A.   I only
   B.   II only
   C.   III only
   D.   Neither I, II, nor III

34. 1.0 mole of HZ is dissolved in 1 L of water. Which one of the following statements is correct?

   A.   The pH of the resulting solution is 0.
   B.   The pH of the resulting solution is 7.
   C.   The pH of the resulting solution is greater than 7.
   D.   The pH of the resulting solution cannot be determined from the data.

35. If equal volumes of the solutions prepared in experiments 1 and 3 are mixed, what would be the pH of the resulting solution?

   A.   3
   B.   5
   C.   7
   D.   9

Questions 36–40 are NOT based on a descriptive passage.

36. Paramagnetism, the ability to be pulled into a magnetic field, is demonstrated by:

   A.   transition elements that have unpaired d-orbital electrons.
   B.   nonmetal elements that have paired d-orbital electrons.
   C.   nonmetal elements that have unpaired p-orbital electrons.
   D.   any substance containing unpaired electrons.

37. The Van der Waals equation is used to describe non-ideal gases. The terms n^2a/v^2 and nb stand for which of the following?

Van der Waals equation

$(P + n^2a/v^2)(V - nb) = nRT$

- **A.** Intermolecular forces and the volume of gas molecules, respectively
- **B.** Nonelastic collisions and the volume of gas molecules, respectively
- **C.** Nonrandom movement and intermolecular forces between gas molecules, respectively
- **D.** Volume of gas molecules and intermolecular forces, respectively

38. What is the oxidation state of sulfur in sulfuric acid (H_2SO_4)?

- **A.** $- 6$
- **B.** $+ 6$
- **C.** $- 4$
- **D.** $+ 4$

39. If X moles of $PbCl_2$ fully dissolve in 1 L of water, the solubility product constant (K_{sp}) product is equivalent to:

- **A.** X^3
- **B.** $2 X^3$
- **C.** $3 X^2$
- **D.** $4 X^3$

40. A galvanic cell is constructed with the two elements and their ions given below. Find E° for the net reaction of the oxidation of Mg(s) and the reduction of Pb(s).

$$Mg(s) \rightarrow Mg^{2+} + 2e^{-} \qquad E^{\circ} = 2.37 \text{ V}$$
$$Pb(s) \rightarrow Pb^{2+} + 2e^{-} \qquad E^{\circ} = 0.126 \text{ V}$$

- **A.** -2.496 V
- **B.** $+ 2.496$ V
- **C.** -2.244 V
- **D.** $+2.244$ V

Answers and Explanations to General Chemistry Practice Test 2

PASSAGE I	1.	**C**	Remember that oxygen is diatomic, so its molecular weight is 32. Its molecular weight is the highest in the list of possibilities. Therefore, oxygen will effuse more slowly through the pores of the balloon, and choice C is correct.
	2.	**B**	The gas that will be depleted first will be the one with the lowest molecular weight. This is because the low molecular weight gases effuse the fastest. Diatomic hydrogen, choice B, has the lowest molecular weight and will effuse the fastest.
	3.	**D**	To arrive at D as the correct answer, use the given choices and work backward. Of the choices, note that nitric oxide (NO) is the only compound in the list that should fall between nitrogen (N_2) and oxygen (O_2).
	4.	**D**	The molecular weights of both hydrogen sulfide (H_2S) and fluoride (F_2) fall between oxygen (O_2) and argon. Therefore, both of these compounds could be unknown 2. Carbon monoxide, with a molecular weight of 28, falls outside the molecular weight range of oxygen (32) and argon (40).
	5.	**B**	Because E_o is proportional to $1/(MW_o)^{1/2}$, and E_u is proportional to $1/(MW_u)^{1/2}$, the ratio is properly described by answer B
	6.	**D**	The overall effusion rate of the mixture should fall between that of the pure compounds. Therefore, choices A and B are incorrect because the mixture is not intermediate in rank. Choice C is incorrect because the hydrogen balloon will not be the smallest. The best answer is choice D (i.e., helium > mixture > hydrogen).
	7.	**A**	The heaviest compound will effuse most slowly, so most of that compound will remain at the end of 3 days. Likewise, the lightest compound will effuse most quickly, so very little of it will remain after 3 days. Therefore, the amount of neon present will be greater than helium, and the amount of helium present will be greater than hydrogen.
PASSAGE II	8.	**A**	In an exothermic reaction, the products are lower in energy than the starting materials. This indicates that energy was given off by progress of the reaction. Reactions B and C demonstrate endothermic (i.e., energy-absorbing) reactions. Note that the energy content of the products is greater than the energy content of the reactants.
	9.	**D**	Both reactions B and C are endothermic (i.e., energy absorbing) [see explanation for question 8], making choice D the best answer. Choice A is incorrect because it is an exothermic reaction, which releases energy.
	10.	**C**	An intermediate is signified by a dip in the energy-versus-reaction progress diagram.
	11.	**A**	Transition states occur at the top of every "hill" in the energy-versus-reaction progress diagram.

ANSWERS AND
EXPLANATIONS
TO GENERAL
CHEMISTRY
PRACTICE TEST 2

318

12. **D** The mechanism has two steps, of which the first is rate-determining. However, the first and only step is rate-determining in the other reactions as well, therefore, this is not a difference. Each step has its own transition state.

13. **D** The addition of a catalyst allows the reaction to proceed more rapidly by allowing it to occur through a lower energy pathway. Lowering the energy of the transition state or providing a new mechanism that may involve new intermediates both allow the reaction to proceed more quickly. Therefore, the statements in B and C are correct, making choice D best.

14. **B** The choice of wavelength affects only the value of ϵ. A larger value of ϵ would give a greater difference in A values for two very dilute solutions. If this does not seem clear, pick some very low concentrations, and calculate A using two different values for ϵ. This decreases the error in the determination of their concentrations.

15. **D** This question tests data interpretation. It is straightforward and can be answered by simply reading the graph in Figure 2. At 0.5 absorbance on the y-axis, 0.1 moles/L is the corresponding value on the x-axis.

16. **D** This is a challenging conceptual question. If a solution strongly absorbs in the blue region, as indicated by the peak absorbance at 500 nm, then the blue light will not be reflected or transmitted to the eyes. The solution will not look blue, although it absorbs blue light. Thus, the best answer is choice D.

17. **A** Absorption spectroscopy works for substances that absorb visible light. If a substance absorbs visible light, it will appear colored. Food dye is colored, but sugar and alcohol are not. Therefore, A is the best choice.

18. **C** Beer's law is a linear relationship ($y = mx + b$) where b, the y-intercept, is equal to zero. Absorbance corresponds to y, concentration corresponds to x, and ϵb corresponds to m, where ϵ is the molar extinction coefficient. To solve for ϵ alone, the slope (m) must be divided by the path length (b).

19. **D** To perform the calculation required to answer correctly, use Beer's law given in the passage. Since $A = \epsilon bc$, $c = A/\epsilon b = 0.5/(100)(1) = 0.005$ M.

20. **D** An equilibrium constant consists of the concentrations of products over the concentrations of reactants. Therefore, any reaction that produces a great deal of products with very small amounts of reactants remaining generally have a very large equilibration constant (K_{eq}).

21. **D** The passage states that the walls are well-insulated to minimize heat exchange with the surroundings. However, a longer reaction time will allow even small rates of heat exchange to cause large errors. The other possibilities depend on the individual case being examined.

22. **C** This question tests understanding of the concept of ΔE. Recall that the definition of ΔE is heat absorbed at constant volume, which is choice C.

23. **B** The definition of ΔH is heat absorbed at constant pressure. Because a bomb calorimeter is designed to keep volume rather than pressure at a constant value, ΔH cannot be directly measured. Thus, choice B is best.

24. **C** Combustion occurs rapidly, it is essentially nonreversible, and it produces two identifiable products without side reactions. These statements are listed in the passage as requirements for the use of a bomb calorimeter for the determination of ΔE. Each of the other types of reactions listed (i.e., acid–base and precipitation reactions, a salt dissolving in water) have some examples that would fit these criteria and some that would not. Thus, choice C is the best choice.

25. **D** Combustion, by definition, is the burning of a substance in oxygen to produce carbon dioxide and water. Therefore, choices A and C are incorrect because the products are not carbon dioxide and water. Choice B is not balanced correctly. That leaves choice D as the best choice.

26. **D** Because heat is lost to the surroundings, ΔE_{comb} must be negative, which eliminates choices A and C. To determine the value, the following calculations should be done:

Heat gained by surroundings = 5.647 K × 10 kJ/K = 56.47 kJ
Heat lost by sucrose = −56.47 kJ
Moles sucrose = 3.42 g × 1 mole/342g = 0.01 mole
Heat lost per mole sucrose = −56.47/0.01 = −5647.

27. **C** This is a question based on information given in the passage and on common sense. The passage indicates that water has a high heat capacity. The passage also states that the heat capacity is the ratio between the amount of energy and the temperature change. Therefore, a high heat capacity would correspond to the description given in choice C, which is a large amount of energy for a small temperature change. Choices A, B, and D describe small ratios.

PASSAGE V

28. **B** To determine the concentration of hydrogen ions in the solution described in experiment 1, one must recall that hydrogen and hydroxide concentration expressions use a logarithmic base-ten scale. Therefore, $[H^+] = 10^{-pH} = 10^{-5}$ M.

29. **B** Recall that HA dissociates into equal amounts of H^+ and A^- by the law of mass action according to the reaction below:

$$HA \rightleftharpoons H^+ + A^-$$

Based on the fact that the $[H^+]$, as determined in question 28, is 10^{-5}, the $[A^-]$ must also equal 10^{-5} M. Again, $[A^-] = 10^{-pH}$. The pH is given in the passage as 5, therefore, the $[A^-] = 10^{-5}$.

30. **D** Recall that the acid ionization constant $(K_a) = [H^+][A^-]/[HA]$. Plugging in the values (see questions 28 and 29, as well as the passage), gives:

$$K_a = (10^{-5})(10^{-5})/0.1 = 10^{-9}.$$

Note that $pK_a = -\log K_a = -\log 10^{-9} = 9$.

31. **C** Remember that ionic solutions are generally good conductors of electricity. The description of experiment 2 states that solution HZ conducts electricity well. Therefore, the results suggest that the HZ molecule dissociates completely into ions in water (choice C). And, if the solution dissociates completely in water, it must be a strong electrolyte (strong acid).

32. **D** This is a difficult question, and the problem involves hydrolysis (salt of a weak acid in water). Recall that $K_a = 10^{-9}$. The reaction is:

$$A^- + H_2O \rightarrow HA + OH^- \qquad K_h = K_w/K_a = 10^{-5}.$$

This relation for K_h can be derived by knowing that the equilibrium constant for the previous reaction would be $[HA][OH^-]/[A^-]$. To obtain this expression in known terms, the expressions for K_w, $[OH^-][H^+]$, and for K_a, $[A^-][H^+]/[HA]$, can be used. Dividing the expression for K_w by the expression for K_a gives us the expression for K_h. Now the value of K_h needs to be used to determine H^+.

At equilibrium, $[A^-] = 0.1$; $[HA] = x$; $[OH^-] = x$.
$K_h = [HA][OH^-]/[A^-] = x^2/0.1 = 10^{-5}$
$x = 10^{-3}$; $pOH = 3$, $pH = 14 - pOH$

Therefore, $pH = 11$.

ANSWERS AND
EXPLANATIONS
TO GENERAL
CHEMISTRY
PRACTICE TEST 2

320

33. **D** This is also a difficult question. HZ is a strong acid. NaA is the salt (conjugate base) of the weak acid HA. The net reaction is:

$$A^- + H^+ \rightarrow HA$$
(Na$^+$ and Z$^-$ are spectator ions)

Because HA forms in the net reaction, the pH of the resulting solution cannot be 7. HA is a weak acid, thus the pH < 7. A buffer is a mixture of HA and A$^-$ in similar (but not necessarily equal) concentrations. To create a buffer solution by mixing HZ and NaA, one would have to mix an excess of NaA with HZ. By doing this, one would use up all of the HZ to make HA and would have some A$^-$ left over in solution. Therefore, the resulting mixture would have both HA and A$^-$ in similar concentrations, thus making a buffer.

34. **A** The data show that HZ is a strong acid, therefore HZ completely dissociates and [H$^+$] = 1.0M. The pH = $-\log$ [H$^+$], and $-\log 1 = 0$.

35. **D** This passage ends with yet another challenging question. This is a buffer problem because there is a mixture of HA and A$^-$ in similar (in this case equal) proportions. The Henderson-Hasselbach equation (i.e., pH = pK_a + log [A$^-$]/[HA]) can be used to solve for the answer. The pK_a value was determined in question 30. If equal volumes of HA and A$^-$ are mixed, the concentration of [HA] = [A$^-$] = 0.05. (The concentration must be divided by two after mixing equal amounts.) Thus, the ratio [A$^-$]/[HA] = 1, and the log of 1 = 0. Therefore, the Henderson-Hasselbach equation reduces to pH = pK_a = 9.

36. **D** Paramagnetic elements are substances that tend to move into a magnetic field. They have one or more unpaired electrons. Most of the transition metals and their compounds in oxidation states that involve incomplete inner electron subshells are paramagnetic.

37. **A** The Van der Waals equation describes the additional factors that must be accounted for when the ideal gas law is used to calculate values for nonideal gases. The terms that affect the pressure and volume terms of the ideal gas law are intermolecular forces and volume of the nonideal gas molecules, respectively.

38. **B** The net charge of sulfuric acid (H_2SO_4) is zero. Hydrogen has a common oxidation state of $+1$, whereas each oxygen atom has an oxidation number of -2.

$$
\begin{array}{ccccc}
H_2 & & S & & O_4 \\
(2)(1) & + & x & + & (4)(-2) = 0 \\
2 + x & + & -8 & = & 0 \\
x & = & 6 & &
\end{array}
$$

39. **D** The equation is:

$$PbCl_2 \rightarrow Pb^{2+} + 2\ Cl^-$$

To solve for the solubility product constant (K_{sp}), one must know that $K_{sp} = [Pb^{2+}][Cl^-]^2$.

Starting with X moles of $PbCl_2$, which fully dissociate, X moles of Pb and 2X moles of Cl$^-$ are produced.

$$K_{sp} \text{ is thus, } (X)(2X)^2 = 4X^3.$$

40.   **D**   To solve this question, leave the magnesium equation as written, and reverse the lead equation.

Oxidation of Mg(s)

$Mg(s) \rightarrow Mg^{2+} + 2e^-$ $E° = 2.37$ V

Reduction of Pb(s)

$Pb^{2+} + 2e^- \rightarrow Pb(s)$ $E° = -0.126$ V

$E°$ net $= +2.244$ V. Thus, the net reaction requires that the $E°$ values be added. Remember that when a reaction is reversed, the sign of $E°$ is changed.

ANSWERS AND
EXPLANATIONS
TO GENERAL
CHEMISTRY
PRACTICE TEST 2

322

GENERAL CHEMISTRY PRACTICE TEST 3

Time: 50 minutes

Directions: This test contains as many general chemistry passages as you may encounter on the real MCAT. The time allotted approximates the time allowed on a real MCAT to solve the given number of questions. Choose one best answer for each question. You may refer to a periodic table as needed.

Passage I (Questions 1–5)

A Lewis acid is any species that can accept an electron pair, and a Lewis base is any species that can donate an electron pair. A Lewis acid–base reaction can create a coordinate covalent bond in the reaction product. In the Lewis system, all cations are acids, and all anions are bases.

Lewis acidity does not always follow the same trends in reactivity toward halide ions as does Brönsted acidity. One class of Lewis acids follows the reactivity order $I^- < Br^- < Cl^- < F^-$. Lewis acids that follow this reactivity order are called Class A. Lewis acids that follow the opposite order $F^- < Cl^- < Br^- < I^-$ are called Class B.

Lewis acids that belong to Class A are known as hard acids because their orbitals lie close to the nucleus and are not very polarizable. Class B acids have orbitals that are much farther from the nucleus and are, therefore, much more polarizable. Thus, hardness and softness tend to follow trends in size. Another way to determine hardness and softness is to consider that hard acids and bases tend to form ionic bonds, whereas soft acids and bases tend to form covalent bonds. Therefore, H^+ is an exception to the bonding trend; it is a hard acid that tends to make covalent rather than ionic bonds. A general rule to follow is that hard acids tend to bind well to hard bases, and the soft acids tend to bind well to soft bases.

1. Which of the following would be the hardest Lewis acid?

    A. Zn^{2+}
    B. Na^+
    C. Ca^{2+}
    D. Li^+

2. Which of the following would be the softest Lewis base?

    A. Te^{2-}
    B. NH_3
    C. F^-
    D. O^{2-}

3. Would Ni^{2+} or Al^{3+} be more likely to be found as an oxide in ores?

    A. Ni^{2+} would be more likely to be found as an oxide because it is harder than Al^{3+}.
    B. Al^{3+} would be more likely to be found as an oxide because it is harder than Ni^{2+}.
    C. Ni^{2+} would be more likely to be found as an oxide because it is softer than Al^{3+}.
    D. More information is needed on oxide ion to answer this question.

4. Determine the magnitude of the equilibrium constant (K_{eq}) for the following reaction using the concepts outlined in the passage.

$$CH_3HgI + HCl \rightleftharpoons CH_3HgCl + HI$$

    A. $K_{eq} > 1$
    B. $K_{eq} < 1$
    C. $K_{eq} = 1$
    D. This reaction is not reversible, therefore it has no K_{eq}.

5. Would the following reaction be a useful method for the synthesis of the silver cyanide ion $[Ag(CN)_2]^-$?

$$[AgCl_2]^-(aq) + 2\ CN^-(aq) \rightarrow [Ag(CN)_2]^-(aq) + 2\ Cl^-(aq)$$

A. Yes, because the Ag^+ ion is hard and will preferentially choose cyanide ion over chloride ion.
B. No, the reaction should go in the opposite direction considering the hardness and softness concepts.
C. Yes, because the Ag^+ ion is soft and will preferentially choose cyanide ion over chloride ion.
D. Yes, because the thermodynamics should favor the formation of the more stable $[Ag(CN)_2]^-(aq)$ over $[AgCl_2]^-(aq)$.

Passage II (Questions 6–12)

Phase diagrams are important because they allow the prediction of the phase of a substance based on its temperature and pressure. Phase diagrams summarize the various states possible for a substance, the transitions that occur between the various states of matter, and key points of interest. These key points of interest include the critical point and the triple point.

The phase diagram allows prediction of the pressure and temperature values at which freezing, melting, and boiling occur. Specifically, the freezing point is the temperature and pressure at which a liquid changes to the solid phase. The melting point is the temperature and pressure at which a solid changes to the liquid phase. Finally, the boiling point is the temperature at which the vapor pressure is equal to the ambient pressure.

Understanding phase diagrams is an important part of general chemistry. The following three figures are phase diagrams for carbon dioxide, water, and sulfur. Answer the following questions based on the diagrams, the information presented in this passage, and your understanding of the concepts.

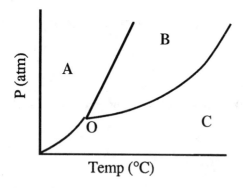

Figure 1   Phase diagram for carbon dioxide.

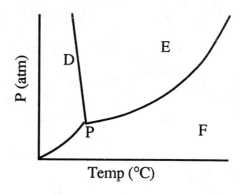

Figure 2   Phase diagram for water.

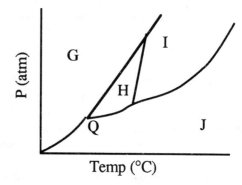

Figure 3   Phase diagram for sulfur.

6. In the phase diagram for carbon dioxide (Figure 1), what region represents the gaseous phase?

A. Region B
B. Region C
C. Region A
D. There is no region; the gaseous phase is represented by point O.

7. In the phase diagram for water (Figure 2), one line has a negative slope. This line represents:

A. the sublimation line.
B. the fusion line.
C. the vaporization line.
D. the triple point.

8. In the phase diagram for carbon dioxide (Figure 1), point O is the:

   A. triple point.
   B. point at which liquid and solid are in equilibrium.
   C. point at which all three phases are in equilibrium.
   D. more than one of the above.

9. In the phase diagram for water (Figure 2), the line with a negative slope is unusual because:

   A. it indicates that as pressure goes up, liquid in equilibrium with solid will begin to freeze.
   B. it indicates that as pressure goes up, solid in equilibrium with liquid will begin to melt.
   C. it indicates that solid in equilibrium with liquid at the freezing point occupies more volume per gram than the liquid.
   D. both B and C are correct.

10. In the phase diagram for sulfur (Figure 3), the line between Q and the origin represents:

    A. equilibrium among the solid phase in region H, the solid phase in region G, and the liquid phase in region J.
    B. the equilibrium between the solid phase in region G and the liquid phase in region J.
    C. the equilibrium between the solid phase in region J and the liquid phase in region G.
    D. the equilibrium between the solid phase in region G and the vapor phase in region J.

11. One atmosphere pressure and 298 K probably intersect in which regions on the phase diagrams for carbon dioxide and water (Figures 1 and 2), respectively?

    A. Region B and region E
    B. Region C and region F
    C. Region A and region D
    D. Region C and region E

12. If regions G and H on the phase diagram for sulfur (Figure 3) represent different crystalline solids, which one is more stable?

    A. The solid represented by region G is more stable because it is present in a much wider range of temperatures and pressures.
    B. The solid represented by region H is more stable because it is present at higher temperatures over a wide range of pressures.
    C. The solid represented by region G is more stable because it is present at much lower pressures.
    D. The most stable compound depends upon the temperature and pressure.

Passage III (Questions 13–19)

An explosive compound called nitroglycerin forms from the reaction of glycerol with nitric acid. It is particularly unstable in liquid form. However, controlled explosions yield much information.

When a glass vial containing 454 g dry nitroglycerin, $[C_3H_5(NO_3)_3]$, explodes stoichiometrically, no solid products are produced. The gaseous products of the explosion are initially collected at STP.

Another vial containing 454 g nitroglycerin is allowed to explode stoichiometrically in a controlled fashion. The gaseous products of this explosion are collected in a special container of unknown volume at an unspecified temperature. The total pressure is determined to be 290 atm.

Analysis of the explosion products led to the identity of the gases present after the explosion. Carbon dioxide gas, nitrogen gas, oxygen gas, and water vapor were identified. This indicates that the balanced chemical equation is:

$$4\ C_3H_5(NO_3)_3 \rightarrow 12\ CO_2 + 10\ H_2O + O_2 + 6\ N_2$$

An information search was conducted and the following data was obtained on nitroglycerin:

Density at 273 K (liquid form) = 2.0 g/ml.
MW = 227 g/mole

Table 1 gives the data collected at 300 K:

TABLE I. Data Collected at 300 K

Compound	Heats of Formation (kJ/Mole)	Absolute Entropies (J/Mole-K)
CO₂ (g)	−400	200
H₂O (g)	−250	200
N₂ (g)	NA	200
O₂ (g)	NA	150
C₃H₅ (NO₃)₃ (l)	100	300

325

13. What is the mole fraction of nitrogen in the gaseous products formed after the explosion?

   A. 12/33
   B. 6/29
   C. 12/47
   D. 10/29

14. What is the total volume in liters of the gases produced at STP after the initial explosion of 454 g nitroglycerin?

   A. (0.5) (29) (22.4)
   B. (0.5) (29) (0.082) (298)/(290)
   C. (0.5) (29) (8.3144) (273)/(290)
   D. More than one of the above is correct.

15. In the second explosion, the total pressure was found to be 290 atm. What is the pressure of oxygen in this special container?

   A. 10 atm
   B. 60 atm
   C. 100 atm
   D. 120 atm

16. What is the free energy change in kJ per mole of nitroglycerin that explodes at 300 K?

   A. $-(750/4) - (300 \times 450/4)$
   B. $-(7700/4) + (300 \times 4.550/4)$
   C. $-(7700/4) - (300 \times 4.550/4)$
   D. $-(7700/4) - (300 \times 4550/4)$

17. Would it be possible to make nitroglycerin at 300 K from the gases produced by its explosion?

   A. Yes, because the free energy change for this reaction would be positive.
   B. Yes, because the free energy change for this reaction would be negative.
   C. No, because the free energy change for this reaction would be positive.
   D. No, because the free energy change for this reaction would be negative.

18. Which of the following would allow the same conclusion as in the previous question without the calculation of the free energy change?

   I. Nitroglycerin is unstable.
   II. Nitroglycerin is explosive.
   III. Nitroglycerin has a higher entropy than any of the gases.

   A. I only
   B. II only
   C. III only
   D. I and II only

19. What is the free energy of formation in kJ/mole of the oxygen gas produced by the stoichiometric explosion of nitroglycerin at 300 K?

   A. +150
   B. −150
   C. +0.150
   D. None of the above

Passage IV (Questions 20–26)

Radiocarbon dating is an important technique in dating previously living material up to 25,000 years old. This technique makes use of the interaction of cosmic rays with nitrogen in the atmosphere, which produces radioactive carbon 14 according to the following equation:

$$^{14}_{7}N + ^{1}_{0}n \rightarrow ^{14}_{6}C + ^{1}_{1}H$$

The carbon 14 produced by this reaction decays by emitting β-particles following first-order kinetics with a half-life of 5730 years. The carbon 14 is oxidized to carbon dioxide in the atmosphere and is converted to sugars by plants. As plants form the bottom of the food chain, all living creatures incorporate this radioactive carbon into their tissues at a constant concentration.

Radiocarbon dating determines the radioactivity in a sample per gram of carbon and calculates the amount of time needed to reduce the original radioactivity to that level. This gives the amount of time that the organic matter has been dead. The equation used to calculate the age of the sample is:

$$\ln(N/N_0) = -\lambda t,$$

where N is the radioactivity at time t, N_0 is the radioactivity at the moment the organism died, and λ is a constant.

Some useful numbers are:
   $\ln(1) = 0$
   $\ln(2) = 0.7$
   $\ln(.5) = -0.7$

20. What species is involved in the rate-determining step of the radioactive decay of carbon 14?

    A. Nitrogen 14
    B. A neutron
    C. Carbon 14
    D. A β-particle

21. Which of the following are assumed by the method described in the passage?

    I. The atmospheric ratio of radioactive-to-nonradioactive carbon dioxide has been constant for 25,000 years.
    II. All animals eat plants.
    III. The atmospheric ratio of radioactive-to-nonradioactive carbon dioxide is the same in China as it is in Bolivia.

    A. I, II, and III
    B. I and II only
    C. II and III only
    D. I and III only

22. What is the value of λ for carbon 14?

    A. $-0.7/5730$
    B. $0.7/5730$
    C. $0/5730$
    D. 0.7×5730

23. What is the best reason for the inability of radiocarbon dating to determine the age of samples older than 25,000 years?

    A. The assumptions made about carbon 14 in the atmosphere fall apart at this age.
    B. There was nothing living on Earth before this date.
    C. There is not enough radioactivity remaining in a sample older than 25,000 years to be measured accurately.
    D. The method has not been verified with samples older than 25,000 years.

24. What is the order of reaction that forms carbon 14 in the atmosphere?

    A. 0
    B. 1
    C. 2
    D. 3

25. Which of the following statements correctly defines the half-life?

    A. The amount of time required for the first half of the sample to react
    B. The amount of time required for half of the sample to react
    C. The amount of time required for the reaction to be half complete
    D. The amount of time required for the reaction to get half way to the point where the radioactivity can no longer be measured

26. If the atmospheric radioactive carbon dioxide were lower compared to the nonradioactive carbon dioxide concentration 4000 years ago, what effect would that have on the experimentally determined age of a tree that died 5000 years ago?

    A. The age would be determined correctly.
    B. The age would be underestimated.
    C. The age would be overestimated.
    D. The age would be incalculable.

Passage V (Questions 27–33)

Consider the following experimental protocol for the synthesis of a sulfide of copper (Cu_xS_y) and the quantitative determination of its formula. The atomic weights of Cu and S are 64 and 32 gm/mole, respectively.

Part I

A clean porcelain crucible with its cover is placed on a ring stand utilizing a wire triangle. It is heated to low redness with a Bunsen burner and allowed to cool to room temperature. The crucible without its cover is then weighed at room temperature on an analytical balance after initially zeroing the balance.

Part II

A piece of copper is clipped from a roll of wire and twisted into a flat spiral sheet that will fit in the bottom of the crucible. This spiraled piece of copper wire then is added to the crucible without its cover, and the crucible containing the copper wire is weighed.

Part III

Excess solid sulfur is added to the crucible containing the copper wire. The cover is put on the crucible, and the mixture is heated vigorously. The excess sulfur evolves as sulfur dioxide when the mixture is heated. The product (Cu_xS_y) is cooled to room temperature and is weighed in the crucible without its cover.

All weights are obtained without the crucible cover, and the same analytical balance is used each time. Results are:

Weight of empty crucible	25.401 g
Weight of crucible w/copper	31.799 g
Weight of crucible with product	33.402 g

27. How many moles of copper were clipped from the roll of wire in part II of the experiment?

    A.   0.01
    B.   0.1
    C.   6.398
    D.   32

28. How many moles of sulfur reacted with the copper wire in part III of the experiment?

    A.   0.05
    B.   0.50
    C.   1.603
    D.   16

29. What does the "x" in Cu_xS_y represent?

    A.   Moles of sulfur
    B.   Moles of copper
    C.   Moles of copper per mole of Cu_xS_y
    D.   Moles of copper per mole of sulfur

30. The formula for the sulfide of copper is best described as:

    A. Cu_2S.
    B. CuS_2.
    C.   dependent on the amount of sulfur dioxide evolved.
    D.   undeterminable from these data.

31. What will happen to the value of "x" in Cu_xS_y if the crucible is accidentally weighed with its cover on in part I, but then weighed normally (without cover) in the other parts of the experiment?

    A.   It will increase.
    B.   It will decrease.
    C.   The value will not change.
    D.   The effect on "x" cannot be predicted.

32. Which measurement below would introduce the largest percentage error in "x" if it were off by 0.200 g?

    A.   The weight of the empty crucible
    B.   The weight of the crucible with copper
    C.   The weight of the crucible with product
    D.   Not enough information to determine

33. If the analytical balance is not zeroed before the experiment, how will this affect the value of "x?"

    A.   It will increase.
    B.   It will decrease.
    C.   It will have no effect.
    D.   It cannot be predicted.

Passage VI (Questions 34–40)

Chemical kinetics is the study of reaction rates and reaction mechanisms. The reaction rate is a measurement of the change in concentration of reactant or product over time. The rate for a chemical reaction depends on the reactants and on external factors, such as temperature, concentration, and the presence of catalysts. Furthermore, concentration effects on reaction rate can only be established by experiment. The experimental results can be reported as a rate equation or a rate law. In rate equations, the reaction rate is expressed as a function of the concentrations of the reactants.

Consider the following scenario in which substance A can decompose by either of two pathways, giving rise to different products B and C as described below. Such reaction mechanisms are often seen in nuclear decay reactions and are called parallel reactions.

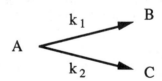

Figure 4

For the following problems, the notation used is summarized as follows:

    [X] = Concentration of X
    k_1 = Rate constant for A → B
    k_2 = Rate constant for A → C

34. Which equation below represents the rate of formation of B?

    A. $dB/dt = k_1[A]$
    B. $dB/dt = k_2[A]$
    C. $dB/dt = k_1[B]$
    D. $dB/dt = (k_1+k_2)[B]$

35. Which equation below represents the rate of formation of C?

    A. $dC/dt = k_1[B]$
    B. $dC/dt = k_2[A]$
    C. $dC/dt = k_1[C]$
    D. $dC/dt = (k_1 + k_2)[C]$

36. Which equation below represents the rate of disappearance of A?

    A. $-dA/dt = k_1[B] + k_2[A]$
    B. $-dA/dt = k_2[A] + k_1[C]$
    C. $-dA/dt = (k_1 + k_2)[B]$
    D. $-dA/dt = (k_1 + k_2)[A]$

37. Under which condition is the following approximation true?

    The rate of disappearance of $A \sim k_1[A]$

    A. If the initial concentration of B is low
    B. If the initial concentration of C is low
    C. If the rate of formation of B is much greater than the rate of formation of C
    D. If the rate of formation of C is much greater than the rate of formation of B

38. Which of the following is true regarding parallel reactions?

    A. They follow zero-order kinetics.
    B. They follow first-order kinetics.
    C. They follow second-order kinetics.
    D. The steps in the mechanism are bimolecular.

39. If an experiment was performed that showed that the decomposition of A was second order, which of the following would explain this?

    I.   The scenario above is not the correct mechanism.
    II. The experiment was flawed.
    III. Substance A decomposes by colliding with a second A molecule.

    A. I only
    B. II only
    C. I and III only
    D. I, II, and III

40. Which of the following statements is NOT true about chemical kinetics?

    A. The rate of a chemical reaction is measured by the change of a reactant or product concentration in a certain period of time.
    B. The exponent (power) of the concentration of each component in the general-rate equation is the order of the reaction with regards to that component.
    C. The rate of a reaction may be increased by a catalyst, which lowers the activation energy and appears in the stoichiometric equation of the reaction.
    D. Concentration effects on reaction rate can be established by experiment.

Answers and Explanations to General Chemistry Practice Test 3

PASSAGE I

1. **D** The lithium cation is the smallest cation present, and it has an empty orbital that allows it to act as a hard Lewis acid.

2. **A** Among isoelectronic species (e.g., I^-, Te^{2-}), the species with the highest negative charge is the largest, and the species with the highest positive charge is the smallest. The largest species will be the softest. The telluride anion does have lone electron pairs, which allow it to act as a soft Lewis base.

3. **B** The aluminum cation is higher on the periodic table than is the nickel cation. In fact, it is in the same period as oxygen, which indicates that aluminum's hardness is more similar to that of oxygen than is nickel's.

4. **B** The equilibrium constant (K_{eq}) is less than 1 because hard ions like to associate and soft ions like to associate. The mercury cation is very soft, as is the iodide anion. The chloride ion is hard, as is the hydrogen cation. These species are associated on the left side of the equation, which will therefore be the favored side.

5. **C** Even without considering the cyanide anion, which is polyatomic and not mentioned in the passage, it can be determined that silver is a soft cation but chloride is a hard anion. These indicate that replacing the chloride is probably favorable. If known compounds, such as hydrogen cyanide (covalent), are also considered, it can be determined that cyanide should be a soft Lewis base, which is another clue in determining that the reaction should be favorable.

PASSAGE II

6. **B** The gas phase is the one that predominates at low pressures and high temperatures. This would be region C in the phase diagram, which makes B the correct choice.

7. **B** The curve between the liquid phase and the solid phase can be called the melting curve or the freezing (fusion) curve. This makes choice B correct. Choice A is incorrect because the sublimation line is found between regions D and F, and this line has a positive slope. Choice C is incorrect because the vaporization line is found between regions E and F, and this line has a positive slope. The triple point is found at point P, where all three phases are in equilibrium.

8. **D** The triple point (choice A) is equivalent to the point at which all three phases are in equilibrium (choice C). This makes both choices A and C correct, so the best choice is D (i.e., more than one statement is correct).

9. **D** If a point on the curve is chosen, and pressure is increased (i.e., moving directly up the diagram), the liquid phase is reached. This indicates that any solid that was in equilibrium with the liquid has melted. This occurs because high pressures favor the more dense phase (which is usually the solid). Therefore, the liquid must occupy less volume per gram than the solid.

ANSWERS AND
EXPLANATIONS TO
GENERAL
CHEMISTRY
PRACTICE TEST 3

330

10. **D** The line between Q and the origin represents the sublimation curve, in which solid G and vapor J are in equilibrium. The other choices are incorrect because they misname the phases of the various sections of the phase diagram.

11. **D** The conditions given (i.e., 1 atm and 298 K) are basically room temperature and atmospheric pressure. Water is known to be a liquid at these conditions (region E), and carbon dioxide is known to be a vapor (region C).

12. **D** The stability of a phase depends upon the conditions. For example, water is not stable as a liquid at 300°K, although it is known to be a stable liquid at room temperature (i.e., 298 K).

PASSAGE III

13. **B** The total relative moles of gaseous products formed after the explosion can be determined by the following equation: $12 + 10 + 1 + 6 = 29$. The numbers for this equation come from the given number of moles on the product side of the balanced equation in the passage. Recall that the passage states that water vapor was a product. Therefore, the moles of water (i.e., 10) are included because water is in its gaseous not liquid state. The mole fraction of nitrogen in the mixture, therefore, is 6/29, which is choice B.

14. **A** Note that in the equation given in the passage, 4 moles of nitroglycerin reacts to give 29 moles of gas. When 2 moles of nitroglycerin (454 g) explode, only $(0.5)(29)$ moles of gas are produced. Using $PV = nRT$, where $RT = 22.4$ at standard temperature and pressure (STP), the volume of the gases is $(0.5)(29)(22.4\text{ L}) = 324.8$ L. The same result can be achieved by using the actual temperature and gas constant. Therefore, $(0.5)(29)(273)(0.082) = 324.8$ L.

15. **A** Because the explosion occurs stoichiometrically, the mole fraction of oxygen in the products is 1/29. If the total pressure is 290 atm, then the partial pressure of oxygen gas is 10 atm.

16. **C** Recall that $\Delta G = \Delta H - T(\Delta S)$. ΔH from the heats of formation $= 12(-400) + 10(-250) - 4(100) = -7700$ KJ/mole. ΔS from the absolute entropies $= 12(200) + 10(200) + 150 + 6(200) - 4(300) = 4550$ J/mole-K, or 4.550 KJ/mole-K. Therefore, ΔG/mole nitroglycerin $= (-7700$ KJ/mole)/4 $- 300K(4.550$ KJ/mole-K)/4.

17. **C** Note that the ΔG for the reverse reaction is positive. Therefore, this process would be nonspontaneous in the reverse direction. ΔH and ΔS are not measures of spontaneity, and they cannot be used to answer this question.

18. **D** The properties of instability and explosiveness imply that the compound has a decomposition pathway with a favorable ΔG. As in question 17, entropy alone cannot be used to determine the spontaneity of a reaction. Thus, statements I and II are correct, statement III is unsupported, which makes D the best choice.

19. **D** Remember that the free energy of formation of an element in its standard state is zero by definition. The standard state of oxygen is gaseous, and oxygen gas is a product in the explosion.

PASSAGE IV

20. **C** The passage states that the decay of carbon 14 is first order. Therefore, the only species appearing in the rate-determining step must be carbon 14.

21. **D** If the ratio of radioactive-to-nonradioactive carbon dioxide were not relatively constant, then material of different ages would have different values of N_0, making determination by this method extremely difficult. It is unnecessary to assume that all animals dated by this method ate only plants, because they could incorporate the same level of radioactivity by eating other animals that ate plants. The decay of carbon 14 is slow relative the lifespan of an animal, so the longer path between carbon 14 from plants to herbivores or from plants to carnivores is unimportant. For the dating technique to be useful, the radioactive carbon 14 ratio must be constant regardless of from where in the world the sample was taken. This is an absolute requirement when dating a sample of unknown origin.

22. **B** The definition of half-life is the amount of time required for half of the material to decay (or react). This definition applies regardless of the starting concentration. Thus, λ can be calculated using the second equation supplied in the passage.

$$\ln(0.5/1) = -\lambda \times 5730$$
$$-0.7 = -\lambda \times 5730$$
$$\lambda = 0.7/5730$$

23. **C** The answer to this question can be determined by a process of elimination. Choice A is incorrect because the invalidity of assumptions could be corrected for by verifying the difference with other methods and applying a correction factor. Choice B is incorrect because life has existed on Earth for significantly longer than 25,000 years. Radiocarbon dating could be used if samples of known age were unavailable for verification of the method; however, results would not be completely reliable. The passage said that the technique could not be used, not that the technique could not be unreliable. Choice D is incorrect because some samples may have fossilized, but the passage stated that the technique could not be used, not that there were no samples on which to use it. Thus, the best choice is C.

24. **C** The first reaction shown indicates the balanced equation and the mechanism as well, so the order can be determined by adding up the reacting species.

25. **B** The half-life is the amount of time required for half of a sample to react (i.e., decay).

26. **C** If the ratio of radioactive carbon dioxide was lower 4000 years ago than believed, then the value of N_0 used in the calculation would be too high. This makes the ratio N/N_0 larger than it actually should be. This also makes the natural log of that ratio larger than the actual value. Thus, the value of the age would be overestimated.

---

27. **B** This question can be answered via a simple calculation. The mass of copper (Cu) = 31.799. Subtracting 25.401, the weight of the empty crucible, leaves 6.398 g of copper clipped from the roll of wire. The moles of copper can be determined by dividing the mass of copper (6.398 g) by the atomic weight (63.55 g/mole) = 0.1 moles.

28. **A** The mass of reacted sulfur (S) = 33.402 g − 31.799 g = 1.603 g. The moles of S can be determined by dividing 1.603 by the atomic weight of S, which is 32 g/mole. Thus, moles of S = 0.05.

29. **C** This question tests understanding of chemical notation. Choices A and B are not specific enough. Choice D is correct only when y = 1. Therefore, choice C is the best answer.

30. **A** The formula for copper sulfide is best described as Cu_2S. Moles of copper per moles of sulfur (determined in questions 27 and 28) = 0.1/0.05 = 2.

31. **B** If the crucible cover is included, then the weight of the crucible will be greater than 25.401 g. The measured mass of copper will be decreased, which will decrease the moles of copper. The mole ratio of Cu/S also decreases; therefore, x decreases.

32. **B** As with most MCAT questions, detailed calculations are not needed to solve this problem but logical thinking is needed. An error involving the weight of the crucible would only affect the weight of copper. An error affecting the weight of the crucible with product would only affect the weight of combined sulfur. However, an error affecting the weight of the crucible with copper would affect both the weight of copper and sulfur, and this would introduce the largest percentage error in x. This would happen if the weight of the crucible with copper were too high or too low by the 0.200 g. If it were too high, then x would be very high. That is, moles of Cu would be increased, and moles of S would be decreased; therefore, the ratio of moles of copper to sulfur would be increased. If

the weight of the crucible with copper were too low, then x would be very low. That is, moles of copper would be decreased, and moles of sulfur would be increased; therefore, the ratio of moles of copper to sulfur would be decreased.

33. **C**   The weight of copper and combined sulfur are both determined by subtraction. If the scale were slightly off, the amount of difference would be subtracted from the total.

---

34. **A**   This question tests the understanding of the definition of the rate of formation of a product. The reaction rate is a measurement of the change in concentration of reactant or product over time. Choice A is correct based on the basic definition, which is the product of the rate constant and the reactant(s).

35. **B**   Again, the formation of a product is determined by the product of the rate constant and the reactant(s). Therefore, $dC/dt = k_2[A]$.

36. **D**   By the law of mass action, the following is true.

$$-dA/dt = dB/dt + dC/dt.$$
$$-dA/dt = k_1[A] + k_2[A] = (k_1 + k_2)[A].$$

37. **C**   Using the equation derived in the explanation to question 36:

$$-dA/dt = k_1[A] + k_2[A],$$

then $-dA/dt = k_1[A]$ is true when $k_2[A]$ is insignificant compared with $k_1[A]$. This occurs if the rate of formation of $B(k_1[A])$ is much greater than the rate of formation of C $(k_2[A])$.

38. **B**   Because there is only one reactant, and it gives rise to different products B and C, the reaction is first order by definition. Note that all nuclear decay reactions are first order by definition. A plot of the log [A] on the ordinate (y-axis) versus time (t) on the abscissa (x-axis) is linear with slope $k_1 + k_2$.

39. **D**   All of the explanations offered would explain experimental observation of a second-order rate law. In fact, one of them must be true. Either the experiment was wrong (statement II) or the mechanism depicted is wrong (statements I and III).

40. **C**   Choices A, B, and D are all true statements regarding chemical kinetics. The first part of choice C is a correct statement; however, the second part of choice C is incorrect. Catalysts do not appear in the stoichiometric equation of a reaction.

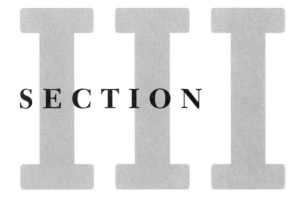

SECTION III

Preparation for the Biological Sciences

....

A. **Biology Review Notes**

B. **Biology Practice Tests**

C. **Organic Chemistry Review Notes**

D. **Organic Chemistry Practice Tests**

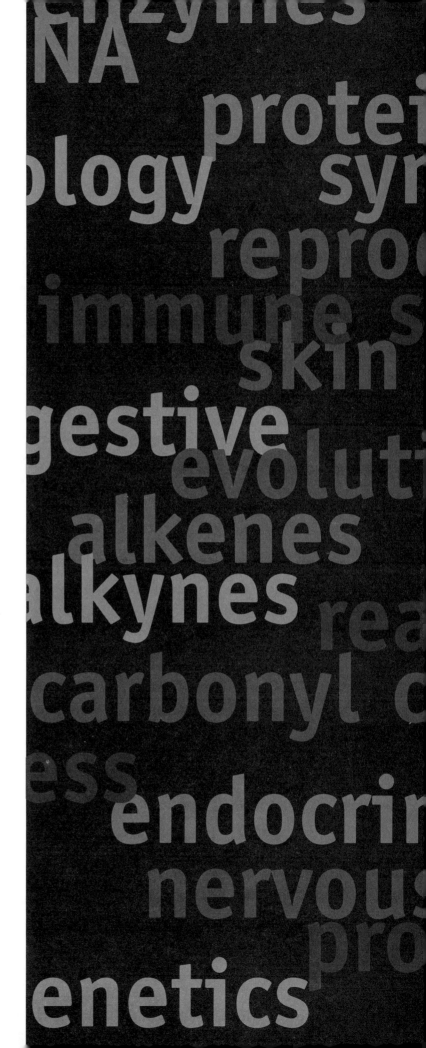

Biology

REVIEW NOTES

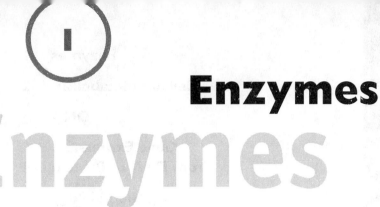

Enzymes

I. Enzyme Structure and Function

A. Introduction to Enzymes

1. **Every activity in a living cell involves chemical reactions.** In these reactions, the chemical bonds in organic molecules are broken so that new bonds can form.

2. The molecules need an **initial input of energy** from their surroundings for a reaction to start. This energy—the **activation energy (E_A)**—can be thought of as an energy "bump" that must be overcome before a reaction can occur (Figure 1-1A).

FIGURE 1-1.
A) Reaction without enzyme. Note that the reaction requires more energy and time (progress) than the reaction in **B)**, a reaction with enzyme. E_A = activation energy.

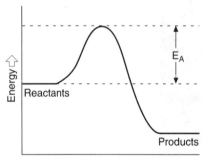

A. Reaction without enzyme

Energy / Reactants / E_A / Products / Progress of reaction

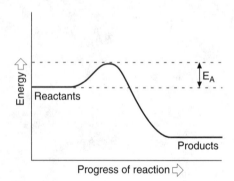

B. Reaction with enzyme

Energy / Reactants / E_A / Products / Progress of reaction

3. **Enzymes** are proteins that lower the E_A of reactions (see Figure 1-1B).

   a. Enzymes **reduce E_A** through various mechanisms. For example, enzymes can bring molecules together in the proper orientation to react or can provide a microenvironment conducive to a reaction.

   b. Enzymes act as **biologic catalysts;** they speed up reactions without being changed themselves.

   c. **Without enzymes,** an E_A could not be overcome at the normal temperature of a cell. The chemical reactions would occur so slowly that the cell would die.

4. **Every cell makes many different types of enzymes,** each of which catalyzes a different and highly specific reaction.

    a. Each type of enzyme has a **specific shape** that exclusively binds a set of other molecules.

    b. **Substrates** are the reactants that are acted on in an enzyme-catalyzed (enzymatic) reaction.

B. Enzyme Structure

1. **Enzymes are proteins** (with a few exceptions). Each enzyme has a different, highly precise conformation resulting from several levels of protein structure.

    a. **Primary structure** is the amino acid sequence of the polypeptide chain (or chains) that makes up the enzyme.

    b. **Secondary structure** results from weak chemical bonds (e.g., hydrogen bonds) formed between atoms along the backbone of the polypeptide chain. These are local interactions that result in repetitive three-dimensional patterns (e.g., alpha-helices, beta-pleated sheets).

    c. **Tertiary structure** involves long-distance interactions between amino-acid side chains. These give the protein a highly precise globular shape.

    d. **Quaternary structure** refers to the interaction between two or more different polypeptide subunits of a functional protein.

2. **Active site.** The active site is the restricted area of the enzyme where the substrate (or substrates) binds and where the enzymatic reaction occurs. An active site may be a pocket or a groove in the enzyme molecule.

C. Enzyme Function

1. **Catalytic cycle** (Figure 1-2)

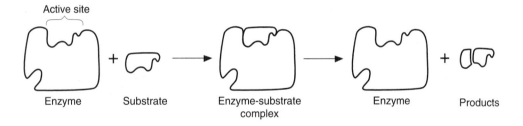

FIGURE 1-2.
The interaction of substrate with enzyme, forming an enzyme–substrate complex. The complex breaks down to reform the enzyme and release the products.

    a. **First step: substrate binds to enzyme.** The substrate or substrates bind to the active site to form the enzyme–substrate complex.

    b. **Second step: induced fit.** Substrate-binding induces a change in the shape of the enzyme so that the substrate fits more snugly in the active site (i.e., induced fit). Induced fit is a reversible change in the enzyme.

    c. **Third step: catalysis.** When the reaction is catalyzed, the substrate or substrates are changed in a specific way, such as by chemical modification, cleavage, or the joining of multiple substrates.

        (1) **Turnover number.** Catalysis occurs so rapidly that a single enzyme molecule can convert more than 1000 substrate molecules per second, which is called the turnover number of an enzyme.

        (2) **Bidirectional.** The same enzyme catalyzes a given reaction in the forward or the reverse direction.

d. **Fourth step: products are released.** The products of the reaction are released from the active site, and the enzyme remains in its original form. The enzyme can then leave the active site and be reused with new substrate.

2. **The rate of a reaction** (i.e., the total amount of product per unit time) depends largely on the relative concentrations of substrate and enzyme molecules. As the substrate concentration increases, the rate of the reaction increases because more molecules of enzyme are occupied.

    a. **Saturation.** At a certain level of substrate, the enzyme becomes saturated (i.e., the active sites of all the enzyme molecules are occupied).

    b. At the point of saturation, the reaction proceeds at its maximum rate. This rate depends only on how fast each enzyme molecule can convert substrate.

D. Factors that affect enzyme activity. Several factors influence the catalytic activity of enzymes.

1. In many reactions, small **nonprotein substances** are needed for proper enzyme activity. These substances "trigger" a reaction by binding in a specific way to the enzyme molecule.

    a. **Coenzymes** are organic substances (e.g., vitamins, coenzyme A, biotin, heme).

    b. **Cofactors** are inorganic substances (e.g., metal atoms of zinc, iron, copper).

    c. **Prosthetic groups.** Coenzymes or cofactors may bind so tightly that they are effectively part of the protein, at which point they are called prosthetic groups.

    d. **The holoenzyme** is the protein and nonprotein portions of an enzyme together.

    e. **The apoenzyme** is the protein portion alone.

2. Each enzyme has **optimal environmental conditions** that favor the most active enzyme conformation.

    a. **Temperature**

        (1) **Effect on reactions.** A mild increase in temperature speeds up reactions; molecules move faster and are therefore more likely to interact. A mild decrease in temperature has the opposite effect.

        (2) **Denaturation.** When a certain temperature is exceeded, chemical bonds are broken, and the enzyme loses its specific shape (i.e., it is denatured). Denaturation is a permanent change that inactivates an enzyme.

    b. **pH.** An environment that is too acidic or too alkaline can denature enzymes. For most enzymes, the optimum pH is neutral (pH 7). There are exceptions. For example, digestive enzymes in the stomach are active at pH 2.

3. **Inhibitors** are molecules that bind selectively to enzymes and inhibit enzyme activity. Some inhibitors bind to enzymes reversibly, and others bind irreversibly.

a. **Competitive inhibitors** resemble the normal substrate and compete with it for binding to the active site of an enzyme (Figure 1-3A). Binding of the inhibitor, therefore, blocks the active site from the substrate (see Figure 1-3B). If the inhibitor is reversible, the effect of competitive inhibition can be overcome by an increase in substrate concentration.

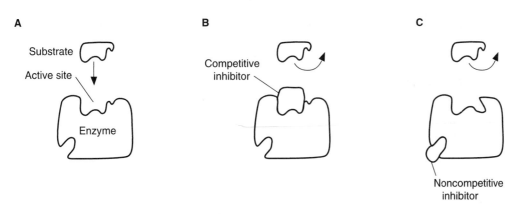

FIGURE 1-3.
A) The binding of normal substrate to the active site. **B)** The binding of competitive inhibitor to the active site. **C)** The binding of a noncompetitive inhibitor to a site other than the active site.

b. **Noncompetitive inhibitors** bind to a part of an enzyme other than the active site (see Figure 1-3C). Inhibitor binding changes the shape of the active site so that it cannot bind substrate.

II. Mechanisms of Enzyme Regulation

A. Allosteric Regulation

1. An **allosteric site** is a specific site on an enzyme other than the active site. Binding of regulatory molecules to an allosteric site stabilizes one or another alternative conformations of the active site of the enzyme.

   a. **Allosteric binding of an activator** stabilizes an active conformation of the enzyme.

   b. **Allosteric binding of an inhibitor** stabilizes an inactive enzyme conformation.

2. **Allosteric enzymes** are usually protein complexes with multiple subunits, with each subunit having its own active site. Binding of a regulatory molecule to an allosteric site between the subunits can cooperatively affect the entire complex.

B. Feedback inhibition.
During feedback inhibition, a metabolic pathway is regulated by the end product of that pathway (Figure 1-4).

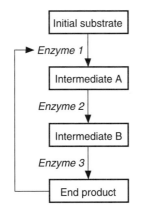

FIGURE 1-4.
The feedback inhibition loop.

1. **When the end product is in excess,** it allosterically inhibits the activity of an early enzyme in the pathway. This negative regulation prevents the unnecessary and potentially harmful accumulation of excess intermediates and end products.

2. **When the end product is no longer in excess,** the enzyme is released from the allosteric inhibition. This results in reactivation of the pathway.

C. **Multienzyme complexes.** Several enzymes acting in the same pathway may be assembled together so that the reactions occur efficiently and in the proper sequence (analogous to an assembly line). Multienzyme complexes may be localized in specific cell compartments or organelles.

I. Introduction to Metabolism

A. Metabolic Pathways

1. The term **metabolism** refers to the entire set of chemical reactions in a living cell or organism. Metabolism is an essential characteristic of all living organisms.

    a. **Metabolic reactions** occur in "chains" or pathways. In a metabolic pathway, the product of reaction 1 would be a reactant in reaction 2, and so forth. Many pathways are branched because particular molecules enter more than one alternative reaction.

    b. **Enzyme regulation.** Each reaction is catalyzed by a different enzyme. Enzyme regulation controls which pathways are involved in a reaction and to what extent (see Chapter 1 of the Biology Review Notes).

2. There are two general types of metabolic pathways in living cells (Figure 2-1A).

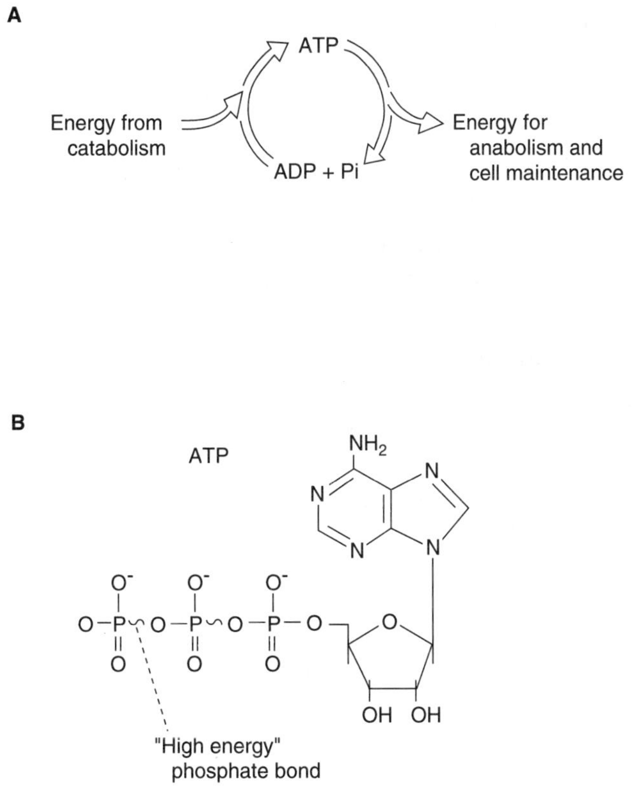

FIGURE 2-1.
A) The relationship between catabolism and anabolism, and **B)** the structure of adenosine triphosphate (ATP). Note the position of the key high-energy phosphate bonds. *ADP* = adenosine diphosphate; *P* = phosphate.

    a.   **Catabolic pathways** result in the decomposition of organic molecules into their simpler components. Catabolism releases the chemical energy stored in the chemical bonds of organic molecules.

    b.   **Anabolic pathways** result in the synthesis of organic molecules from their simpler components. Anabolism requires an input of chemical energy, storing the energy in organic molecules.

3.   **Coupled processes.** In cells, catabolic pathways provide the chemical energy needed to drive anabolic pathways.

B. Chemical Energy and Adenosine Triphosphate

1.   **Obtaining organic molecules.** Only plants and other photosynthetic organisms can synthesize their own organic molecules using energy absorbed from sunlight. All other organisms obtain organic molecules from their surroundings.

2.   **Decomposition of organic molecules releases energy.** In all living cells, the chemical energy that is stored in organic molecules is released when these molecules are broken down in catabolic pathways. Some of this energy is lost as heat. The rest of the energy released by catabolism is used to synthesize adenosine triphosphate (ATP; see Figure 2-1B). ATP is the immediate energy source for cellular work (i.e., energy-requiring processes such as synthesis, movement, transport).

    a.   **ATP is synthesized** from adenosine diphosphate (ADP) and inorganic phosphate (Pi) with an input of cellular energy. This phosphorylation reaction stores chemical energy in the unstable ("high-energy") phosphate bond of ATP.

$$ADP + Pi + energy \rightarrow ATP$$

    b.   **ATP is hydrolyzed** when the phosphate bond breaks, releasing the stored energy. The energy released by ATP hydrolysis is captured by the transfer of the phosphate to another molecule. This activates the other molecule to do work.

$$ATP \rightarrow ADP + Pi + energy$$

3.   **ATP synthesis** is driven by catabolism of the six-carbon sugar glucose. The energy in glucose is released by either of two catabolic pathways.

    a.   **Cellular respiration** is the most prevalent and efficient catabolic pathway. Respiration requires the presence of oxygen (i.e., aerobic conditions).

    b.   **Fermentation** is a less efficient pathway and does not require oxygen. Fermentation occurs in many microorganisms, and it occurs under anaerobic conditions in some cells of higher organisms.

4.   **Glucose catabolism** involves electron transfer reactions. The stepwise transfer of high-energy electrons from glucose releases energy to drive ATP synthesis.

    a.   **Coupled oxidation-reduction reactions** ("redox" reactions) involve the transfer of electrons from one compound to another.

       (1)   **Oxidation** occurs when an organic compound loses (donates) electrons. **Reduction** occurs when a compound gains (accepts) electrons.

(2) In a redox reaction, one molecule donates electrons, and the other accepts electrons. The electron donor is oxidized and the electron acceptor is reduced. Xe^- is oxidized to X, Y is reduced to Ye^-.

$$\overset{\text{oxidation}}{Xe^- + Y \rightarrow X + Ye^-} \atop \underset{\text{reduction}}{}$$

(3) Hydrogen ions (protons) are transferred along with electrons in many redox reactions.

b. **High-energy electrons** are released from glucose and transferred to special molecules called **electron carriers,** which include the coenzymes nicotinamide adenine dinucleotide (NAD^+) and flavin adenine dinucleotide (FAD^+).

$$\overset{\text{oxidation}}{X - H_2 + NAD^+ \rightarrow X + NADH + H^+} \atop \underset{\text{reduction}}{}$$

II. Cellular Respiration and Fermentation

A. Overview

1. The **overall reaction** for cellular respiration is:

$$C_6H_{12}O_6 + 6O_2 \rightarrow 6CO_2 + 6H_2O + \text{Energy}$$

2. **Respiration**

   a. During respiration, **glucose is completely oxidized to carbon dioxide.** Stepwise redox reactions release a substantial amount of energy for ATP synthesis. Overall, approximately 40% of the energy released from glucose is captured as ATP, and the rest is lost as heat.

   b. In respiration, oxygen is the final electron acceptor. **Oxygen is reduced to water.**

   c. **The respiration pathway includes three stages:** glycolysis, Krebs cycle, and the electron transport chain (ETC).

   d. Most of the ATP production occurs in the final stage of respiration.

   e. Glycolysis occurs in the cytoplasm of the cell, whereas the last two stages occur in the mitochondria.

3. **Fermentation.** During fermentation, glucose is only partially oxidized, and an organic molecule is reduced. Only a small amount of ATP is produced because the Krebs cycle and the ETC do not take place.

B. Glycolysis

1. Glycolysis can be summarized in the following equation:

$$\text{Glucose} + 2NAD^+ + 2ADP + 2Pi \rightarrow 2 \text{ pyruvic acid} + 2NADH + 2H^+ + 2ATP$$

2. **The reactions of the glycolysis pathway** (Figure 2-2A) are catalyzed by enzymes in the cytoplasm.

   a. In the first part of glycolysis, the **preparatory phase,** two molecules of ATP are consumed. Each molecule of glucose is split to form two molecules of a three-carbon compound, glyceraldehyde-3-phosphate (G3P).

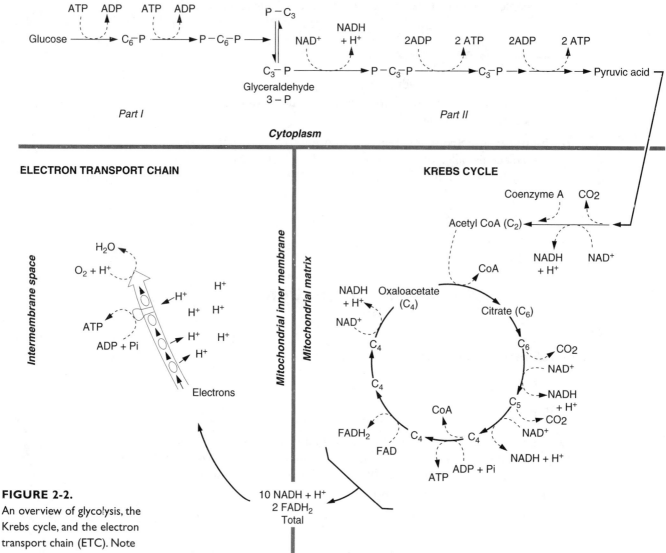

GLYCOLYSIS

Part I

Part II

Cytoplasm

ELECTRON TRANSPORT CHAIN

Intermembrane space

Mitochondrial inner membrane

Mitochondrial matrix

KREBS CYCLE

FIGURE 2-2.
An overview of glycolysis, the Krebs cycle, and the electron transport chain (ETC). Note the interrelation of the pathways and the flow of products from one pathway to the next. Also note that in Part II of glycolysis, the pathway is shifted to the right, because only glyceraldehyde-3-phosphate (G3P) directly continues the glycolytic pathway. *ADP* = adenosine diphosphate; *ATP* = adenosine triphosphate; *FAD* = flavin adenine dinucleotide; *FADH₂* = reduced flavin adenine dinucleotide; *Pᵢ* = inorganic phosphate; *NAD⁺* = oxidized nicotinamide adenine dinucleotide; *NADH* = reduced nicotinamide adenine dinucleotide.

346

b. In the second part of glycolysis, the **oxidative phase,** four molecules of ATP are synthesized by the direct transfer of a phosphate group from an intermediate molecule to ADP. This method of ATP synthesis is referred to as **substrate-level phosphorylation:**

$$X - P + ADP \rightarrow X + ATP$$

where X is an organic molecule.

(1) G3P is oxidized and two molecules of NAD⁺ are reduced to NADH.

(2) Two molecules of the three-carbon compound pyruvic acid are produced.

3. **The main outcomes of glycolysis** are as follow:

a. **A net gain of two molecules of ATP per one molecule of glucose**

b. **Transfer of high-energy electrons from glucose to NADH**

    c. **Partial oxidation of glucose to form pyruvic acid** (most of the chemical energy from glucose is in this organic compound)

        (1) **Pyruvic acid is converted to acetyl coenzyme A (acetyl CoA).**

            (a) In the presence of oxygen, pyruvic acid is transported from the cytoplasm into the mitochondria and converted to a two-carbon compound, **acetyl CoA.**

            (b) One carbon is cleaved from pyruvic acid and released as carbon dioxide, pyruvic acid is oxidized, and NAD^+ is reduced. The resulting two-carbon compound is then attached to coenzyme A to form acetyl CoA.

        (2) **For each molecule of glucose that enters glycolysis, two molecules of acetyl CoA enter the next stage of respiration, the Krebs cycle.**

C. The **Krebs cycle** (see Figure 2-2B) is also known as the citric acid cycle or the tricarboxylic acid (TCA) cycle.

    1. The Krebs cycle occurs in the **inner compartment or matrix of the mitochondria.**

    2. This **series of reactions** can be summarized as follows:

        a. Each molecule of acetyl CoA (a two-carbon compound) enters the Krebs cycle by combining with a four-carbon compound (i.e., oxaloacetate). This results in a six-carbon compound (i.e., citrate).

        b. In subsequent steps, two carbon dioxide molecules are removed from citrate, leaving a four-carbon compound. Stepwise redox reactions oxidize the organic intermediates and reduce three molecules of NAD^+ and one of FAD^+ to NADH and $FADH_2$, respectively.

        c. One molecule of ATP is synthesized by substrate-level phosphorylation.

        d. The four-carbon oxaloacetate is regenerated and is ready to combine with another incoming molecule of acetyl CoA.

    3. The **main outcomes** of the Krebs cycle are as follow:

        a. **Production of two molecules of ATP per glucose molecule**

        b. **Transfer of high-energy electrons to NADH and $FADH_2$**

D. **Electron transport chain** (see Figure 2-2C)

    1. The ETC is composed of a series of electron carriers located in the inner mitochondrial membrane (i.e., cristae). These carriers are mainly proteins with prosthetic groups (e.g., cytochrome with attached iron).

    2. The reduced coenzymes produced by glycolysis and the Krebs cycle (10 NADH and 2 $FADH_2$ per glucose molecule) donate high-energy electrons to the ETC. The electrons are transferred from one carrier to the next in a series of redox reactions.

        a. **The final acceptor is oxygen.** Oxygen has such a high affinity for electrons that it essentially pulls them down the chain.

        b. **Oxygen is reduced to water** when, at the end of the chain, oxygen accepts the electrons combined with hydrogen ions (protons).

3. **Proton pumps and the proton gradient.** As electrons flow down the chain, NADH and FADH₂ release protons into the mitochondrial matrix. Some of the inner membrane proteins can pump protons into the intermembrane space (i.e., space between the inner and outer mitochondrial membranes). These **pumps generate an electrochemical concentration gradient** across the inner membrane, which is impermeable to protons. The proton gradient is a source of potential energy.

4. **Energy is released as protons flow down their concentration gradient across the inner membrane.** Protons can cross the membrane only by passing through a membrane-spanning protein complex called ATP synthase. This enzyme uses the released energy to phosphorylate ADP.

   a. **Chemiosmosis** is the term for the coupling of proton flow to ATP synthesis.

   b. During chemiosmosis, three molecules of ATP are generated for each molecule of NADH. Also, two molecules of ATP are generated for each molecule of FADH₂, which donates electrons at a later point in the ETC (Table 2-1; Figure 2-3).

TABLE 2-1. Cellular respiration summary.

Process	Location	Input	Output (per glucose)
Glycolysis	Cytoplasm	Glucose	2 Pyruvic acid, 2 NADH, 2 ATP
Krebs cycle	Mitochondria— inner space (matrix)	2 Pyruvic acid converted to 2 acetyl CoA	2 NADH⁺ (pyruvic acid conversion step), 6 NADH⁺, 2 FADH₂, 2 ATP
Electron transport chain and oxidative phoshorylation	Mitochondria— inner membrane (cristae)	10 NADH, 2 FADH₂	32 ATP (12 H₂O)
			*Total: 36 ATP/glucose

Acetyl CoA = acetyl coenzyme A; ATP = adenosine triphosphate; FADH₂ = reduced flavin adenine dinucleotide; NADH = reduced nicotinamide adenine dinucleotide.

FIGURE 2-3.
Summary of respiration and fermentation.

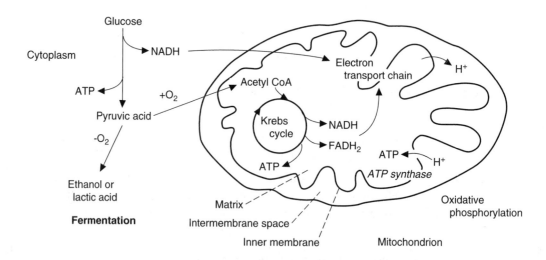

5. **Oxidative phosphorylation** is the term used to describe the production of ATP using energy from the redox reactions of the ETC. Most of the ATP output of respiration is produced by oxidative phosphorylation.

E. Anaerobic Pathways

1. **Anaerobic pathways** allow glucose catabolism to occur in the absence of oxygen. Table 2-2 compares cellular respiration and fermentation.

TABLE 2-2. Comparison of respiration and fermentation

	Cellular Respiration	Fermentation
Growth conditions	Aerobic	Aerobic or anaerobic
Electron transport chain	Yes	No
Final electron and hydrogen acceptor	Oxygen	Organic (e.g., acetaldehyde or pyruvic acid)
Method of making ATP	Mostly oxidative phosphorylation; some substrate-level phosphorylation	Substrate-level phosphorylation

ATP = adenosine triphosphate.

2. Certain microorganisms are capable of **anaerobic respiration,** in which an inorganic compound is the final electron acceptor instead of oxygen. (For example, some bacteria reduce sulfates or nitrates in soil.)

3. **Fermentation** is an anaerobic pathway that occurs in many different microorganisms as well as in certain cell types in higher organisms (e.g., human muscle cells). The entire pathway occurs in the cytoplasm, and there is no ETC.

   a. **Fermentation pathways start with glycolysis, followed by production of fermentation waste products** (Figure 2-4). This process partially oxidizes glucose to an organic molecule, which is then reduced by NADH. Most of the energy in glucose remains in an organic molecule.

A. Alcohol fermentation

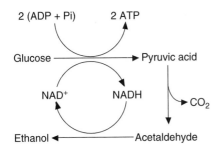

B. Lactic acid fermentation

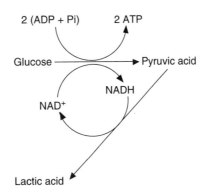

FIGURE 2-4.
A) Alcohol fermentation.
B) Lactic acid fermentation.

   b. A total of two molecules of ATP per one molecule of glucose are produced by **substrate-level phosphorylation** during glycolysis.

4. The various **types of fermentation pathways** differ in the waste products produced (see Figure 2-4).

   a. In **alcohol fermentation,** pyruvic acid releases carbon dioxide and forms a two-carbon compound, **acetaldehyde.** Acetaldehyde is reduced to form **ethanol,** and NADH is oxidized to regenerate NAD$^+$.

   b. In **lactic acid fermentation,** pyruvic acid is reduced to lactic acid, and NADH is oxidized. Some cells, such as human muscle cells, can switch from cellular respiration to lactic acid fermentation when oxygen is depleted.

F. Regulation of Respiration

1. **Respiration is interconnected with the metabolism of all the organic molecules in cells** (Figure 2-5A).

    a. Carbohydrates, proteins, and fats from food can enter respiration at different points. For example, complex carbohydrates are converted into glucose, proteins are converted into pyruvic acid or Krebs cycle intermediates, and fats are converted into glycolytic intermediates or acetyl.

    b. Conversely, organic intermediates can leave respiration to enter synthesis pathways (anabolism). In this way, carbohydrates can be converted to fats, fats can be converted to proteins, and so forth.

2. The **rate of respiration** is controlled by the enzymes that catalyze the various reactions along the pathway. Many of these are allosteric enzymes with sites for binding activators and inhibitors. **One of the main rate-limiting reactions is the third step of glycolysis, which is catalyzed by the enzyme phosphofructokinase** (see Figure 2-5B). This step is sometimes referred to as the "pacemaker" of respiration.

    a. Phosphofructokinase is inhibited by ATP and is activated by ADP. Thus, when ATP is high, respiration slows down.

    b. When ATP is depleted, the ADP concentration increases, and the enzyme is reactivated. This accelerates the rate of respiration.

FIGURE 2-5.
A) The metabolism of organic molecules and **B)** an example of metabolic regulation by phosphofructokinase, the key rate-limiting step of glycolysis.

A

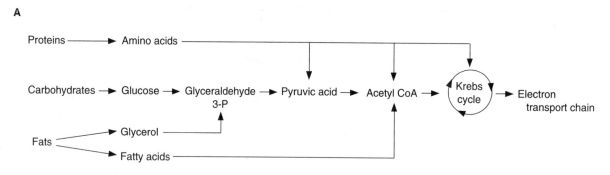

B

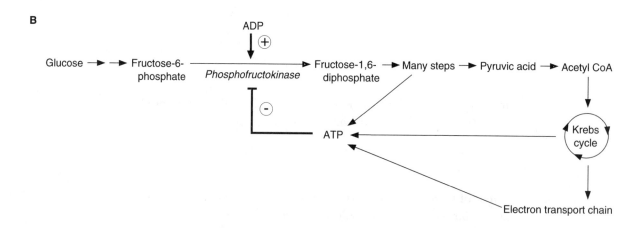

3

DNA Functions and Structure

I. DNA Functions and Structure

A. Functions

1. **Deoxyribonucleic acid (DNA)** is the heritable (genetic) material in all cells. DNA is precisely replicated during each cell generation. When the cell divides, an identical copy of the parental DNA is distributed to each daughter cell. Thus, DNA provides instructions for all future generations of single cells and entire multicellular organisms.

2. **DNA controls the activities of cells** by specifying the synthesis of enzymes and other proteins. Proteins are the class of molecules with the greatest diversity of essential cellular functions; they catalyze and regulate metabolic reactions, provide raw materials for cell structures, allow movement, interact with the environment and other cells, and control growth and cell division.

3. **A gene is the unit of information in DNA.** Each gene specifies the amino acid sequence of a particular protein. Thousands to millions of different genes are needed to make all the necessary proteins in a single cell.

B. DNA Structure

1. DNA belongs to a class of organic molecules called **nucleic acids.** The subunits of nucleic acids are called **nucleotides** (Figure 3-1A). Each nucleotide is composed of the following:

   a. **Deoxyribose,** which is a five-carbon sugar

   b. **A phosphate group,** which is attached to the 5′ carbon of deoxyribose

   c. **A nitrogenous base,** of which there are four different types—two purines and two pyrimidines (see Figure 3-1B).

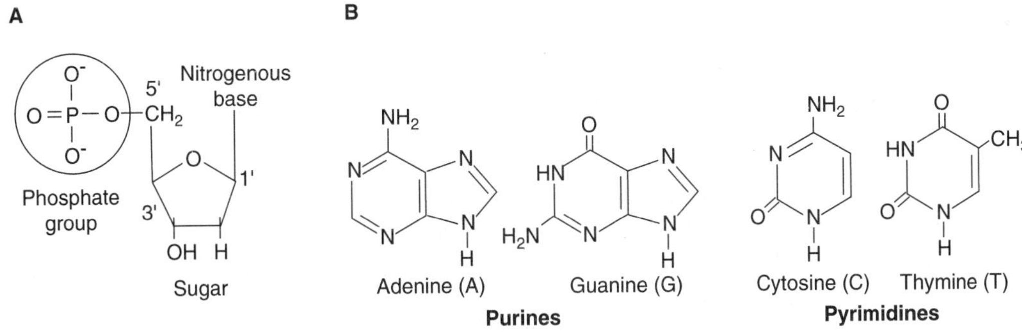

FIGURE 3-1.

A) The structure of a nucleotide. **B)** The structure of the nitrogenous bases—the purines and pyrimidines. The structure of uracil, a pyrimidine found in RNA, is not shown. Note the presence of a hydroxyl group on the 3′ carbon of the nucleotide.

A

Phosphate group

Sugar

Nitrogenous base

B

Adenine (A)   Guanine (G)

Purines

Cytosine (C)   Thymine (T)

Pyrimidines

2. **Nucleotides are linked together by phosphodiester bonds** between the phosphate of one nucleotide and the sugar of the next nucleotide (Figure 3-2A). Alternating sugars and phosphates make up the long "backbone" of the nucleotide chain, or polynucleotide. The bases extend from the 1' carbon of each sugar in the chain.

3. The two ends of a polynucleotide differ from each other, making it a **polar molecule.** The ends are designated according to the numbered carbon in the sugar. A phosphate group is at the 5' end, and a hydroxyl group is at the 3' end.

4. **The DNA double helix** (see Figure 3-2B)

   a. The structure of DNA was deduced in the early 1950s by James Watson and Francis Crick. They built a model of DNA using information from experiments by Rosalind Franklin and other scientists.

   b. DNA is a **double-stranded molecule,** or duplex, composed of two paired polynucleotides. The pairing results from specific interactions between the bases in each DNA strand. The structure is like a rope ladder in which the sugar-phosphate backbones form the "sideropes" and the pairs of bases form rigid "rungs."

   c. The DNA molecule twists to form a **helix** with 10 bases per helical turn.

   d. The two DNA strands are paired with opposite 5'-to-3' polarity. In other words, the two strands are **antiparallel.** The 5' end of one strand is paired with the 3' end of the other, and they run in opposite directions.

FIGURE 3-2.
A) The backbone of DNA is comprised of sugars and phosphates. **B)** Details of DNA at the molecular level.

A

B

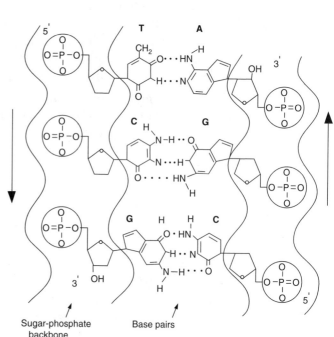

Sugar-phosphate backbone   Base pairs

5. The two strands of a DNA molecule are paired by **complementary base pairing.** Each nucleotide in one strand pairs with a specific (complementary) nucleotide in the other strand.

   a. **Purines and pyrimidines.** Purine bases (i.e., adenine, guanine) are larger and always pair with pyrimidines (i.e., thymine, cytosine), which are smaller. Specifically, **adenine (A) always pairs with thymine (T), and guanine (G) always pairs with cytosine (C).**

CHAP. 3
DNA
FUNCTIONS
AND
STRUCTURE

352

b. **Complementary base pairing** results from the formation of hydrogen bonds (weak, noncovalent bonds) between the specific pairs. Each A–T pair forms two hydrogen bonds, whereas each G–C pair forms three hydrogen bonds. A DNA molecule is stabilized by the large number of hydrogen bonds along its length.

6. The variation in DNA is found in the linear sequence of base pairs along the lengths of the molecules. Amazing sequence diversity is generated in DNA molecules thousands to millions of base pairs (bp) long.

II. DNA Replication

A. Overview

1. **Templates.** One key feature of DNA is its ability to be replicated, so that identical copies of the genes can be passed on to the next generation. Each DNA molecule provides its own templates for replication.

   a. **Each strand serves as a template** for the synthesis of a new complementary DNA strand according to the rules of specific base pairing.

   b. An enzyme called **DNA polymerase** synthesizes DNA by linking each newly paired nucleotide to the 3′ end of a growing DNA strand.

   c. **Semiconservative replication.** In each daughter DNA molecule, one parental (old) DNA strand is conserved, and it is paired with one newly synthesized strand. This pattern of replication is referred to as semiconservative (Figure 3-3). In contrast, a **conservative pattern** would result in one intact parental DNA molecule and one completely new DNA molecule. DNA replication has been found to be semiconservative.

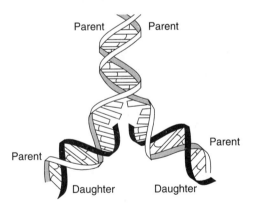

Parent   Parent

Parent

Parent

Daughter   Daughter

FIGURE 3-3.
The semiconservative replication of DNA.

   d. **DNA replication is extremely fast and accurate.** Approximately 500 nucleotides are replicated per second, and there is approximately one mistake in 1 billion bp. This is an amazing feat, considering the size of a eukaryotic genome (i.e., approximately 3 billion bp of DNA) within a single cell nucleus.

B. The mechanism of DNA replication was initially observed in the bacteria *Escherichia coli*. A similar process occurs in eukaryotes.

1. **Initiation.** Replication is initiated when specific proteins recognize and bind to special sites on a chromosome called **replication origins.** There are multiple origins on each linear eukaryotic chromosome, but only one origin on the single circular *E. coli* chromosome.

2. **Processing.** Replication proceeds at structures called **replication forks.** Each fork moves in one direction as more parental sequences are made available for replication. Several processes go on at the replication fork (Figure 3-4).

FIGURE 3-4.
The replication of DNA occurring at replication forks.

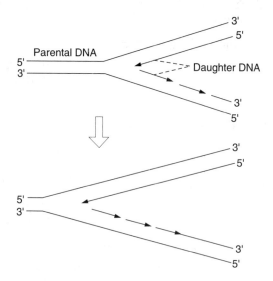

a. **5′ to 3′ direction.** Base pairing with a parental template strand determines the sequence of nucleotides in each new DNA strand. The complementary nucleotide is linked to the 3′ end of the new strand by a molecule of DNA polymerase, which moves along the template. Thus, a new DNA strand is always synthesized in the 5′ to 3′ direction.

b. **Continuous elongation.** At the replication fork, one new strand is elongated continuously in the leading 5′ to 3′ direction toward the moving fork. This is called **leading strand synthesis.**

c. **Lagging strand synthesis** describes the mechanism of discontinuous elongation, which occurs in the nonleading template strand. Because one template strand is antiparallel, one new strand must be formed in an overall 3′ to 5′ direction, which is not the leading direction.

(1) **Okazaki fragments,** which are short DNA fragments, are synthesized in a 5′ to 3′ direction, which is away from the replication fork.

(2) As the fork moves, additional Okazaki fragments are added in a 3′ to 5′ direction, which is toward the moving replication fork, so that overall growth is in this direction.

d. Different molecules of DNA polymerase synthesize the leading and lagging strands at the replication fork.

C. Enzymes Involved in DNA Replication

1. **Replication complex.** The replication process involves many different enzymes. A replication complex is formed when several of the different enzymes join with DNA polymerase.

2. **Enzymes at the replication fork** (Figure 3-5)

a. **DNA helicase** unwinds the two parental DNA strands in front of the replication complex.

b. **Single-strand binding proteins** bind to the separated parental strands to keep them from reannealing (i.e., repairing).

CHAP. 3
DNA
FUNCTIONS
AND
STRUCTURE

354

c. **RNA primase** starts de novo synthesis of each new Okazaki fragment of the lagging strand. The primase synthesizes a short RNA primer complementary to the newly exposed DNA template. The RNA primer provides the 3′ end that DNA polymerase needs to start adding DNA nucleotides.

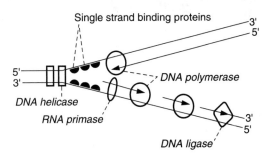

FIGURE 3-5.

The enzymes involved at the replication fork.

3. An **exonuclease** removes the RNA primer between fragments.

4. **DNA ligase** joins the Okazaki fragments together to elongate the new continuous DNA strand.

Gene Expression: From DNA to Protein

I. Overview

A. Deoxyribonucleic Acid (DNA). The information in a gene is specified by the linear sequence of nucleotides in the DNA. A single gene may be hundreds to hundreds of thousands of nucleotides in length.

B. Ribonucleic Acid (RNA). DNA does not build a protein directly; it sends instructions to the protein synthesis "machinery" in the form of RNA.

   1. **Transcription** is the process by which RNA is copied from the DNA. After the DNA is transcribed in the nucleus, the RNA moves into the cytoplasm.

   2. **Translation** is the process by which the information in RNA is used to synthesize proteins. Translation occurs in the cytoplasm.

C. Gene Expression. A gene undergoing transcription and translation is said to be expressed (i.e., the information in DNA is used to make a protein).

D. The central dogma of molecular biology is the scheme DNA $\rightarrow$ RNA $\rightarrow$ protein.

II. Transcription

A. Mechanism of Transcription

   1. **RNA structure.** RNA is a nucleic acid with a structure similar to that of DNA. However, there are several important differences (Table 4-1).

TABLE 4-1. Comparison of deoxyribonucleic acid (DNA) and ribonucleic acid (RNA).

Characteristic	DNA	RNA
Sugar	Deoxyribose	Ribose
Bases	A, G, C, T	A, G, C, U
Structure	Double-stranded	Single-stranded
Synthesis process	Replicated from DNA template	Transcribed from DNA template
Functions	Storage and inheritance of information for proteins	Transmittance of DNA information to cytoplasm for translation

A = adenine; C = cytosine; G = guanine; T = thymine; U = uracil.

a. In RNA, a **hydroxyl group** instead of a hydrogen molecule is attached to the 2′ carbon of the five-carbon sugar.

b. RNA contains the nitrogenous base **uracil (U)** instead of thymine. Uracil pairs with adenine.

c. RNA molecules are **single-stranded** rather than double-stranded **polynucleotides.**

2. **Transcription of a gene** involves synthesis of a complementary strand of RNA from a DNA template strand (Figure 4-1).

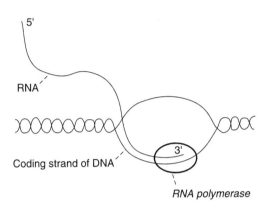

FIGURE 4-1.
The transcription of ribonucleic acid (RNA) from a deoxyribonucleic acid (DNA) template.

a. **RNA polymerase** is the enzyme responsible for RNA synthesis.

b. **Promoter sequence.** Transcription starts when RNA polymerase binds to a specific DNA sequence found near the start of the gene. This transcription start site is called the promoter. Only one strand of the DNA duplex contains the promoter sequence, so only that strand is transcribed.

c. **Processing.** Transcription proceeds as RNA polymerase moves along the DNA template, linking complementary RNA nucleotides into a growing chain. The only change in the base pairing rules (compared with DNA replication) is that uracil is incorporated into the RNA opposite adenine in the DNA template.

d. **Elongation.** As in DNA synthesis, the new RNA strand is elongated in the 5′ to 3′ direction. The "start" of a gene (the promoter) is therefore called the 5′ end of the gene. Accordingly, the end of a gene is its 3′ end.

e. **The DNA duplex "opens up"** during active transcription, which allows many molecules of the RNA polymerase to transcribe the gene at the same time.

f. **Termination sequence.** Transcription stops at a termination sequence in the DNA. Here, the RNA polymerase leaves the DNA template and releases the newly synthesized RNA.

3. **Coding and noncoding regions.** An entire gene is transcribed into one continuous RNA molecule. However, most eukaryotic genes contain stretches of DNA that do not code for amino acids. The protein-coding regions of a gene are called **exons** (they are expressed as protein), and the noncoding regions are called **introns** (intervening sequences).

a. **RNA splicing.** While a newly synthesized RNA molecule is still in the nucleus, the introns are removed (spliced), and the exons are joined together (Figure 4-2). This process results in a continuous protein-coding sequence.

FIGURE 4-2.
Posttranscriptional modification of RNA. Note the RNA
splicing and the placement of
a "cap" and a polyadeny-
late (poly A) "tail."

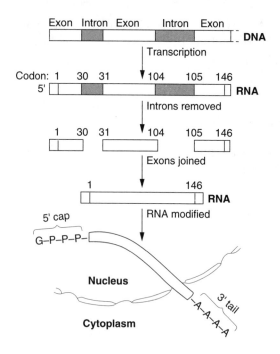

b. **5′ Cap and poly A tail.** The RNA is also modified at its 5′ and 3′ ends to protect it from degradation. These modifications include a 5′ cap, which is modified guanosine triphosphate (GTP), and a 3′ polyadenylate (poly A) tail.

4. **Nontranscribed regions.** Genes make up only a small fraction of the DNA in a eukaryotic cell. The genes are often separated by large regions of noncoding DNA that are never transcribed.

B. Regulation of Transcription

1. Transcription is a highly regulated process. Many of the genes in the genome of an organism are not expressed in all cells or at all times.

   a. **Unicellular organisms** are short-lived and vulnerable to their surroundings; they must reproduce rapidly to ensure population survival. In these cells, gene regulation avoids producing unneeded gene products (which would be a waste of energy) and allows rapid adaptation to changes in the surroundings.

   b. In **multicellular organisms,** many genes are expressed only at specific developmental stages and only in specific cells. This **differential gene expression** produces the many specialized cell types of the tissues, organs, and organ systems that make up the entire organism.

2. Transcription is generally controlled by the **binding of regulatory proteins to specific regulatory DNA sequences** located near or within a gene. This molecular interaction either stimulates or inhibits the ability of RNA polymerase to transcribe the gene.

3. **Transcriptional regulation in prokaryotic cells** (bacteria)

   a. **Constitutive expression** describes the fact that some genes are always transcribed (not regulated).

   b. Genes that code for proteins with related metabolic functions are clustered together in **operons** (Table 4-2). The **structural genes** are the genes that code for the polypeptide products of the operon. When expressed, these genes are transcribed into one continuous RNA.

TABLE 4-2. Operon summary.

Operon Function	Example	Transcription	Control
Synthesis of a product	Trp operon	On unless the product is in excess	Repressible
Catabolism (break down) of a nutrient	Lac operon	Off unless nutrient is available	Inducible

Lac = lactose; *Trp* = tryptophan.

(1) An operon allows coordinated control over the expression of multiple gene products by having **one regulatory system** for all of its structural genes.

(2) The **promoter sequence** binds RNA polymerase to start transcription. This DNA sequence is located at 5′ to the structural genes.

(3) The **operator sequence** is a specific DNA sequence located between the promoter and the structural genes. A regulatory protein called the **repressor** can bind to the operator and block RNA polymerase from transcribing the genes. The repressor–operator interaction is an "on–off switch" that controls whether the operon is transcribed.

   c. A **repressible operon** is turned off (repressed) by activation of the repressor. An example is the **tryptophan (Trp) operon,** which codes for enzymes in the tryptophan synthesis pathway. Tryptophan serves as the corepressor of the Trp operon: when the amino acid tryptophan begins to accumulate, it binds to and activates the repressor. This turns off the operon, thereby preventing synthesis of excess tryptophan.

   d. An **inducible operon** is turned on (induced) by inactivation of the repressor. An example is the **Lac operon** (Figure 4-3), which codes for enzymes in the lactose catabolism pathway (e.g., β-galactosidase). When

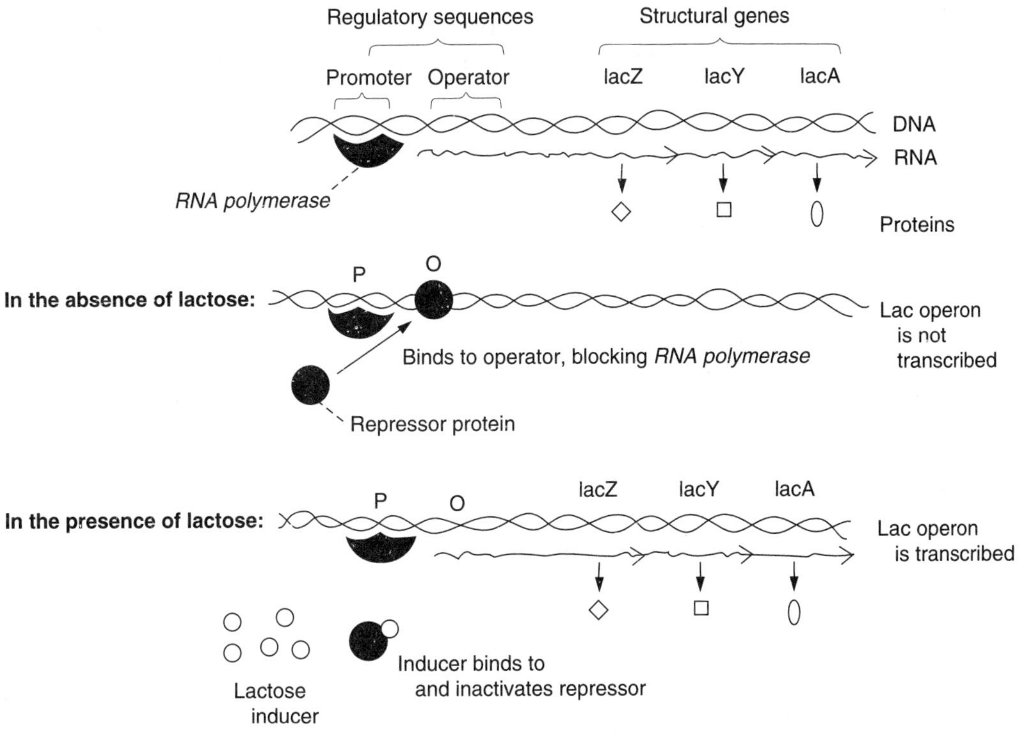

FIGURE 4-3.
The lactose (Lac) operon is a classic example of transcriptional regulation.

lactose is present, it binds to and inactivates the repressor. This turns on the operon, thereby allowing breakdown of the nutrient lactose.

4. The examples in Figure 4-3 illustrate **negative control,** which involves a **repressor protein** that turns transcription off. **Positive control** involves an **activator protein,** which stimulates transcription. An example from the Lac operon is the activity of the catabolite activator protein (CAP). CAP stimulates transcription by interacting with RNA polymerase at the promoter region.

  a. **CAP** is activated when lactose is needed as an energy source because glucose is unavailable.

  b. CAP is activated by interacting with **cyclic adenosine monophosphate (cAMP),** which increases in concentration as glucose levels decrease.

5. **Transcriptional regulation in eukaryotic cells** (Table 4-3)

TABLE 4-3. Comparison of gene regulation in prokaryotes and eukaryotes

	Prokaryotes	Eukaryotes
General emphasis	Economy, efficiency (rapid growth, short life span)	Cell specificity and cooperation (multicellular organisms)
Gene organization	Approximately 2500 genes; no introns; few DNA-associated proteins; genes cotranscribed in operons	Approximately 100,000 genes, introns, and exons. DNA packaged with proteins; genes transcribed separately
Regulatory mechanisms	Genes have shared regulatory regions for rapid, coordinated control (repression and induction mechanisms)	Many levels of regulation (e.g., chromosome packaging, transcription factors, mRNA processing, translation, protein processing)
Transcription and translation	Simultaneous; both occur in the cytoplasm	Separated in time and space
mRNA	Rapidly degraded	Controlled stability

  a. **Packaging of DNA.** Transcriptional activity is influenced by the organization of the DNA in the chromosomes. Each unreplicated chromosome is composed of a single, linear DNA molecule associated with special proteins called **histones.** The histones serve to package enormous amounts of DNA into the nucleus. The ability of a gene to be transcribed is influenced by the condensation or packaging of the DNA. Examples include the following:

    (1) **Heterochromatin** describes certain permanently condensed regions of the chromosome. Few or no actively transcribed genes are located in heterochromatin.

    (2) **Open or looped regions** of chromosomes often contain actively transcribed genes.

  b. **Eukaryotic regulation.** As in bacteria, transcription is regulated by binding specific proteins to DNA sequences at or near the promoter of the gene. For example, transcription factors are proteins that help RNA polymerase bind to the promoter.

  c. The binding of specific proteins to regions called **enhancers** increases the rate of transcription. Enhancer sequences may be located at 5′ or 3′ to a gene, near a gene, distant from a gene, or even within the gene.

C. Types of RNA (Table 4-4)

TABLE 4-4. RNA summary.

Type of RNA	Function
mRNA	Carries information for amino acid sequence from the DNA to the ribosomes
tRNA	Carries amino acids to the mRNA on the ribosome (interpreter in protein synthesis)
rRNA	Structural component of ribosomes (also some enzymatic activity)

1. **Messenger RNA (mRNA)** is transcribed from a gene and contains the information for the amino acid sequence of a protein. The mRNA is the essential link between a gene and its protein product. After being synthesized in the nucleus, mRNA molecules move out into the cytoplasm where they are translated by the protein synthesis machinery.

   a. **Genetic code** (Table 4-5). The mRNA specifies a sequence of amino acids according to the genetic code. In this code, each continuous set of three nucleotides specifies one amino acid.

TABLE 4-5. An example of the genetic code.

DNA codon	TAC	CAG	TTC	ATG
mRNA codon	AUG	GUC	AAG	UAG
Anticodon	UAC	CAG	UUC	None
Amino acid	Methionine	Valine	Lysine	Stop

   (1) Each nucleotide triplet is called a **codon.** For example, the following mRNA sequence:

$$\overbrace{AUG}\overbrace{CCA}\overbrace{GGC}\overbrace{AAA}\overbrace{UUU}$$

   specifies the following amino acid sequence:

   met—pro—gly—lys—phe

   (2) There are a total of 61 codons that specify amino acids, including the "start" codon AUG, which codes for methionine. There are three "stop" codons (UAA, UAG, UGA) that signal the protein synthesis machinery to stop translation. The stop codons do not code for any amino acid.

   b. **Properties of the genetic code**

   (1) **The code is redundant.** There are more than 60 different codons, but only 20 different amino acids. Two or more codons may specify the same amino acid. These redundant codons differ in the second or third position. For example, CUU, CUC, CUA, and CUG all specify the amino acid leucine.

   (2) **The code is unambiguous.** Each codon specifies one and only one amino acid.

   (3) **The code is nearly universal.** Almost all organisms share the same genetic code.

2. **Ribosomal RNA (rRNA)** does not code for a polypeptide product. The rRNA functions as a structural component of the ribosomes, the structures on which proteins are synthesized (see III).

3. **Transfer RNA (tRNA)** also does not code for protein. The tRNA functions in protein synthesis as an "interpreter" between the mRNA and amino acids. A different tRNA matches each mRNA codon with the correct amino acid.

   a. **Structure.** tRNA molecules have a distinctive cloverleaf-like structure (Figure 4-4).

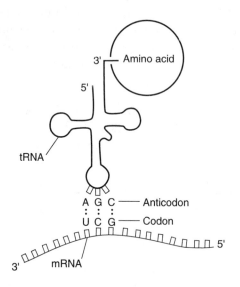

   b. **Types.** There are many types of tRNA, each with a different nucleotide triplet, called the **anticodon,** in a specific region of the molecule.

      (1) The anticodon of each tRNA can recognize a specific codon in the mRNA by complementary base pairing.

      (2) Some tRNAs can bind to two or three redundant codons because of inaccurate pairing or "wobble" in the third nucleotide position of the tRNA.

   c. **Aminoacyl-tRNA synthetase,** an enzyme that **activates amino acids,** attaches a specific amino acid to the 3′ end of each tRNA. There is a specific aminoacyl-tRNA synthetase for each amino acid, enabling it to participate in protein synthesis.

III. Translation (Table 4-6)

A. The Structure and Function of Ribosomes

1. **Structure**

   a. **Ribosomes are present as two subunits (large and small) in the cytoplasm.** Ribosomes are composed of approximately 60% rRNA and approximately 40% protein. The two subunits come together and bind the mRNA as it exits the nucleus.

   b. Each ribosome has **one binding site for mRNA** and **two binding sites for tRNA.**

TABLE 4-6. Comparison of transcription and translation.

	Transcription	Translation
Template	DNA	RNA
Location	Nucleus (cytoplasm in prokaryotes)	Cytoplasm; ribosomes free or on endoplasmic reticulum
Molecules involved	RNA nucleotides, DNA, RNA polymerase, transcription factors	Amino acids, tRNA, mRNA, ribosomes, enzymes, ATP, GTP, initiation/elongation factors
Enzymes needed	RNA polymerase, RNA processing enzymes	Aminoacyl-tRNA synthetase, peptidyl transferase
Control: start and stop	Transcription factors at promoter region, (TATA box), terminator region	Initiation factors, AUG, stop codons, release factors
Product	mRNA	Protein
Processing involved	RNA processing: 5′ cap and poly A tail, RNA splicing (introns removed, exons joined)	Spontaneous folding, disulfide bridges, some polypeptide trimming and modifications

GTP = guanosine triphosphate.

    (1)   The **P site** holds the tRNA carrying the growing polypeptide chain.

    (2)   The **A site** holds the tRNA carrying the next amino acid to be added to the chain.

  2.   **Function.** The ribosomes hold the tRNA and mRNA molecules together, and enzymes catalyze the addition of a new amino acid to a growing polypeptide chain.

B. The Mechanism of Protein Synthesis

  1.   **Initiation** (Figure 4-5A). With the help of proteins called initiation factors, the ribosome subunits come together and bind the mRNA at the "start" codon, AUG. The initiator tRNA (carrying methionine) binds to the start codon in the P site on the ribosome.

  2.   **Elongation** occurs by addition of amino acids one by one to the initial amino acid. Elongation is a three-step process that requires an input of energy from GTP hydrolysis.

    a.   The anticodon of a new activated tRNA binds to the complementary codon in the A site of the ribosome (see Figure 4-5B).

    b.   The first amino acid in the P site (met) forms a peptide bond with the new amino acid, and the bonded amino acids are then transferred to the tRNA in the A site (see Figure 4-5C). In subsequent elongation steps, the growing polypeptide chain is transferred to the A site tRNA as each new amino acid is added.

    c.   The empty tRNA is released from the P site. Then the tRNA, along with the bound mRNA, moves from the A site into the P site. This is the **translocation step** (see Figure 4-5D).

        (1)   The next codon is brought into the A site, available for the correct incoming tRNA.

        (2)   The mRNA moves through the ribosome in the 5′ to 3′ direction.

3. **Termination of the polypeptide chain** occurs when any one of the three stop codons reaches the A site (see Figure 4-5E). With the help of a release factor, the completed polypeptide chain is released from the tRNA in the P site and from the ribosome (which disassembles).

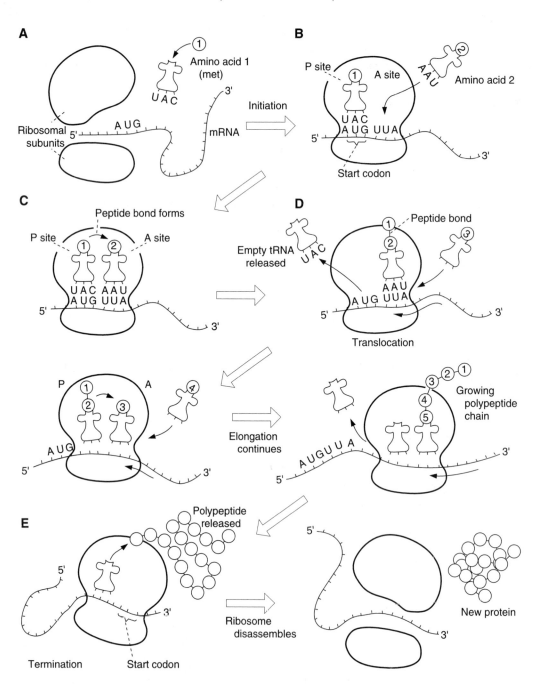

FIGURE 4-5.

The mechanism of protein synthesis (translation). **A)** Initiation. **B) through D)** Elongation. **E)** Termination.

4. **Processing** during and after synthesis is usually required to render a polypeptide functional. Processing events include specific folding of the polypeptide, formation of disulfide bonds (tertiary structure), chemical modifications, or combining with other polypeptides.

5

Microbiology

I. Viruses

A. Viral Structure

1. Viruses are particles of genetic material surrounded by protein. A complete viral particle is called a **virion.**

   a. **Viral genomes** differ for different viruses. The genetic material may be DNA or RNA, double-stranded or single-stranded, linear or circular. Genome sizes range from just a few genes to hundreds of genes.

   b. The protein **capsid** is the outer covering of the virion.

      (1) Capsids come in various shapes, including helical, polyhedral, or complex. Some simple capsids are composed of repetitive subunits of only a single type of protein.

      (2) In some viruses, the capsid is surrounded by a lipid-membrane **envelope.** The envelope is usually derived from a host cell.

   c. **Size.** Viruses range from 20–300 nm in diameter. The smallest is approximately 500 times smaller than a human red blood cell; the largest is approximately the same size as the smallest bacterial cells.

B. Viral Life Histories

1. **Viruses are obligate intracellular parasites;** that is, they can reproduce only inside a living cell (the host).

   a. **Different types of viruses infect different types of cells,** including bacterial, animal, or plant cells. Once they enter a cell, viruses can command the cellular machinery to produce new virions (reproduce).

   b. **Some viruses can integrate into the genome of the host** instead of reproducing immediately after infection. The integrated viral genome can then replicate with the host's DNA. During this time, the viral infection may remain undetected.

   c. After viral reproduction, the new viruses leave the host cell to infect more cells.

2. **Bacteriophages** are viruses that infect bacterial cells. The most well studied are the T-even phages and phage lambda, which infect *Escherichia coli.*

a. Structure. Bacteriophages have a complex structure composed of many types of proteins (Figure 5-1). They have an icosahedral head that encloses the genetic material (DNA), a sheath, and tail fibers.

FIGURE 5-1.
The structure of a bacteriophage.

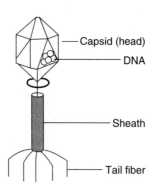

— Capsid (head)

— DNA

— Sheath

— Tail fiber

b. Mechanism of infection. A bacteriophage infects a cell by binding with its tail fibers to specific cell membrane receptors. The sheath contracts and the DNA is injected into the cell, leaving the protein component outside.

3. The **lytic cycle** is one of two alternative life cycles for bacteriophages (Figure 5-2A). **Phage lambda** illustrates the lytic cycle.

    a. Once the viral DNA is inside the cell, it is transcribed and translated by the host cell machinery. A viral enzyme degrades the host's DNA.

    b. When the viral DNA has been replicated and proteins have been synthesized, the new virions are assembled.

    c. The host cell lyses and releases the phage. This entire cycle can occur in only 20–30 minutes, and it can result in a 100-fold increase in the number of phages.

FIGURE 5-2.
A) The lytic and **B)** lysogenic cycles for bacteriophages.

4. The **lysogenic cycle** is the life cycle of temperate bacteriophages (see Figure 5-2B). These phages can reproduce without killing the host cell.

A

B

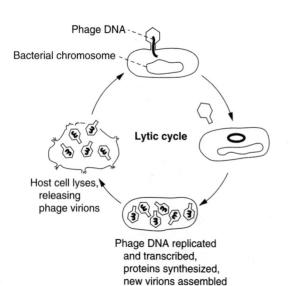

Phage DNA

Bacterial chromosome

Lytic cycle

Host cell lyses, releasing phage virions

Phage DNA replicated and transcribed, proteins synthesized, new virions assembled

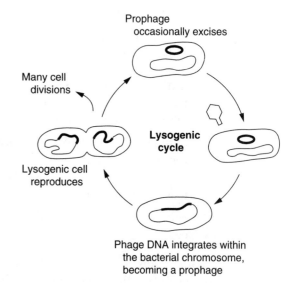

Prophage occasionally excises

Many cell divisions

Lysogenic cycle

Lysogenic cell reproduces

Phage DNA integrates within the bacterial chromosome, becoming a prophage

a. Once inside, the viral DNA is integrated into the host's DNA and becomes a **prophage.** During this stage, the viral genes are kept inactive by a viral repressor protein.

b. The prophage replicates with the host chromosome and is transmitted to progeny cells during cell division. A prophage may be carried in the chromosome of the host cell for many generations. During this time, the host cell may express new properties because of the presence of the prophage.

c. Excision of the prophage and induction of the lytic cycle may occur spontaneously or may be caused by environmental stress.

5. **Animal viruses** are viruses that infect animal cells (including human cells).

    a. **Structure.** Many animal viruses have an envelope with protruding protein spikes that bind to cell receptors. Once bound, the viral envelope fuses with the cell membrane and the entire virus (capsid and genome) enters the cell. Then, the protein capsid is removed.

    b. In the **productive cycle,** the virus reproduces soon after infection. If the genome is RNA, viral enzymes are used to replicate it and transcribe mRNA. After the host's machinery synthesizes new capsids, the new virions are assembled. They exit the host cell by budding off from its membrane, which may occur without lysing the cell.

    c. Some animal viruses with DNA genomes can integrate into the host's genome as a **provirus.** After a latent period, the virus may enter a productive cycle.

II. Prokaryotic Cells

A. General Characteristics of Prokaryotes (Table 5-1)

TABLE 5-1. Summary of prokaryotic cell characteristics.

Characteristic	Description
Cell shape and size	Spheres, rods, or spirals; $\approx$1–5 μm (1/10th the size of eukaryotic cells)
Cell surface	Cell wall of peptidoglycan; may have capsule for adherence or protection; may have pili for adherence or conjugation
Motility	Move with flagella; show taxis to stimuli
Genome	Single circular DNA molecule with little associated protein; may have plasmids (1/1000th the DNA of eukaryotes)
Growth and reproduction	Divide by binary fission; some genetic exchange by conjugation

1. **Classification.** Prokaryotes make up the kingdom *Prokaryotae* or *Monera*. All prokaryotes are bacteria (and all bacteria are prokaryotes). Bacteria are simple, unicellular organisms, and they are the most abundant organisms on Earth. All organisms other than bacteria are eukaryotes (see Chapter 6 of the Biology Review Notes for a description of eukaryotic cells).

2. **Structure.** Prokaryotic cells have **no membrane-enclosed nucleus.** Thus, the DNA is not in a separate compartment as it is in eukaryotic cells. This is the most fundamental structural difference between the two general types of cells.

3. The **diameter** of most prokaryotes ranges from approximately 1–10 μm, although some types can be as small as 0.1 μm. In comparison, the diameter of eukaryotic cells ranges from approximately 10–100 μm.

4. Each type of bacteria has a distinctive **cell shape.** The various shapes include rods (bacilli), spheres (cocci), and spirals (spirilla). Some bacterial cells arrange themselves in chains, clusters, or filaments of cells.

B. Prokaryotic Cell Structure (Figure 5-3)

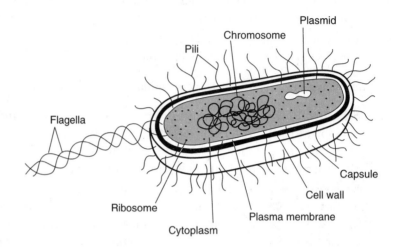

FIGURE 5-3.

The structure of a prokaryotic cell.

1. The **prokaryotic genome** contains less DNA (approximately 1000-fold less) than the eukaryotic genome.

   a. The **bacterial chromosome** is a single, circular DNA molecule. There is very little protein associated with the DNA.

   b. **Plasmids.** Many bacterial cells also contain small, circular DNA molecules that replicate separately from the chromosome. These plasmids carry a few nonessential genes and can be transferred between bacterial cells during mating (conjugation).

2. A semipermeable **plasma membrane** surrounds the intracellular gel-like substance (cytoplasm). The plasma membrane mediates selective exchange between the cell and its external environment.

   a. Infoldings of the plasma membrane provide extra surface area for chemical reactions.

   b. There are no separate intracellular membranes or membrane-enclosed organelles in prokaryotes.

3. Most bacteria have a rigid, nonliving **cell wall** outside the plasma membrane. Bacterial cell walls usually contain a chemical called peptidoglycan, which is not found in eukaryotes. The external wall maintains cell shape and protects the cell from the effects of osmotic changes in the environment. Some antibiotics work by damaging bacterial cell walls.

4. Some bacteria have a flexible outer covering called a **capsule,** which is exterior to the cell wall. The capsule protects cells from attackers, prevents dehydration, and allows attachment to surfaces.

5. **Pili** are short thin extensions from bacterial cells.

   a. **Common pili,** or fimbriae, are used for attachment.

   b. **Sex pili** are used for genetic transfer during conjugation.

6. **Flagella** are long structures used for motility that are attached to bacterial cells. One or many flagella may be located at one or both poles or all around the cell. Rotation of each flagella propels the cell through its fluid environment.

    a. **Taxis** is the movement response by which bacteria move toward or away from stimuli in their environment. An example is chemotaxis, which is movement toward or away from chemicals.

    b. A change in the direction of flagellar rotation (clockwise or counterclockwise) causes the cell to change its direction of movement.

7. **Endospores** are tough, metabolically inactive structures formed by some bacteria. These resting bodies are resistant to environmental stress and can survive for long periods of time. At some point, endospores can germinate to reform the vegetative (dividing) cell.

C. Prokaryotic Life Histories

1. **Binary fission** is a type of cell division by which single bacterial cells generally reproduce asexually. In this process, the single replicated chromosome is partitioned into each of the two daughter cells, which are separated by pinching in of the plasma membrane. A single cell can rapidly form an entire population of identical cells by binary fission. Most of the variation in a bacterial population results from mutations in the DNA.

2. **Conjugation** is a type of mating that bacteria undergo in which DNA is transferred between two cells that are temporarily joined (Figure 5-4). In conjugation, one cell is the donor, and the other is the recipient of genetic information.

FIGURE 5-4.
The process of conjugation in bacteria, in which DNA is transferred between two cells that are temporarily joined. F = fertility factor (+ = present; − = absent); Hfr = high-frequency recombination.

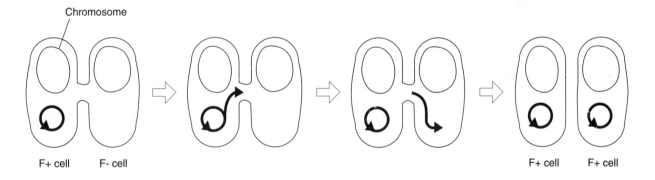

Chromosome

F+ cell   F- cell   F+ cell   F+ cell

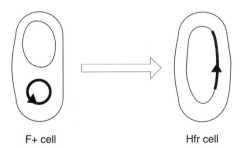

F+ cell   Hfr cell

a. **The donor is an F+ cell** (i.e., a cell that contains a plasmid called the fertility, or F, factor). The F factor enables the F+ cell to form sex pili. **The recipient is an F− cell** (i.e., the cell lacks the F factor). The F+ cell attaches to the F− cell by its sex pili.

b. A copy of the F factor is transferred from the donor to the recipient cell through the **cytoplasmic bridge** in the pilus. This converts the F− cell to F+. (The F+ cell remains F+.)

c. **The F factor is an episome,** which is a plasmid that can integrate into the bacterial chromosome. When this happens, the cell becomes a **high-frequency recombination (Hfr) cell.** Chromosomal genes can then be transferred with the integrated F factor during conjugation.

d. By timing the transfer of chromosomal genes during Hfr conjugation, scientists have mapped the relative locations of different genes on the bacterial chromosome.

3. There are **two other processes that involve the transfer of DNA** in bacteria.

a. **Transformation** occurs when bacterial cells take up DNA directly from their surroundings. Bacterial transformation is commonly used for research and biotechnology purposes.

b. **Transduction** occurs when bacteriophages incorporate bacterial DNA into their genomes, then carry that DNA to the next host cell. There are two types of transduction.

(1) In **general transduction,** random pieces of host DNA are picked up during the lytic cycle.

(2) In **specialized transduction** (by temperate phages only), excision of a prophage from the host chromosome brings with it some adjacent bacterial genes.

III. Fungi

A. Characteristics of Fungi (Table 5-2)

TABLE 5-2. Summary of fungal characteristics.

Group	Examples	Morphology	Asexual Reproduction	Sexual Reproduction	Miscellaneous Information
Zygomycota	Black bread mold	Aseptate hyphae	Sporangia on aerial hyphae	Zygosporangia	In soil and decaying matter
Ascomycota	Sac fungi, yeasts	Septate hyphae	Conidia	Ascosporangia, asci	Plant parasites, lichens, decomposers
Basidiomycota	Club fungi, mushrooms, shelf fungi	Dikaryotic hyphae	Uncommon	Basidia	Some edible, plant parasites
Deuteromycota	Penicillium	Molds	Conidia	None known	Some produce antibiotics

1. Fungi are eukaryotes; most are multicellular.

2. All fungi obtain their organic nutrients by **absorption.** Fungi get their nutrients from various sources.

a. Most fungi are **parasitic**—they absorb nutrients from the body of a living host.

b. Some fungi are **saprophytic**—they absorb nutrients from dead organic matter (i.e., the fungi are decomposers).

c. Some fungi are **mutualistic**—they absorb nutrients from a host but reciprocate to benefit the host.

3. There are three major **types of fungi** that are distinguished by their structure.

a. **Molds** are multicellular, filamentous organisms, such as mildew, rust, and smut.

b. **Fleshy fungi** are multicellular, filamentous organisms that produce a thick (fleshy) reproductive body. The fleshy fungi include mushrooms, puffballs, and coral fungi.

c. **Yeasts** are nonfilamentous, unicellular organisms, typically spherical or oval in shape.

B. Fungal Structures

1. **Vegetative structures** are composed of cells involved in catabolism and growth.

a. **Hyphae** are long filaments of cells joined together to form the body (thallus) of a mold or fleshy fungus. A hyphae grows at its tips to form an intertwined mass of hyphae called a **mycelium.** Each part of the vegetative mycelium is capable of growth.

b. **Septa** are the crosswalls that divide the hyphae of most fungi into uninucleate cells. However, the hyphae of a few fungi do not contain septa (i.e., they are aseptate). These **coenocytic hyphae** are composed of long, continuous, multinucleate cells.

c. Most nuclei of fungal mycelia are **haploid.**

d. Fungi have no flagellated structures and are **nonmotile.**

2. The **reproductive or aerial mycelium** is the part of the fungus concerned with reproduction. The aerial mycelium produces **spores,** the reproductive structures in both asexual and sexual reproduction.

a. Spores are generally produced asexually in favorable conditions and asexually in unfavorable conditions (e.g., stress).

b. Spores are dispersed by wind or water. They germinate in favorable conditions to reform the vegetative body.

C. General Life Histories of Fungi

1. **Asexual spores** are most frequently produced by the aerial mycelium of one haploid organism. The spores are produced through mitosis and subsequent cell division. When these spores germinate, they become organisms that are genetically identical to the parent. Note that each of the three divisions of fungi form their haploid, asexual spores in different ways.

a. The *Zygomycota* division produces asexual spores in sacs called **sporangia** at the tips of aerial hyphae.

b. Most fungi of the *Ascomycota* division produce chains of spores called **conidia.**

c. The *Basidiomycota* division does not undergo asexual reproduction.

2. **Budding** is a type of asexual reproduction in which the parent cell forms a protuberance (bud) that elongates and eventually breaks away as an independent daughter cell. **Yeasts** belong to the *Ascomycota* fungi group, but differ in their reproduction. Yeasts are colonies of unicellular organisms that do not form asexual spores but reproduce asexually by budding.

3. **Fungal sexual spores** are formed by sexual reproduction.

   a. The following steps are involved.

      (1) Two opposite mating strains of the same species of fungus conjugate by fusion of hyphae from each of the organisms.

      (2) A haploid nucleus of the donor cell enters the recipient cell, and the two nuclei fuse. This step is delayed in some fungi, which results in cells with two nuclei (dikaryons). Fusion of the nuclei results in a diploid sexual spore.

      (3) The sexual spore divides by meiosis to form new haploid spores. The spores can then form new haploid mycelia.

   b. **Methods of sexual spore production.** The various fungi produce sexual spores in different ways.

      (1) *Zygomycota,* such as black bread mold, form resistant bodies (**zygosporangia**) that can remain dormant in unfavorable environmental conditions.

      (2) *Ascomycota* (sac fungi) produce sexual spores in a saclike structure called an **ascus.**

      (3) *Basidiomycota* (club fungi), such as mushrooms, produce sexual spores externally on a base pedestal called a **basidium.**

4. *Deuteromycota,* or **imperfect fungi,** is a group of fungi with no known sexual reproduction. Their asexual reproduction is by conidia. An example is *Penicillium.*

5. **Lichens** are symbiotically associated fungi and algae. They have a mutualistic relationship in which each benefits the other.

The Eukaryotic Cell

6

I. Overview

A. All Organisms Other Than Bacteria Have Eukaryotic Cells. Eukaryotic organisms may be unicellular or multicellular. Eukaryotic cells range in size from approximately 10–100 μm in diameter (approximately 10 times larger than prokaryotic cells).

B. Eukaryotes Are More Advanced in An Evolutionary Sense Than Prokaryotes (see Chapter 20 of the Biology Review Notes). The fundamental difference between the two cell types is that **eukaryotic cells have a membrane-bound (true) nucleus.**

   1. The nucleus is the information center of the cell. It contains the **genes,** which are encoded in DNA, that control all of the cell activities.

   2. The **cytoplasm** of the cell includes the entire region outside the nucleus. Cytoplasmic structures are suspended in a gel-like fluid called **cytosol.**

   3. **Membranes** are important components of most eukaryotic cell structures.

      a. **Organelles** are intracellular structures surrounded by one or more membranes. The normal function of a cell involves several types of membrane-bound organelles.

      b. **Intracellular membranes** provide internal surface area and partition the cell into separate compartments. Specific chemical reactions occur at the membrane surfaces and within the compartments.

C. Cell Structure Can Only Be Studied By Microscopic Observation.

   1. **Light microscopes** are used for magnification of living cells up to 1500-fold.

   2. **Electron microscopes** are used to magnify specially prepared (dead) cells up to 250,000-fold.

II. The Eukaryotic Cell: Structures and Functions (Figure 6-1; Table 6-1)

A. Nucleus

   1. The nucleus is a membrane-bound organelle containing most of the genetic material of the cell.

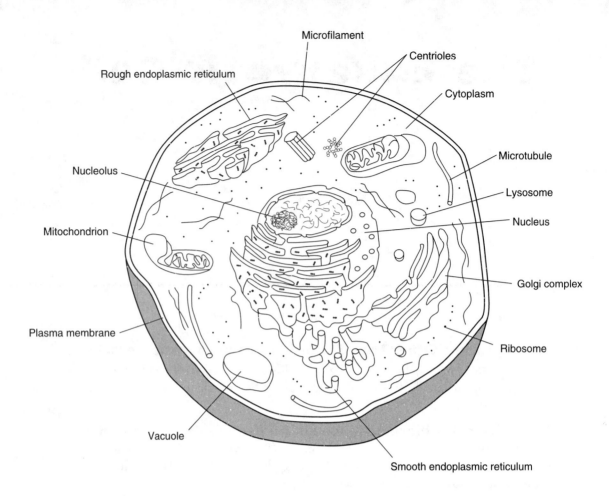

Microfilament

Centrioles

Rough endoplasmic reticulum

Cytoplasm

Microtubule

Lysosome

Nucleolus

Nucleus

Mitochondrion

Golgi complex

Plasma membrane

Ribosome

Vacuole

Smooth endoplasmic reticulum

FIGURE 6-1.

The structure of a eukaryotic cell.

2. **Genetic material** resides in the nucleus in the form of **chromatin,** which is a complex of DNA and associated histone proteins. Chromatin appears as wispy, indistinct material in the nucleus of nondividing cells.

    a. **Chromosomes** become visible when a cell prepares to divide and the chromatin condenses. Chromosomes are the distinct, linear structures that carry the genes. Each species of organism has a characteristic number of chromosomes in the nucleus (e.g., humans have 46).

    b. During **mitosis,** the two copies of each chromosome are separated into two sets, which are segregated into the daughter cells.

3. The **nucleolus** is the most conspicuous structure in a nondividing cell. This is a special region of DNA where the genes for ribosomal RNA (rRNA) are located. The nucleolus is also where the rRNA and ribosomal proteins assemble to form the ribosomes.

4. The **nuclear envelope** surrounds the nucleus with a double membrane. Molecules are exchanged between the nucleus and the cytoplasm through **pores** in the nuclear envelope. A complex of proteins is organized around each pore.

B. Membrane-Bound Organelles

1. The **mitochondria** serve as the sites of cellular respiration, the oxygen-requiring catabolic process that extracts energy from organic molecules to produce adenosine triphosphate (ATP). The mitochondria are sometimes referred to as the "powerhouse of the cell." Mitochondria are found in nearly

TABLE 6-1. Summary of eukaryotic cell structures

Structure	Description	Functions
Membrane-bound nucleus	Large orangelle surrounded by double membrane with pores; contains chromosomes (DNA and histones)	Information storage and transfer
DNA	Multiple, linear chromosomes associated with histone proteins; usually in dispersed form (chromatin)	Heritable material
Mitochondria	Double-membrane bound with highly folded inner membrane, ETC	Cellular respiration (ATP production)
Lysosomes	Membrane sacs with hydrolytic enzymes	Digestion, organelle recycling
Vacuoles/Vesicles	Membrane sacs (various sizes and compositions)	Transport, chemical reactions, water balance, food intake
Endoplasmic reticulum (rough and smooth)	Membrane sacs and tubules	Manufacture of export proteins, membrane proteins and lipids
Ribosomes	Two protein/RNA subunits; free in cytoplasm or attached to ER membrane	Protein synthesis
Golgi apparatus	Stacked, flattened membrane sacs	Product modification, packaging & transport
Plasma Membrane	Phospholipid bilayer with proteins, also cholesterol and carbohydrates	Selective exchange with environment
Cytoskeleton	Complex network of three filament types	Structural support, shape , movement
Cilia and flagella	Cytoplasmic extensions with a "9 + 2" arrangement of microtubules	Cell motility
Centrioles	Self-replicating microtubule structures	Cell division

*Structure is not found in all cell types.
ATP = adenosine triphosphate; DNA = deoxyribonucleic acid; ETC = electron transport chain.

all eukaryotic cells, in varying numbers depending on the metabolic activity of the cell. They are dynamic organelles, capable of growth and division.

a. **Membranes.** Mitochondria are surrounded by two membranes—one inner and one outer.

   (1) The **inner membrane** is highly convoluted, forming many infoldings called **cristae.** The cristae provide surface area for the chemical reactions of respiration. Electron transport occurs here.

   (2) The **outer membrane** is smooth and is in contact with the cellular cytoplasm.

   (3) The **intermembrane space** exists between the inner and outer membranes. This space is important in separating and insulating inner mitochondrial structures.

   (4) The **matrix** is the compartment that is internal to the inner membrane. This compartment contains many metabolic enzymes. The Krebs cycle occurs here.

b. **Enzymes.** Specific mitochondrial enzymes and other proteins are localized in each compartment of the cell and are embedded within the membranes. Mitochondria contain some DNA and ribosomes to program and carry out the synthesis of some of their own proteins.

2. **Lysosomes** are membrane-bound organelles that contain hydrolytic (digestive) enzymes. The inside of the lysosome is highly acidic, which is the optimal environment for hydrolytic enzymes. Lysosomes serve several important functions in cells.

   a. Lysosomes are needed for **digestion** of food or other substances that are engulfed by the cell. These substances are pinched off into a membrane-bound **food vacuole.** When a lysosome fuses with the vacuole, the lysosomal enzymes digest the food.

   b. **Recycling of organic materials** involves lysosomal destruction of old or damaged organelles. In "storage diseases," such as Tay-Sachs disease, defects in lysosome function result in the accumulation of substances that interfere with cell function.

   c. **Programmed cell destruction** occurs during embryonic development to give body parts their proper form (e.g., separated fingers).

3. **Vacuoles and vesicles** include various types of membranous sacs, which differ in size (vacuoles are larger than vesicles) and function.

   a. **Transport vesicles** carry enclosed substances from place to place in the cell.

   b. **Food vacuoles** contain solid materials that are brought into the cell from its surroundings.

   c. **Water vacuoles,** also called contractile vacuoles, are found in many freshwater protozoa. These organelles pump out excess water so that the cell does not burst.

   d. **Central vacuoles** are found in plant cells, where they function in storage, digestion, pigment localization, and water absorption. They are the most conspicuous organelle in a plant cell.

C. Intracellular Membranes

1. **Membranous structures** are a complex, constantly changing network found within the cytoplasm of the eukaryotic cell. These structures interact either directly through physical contact or indirectly through the exchange of vesicles. Each type of membranous structure provides a distinct local environment for specific chemical reactions.

2. The **endoplasmic reticulum (ER)** is an organization of membranous sacs and tubules that is connected to the nuclear envelope. The ER compartments or **cisternae** sequester an internal lumen (the cisternal space) from the cytosol. There are two types of ER—rough and smooth.

   a. The **rough ER** is made up of sacs and folds of membrane, which is studded with attached ribosomes. The rough ER is involved in the manufacture and transport of proteins that are secreted from the cell (export proteins) or used in cell membranes.

      (1) A **signal sequence** is a specific sequence that starts the messenger RNAs, which code for export proteins. The signal sequence makes it possible for the ribosomes translating these RNAs to link to specific receptors on the rough ER. All other ribosomes remain free in the cytoplasm. As the export protein is being synthesized, it enters the cisternal space, and the signal sequence is enzymatically removed.

(2) **Glycoproteins** used in the plasma membrane are also produced in the ER by enzymatic attachment of a sugar to specific proteins.

(3) ER products eventually depart in **transport vesicles** that are pinched off from the membrane. These vesicles carry the materials out of the cell, to the plasma membrane, or to intracellular destinations.

b. The **smooth ER** is made up of tubules of naked membrane. The reactions in the smooth ER are involved in **lipid metabolism.**

(1) **Phospholipids, fats, and steroids are synthesized** in the smooth ER.

(2) The smooth ER is also where certain drugs, such as alcohol and barbiturates, are **detoxified.** Chemical modification by enzymes in the smooth ER allows these drugs to be flushed from the body.

3. The **Golgi apparatus** is a series of flattened and stacked membrane sacs. These structures are involved in the chemical modification, storing, and distribution of products made in the ER.

a. The *cis* face of the Golgi apparatus **receives transport vesicles from the ER.** Golgi enzymes chemically modify the received materials (e.g., by adding an oligosaccharide to some glycoproteins). Other compounds are synthesized in the Golgi apparatus itself.

b. The **chemical modifications** in the Golgi apparatus provide organic materials with "address tags" for their transport to a particular destination in the cell. The products are enclosed in vesicles that pinch off into the cytoplasm from the *trans* face of the Golgi apparatus.

D. Production of a Secretory Product. The following summarizes the production of a secretory product.

	Moves into cytoplasm		
	and complexes with	Attaches to	
Transcription of gene			
DNA ———————→ **mRNA** ———————→ **Ribosome** ———→ **Rough ER**			

Polypeptide moves into lumen;
Carbohydrate added
to form glycoprotein;
↓ Pinched off into

| **Plasma** | | | |
| **membrane** ←——————— **Golgi Apparatus** ←——— **Transport vesicles** | | | |

Polypeptide may be modified;   Joined to
Leaves from *trans* face;   *cis* face
Fuses with

E. Plasma Membrane

1. **Protective function.** The plasma membrane surrounds the entire cell, providing a physical barrier between the cytoplasm and the extracellular environment. The membrane is **selectively permeable,** so that only certain substances can cross it. This allows for controlled cell–cell and cell–environment communication and exchange (see II D 3).

2. **Plasma membrane structure** (Figure 6-2)

a. **The plasma membrane is a phospholipid bilayer** (as are the intracellular membranes). The membrane is a very thin sheet composed of

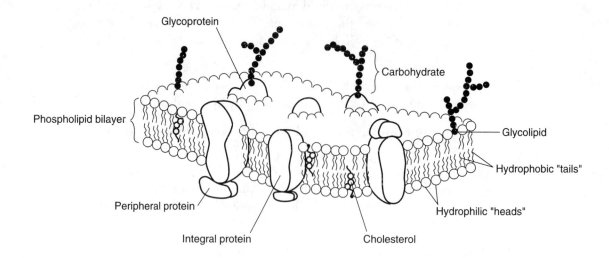

FIGURE 6-2.

The structure of a plasma membrane.

two layers of organic molecules called phospholipids. Each phospholipid has a polar "head" at one end (a negatively charged phosphate group) and a nonpolar "tail" at the other end (a long, hydrocarbon chain). These chemical properties lead to spontaneous formation of the bilayer structure in aqueous fluids.

(1) **The polar head is hydrophilic** (i.e., water loving) and points toward the exterior of the bilayer. This surface comes in contact with the aqueous cytoplasm and extracellular fluids.

(2) **The nonpolar tail is hydrophobic** (i.e., water hating) and points toward the interior of the bilayer. This region is sequestered away from the cytoplasm and extracellular fluids.

b. The **fluid consistency** (much like salad oil) of the membrane is caused by the weak hydrophobic interactions of the bilayer.

(1) **Phospholipid molecules can drift laterally** in the membrane and change places with their neighbors.

(2) **Cholesterol and unsaturated fatty acids** are included in the membrane bilayer. These bulky lipids prevent the plasma membrane from hardening in cold environments.

c. **Proteins** make up approximately 60% of the plasma membrane (40% is lipid). Proteins are inserted individually into the bilayer and are capable of some lateral drift. This structural design of the membrane is described by the **fluid mosaic model.**

(1) **Types**

(a) **Integral proteins** penetrate the interior hydrophobic zone of the membrane. Most integral proteins span the membrane, with their hydrophilic regions protruding from one or both surfaces.

(b) Peripheral proteins are located on the membrane surface, anchored by attachment to integral proteins. Some peripheral proteins are on the extracellular side of the plasma membrane and some are on the intracellular side.

(2) Synthesis. Plasma membrane proteins are synthesized on the rough ER, where they are inserted directly into the ER membrane. After being transported in vesicles to the cell surface, the rough ER membrane (including proteins) fuses with the plasma membrane. The proteins that face the cytoplasmic side of the ER membrane are destined to face the cytoplasmic side of the plasma membrane as well. Likewise, the proteins that face the lumen of the ER will face the extracellular side of the plasma membrane.

3. Movement across the membrane

a. Overview

(1) The plasma membrane is **selectively permeable,** allowing some substances to cross more easily than others.

(2) Nonpolar molecules and **small polar molecules** can pass through the phospholipid bilayer via passive transport. Examples include oxygen, carbon dioxide, and water molecules.

(3) Large molecules and polar molecules cannot pass through the hydrophobic zone of the phospholipid bilayer. Examples include glucose and charged molecules, such as ions. These substances must be carried across the membrane by selective transport proteins or **carrier proteins.**

b. Passive transport

(1) A **concentration gradient** is the driving force for movement of a substance by passive transport. When molecules of a solute are more concentrated on one side of the membrane than on the other, they move spontaneously from the area of higher concentration to the area of lower concentration (i.e., down the concentration gradient).

(a) The **rate of movement** is regulated by the permeability of the membrane to the particular substance. Water diffuses freely across most cell membranes.

(b) Cellular energy is not needed for passive transport.

(2) Osmosis is a special case of passive transport. Osmosis allows the diffusion of water molecules across a membrane that is permeable to water but not to the solutes in the water. Cytoplasm and extracellular fluids are both aqueous solutions.

(a) Water diffuses from an area of lower solute concentration to an area of higher solute concentration. The net movement of water is **down its concentration gradient.**

(b) Osmotic pressure is the tendency for a solution, regardless of the type of solute, to take up water by osmosis. Osmotic pressure depends on the total solute concentrations, regardless of whether there are different solutes on each side of a membrane.

(c) **Tonicity** concerns the relation of a cell with its environment.

  (i)   An extracellular environment is **hypertonic** to a cell when the concentration of solutes outside the cell is greater than inside. In a hypertonic environment, the cell loses water and shrinks (Figure 6-3A).

  (ii) An environment is **hypotonic** to a cell when the solute concentration outside is **less** than inside. In a hypotonic environment, water enters the cell, causing it to swell and even to pop (see Figure 6-3B).

  (iii) A cell and its environment are **isotonic** when the solute concentration is the same both inside and outside the cell. In this case, water molecules move across the membrane at the same rate in both directions (see Figure 6-3C). The system is in **dynamic equilibrium.**

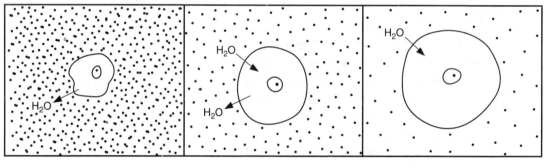

A. Hypertonic environment   **B. Isotonic environment**   **C. Hypotonic environment**

FIGURE 6-3.

A) The effects on water movement and cell size of a hypertonic environment. **B)** An isotonic environment. **C)** A hypotonic environment.

FIGURE 6-4.

In facilitated diffusion, a passive process, a carrier protein specifically transports molecules across cell membranes.

(3) **Facilitated diffusion** is a type of passive transport in which solute molecules are moved down a concentration gradient by **carrier proteins** in the membrane. A carrier protein picks up a molecule, then shifts to an alternative conformation to deposit the molecule on the other side of the membrane (Figure 6-4). **No input of energy** is required.

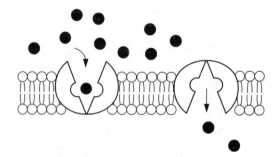

c. **Active transport**

(1) Active transport moves small molecules up a concentration gradient. The driving force for movement by active transport is an **input of cellular energy.**

(2) Active transport involves **carrier proteins** that are linked to a source of energy, such as ATP hydrolysis.

(3) Certain carrier proteins called **ion pumps** use active transport to generate and maintain gradients of ion concentrations across a membrane.

   (a) An example of an ion pump is the **sodium–potassium pump—ATPase** (Figure 6-5). This protein (i.e., ATPase) uses ATP to pump sodium out of the cell and potassium into the cell. For every three sodium ions pumped out, two potassium ions are pumped in. This results in a **voltage gradient** caused by the net negative charge (voltage) inside the cell. The sodium–potassium pump also regulates intracellular solute concentration by keeping the intracellular sodium low. This function helps to maintain osmotic balance with the environment.

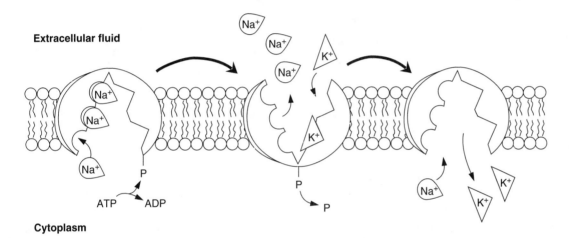

Extracellular fluid

Cytoplasm

   (b) Each type of ion moves down its electrochemical gradient by passing through specific **ion channels** in the membrane. Electrostatic attractions favor movement of cations into the cell and movement of anions out of the cell.

   (c) **Membrane potential** is generated by the differences in ion concentrations across a membrane. This is an essential property for electrically excitable cells such as nerve and muscle cells (see Chapter 7 of the Biology Review Notes).

FIGURE 6-5.
The sodium–potassium ATPase. Three sodium ions are pumped out of the cell for every two potassium ions molecules pumped into the cell. This process requires the input of adenosine triphosphate (ATP) for energy.

d. **Endocytosis.** Large molecules are brought into cells by endocytosis, in which the **plasma membrane buds inward to form vesicles that pinch off into the cytoplasm.** There are three types of endocytosis.

(1) In **phagocytosis** ("cell-eating"), an extension of the plasma membrane brings in solid particles, such as food, enclosing them in a food vacuole (Figure 6-6A). The vacuole must fuse with a lysosome for digestion to occur.

(2) In **pinocytosis** ("cell-drinking"), droplets of extracellular fluid are incorporated into small vesicles (see Figure 6-6B). This is a nonspecific process in which all the solutes in the droplets are taken in.

(3) **Receptor-mediated endocytosis** is the specific uptake of molecules that bind to clusters of receptors in specific regions of the membrane, called coated pits (see Figure 6-6C). The "budding in" of a coated pit forms a vesicle (reinforced by a fibrous protein called clathrin), which then releases the ingested material. This process allows cells to take in large amounts of a specific substance, even if that solute has a low extracellular concentration.

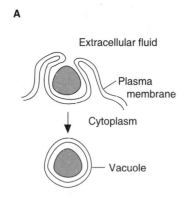

A

Extracellular fluid

Plasma membrane

Cytoplasm

Vacuole

B

Cytoplasm

C

Cytoplasm

FIGURE 6-6.
The process of **A)** phagocytosis, **B)** pinocytosis, and **C)** receptor-mediated endocytosis.

e. **Exocytosis.** Large molecules are removed from a cell by fusion of cytoplasmic vesicles with the plasma membrane. This process is used by secretory cells to export products to the extracellular environment.

4. **Receptors** are specific membrane proteins that face the outside of the cell and bind substances in the cell surroundings. Different cell types have distinct sets of membrane receptors. Each type of receptor binds and responds to a specific set of molecules (the ligands) in a characteristic way. Substances that bind receptors include hormones, viruses, bacteria, antibodies, and the surface proteins of other cells.

5. **Cell–cell recognition and adhesion** are also mediated by components of the plasma membrane.

(a) **Glycoproteins** are proteins with attached carbohydrates, such as branched polysaccharides. Glycoproteins identify cells as belonging to a particular organism or tissue rather than to a foreign invader. For example, glycoproteins are the blood-type determinants that prevent an immune response against a person's own red blood cells.

(b) **Intercellular junctions** formed between adjacent cells mediate direct cell–cell interactions in multicellular organisms. There are three major types.

(1) **Tight junctions** are connections between the adjacent plasma membranes that do not leave enough space for substances to cross the cell surfaces (Figure 6-7A).

(2) **Desmosomes,** or spot welds, are rigid junctions that allow transport of substances through the space between adjacent cells and across the cell surfaces (see Figure 6-7B).

(3) **Gap junctions** are pores between adjacent cells that allow transfer of small molecules between the two cytoplasms (see Figure 6-7C).

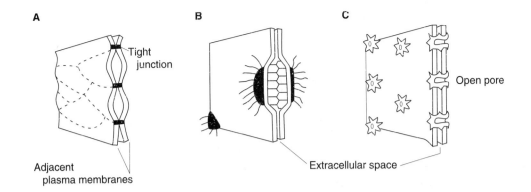

F. Cytoskeleton (Table 6-2)

TABLE 6-2. Cytoskeleton summary.

Element	Structure/Size	Protein	Functions
Microtubules	Hollow tubes largest (25 nm diameter)	Tubulin (dimers)	Motility, cell shape, chromosome & organelle movement, intracellular organization
Microfilaments	Twisted strands smallest (7 nm diameter)	Actin	Muscle cell contraction, cytoplasmic streaming, amoeboid movement, division furrow, cell shape changes
Intermediate filaments	Hollow Tubes medium (8-10 nm diameter)	Varies	Structural support, tension, cell shape maintenance

1. **Structure.** The cytoskeleton of the cell is composed of a dynamic network of fibers organized throughout the cytoplasm. The cytoskeleton is important for structural support, control of cell shape, cell motility, and intracellular movement.

2. **Types.** There are three major types of cytoskeletal elements.

    a. **Microtubules** are long hollow tubes composed of subunits of the protein **tubulin.** Microtubules have the largest diameter of the various cytoskeletal fibers. Microtubule structures are organized by regions called microtubule-organizing centers (Figure 6-8).

        (1) **Microtubules can move objects.** Microtubules can be lengthened or shortened by the spontaneous addition or removal of tubulin subunits at their ends. This process can cause objects attached to the microtubules to move. An example of this type of movement occurs during chromosome segregation in mitosis.

        (2) **Microtubules provide transportation "tracks"** in the cytoplasm. Objects move by attaching to specific proteins that can slide along these microtubule tracks. An example of this is the movement of transport vesicles from the Golgi apparatus to the plasma membrane for protein export.

        (3) **Cell motility** is another important function of microtubules.

    b. **Microfilaments** are solid fibers made of two intertwined chains of the protein **actin.** Microfilaments have the smallest diameter of the cytoskeletal fibers. Microfilaments are important for cellular movement that involves **contractions.** Examples include:

(1) Contraction of muscle cells

(2) Ameboid movement, involving extension and contraction of a part of a cell

(3) Cytoplasmic streaming, involving mass movement of cytoplasm (seen in large plant cells)

(4) Formation of the cleavage furrow during cell division

   c. **Intermediate filaments** have varying protein compositions and sizes in different cell types. **Cellular stability** is thought to be the main function of intermediate filaments. For example, intermediate filaments hold organelles in place and help maintain cell shape.

3. **Cilia and flagella.** The cilia and flagella are the microtubule structures responsible for cell motility. These structures are long, thin cell protrusions that are continuous with the plasma membrane (see Figure 6-8).

FIGURE 6-8.
A cross section demonstrating cilia and flagella structure.

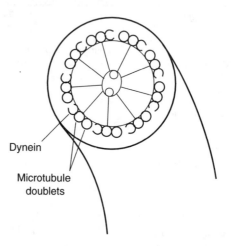

Dynein

Microtubule doublets

   a. **Structure.** Cilia and flagella are composed of nine sets of microtubule triplets arranged in a ring with a pair of microtubules in the center ("9 + 2 arrangement"). The base or anchor of the structure is called the **basal body,** which is composed of nine sets of microtubules, with no additional pair in the center.

     (1) Flagella are longer than cilia.

     (2) There is usually only one or a few flagella per cell, whereas cilia are much more numerous.

     (3) Eukaryotic cilia and flagella move in a wavelike motion.

   b. **Function.** The most common function of the cilia or flagella is to propel a cell through its fluid environment. However, some ciliated cells in multicellular organisms are nonmotile; they use their cilia to sweep materials across the surface of a tissue.

   c. **Movement.** Movement of cilia or flagella involves a protein called **dynein,** which is associated with the microtubules. Dynein attaches to one microtubule and causes it to slide in a ratchet-like motion along an adjacent microtubule. This process requires an input of energy (ATP).

4. **Centrioles.** Centrioles have essentially the same microtubular structure as basal bodies, but they are not associated with cilia or flagella. A pair of centrioles is associated with each of two microtubule-organizing centers in dividing cells. Nondividing cells have only one pair of centrioles.

a. Animal cells have centrioles, but plant cells do not.

b. Centrioles are involved in the movement of chromosomes during mitosis (see III).

III. The Eukaryotic Cell Cycle and Mitosis.

In **multicellular organisms,** cell division plays a primary role in **growth, reproduction, and repair.** Many cells divide during a period of growth, but they lose that ability as they become specialized for a particular function in the mature organism. In **unicellular organisms,** cell division is the **means for the organisms to reproduce themselves.** The **cell cycle** is the interval between formation of a cell and division of that cell to form two new daughter cells (Figure 6-9). Typical cell cycles range from 1–24 hours, depending on cell type, age, and conditions. The cell cycle includes two phases: **interphase** and **mitosis.**

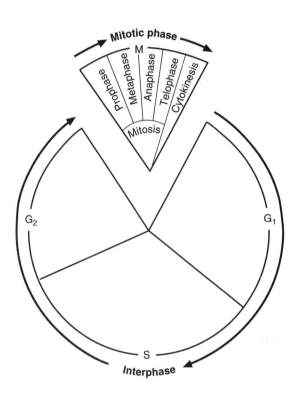

FIGURE 6-9.
The cell cycle.

A. **Interphase** accounts for approximately 90% of the cell cycle. Growth and metabolic activities occur continuously during interphase. The nuclear genetic material is dispersed as chromatin.

1. During interphase, **cells grow** by increasing in size and by increasing the number of organelles in preparation for division.

2. Interphase is composed of a **continuous succession of three phases.**

   a. During the **gap 1 (G1) phase,** metabolic activities resume at a high rate after having slowed during mitosis.

   b. **DNA synthesis** occurs in **synthesis (S) phase.** At the end of S phase, the DNA content of the cell has doubled and all the chromosomes are replicated. The single pair of centrioles has also duplicated, forming two pairs.

   c. During **gap 2 (G2) phase,** the cell makes final preparations for division.

B. **Mitosis (M) Phase** is the process by which the chromosomes are compacted then separated into two equal sets. Mitosis is usually followed by cytokinesis, which is division of the cytoplasm to form the two identical daughter cells. Mitosis is composed of a continuous succession of several stages: **prophase, metaphase, anaphase, and telophase** (Figure 6-10).

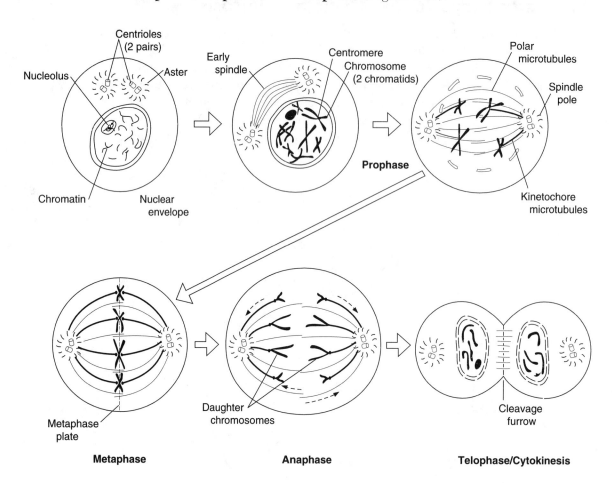

FIGURE 6-10.

The process of mitosis. Note that in anaphase, microtubules shorten and slide apart, which separates daughter chromosomes.

1. **Early prophase**

   a. **The DNA condenses to form discrete, visible chromosomes.** Having been duplicated during S phase, each chromosome is composed of two identical copies called **sister chromatids.** Each chromatid is one continuous DNA molecule (with associated histones). The two chromatids are joined at a constricted region of the chromosome called the **centromere.** The chromosome "arms" extend from the centromere and terminate at structures called **telomeres.**

   b. **The nucleoli** (dark regions) in the nucleus **disappear.**

   c. **The mitotic spindle,** which is a bipolar organization of the cytoskeleton, forms in the cytoplasm. The spindle starts to form at the **centrosome,** which is the microtubule-organizing center. The centrosome is initially composed of bundles of microtubules plus associated proteins assembled around the two pairs of **centrioles.** The centrosome then splits, forming two star-like microtubule bundles called **asters** surrounding each pair of centrioles.

2. **Late prophase**

   a. The **nuclear envelope breaks into membrane vesicles** that look like bits of ER.

b.   The **microtubules** in each aster **elongate,** moving the centrosomes toward opposite poles of the cell. The spindle is then bipolar, each consisting of two microtubule components. The **polar microtubules** extend from each pole toward the cell equator. The **kinetochore microtubules** extend from each pole and attach to the kinetochore, which is a special structure associated with each sister chromatid at the centromere. The kinetochores of sister chromatids attach to kinetochore microtubules extending from opposite poles.

3.   **Metaphase**

a.   The **chromosomes align along the metaphase plate** (the equator), with balanced forces from opposite kinetochore microtubules. The sister chromatids of each chromosome are held together at the centromere.

b.   **Each chromosome is oriented perpendicular to the spindle,** with the kinetochores facing opposite poles. Each sister chromatid faces one pole or the other at random. When metaphase is seen from a polar viewpoint, the chromosomes appear to be spread out on a plate.

4.   **Anaphase**

a.   The **centromere disconnects the two sister chromatids,** which separate to become identical daughter chromosomes. Each daughter chromosome moves centromere first toward its respective pole.

b.   One force for chromosome movement during anaphase is the **shortening of kinetochore microtubules at the chromosome end.** As the chromosome maintains its attachment just ahead of the shortening microtubule end, it moves toward the pole.

c.   Another force for chromosome movement is the **sliding apart of polar microtubules extending from opposite poles.** This moves the poles further apart, thereby separating the chromosomes.

d.   At the end of anaphase, each pole has the same set of chromosomes (now single DNA molecules).

5.   **Telophase**

a.   **Daughter nuclei are reformed** from the fragments of the nuclear envelope and other membrane vesicles of the parent cell.

b.   **The nucleoli reappear** and **the chromosomes condense** back into chromatin.

c.   Most cells undergo **cytokinesis** at the end of telophase. This process **divides the cytoplasm,** thereby partitioning nuclei and organelles into two separate cells. In animals, contraction of a ring of microfilaments forms the **cleavage furrow** and eventually pinches the cell in half. (In plants, convergence of vesicles forms a cell plate, which gives each daughter a plasma membrane. Substances are secreted between the membranes to form the new cell walls.)

d.   **If mitosis occurs without cytokinesis,** the result is a cell with **multiple nuclei** in the same cytoplasm. Such cells are characteristic of muscle tissue, slime molds, and filamentous fungi.

7

Specialized Eukaryotic Cells and Tissues

I. Overview

A. Specialization. During animal development, cells become specialized in structure and function (see Chapter 18 of the Biology Review Notes). Individual cells are the basic unit for hierarchies of higher order structures.

B. Tissues. Tissues are groups of cells with a common structure and function. Each tissue also has its own distinctive characteristics (Table 7-1). This chapter describes the specialized cell types that make up various tissues in the animal body.

TABLE 7-1. Summary of specialized tissues.

Tissue	Structure	General Functions	Examples
Nerve	Neurons with cell body, axons, dendrites	Sense stimuli, conduct impulses	Brain, spinal cord, peripheral nerves
Muscle	Long cells with actin and myosin microfilaments	Contract, move	Skeletal, visceral, cardiac tissue
Epithelial	Packed cells with basement membrane; cuboidal, columnar, squamous; simple or stratified	Protect, absorb, secrete, line body surfaces	Mucous membranes, glands
Connective	Few cells, secrete extra-cellular matrix with fibers	Connect and support other tissues	Loose, adipose, fibrous tissue; cartilage, bone, blood

1. **Organs** are different tissues organized into specialized centers of function.
2. **Organ systems,** which are present in higher order animals, involve several organs that perform a major body function together. All the organ systems must be coordinated for the organism to survive.

II. Neural Cells and Tissues

A. Nervous System. Two internal communication systems coordinate the activities of the specialized parts of an animal—the nervous system and the endocrine system.

B. Cells of the Nervous System. The cells of the nervous system are specialized for quick reactions and direct control of target cells. These cells lay the foundation for building the highly ordered and complex structures of the nervous system. There are **two main classes of cells** in the nervous system—**neurons** and **supporting cells** (Figure 7-1).

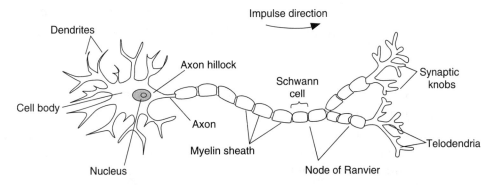

FIGURE 7-1.

The structure of a myelinated neuron. Note the direction of impulse transmission.

1. **Neurons** transmit signals along the pathways of the nervous system. Neurons are the fundamental units of the nervous system, and all neurons have certain structures in common.

    a. The large **cell body** of the neuron contains the nucleus and most of the cytoplasm and organelles.

    b. **Processes** are long, fiber-like extensions from the cell body that enable the neuron to conduct signals over long distances. There are two types of neuron processes—**dendrites** and **axons.**

        (1) **Dendrites** are short, branched processes that transmit signals toward the cell body. Most neurons have numerous dendrites.

        (2) **Axons** are long processes that transmit signals away from the cell body. Most neurons have only a single axon, extending from a part of the cell body called the **axon hillock.**

            (a) **Telodendria** and the **synaptic knob.** An axon may be branched, with each branch ending in numerous branchlets called telodendria. A synaptic knob is a bulbous structure at the tip of each telodendria.

            (b) **Neurotransmitters.** Nervous signals are transmitted by chemicals released from the synaptic knobs, known as neurotransmitters.

            (c) **Synapse.** The gap between the synaptic knob and the dendrite or cell body that receives the signal is the synapse. Neurotransmitters diffuse across the synapse. Communication between two neurons in a neuronal pathway occurs at the synapse between the cells.

2. **Supporting cells** provide structural support, protection, and assistance to neurons. There are many more supporting cells than there are neurons.

    a. **Schwann cells** are supporting cells arranged in chains along the axons of many neurons. Together, Schwann cells coat the axon with an insulating layer called the **myelin sheath.**

    b. The **nodes of Ranvier** are small gaps in the myelin sheath that occur between the serially arranged Schwann cells along the axon.

C. Transmission Along the Neuron

1. The **impulse transmitted along a neuron** depends on ionic changes (currents) across the plasma membrane of the cell. The cytoplasm of most cells is negatively charged relative to the extracellular fluid (see Chapter 6 of the Biology Review Notes). Because of this ionic difference (voltage), the cell membrane has an electrical potential or **membrane potential.**

2. **Resting potential** is the membrane potential of a neuron that is not conducting an impulse.

   a. Most neurons have a resting potential of approximately -70 **mV.** The negative value indicates that the inside of the cell is negative relative to the outside.

   b. The resting potential results from the combined effects of **ion pumping** by the sodium–potassium pumps in the membrane and by **diffusion of ions** down their electrochemical gradients.

      (1) Ion pumping generates and maintains steep gradients of ion concentration, with sodium ions more concentrated on the outside and potassium ions more concentrated on the inside of the cell.

      (2) These ions can diffuse down their gradients through ion channels in the membrane: sodium ions tend to reenter the cell, and potassium ions tend to exit the cell.

      (3) The membrane is more permeable to potassium ions than to sodium ions, but the force on sodium ions is greater because they have an electrostatic attraction to the negative charge inside the cell.

3. **Graded potentials** are local changes in voltage induced by a stimulus. Such a stimulus might be physical pressure on the cell, an abrupt chemical change in the extracellular fluid, an electric shock, or a change in temperature. When a stimulus causes a local change in ionic differences across the membrane, it alters the membrane potential of the cell and affects the permeability of the plasma membrane. **Depolarization** and **hyperpolarization** are referred to as graded potentials. The strength of a graded potential decreases with distance from the point where the neuron was stimulated.

   a. **Depolarization** occurs when the resting potential becomes less negative, for example, from -70 to -50 mV, and the inside of the cell becomes more positive. Depolarization increases the chances that a nerve impulse will be triggered.

   b. **Hyperpolarization** occurs when the resting potential becomes more negative. In other words, the inside of the cell becomes more negative in relation to the outside of the cell. Hyperpolarization decreases the chances that a nerve impulse will be triggered.

4. **Action potential.** Neurons transmit ("fire") electrical impulses when graded potentials are converted to a larger depolarization called an **action potential** (Figure 7-2). An action potential occurs near the point of stimulation and makes the inside of the cell positive compared with the outside (e.g., a change from -70 to $+35$ mV).

   a. **Voltage-sensitive gates** are membrane channels through which ions flow to generate the action potential. These channels open and close in response to changes in the membrane potential.

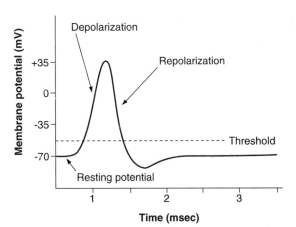

FIGURE 7-2.

An action potential. Note the upsloping depolariza-tion and the downsloping repolarization.

(1) Stimulus causes depolarization; amplification is possible. A stimulus causes a local increase in the permeability of the membrane to sodium ions, which flow into the cell and depolar-ize the membrane. If this depolarization is large enough, the voltage-sensitive sodium ion gates open, increasing the perme-ability further. This amplification of a small depolarization gen-erates the larger change in voltage of the action potential.

(2) Gates close; refractory period follows. An action potential is a local and transient event because the sodium ion gates close quickly. After an action potential is triggered, there is a period of insensitivity to depolarization, during which time the sodium ion gates are inactivated. This refractory period lasts until the mem-brane is returned to its resting potential by repolarization of the membrane.

b. **The membrane is repolarized** when the potassium ion gates open as the sodium ion gates close. Flow of potassium ions out of the cell makes the membrane potential more negative, even to the point of hyperpolarization, before the resting potential is restored.

c. An action potential is triggered only when a stimulus is intense enough to cause a certain minimum depolarization (the **threshold potential**). A greater frequency of action potentials (i.e., repeated "firing") results from strong stimuli rather than from weak stimuli, but the magnitude of depolarization is the same.

5. **Propagation of the action potential.** The **axon hillock** is the zone where action potentials are usually generated. Thus, the chance of trigger-ing an action potential depends on the distance from the point of stimula-tion (usually the dendrites or cell body) to the axon hillock. An action po-tential is transmitted, or propagated, from the axon hillock along the length of the axon (Figure 7-3).

a. **Nerve impulse.** When an initial action potential occurs, sodium ions flowing into the cell also diffuse laterally, triggering an action potential at a site a little farther along the axon. Thus, the action po-tential is transmitted along the axon. The nerve impulse is the self-propagating wave of depolarization.

b. **Serial transmission.** Nerve impulses are serially transmitted in one direction along the axon. Just behind a local depolarization, the re-fractory period from the previous action potential prevents a new one from being triggered.

c. **Saltatory conduction.** Instead of being propagated continuously over the length of the axon, an action potential **"jumps" from one node of Ranvier to the next,** skipping the insulated regions in between. This saltatory conduction results in faster transmission of the nerve impulse. Saltatory conduction occurs because the nodes of Ranvier are where the voltage-sensitive ion channels are concentrated and where ions in the extracellular fluid are in direct contact with the neuron membrane.

FIGURE 7-3.

The sodium and potassium ion flows associated with a propagating action potential. Note the influx of sodium into the cell and the outflow of potassium from the cell.

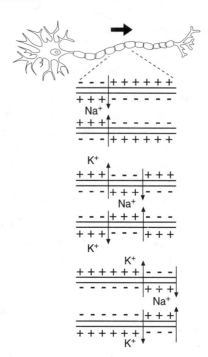

D. Transmission Across the Synapse

1. **Presynaptic and postsynaptic cells.** Signals are transmitted between two neurons in a pathway at the synapse between the two cells. The cell **transmitting** the signal is called the presynaptic cell and the cell **receiving** the signal is called the postsynaptic cell.

2. **Types of synapses.** There are two types of synapses, electrical and chemical. Chemical synapses are much more common.

   a. **Electrical synapses** allow action potentials to spread directly from the presynaptic cell to the postsynaptic cell. The cells are connected by gap junctions, which are intercellular channels that allow ions to flow between the cells. Because of this electrical coupling, an impulse can be transmitted quickly from neuron to neuron.

   b. **Chemical synapses** (Figure 7-4) are narrow gaps (i.e., **synaptic clefts**) between the presynaptic cell and postsynaptic cell. The presynaptic cell converts the electrical signal of the action potential into a chemical signal that travels across the synapse to the postsynaptic cell. There, the signal is converted back into an electrical signal. Nerve impulses are transmitted in only one direction at a chemical synapse.

      (1) **Synaptic vesicles** exist within the synaptic knob of the presynaptic cell. The synaptic vesicles contain thousands of molecules of neurotransmitters, the chemical intercellular messenger in the synaptic cleft. One of the most common neurotransmitters is

acetylcholine (ACh), which stimulates contractions at synapses between motor neurons and skeletal muscle cells.

(2) **The presynaptic membrane is depolarized** when an action potential being propagated along an axon reaches the synaptic knob. Calcium ions rush into the cell through voltage-sensitive calcium ion channels, stimulating the synaptic vesicles to fuse with the presynaptic membrane. The **neurotransmitter is released by exocytosis** into the synaptic cleft, where it diffuses to the postsynaptic membrane.

(3) The postsynaptic membrane has **neurotransmitter receptors** for specific neurotransmitter molecules. Binding of a neurotransmitter to its receptor opens the ion channels associated with the receptor. The resulting flow of a particular ion (e.g., Na^+, K^+, or Ca^{2+}) alters the membrane potential.

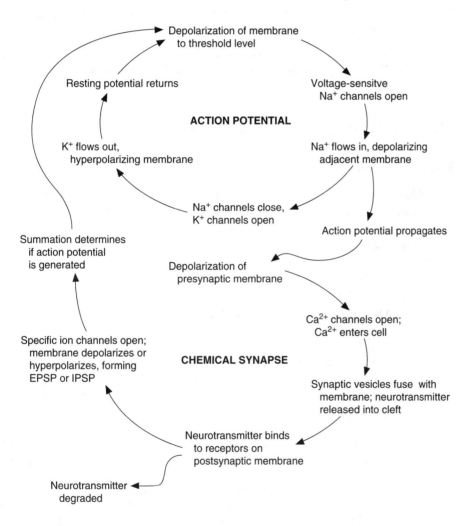

FIGURE 7-4.
Summary diagram showing the flow of an action potential. *EPSP* = excitatory postsynaptic potential; *IPSP* = inhibitory postsynaptic potential.

3. **Types of receptors.** Whether the membrane is depolarized (excited) or hyperpolarized (inhibited) by neurotransmitter binding depends on the type of receptors and the ion gates they control. **Excitatory** and **inhibitory signals** from many neurons often converge on a single neuron. The synapse is where all this information is integrated.

a. At an **excitatory synapse,** the open gates allow flow of sodium ions into the cell, which depolarizes the membrane. This electrical change is called an excitatory postsynaptic potential (EPSP).

b. At an **inhibitory synapse,** the open gates allow flow of potassium ion out of the cell (or chloride ion into the cell), which hyperpolarizes the membrane. This change is called an inhibitory postsynaptic potential (IPSP).

4. **Neurotransmitter degradation.** Degradation of the released neurotransmitter quickly silences each signal at a chemical synapse. The smaller chemical components are recycled to the presynaptic cell for synthesis of more neurotransmitter.

5. **Summation.** Postsynaptic potentials have an additive effect at the axon hillock called summation. The process makes the postsynaptic potentials strong enough to depolarize the region of the axon hillock to threshold potential. This allows an action potential to be triggered. There are two mechanisms of summation.

   a. In **temporal summation,** synaptic knobs release neurotransmitters in rapid-fire succession.

   b. In **spatial summation,** several different synaptic knobs, usually from different presynaptic neurons, stimulate a postsynaptic cell at the same time.

III. Contractile Cells and Tissues

A. Muscle Tissue

1. **Contraction.** Animal movement involves contraction of muscles. This contractile ability is characteristic of the long, excitable cells that make up muscle tissue, the most abundant tissue in the body. Contraction is the only action of a muscle (extension occurs passively).

   a. **Actin and myosin** are the longitudinally arranged microfilaments that comprise muscle cells.

   b. **All muscle cells require electrical stimulation** (action potentials) to contract.

2. **Types.** There are three types of muscle tissue that differ in structure and function: **skeletal, cardiac, and visceral (smooth) muscle.** The cells that make up these muscles have different innervating neurons, membranes, and electrical properties.

   a. **Skeletal muscle** is generally responsible for the **voluntary movements** of the body. Skeletal muscle is attached to the bones by tendons.

      (1) **Myofibrils.** A skeletal muscle is a bundle of long fibers that extends the entire length of the muscle. Each muscle fiber is a single long cell with many nuclei, composed of bundles of smaller myofibrils.

      (2) **Myofilaments.** The longitudinally arranged myofibrils are composed of two types of myofilaments.

         (a) **Thin filaments** consist of coils of two strands of **actin** and one strand of a regulatory protein, **tropomyosin.**

         (b) **Thick filaments** consist of linear arrays of **myosin** molecules.

(3) Sarcomeres. Skeletal muscle is also called **striated** muscle because of its striped appearance under the light microscope. This repeating pattern of light and dark bonds results from the regular arrangement of thin and thick filaments along the length of the fiber. Each repeating unit is called a sarcomere. The special arrangement of myofilaments in the sarcomere is the basis for the ability of the muscle to contract.

b. **Cardiac muscle** forms the contractile wall of the heart. Cardiac muscle is also striated, but, unlike skeletal muscle, the cells are branched.

   (1) Intercalated disks. Special gap junctions that electrically couple (interconnect) all the muscle cells of the heart are called intercalated disks. Thus, action potentials generated in one cell can spread to all the cells, causing the entire heart to contract.

   (2) Involuntary contractions. In contrast to other muscles, cardiac muscle cells do not require stimulation by neurons, but can generate action potentials on their own. These action potentials last a long time because of a relatively high permeability of the membrane to sodium. Thus, contractions of the heart last a long time, with long periods of relaxation (refractory period) in between.

c. **Visceral (smooth) muscle** is generally responsible for **involuntary movements.** Visceral muscle is found in the walls of the digestive tract, bladder, arteries, and other internal organs. The cells have a distinctive spindle shape.

   (1) Nonstriated. Visceral muscle is also called **smooth muscle** because of its lack of cross striations. Rather than being aligned along the length of the cell, the myofilaments are arranged spirally within smooth muscle fibers.

   (2) Weaker contractions. The contractions of smooth muscle are weaker than those of striated muscle because the actin and myosin are organized differently. However, smooth muscle has a much greater range of lengths over which the cells can contract. Smooth muscles contract more slowly than striated muscle, but they can retain a contraction for a greater period of time.

B. The Sarcomere: Structure and Mechanism of Contraction
(Figure 7-5)

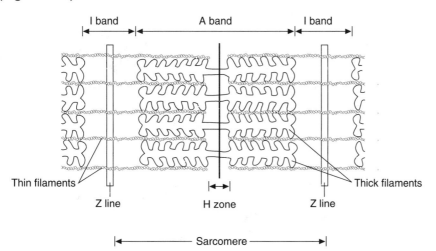

FIGURE 7-5.
The structure of a sarcomere.

1. **Structure**

   a. **Z lines.** The striations in skeletal muscle result from the lining up of Z lines, which are the edges of each sarcomere, of numerous myofibrils.

   b. **I band.** The thin filaments are attached to the Z lines and extend inward toward the center of the sarcomere. The thick filaments are centered within the sarcomere. In a resting muscle, there is an area near the edges of the sarcomere where the thin and thick filaments do not overlap. This region of only thin filaments is the I band.

   c. **A band.** The broad central region where the thin and thick filaments overlap is the A band.

   d. **H zone.** The narrow region in the center of the A band where there are only thick filaments is the H zone. (The thin filaments extend only partially across the sarcomere.)

2. **Sliding filament model.** In the sliding filament model, which is the mechanism of muscle contraction, the thin filaments slide across the thick filaments to pull the Z lines together and shorten the sarcomere. The I bands shorten and the H zone disappears, but the length of the A bands does not change. Shortening of all the sarcomeres in a myofibril allows the muscle to contract to approximately half its resting length.

   a. **Actin and myosin interactions** allow the filaments within the sarcomere to slide by each other (Figure 7-6). The myosin molecules of the thick filaments have "heads" that can bind to specific sites on the actin molecules of the thin filaments, resulting in **cross-bridges** between the thick and thin filaments. When cross-bridges form, the bent position of the myosin head pulls the thin filament toward the center of the sarcomere.

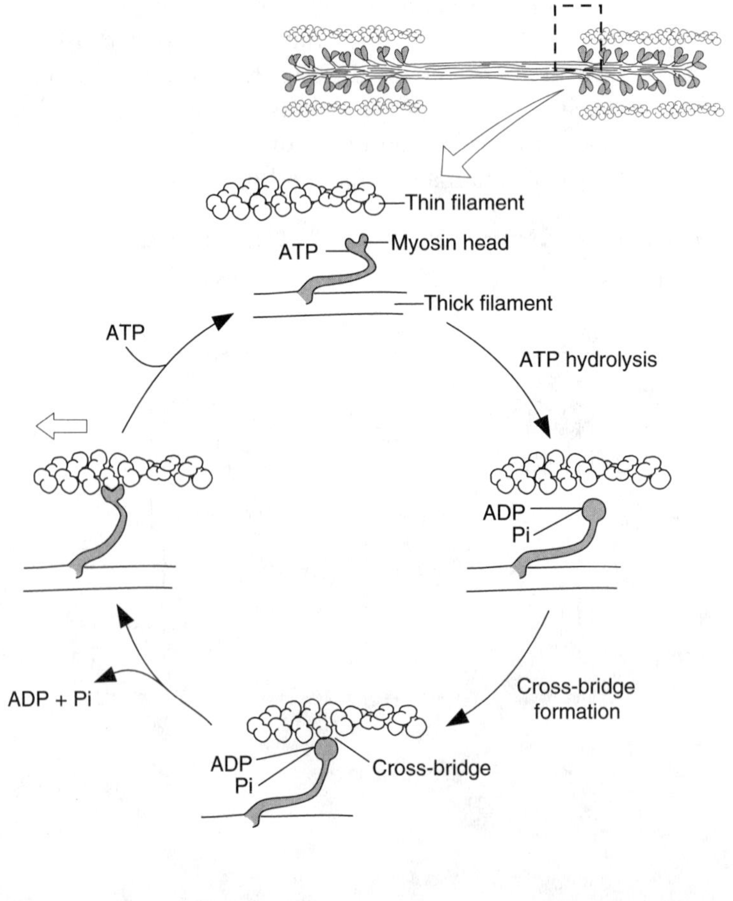

FIGURE 7-6.
The mechanism of muscle contraction. Note the involvement of adenosine triphosphate (ATP) in this process. *ADP* = adenosine diphosphate.

    b.   **Cross-bridges can be broken only with an input of energy.** Adenosine triphosphate (ATP) is hydrolyzed by the myosin head, which breaks its attachment to the thin filament and returns to its original position.

    c.   **To repeat the cycle,** the free myosin head binds to another site farther along the thin filament. Approximately five cross-bridges are formed and reformed every second by each of the approximately 350 myosin heads of a thick filament.

C. Regulation of Muscle Contraction

1.   **Rest.** At rest, the myosin-binding sites on the actin molecules are blocked by the regulatory protein **tropomyosin** in the thin filament. A complex of regulatory proteins, called **troponin,** is also attached to the thin filament.

    a.   **Troponin binds calcium.** Calcium ions are the key regulators of contraction. When troponin binds calcium, the troponin-tropomyosin interaction is altered, and the tropomyosin is displaced from the myosin-binding sites. Thus, muscle contraction occurs in the presence of calcium. When calcium levels drop, the myosin-binding sites are covered again, and contraction stops.

    b.   The **sarcoplasmic reticulum** is a membrane system that accumulates and releases calcium ions.

2.   **Motor neurons.** A muscle contracts only when stimulated by a motor neuron. The coupling of electrical excitation with muscle contraction occurs as follows:

    a.   An **action potential** occurs in the motor neuron, innervating a muscle cell, and the neuron releases ACh into the neuromuscular junction. This results in a graded depolarization of the plasma membrane of the muscle cell. If the depolarization is sufficiently large, it triggers an action potential that spreads across the muscle cell membrane.

    b.   **Transverse (T) tubules** are infoldings of the plasma membrane that carry the action potential into the muscle cell. Where the T tubules contact the sarcoplasmic reticulum, the action potential depolarizes the sarcoplasmic reticulum membrane and stimulates it to release calcium ions. Binding of calcium to troponin allows the muscle to contract.

    c.   **To safeguard against excessive contraction,** the sarcoplasmic reticulum pumps calcium back out of the cytoplasm as soon as the action potential passes, preventing further contraction.

    d.   The **energy** for this process comes from **ATP,** which is produced by the transfer of phosphate from a molecule called creatine phosphate to adenosine diphosphate.

3.   **Muscle fiber innervation**

    a.   Some **small muscles,** such as those controlling eye movements, require a fine degree of control. In such a case, each motor neuron innervates only one fiber.

    b.   In **larger muscles,** each motor neuron may innervate hundreds of fibers, which are scattered throughout the muscle.

    c.   A **motor unit** is a single motor neuron plus all the muscle fibers it controls.

4. **Graded response.** Muscle contraction is a graded response, meaning that the **extent and strength of contraction can be varied.** There are two mechanisms responsible for the graded response.

   a. The **number of motor units varies.** The strength of a contraction depends on the number of motor units that are stimulated. **Recruitment** of additional motor units results in gradually stronger contraction.

   b. The **rate of successive contractions varies.** Whereas a single stimulus results in a muscle twitch, two stimuli in succession results in two twitches, the second of which is stronger than the first. This **wave summation** occurs because the second contraction starts before the muscle has completely relaxed from the first contraction. Although the muscle is still shortened, it contracts even further. Because motor neurons usually transmit stimuli in rapid succession, wave succession results in smooth, continual muscle contraction, called **tetanus.**

IV. Epithelial Cells and Tissues

A. Structure and Function

1. **Function.** Epithelial tissue **covers the outside of the body** and **lines organs and body cavities** inside the body. Epithelium provides an effective **barrier** and **protects a surface** against invading microorganisms, water loss, and physical injury.

2. **Structure.** Epithelial tissue consists of **sheets of tightly packed cells.** Epithelial cells are joined closely, in many cases, by tight junctions between the cells. Little if any material can pass between epithelial cells. An epithelium has **two surfaces.**

   a. The cells at the **free surface** are exposed to air or fluid.

   b. The cells at the **base** of the barrier are attached to a **basement membrane.**

3. **Cell shapes.** One criterion for grouping different types of epithelia is the shape of the cells on the free surface. The different cell shapes are **cuboidal** (like dice), **columnar** (like bricks on their ends), and **squamous** (like flat tiles).

4. **Specialized epithelia.** In addition to protecting the organs that they line, some epithelia are specialized for absorbing or secreting fluids. These epithelia are usually made up of cells with large cytoplasmic volumes (i.e., columnar or cuboidal epithelia).

   a. **Absorbing.** Nutrients are absorbed by the columnar epithelial cells that line the stomach and small intestine.

   b. **Secreting.** Substances are secreted by the cuboidal epithelia of the thyroid gland and kidney tubules.

5. **Mucous membrane.** Another type of epithelium is the mucous membrane, which secretes a solution that keeps a surface moist and lubricated. The free surfaces of some mucous membranes have cilia that move the thin layer of mucus along the surface. In the respiratory tubes, for example, the ciliated epithelium sweeps dust and other particles back up the windpipe to help keep the lungs clean.

B. **Types** (Figure 7-7). In addition to shape, epithelia are classified by **number of cell layers.** The cells at the free surface may be cuboidal, columnar, or squamous, regardless of whether the epithelia has one or more layers.

FIGURE 7-7.
Various types of important epithelia, which are named based on cellular shape. Squamous means flat; columnar means column-like; cuboidal means cube-like ; and stratified means layered. Pseudostratified cells are in a unique layered structure.

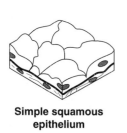

Simple squamous epithelium

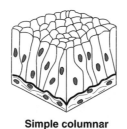

Simple columnar epithelium

Simple cuboida epithelium

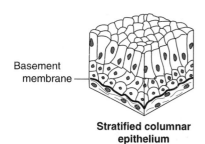

Basement membrane

Stratified columnar epithelium

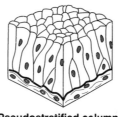

Pseudostratified columnar epithelium

1. A **simple epithelium** has a **single layer** of cells.

    a. **Simple squamous epithelia** are relatively leaky, allowing materials to move across the cell by diffusion. Epithelia specialized for this function are found lining the blood vessels and air sacs of the lungs.

    b. **Simple columnar epithelia** are specialized for absorption or secretion.

2. A **stratified epithelium** has **multiple layers** of cells. This type of epithelium can regenerate relatively easily. As old cells are sloughed off the free surface, cells near the basement membrane divide and push new cells to the free surface. Such epithelia are found on surfaces that are continually exposed to abrasive conditions, such as the outer skin and the linings of certain body passages and cavities.

3. A **pseudostratified epithelium** appears stratified because the cells vary in shape. It is actually a **single layer** of cells.

V. Connective Cells and Tissues

A. Structure and Function (Figure 7-8)

1. **Function.** Most connective tissues **bind and support other tissues.**

2. **Structure.** Unlike epithelia, connective tissues are composed of small numbers of cells dispersed in a matrix of extracellular material. This **extracellular matrix** is composed of a network of fibers in a homogeneous ground substance. The ground substance may be liquid, gel, or solid, depending on the type of connective tissue.

FIGURE 7-8.
The microscopic appearance
of various tissue types.

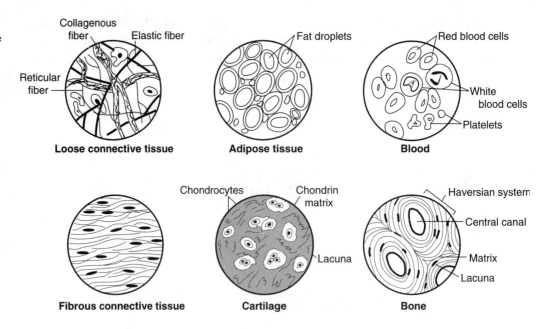

3. **Types**

    a. **Loose connective tissue** is the most abundant connective tissue,
        named for its loose web of fibers. Loose connective tissue **binds
        epithelia to underlying tissues and holds organs in place.** There
        are several kinds of loose connective tissue. Three types of loose
        connective tissue are distinguished by the proteins that make up
        the extracellular fibers. These fibers are secreted by cells called
        fibroblasts.

        (1) **Collagenous fibers** are bundles of fibrils, each of which is
            made of a coiled arrangement of the protein collagen. A distinc-
            tive property of collagenous fibers is their great strength along
            the length of the fiber **(tensile strength).** These fibers are re-
            sistant to stretching, which is important for holding body parts
            together (e.g., keeping skin attached to bone).

        (2) **Elastic fibers** are long thread-like fibers made of the protein
            elastin. These stretchy fibers give the connective tissue **great
            resilience** to insult (e.g., the elasticity of skin).

        (3) **Reticular fibers** are branched and form a tight network of fibers.
            Reticular fibers **join connective tissue to adjacent tissues.**

    b. **Adipose cells** are specialized for fat storage. They are scattered
        throughout **adipose tissue,** which is a type of loose connective tissue.
        Adipose tissue provides padding and insulation for the body, as well as
        storage for fuel molecules. Each adipose cell swells when fat is stored
        and shrinks when the fat is used as fuel.

4. **Blood** is composed of several types of cells suspended in a liquid extracel-
    lular matrix called plasma. It differs from other connective tissues by its
    function in circulation, rather than in binding and support.

    a. **Plasma** consists of water, salts, and various dissolved proteins.

    b. **Three types of cells** are suspended in plasma.

    (1)   **Erythrocytes** (red blood cells) carry oxygen throughout the body.

    (2)   **Leukocytes** (white blood cells) function in the immune system.

    (3)   **Platelets** are involved in blood clotting.

5.   **Fibrous connective tissue.** Dense or fibrous connective tissue has a greater proportion and degree of organization of collagenous fibers than loose connective tissue. The dense fibers are arranged in parallel bundles, which give them greater tensile strength. The **tendons** that attach muscles to bones and the **ligaments** that join bones together at joints are both composed of dense connective tissue.

B. Cartilage and Bone

1.   **Cartilage** is a dense mesh of collagenous fibers in a ground substance called **chondrin,** which is a protein-carbohydrate complex with a rubbery consistency. Chondrin is secreted by cells called **chondrocytes,** which are localized in spaces called **lacunae** that are scattered through the ground substance. The combination of collagenous fibers and chondrin makes cartilage a strong yet flexible material. The main function of cartilage is **support and reinforcement** (e.g., for the nose, ears, vertebral disks).

2.   **Bone,** which is a mineralized connective tissue, forms the skeleton that supports the body of most vertebrates.

    a.   **Osteocytes** are cells that secrete a collagenous matrix and release calcium phosphate, which forms deposits of the mineral **hydroxyapatite** within the matrix. Bone is hardened without becoming brittle by this combination of hard mineral and flexible collagen.

    b.   **Haversian systems** are the repeating units that make up hard bone. Each system is composed of **lamellae,** which are concentric layers of the mineralized matrix. The lamellae are deposited around a central area that contains blood vessels and nerves that provide materials to the bone.

    c.   **Lacunae** are the small spaces that contain osteocytes. The lacunae are surrounded by the hard matrix and are interconnected by cellular extensions called **canaliculi.**

    d.   **Marrow** is spongy bone tissue that forms the interior of long bones. The long bones have a hard outer region made of Haversian systems. The **red marrow** near the ends of long bones are where blood cells are produced.

8

The Nervous System

I. Introduction

A. Function. The human nervous system allows the body to respond to its environment by monitoring sensory stimuli, interpreting the information provided by the senses, and suggesting an appropriate response. The mechanism of the nervous system is complex, with multiple levels of regulation and millions of interconnecting networks. Therefore, when studying this complex system, it is important to understand the anatomic organization of the nervous system with all of its multiple subdivisions (Figure 8-1).

FIGURE 8-1.
A flow diagram of the nervous system.

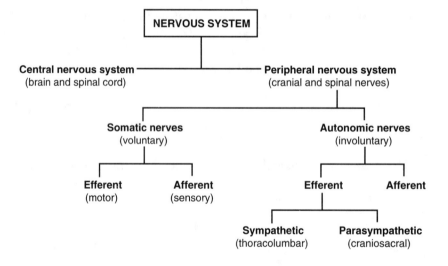

B. Structure. The human nervous system has two anatomic subdivisions. The **peripheral nervous system (PNS)** includes both the cranial nerves and the spinal nerves, as well as their associated ganglia. The **central nervous system (CNS)** is composed of the brain and the spinal cord.

II. Peripheral Nervous System

A. Structure

1. There are **12 pairs of cranial nerves** (Table 8-1) that exit the brain directly; there are **31 pairs of spinal nerves** that exit from the spinal cord.

TABLE 8-1. The cranial nerves.

Number	Cranial Nerve	Components	Innervation and Function
I	Olfactory	Sensory	Nasal epithelium (olfaction)
II	Optic	Sensory	Rods and cones of retina (vision)
III	Oculomotor	Motor	Eye muscles (movement of eye); pupil constriction; ciliary muscle (accommodation)
IV	Trochlear	Motor	Eye muscle (movement of eye)
V	Trigeminal	Sensory	Skin of face and mucosal surfaces of mouth and nose (sensation)
		Motor	Muscles of mastication (chewing)
VI	Abducens	Motor	Eye muscle (movement of eye)
VII	Facial	Sensory	Taste for the anterior two thirds of the tongue
		Motor	Muscles of facial expression
VIII	Vestibulocochlear	Sensory	Cristae of semicircular canals (balance and equilibrium); hair cells of organ of Corti (hearing)
IX	Glossopharyngeal	Sensory	Taste for posterior one third of the tongue; sensation for pharynx
		Motor	Parotid gland (secretion)
X	Vagus	Motor	Constrictors of pharynx (swallowing); muscles of larynx (phonation); heart smooth muscle, and glands of gastrointestinal tract and pulmonary system (autonomic control)
XI	Spinal Accessory	Motor	Trapezius and sternomastoid muscles (elevation of shoulders and movement of head)
XII	Hypoglossal	Motor	Muscles of tongue (movement of tongue)

2. The **spinal, or peripheral, nerves** exit through the vertebral column through the intervertebral foramina and are named according to the vertebral level from which they exit.

3. The cell bodies of spinal nerve sensory fibers are located in the **dorsal root ganglia** (Figure 8-2), and those of motor fibers are present within the **ventral horns.**

4. Normally, **sensory impulses travel to the brain,** where the sensory impulses are processed and motor impulses send information to the periphery to dictate the desired response.

5. In the case of a **reflex arc,** the CNS is bypassed. In the simplest scenario, a sensory receptor stimulates a sensory nerve, which then synapses either directly or indirectly (via interneurons) to a motor nerve. The motor nerve then stimulates the effector tissue, completing the circuit.

B. Function

1. **Voluntary and involuntary functions**

   a. The **voluntary** components of the PNS are the **somatic nerves,** which innervate skeletal muscle.

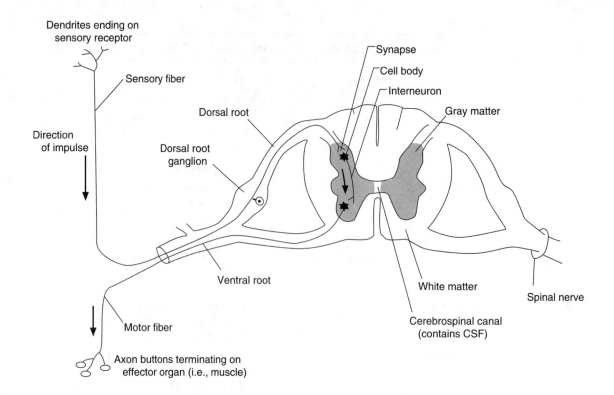

Dendrites ending on
sensory receptor

Sensory fiber

Direction
of impulse

Dorsal root

Dorsal root
ganglion

Synapse

Cell body

Interneuron

Gray matter

Ventral root

Motor fiber

Axon buttons terminating on
effector organ (i.e., muscle)

White matter

Spinal nerve

Cerebrospinal canal
(contains CSF)

FIGURE 8-2.
Cross section of a
spinal cord with a
reflex arc. *CSF* =
cerebrospinal fluid.

  b. The **involuntary** components are the **autonomic nerves,** which are grouped together under a functional unit also known as the **autonomic nervous system (ANS).**

 2. **Efferent and afferent nerve networks** are contained in both the somatic and autonomic branches of the PNS.

  a. The **efferent,** or **motor,** nerves carry nerve impulses from the CNS into the body.

  b. In contrast, the **afferent,** or **sensory,** nerves monitor sensory inputs and carry this information from the periphery to the CNS.

 3. The **ANS** is involved in controlling the maintenance of **internal homeostasis.** The ANS **innervates all smooth muscle, cardiac muscle, and glandular tissue.**

 4. The **motor division of the ANS** is divided once again into **sympathetic** (thoracolumbar) and **parasympathetic** (craniosacral) components (Figure 8-3). The **nerves** that comprise these two components have important anatomic distinctions.

  a. **Sympathetic nerves** arise from the **thoracic and lumbar regions** of the spinal cord.

  b. **Parasympathetic nerve fibers** originate in the **cranial and sacral regions.**

  c. There are differences in the location of the ganglia where the sympathetic and parasympathetic nerves synapse.

 5. A **ganglion** is a collection of nerve cell bodies that usually contains multiple synapses.

  a. In the **sympathetic** nervous system, chains of ganglia are found on **either side of the spinal cord.**

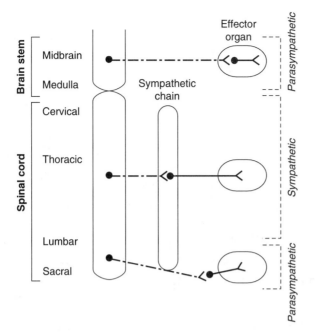

FIGURE 8-3.
The sympathetic and para-sympathetic nervous systems. Parasympathetic fibers arise in the brain stem or the sacral spinal cord, have a synapse in a ganglion close to the target, and finally synapse in the target organ or tissue. Sympathetic fibers originate in the thoracic or lumbar spinal cord, synapse nearby in the sympathetic chain, and finally synapse a distance away in the target organ or tissue. *CSF* = cerebrospinal fluid.

Preganglionic nerves — · — · — · —·
Postganglionic nerves ————————

    b.   In the **parasympathetic** nervous system, the ganglia are located **in or near the innervated organs.**

    c.   As a consequence of this differing ganglial placement, a **third distinction** is made between the two systems.

        (1) **Efferent autonomic circuits** are composed of two nerves. **Preganglionic nerves** arise from the CNS and synapse in the ganglion. **Postganglionic nerves** then complete the circuit, carrying the impulse from the ganglion to the target tissue.

        (2) **Sympathetic circuits** have short preganglionic and long postganglionic fibers. **Parasympathetic pathways are the opposite,** having long preganglionic and short postganglionic nerve fibers.

            (a) **Sympathetic preganglionic nerves tend to synapse with many postganglionic nerves.** This arrangement is contrasted by few synaptic connections in the parasympathetic system.

            (b) Therefore, **the effects of sympathetic activation tend to be more widespread than those of parasympathetic stimulation,** in which the effects are more localized.

6. **The sympathetic and parasympathetic divisions of the ANS exert opposing effects on the body.** See Table 8-2 for a list of autonomic influences on the body.

    a.   The **sympathetic nerves** prepare the body for **"fight or flight,"** raising blood pressure, increasing respiration, and reducing energy expelled on digestive activities.

TABLE 8-2. Effects of autonomic innervation on effector organs.

Effector Organ	Parasympathetic Action	Sympathetic Action
Heart	Decreases rate; no effect on strength of contraction	Increases the rate and the strength of contraction
Blood vessels	Dilates	Constricts
Bronchial tubes	Constricts	Dilates
Pupils	Constricts	Dilates
Bladder	Constricts	Relaxes
Kidney	Increases urine production	Decreases urine production
Gastrointestinal tract	Stimulates smooth muscle contraction and secretion of enzymes	Inhibits smooth muscle contraction and gastrointestinal motility
Sexual function	Dilates blood vessels; erection	Constricts blood vessels; ejaculation
Salivary glands	Stimulates thin, watery secretions	Stimulates thick, viscous secretions
Energy mobilization: liver and adipose tissue	No effect	Stimulates glycogenolysis and fatty acid release respectively
Neurotransmitter	Acetylcholine	Epinephrine and norepinephrine

b.   The **parasympathetic nerves** encourage homeostatic activities (**"rest and digest"**), such as decreasing blood pressure, reducing respiration, and stimulating the glandular secretions necessary for digestion.

III. The Central Nervous System

A. The Spinal Cord (see Figure 8-2)

1.   In the **center of the spinal cord** is a butterfly-shaped mass composed of the cell bodies of the spinal cord neurons. This area is known collectively as the **gray matter** because the cell bodies stain gray whereas the surrounding axons remain white. (The white matter does not stain with the laboratory dye because of its high lipid content.)

2.   The cell bodies that conduct **sensory functions** are located in the **dorsal horns.**

3.   The cell bodies involved in **motor activities** are in the **ventral horns.**

4.   Surrounding the gray matter is the **white matter,** which is composed primarily of myelinated nerve fibers. This arrangement of gray and white matter extends the length of the spinal cord, differing only with respect to the ratio of gray matter to white matter.

5.   The fibers of the white matter travel through the spinal cord in **tracts, or columns.** Each tract contains groups of fibers that share a common function (e.g., pain sensation for the right index finger) in addition to "sharing" similar sites of origin and termination.

a.   These nerve fibers enter or exit the spinal cord via the **dorsal or ventral roots,** depending on whether they are sensory or motor nerves, respectively.

b.   The dorsal and ventral roots then join to form a **spinal nerve** that **carries both sensory and motor fibers.**

6.   The **spinal cord is protected** by the surrounding **vertebral column** as well as by three connective tissue sheaths known as the **meninges** of the brain.

a. From exterior to interior, the meninges are called the **dura mater,** the **arachnoid membrane,** and the **pia mater.**

b. **Cerebrospinal fluid (CSF)** fills the subarachnoid space between the arachnoid membrane and pia mater, **cushioning the spinal cord** from shock.

c. In some **diseases** (e.g., malaria), the meninges become inflamed (meningitis) and a sample of the CSF is needed to determine the appropriate therapy. To prevent injury to the spinal cord, lumbar punctures or spinal taps are performed below the second lumbar vertebra (L2). The spinal cord terminates below L2 into nerve roots termed the **cauda equina.**

B. **The Brain.** The human brain can be divided into distinct **anatomic regions** with different functional domains (Figure 8-4).

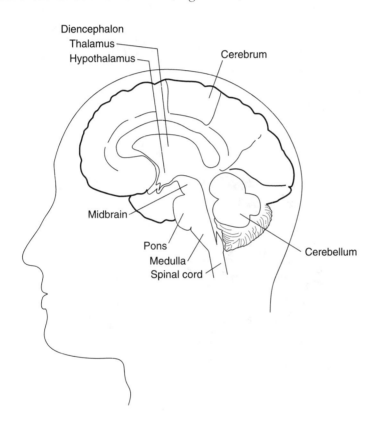

FIGURE 8-4.
Structure of the human brain.

1. The **medulla oblongata,** which is continuous with the spinal cord, is at the **caudal end** of the brain stem. Major activities controlled in this region of the brain include regulation of heart rate, respiration, and blood pressure. The reflex centers that control blinking, coughing, sneezing, swallowing, and vomiting are also in the medulla oblongata.

2. The **pons** is a bulged area on the anterior surface of the brain stem, just superior to the medulla oblongata. The pons aids the medulla in the control of respiration. It relays information between the cerebral cortex and the cerebellum, and it contains the cell bodies that control facial expression, mastication, lacrimation, and salivation.

3. Traveling up the brain stem, the **midbrain** is the next area. The midbrain contains the **red nucleus** (integrates information concerning muscle tone and posture), the **superior colliculi** (mediates visual reflexes), and the **inferior colliculi** (mediates auditory reflexes). The midbrain also controls pupillary constriction and accommodation.

4. The **cerebellum** is a bihemispheric structure located posterior to the brain stem. It is the second largest part of the brain and controls balance, maintenance of muscle tone and posture, and smooth, coordinated movement.

5. The **diencephalon** is the interior of the brain proper. There are three major components of this region.

   a. The **thalamus** acts as the main relay center, conducting information between the cerebral cortex and the rest of the nervous system.

   b. The **hypothalamus** controls body temperature, appetite, sleep, and blood pressure, it secretes releasing factors that regulate pituitary gland function, and it modulates some emotional and sexual responses (e.g., hostility, pain, pleasure). The hypothalamus is a member of the final component of the diencephalon known as the limbic system.

   c. The **limbic system** is concerned with emotion, including interpretation of emotional stimuli and behavioral responses to these stimuli.

6. The **cerebrum** is the largest and most prominent part of the brain. A central, longitudinal fissure divides the cerebrum into left and right hemispheres, which communicate with each other via the **corpus callosum.** Each hemisphere of the cerebrum is further subdivided into four main lobes (Figure 8-5).

FIGURE 8-5.
The lobes of the brain.

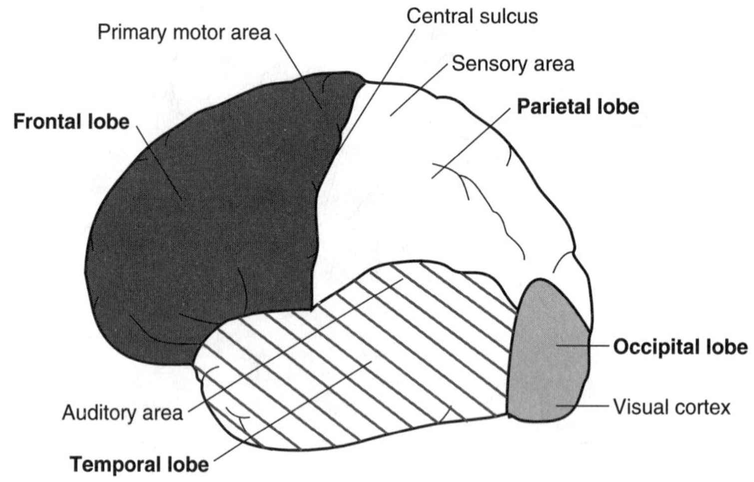

Primary motor area — Central sulcus
Sensory area
Frontal lobe — **Parietal lobe**
Occipital lobe
Visual cortex
Auditory area
Temporal lobe

   a. The **frontal lobe** controls voluntary movement (**motor cortex**), behavior, learning, thought, judgment, and personality.

   b. The **temporal lobe** interprets auditory stimuli and aids in spoken language.

   c. The **parietal lobe** senses heat, cold, touch, and pressure stimuli.

   d. The **occipital lobe** contains the visual cortex, which interprets visual stimuli.

IV. Special Sensory Reception and Processing

A. Vision

1. **Structure** (Figure 8-6)

   a. The outermost layers of the eyeball, the **sclera** and the **cornea,** are composed of fibrous connective tissue.

FIGURE 8-6.
The structure of the eye.

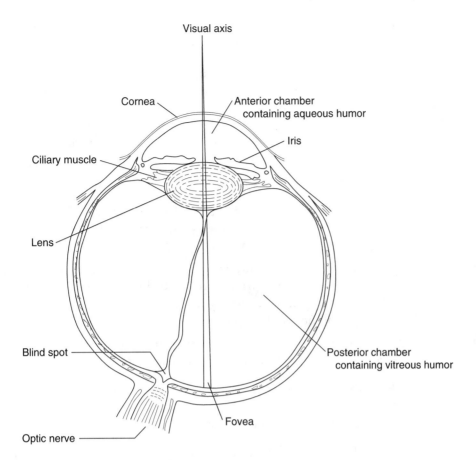

Visual axis

Cornea

Anterior chamber
containing aqueous humor

Iris

Ciliary muscle

Lens

Blind spot

Posterior chamber
containing vitreous humor

Optic nerve

Fovea

b. Just interior is a vascular, pigmented layer that makes up the **choroid,** the **ciliary body,** and the **iris.**

c. The innermost layer—the **retina**—contains photoreceptor cells, namely the **rods** and **cones,** and other neural cells that aid in the transmission and integration of visual stimuli.

d. The visual inputs are then carried via the **optic nerve** to the occipital lobe, where they are processed further.

2. **Mechanism of vision.** The mechanism of vision involves stimulation of the retina by light and the conversion of photon energy to electrical energy by photoreceptor cells.

a. **Photons** of light travel through the cornea, the anterior chamber containing **aqueous humor,** the pupil, and ultimately the lens, where they become refracted, creating an inverse image.

b. Once refracted, the photons pass through the **vitreous humor** until they reach the layers of the retina, causing stimulation of both rod and cone cells (photoreceptor cells).

c. Most of the surface of the **retina** contains photoreceptors; however, there are **special regions.** The **optic disk,** the site where the optic nerve exits from the back of the eye, contains no photoreceptors, which creates an anatomic blind spot. The area of highest visual acuity (i.e., it has the highest density of cone cells) is the **fovea.**

d. **Photopigment ultimately creates electrical energy.** When photons strike the photoreceptor cells, a photopigment absorbs the light and undergoes structural changes that cause the generation of ionic potentials. Therefore, photon energy is first converted into chemical energy and then into electrical energy.

(1) Rod cells contain the photopigment **rhodopsin.** This photopigment contains a protein called opsin, that is chemically joined to a vitamin A derivative called retinal. **Rods** differentiate light intensities (white/black) because they are sensitive and spread out over the surface of the retina. Thus, rods control vision in dim light (e.g., night vision).

(2) **Cones** contain **iodopsin** as their photopigment.

(a) There are **three types of cone cells,** each containing a different form of photopigment to discriminate red, green, and blue wave forms.

(b) Because they are less sensitive than rod cells, cones enable **color perception and bright light vision.** Cones are best for good visual acuity function because they have great resolution ability.

(c) Cones are **grouped together over the retinal surface,** which aids in their discrimination of fine detail.

e. **Photoreceptor cells transmit electrical impulses.** After stimulation of the photoreceptor cells, the generated electrical impulses are received by neurons that are found in layers of the retina.

(1) The photoreceptors transmit the electrical information to the **bipolar cells,** which then transmit the information to the **ganglion cells.**

(2) The axons of ganglion cells give rise to the **optic nerves.**

B. Hearing

1. **Functions of the ear** include receiving auditory stimuli and helping to control equilibrium and balance.

2. The **three major anatomic divisions** of the ear (Figure 8-7) are the **outer ear,** composed of the pinna, the external auditory canal, and the tympanic

FIGURE 8-7.
The structure of the human ear. (Reproduced with permission from Ville CA, Solomon EP, Davis PW: *Biology.* Philadelphia, Saunders College Publishing, 1985, p 887.)

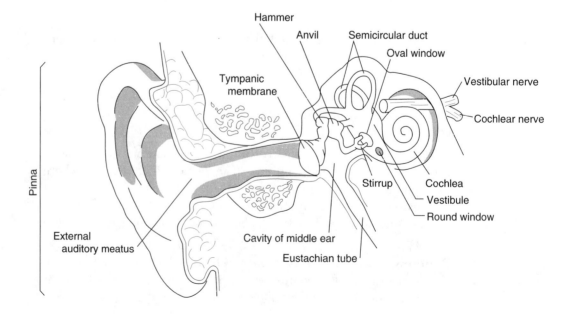

membrane; the **middle ear,** composed of the eustachian tube, the ossicles (i.e., malleus, incus, and stapes), the oval window, and the round window; and the **inner ear,** containing the bony and membranous labyrinths as well as the organ of Corti. For the structures of the cochlea and the organ of Corti, refer to Figures 8-8 and 8-9.

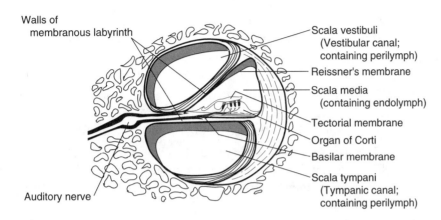

FIGURE 8-8.
The cochlea. (Reproduced with permission from Ville CA, Solomon EP, Davis PW: *Biology*. Philadelphia, Saunders College Publishing, 1985, p 888.)

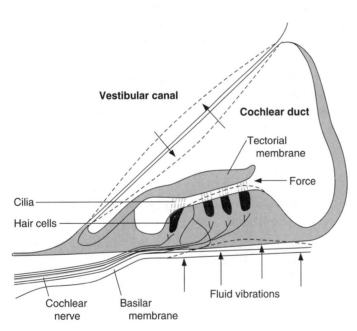

FIGURE 8-9.
The organ of Corti. (Reproduced with permission from Ville CA, Solomon EP, Davis PW: *Biology*. Philadelphia, Saunders College Publishing, 1985, p 888.)

3. The **mechanism of hearing** is complex. The basics of the hearing mechanism are presented here.

    a. **Sound enters the external auditory canal** in the form of waves of air molecules. As these molecules strike the tympanic membrane, unique oscillations are created over the surface of the membrane.

    b. **Oscillations of the tympanic membrane cause movement of the ossicles,** or middle ear bones, which amplify the signal and translate the displacement of the tympanic membrane into mechanical energy.

    c. At the end of the three-bone chain (i.e., the ossicles), **the stapes covers the oval window of the cochlea,** which is a fluid-filled system of canals. When the stapes moves against the oval window, **perilymph** fluid within the **scala vestibuli (bony labyrinth)** of the cochlea creates wave forms of varying amplitudes. This generates pressure changes, which are translated to the **endolymph** of the **scala media (membranous labyrinth)** via distortions of the **Reissner membrane.**

    d.   Movement of the endolymph, varying with the pitch and volume of the eliciting sound, causes **movement of stereocilia** located on the hair cells of the organ of Corti.

    e.   Movement of the stereocilia is coupled with the **opening and closing of ion channels,** which, in turn, can lead to local depolarizations. The mechanical energy of the fluid and the movement of the stereocilia are **translated into electrical energy** via the migration of ions.

    f.   These **electrical depolarizations are transmitted to the cochlear nerve,** ultimately reaching the temporal lobe where they are processed and interpreted as sound.

    g.   **High-frequency sounds** stimulate hair cells near the base of the cochlea, and **low-frequency sounds** stimulate hair cells near the apex. This arrangement of frequency detection is termed **tonotopic organization.**

    h.   Because liquids are not easily compressed, the **pressure changes** of the scala vestibuli need a way to escape. The **flexible round window at the end of the scala tympani** absorbs these pressure changes, acting as a pressure release valve. The pressure can either be **transferred directly,** because the scala vestibuli and scala tympani communicate at the apex at a point referred to as the **helicotrema,** or they can be **transmitted indirectly** from the endolymph via movement of the Reissner membrane and the basilar membrane.

    4.   In addition to its role in hearing, the ear also enables the body to control its position in space via a vestibular function controlling **balance.**

        a.   The **vestibular organ** of the ear comprises the **three semicircular canals, the utricle, and the saccule.**

        b.   Together, these canals monitor the effects of **gravity, body movement, and head position.**

        c.   Displacement of the head causes **movement of endolymph within the semicircular canals.** Each canal responds to a different three-dimensional plane because the three canals are connected to the utricle at right angles to one another.

        d.   As the endolymph moves, the stereocilia on hair cells located at the **crista ampullaris** respond in much the same manner as discussed for hearing. The information is transmitted to cranial nerve VIII and ultimately to the cerebellum.

        e.   **Gravity positional sense** is achieved by the movement of calcium carbonate crystals on hair cells of the macula of both the utricle and the saccule.

C. Olfaction

    1.   **Smell** is a response of specialized cells called **bipolar ganglion cells** to gaseous stimuli.

    2.   The **mechanism of smell** is mediated via a receptor–ligand signal transduction mechanism.

3. There are **four primary types of olfactory stimuli:** acidic, burnt, fragrant, and rancid.

   a. Olfactory stimuli affect the bipolar ganglion cells located in a highly specialized mucous membrane in the **roof of each nasal cavity.**

   b. The ganglion cells terminate in knobs that have several **olfactory hairs.** The hairs contain receptors that bind to the olfactory ligands. This creates **electrical impulses** inside the cells, which are then referred to cranial nerve I.

D. Taste. The mechanism of taste is analogous to that of smell.

1. **Neuroepithelial cells on taste buds** of the tongue act as receptors for substances in solution.

2. The **four types of taste receptors**—bitter, salt, sour, and sweet—are ligand-specific and are distributed over specific areas of the tongue.

   a. **Areas of the tongue.** Sour is perceived on the back part of the tongue. Salt and sour are perceived on the sides of the tongue, and sweet is perceived on the tip of the tongue.

   b. **Innervation and transmission.** Information regarding taste is relayed by cranial nerve VII for the anterior two thirds of the tongue, whereas the posterior one third is innervated by cranial nerve IX.

E. Touch

1. The **skin** functions in sensory reception; it contains nerve endings and specialized receptors that detect pain, touch, temperature, pressure, vibration, and proprioception (joint position sense in space).

2. **Free nerve endings** are stimulated directly by contact with an object on the surface of the body.

3. **Receptor organs** discriminate between different types of stimuli (Figure 8-10).

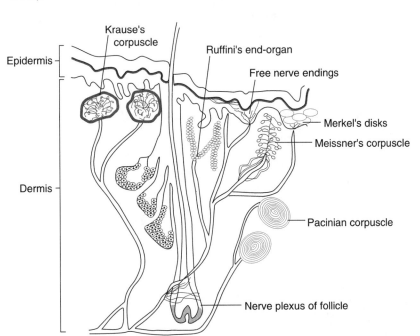

FIGURE 8-10.

Sensory structures of the skin. (Reproduced with permission from Ville CA, Solomon EP, Davis PW: *Biology.* Philadelphia, Saunders College Publishing, 1985, p 880.)

a. **Pacinian corpuscles** respond to pressure changes and are therefore able to detect vibration.

b. **Meissner's corpuscles** are located primarily in hairless regions of the body (especially the hands and feet) and are sensitive to fine touch, as are **Merkel's disks.**

c. **Ruffini's end-organs** are found in subcutaneous tissue. They respond to heat and touch.

d. **Krause's corpuscles** are activated by changes in temperature. For further information on the anatomy of skin, refer to Chapters 7 and 16 of the Biology Review Notes

The Endocrine System

9

I. Function of the Endocrine System

A. Introduction. Like the nervous system, the endocrine system is involved in maintaining homeostasis. Both the nervous system and the endocrine system modulate, integrate, and control the activities of the body. Both systems also enable the body to respond to the environment. However, whereas the effects of the nervous system are rapid and short lived, those of the endocrine system are slower and longer lasting. To control homeostasis, the endocrine system involves feedback loops that are similar to those in the nervous system. Hormones secreted by the endocrine glands regulate organ physiology, and the functioning of the organ systems regulates the secretion of hormones. These feedback loops can be positive or negative, and they are constantly monitored and adjusted.

B. Hormones. Hormones are controlled substances, produced by ductless glands or a collection of cells, which are transported in the circulation to target cells.

1. **Chemical classes**

   a. **Amines** are hormones derived from the amino acid tyrosine. Examples include epinephrine, norepinephrine, and the thyroid hormones triiodothyronine (T_3) and thyroxine (T_4).

   b. **Peptides or glycopeptides** are hormones that are short chains of amino acids. Examples include oxytocin and vasopressin.

   c. **Lipid hormones** are highly hydrophobic, which enables them to easily cross biologic membranes.

      (1) **Prostaglandins** are lipid hormones synthesized from fatty acid precursors. Some of their functions include:

         (a) Decreasing blood pressure

         (b) Inducing labor

         (c) Suppressing gastric secretions

         (d) Mediating inflammation

      (2) **Steroids** are hormones synthesized from a cholesterol precursor. Examples include cortisol and the reproductive hormones estradiol and testosterone.

      d.   **Iodinated hormones** are coupled to inorganic iodine. The thyroid hormones T_3 and T_4 are examples.

2.   Mechanisms of action

      a.   **Target specificity** of the endocrine system is a function of specific **receptors** expressed by cells in the body. Hormones released from cells of the endocrine system bind to these receptors, thereby causing a change in the physiology of that cell. This change often includes the activation of specific genes and an induction of protein synthesis.

      b.   **Hormone receptors** can be in one of **three locations.**

        (1)   The **plasma membrane of the target cell** contains receptors to which amino acid–containing hormones (e.g., amine, peptide, protein classes) bind (Figure 9-1A). This ligand–receptor interaction triggers activation of a second messenger, such as cyclic adenosine monophosphate (cAMP) or guanosine triphosphate (GTP)-binding proteins, which initiates a cascade of events with multiple physiologic outcomes.

        (2)   Hormone receptors can also be **inside a cell.** For instance, steroid hormones cross the plasma membrane and bind to receptors in the **cytoplasm of the target cell** (see Figure 9-1B). This ligand–receptor complex then travels into the nucleus and activates gene transcription.

        (3)   Receptors can also be present **within the nucleus** directly. Thyroid hormones bind to receptors localized in the nucleus, activating gene transcription (see Figure 9-1B).

A

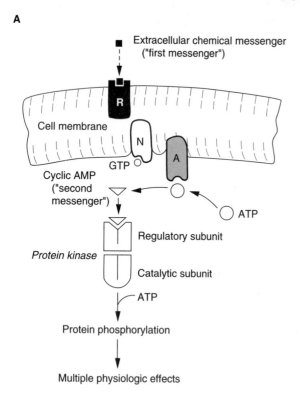

B

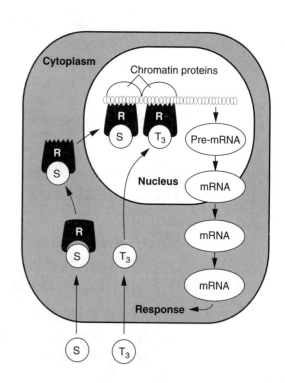

3.   Transport and elimination

      a.   **Many hormones are only active when in a free state.** When hormones are bound to protein, they oftentimes become inactive.

b. **Free hormones are constantly removed** by target tissues, the liver (which degrades them), and the kidneys (which excrete them). As a result, hormones are **continuously secreted** in small amounts so that enough free hormone is available to activate the necessary target cells (because protein-bound hormone is inactive).

II. Major Endocrine Glands

A. **Pituitary Gland.** The master gland of the endocrine system, the pituitary gland, is divided into two lobes, anterior and posterior. The functions of the pituitary are closely linked to hypothalamic regulation.

1. The **anterior pituitary** (Figure 9-2A) develops from oral ectoderm and is connected to the hypothalamus by a portal circulatory system, which is a network of blood vessels containing two capillary beds.

   a. The **normal circulatory pathway** involves blood flowing from an artery, through a capillary bed, and into a vein.

   b. A **portal system** involves blood flowing from an artery, through a capillary bed, into a vein, into a second capillary bed, and into a second vein. The **hypothalamus** secretes peptide-releasing factors into this portal system of blood, which stimulates the cells of the anterior pituitary to secrete the following hormones:

      (1) **Growth hormone (GH)** is a glycoprotein that stimulates growth of bone and muscle and increases blood sugar.

      (2) **Follicle-stimulating hormone (FSH)**

         (a) In **women,** FSH stimulates the growth of follicles and the maturation of oocytes.

         (b) In **men,** FSH stimulates spermatogenesis.

      (3) **Luteinizing hormone (LH)**

         (a) In **women,** LH stimulates ovulation and the formation of the corpus luteum. It also regulates the production of estrogen and progesterone by the follicular cells.

         (b) In **men,** LH stimulates testosterone production by the Leydig cells.

      (4) **Thyroid-stimulating hormone (TSH)** stimulates production of thyroid hormones T_3 and T_4 by the thyroid gland. It also regulates iodination of thyroid hormones.

      (5) **Adrenocorticotropic hormone (ACTH)** stimulates growth of the adrenal cortex. ACTH stimulates the release of glucocorticoids and adrenal androgens but not mineralocorticoids.

      (6) **Prolactin** stimulates the production of breast milk by the mammary glands.

      (7) **Melanocyte-stimulating hormone (MSH)** stimulates melanocytes to produce melanin (skin pigment).

2. The **posterior pituitary gland** (see Figure 9-2B) develops from neural ectoderm and is connected to the hypothalamus by a series of neurons. Two hormones are produced by neurons in the hypothalamus. These neurons transport the two neuropeptides down their axons into the area of the posterior pituitary gland, where they are released into the **systemic circulation.**

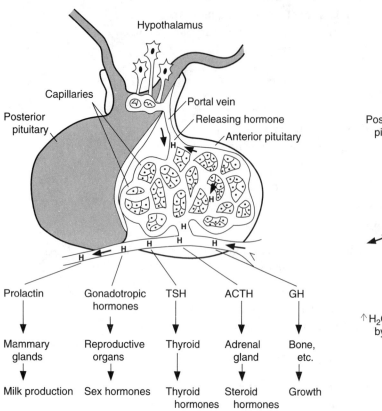

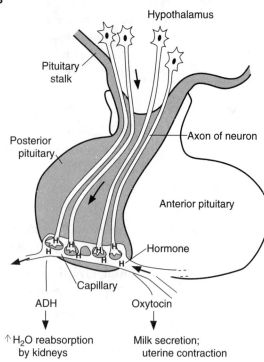

Prolactin — Mammary glands — Milk production

Gonadotropic hormones — Reproductive organs — Sex hormones

TSH — Thyroid — Thyroid hormones

ACTH — Adrenal gland — Steroid hormones

GH — Bone, etc. — Growth

ADH — ↑H₂O reabsorption by kidneys

Oxytocin — Milk secretion; uterine contraction

FIGURE 9-2.

The anatomy of the pituitary gland. **A)** The cells of the hypothalamus produce releasing factors that travel through a portal system to reach the anterior pituitary. The anterior pituitary gland synthesizes its hormones after being stimulated by the releasing factors. **B)** The posterior pituitary gland acts as a storage and release site only. Neurons in the hypothalamus produce the posterior pituitary gland hormones and transport them to the posterior pituitary gland by axonal transport. *TSH* = thyroid-stimulating hormone; *ACTH* = adrenocorticotropic hormone; *GH* = growth hormone. (Reproduced with permission from Ville CA, Solomon EP, Davis PW: *Biology.* Philadelphia, Saunders College Publishing, 1985, p 919.)

418

a. **Antidiuretic hormone (ADH),** or **vasopressin,** stimulates renal tubules to reabsorb water from the collecting ducts of the nephron.

b. **Oxytocin** stimulates smooth muscle contraction during labor and lactation.

B. Thyroid

1. **Structure.** Located on either side of the trachea, the thyroid gland contains **two lobes** connected by an isthmus.

2. **Types.** Two types of hormones are produced by the thyroid gland.

   a. **Thyroid hormones** T_3 and T_4 have the following functions:

      (1) Control metabolic rate

      (2) Regulate growth, differentiation, and maturation

      (3) Modulate the nervous system

   b. **Calcitonin** causes bone absorption of calcium with a subsequent decrease in serum calcium levels. It also inhibits the activity of osteoclasts, which also lowers serum calcium.

C. Parathyroid Gland

1. **Structure.** There are usually **two pairs of parathyroid glands** embedded within the tissue of the thyroid gland.

2. **Parathyroid hormone.** Parathyroid hormone (PTH) is the only hormone made in the parathyroid glands. PTH **increases blood calcium levels** via:

   a. Bone reabsorption by osteoclasts

    b. Decrease in calcium excretion and increase in calcium reabsorption in the kidneys

    c. Activation of vitamin D

D. Pancreas. The pancreas has both an **exocrine** and an **endocrine** function. The exocrine activities are discussed in Chapter 12 of the Biology Review Notes; endocrine activities are conducted through the **islets of Langerhans,** which secrete the following substances.

    1. Glucagon is made by alpha cells. It raises the blood sugar level by stimulating glycogenolysis and gluconeogenesis in the liver. Glucagon also mobilizes fat from adipose tissue.

    2. Insulin is made by beta cells. It lowers the blood sugar level by stimulating glycogenesis in the liver. It facilitates glucose uptake and use of glucose by cells, and it stimulates fat storage and protein synthesis.

    3. Somatostatin is made by delta cells. It inhibits secretin production by the stomach and pancreas, and it slows gastrointestinal motility. Somatostatin also inhibits the release of GH.

E. Adrenal Glands. The adrenal glands are a set of structures resting on the superior border of the kidneys. They are composed of both an outer cortex derived from mesoderm and an inner medulla derived from ectoderm (Figure 9-3).

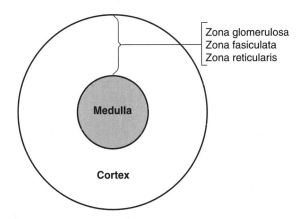

Zona glomerulosa
Zona fasiculata
Zona reticularis

Medulla

Cortex

FIGURE 9-3.
Cross section of an adrenal gland. The outer layer of the gland is the cortex. The inner layer is the medulla.

    1. The **adrenal cortex** is subdivided into three layers: **zona glomerulosa, zona fasciculata, and zona reticularis.** Each zona produces different hormones.

        a. Aldosterone is produced by the **zona glomerulosa.** It is a mineralocorticoid that **regulates ion balance** in the kidney via:

            (1) Stimulation of sodium and chloride reabsorption

            (2) Potassium and phosphorus secretion

            (3) Water retention in the distal convoluted tubule of the nephron

        b. Cortisol is produced by the **zona fasciculata.** It is a glucocorticoid "stress" hormone that:

            (1) Increases blood sugar via conversion of amino acids into sugar instead of protein

            (2) Depresses the immune system

            (3) Inhibits the inflammatory response

     c.   **Sex steroids (androgens and estrogens)** are produced by the **zona reticularis.** They mediate secondary sex characteristics and regulate reproductive functions.

2.   The **adrenal medulla** contains neurons that synapse within the gland and release **epinephrine** and **norepinephrine.** These hormones help the body cope with stress by:

     a.   Increasing heart rate and blood pressure

     b.   Increasing blood sugar concentration

     c.   Increasing metabolic rate

     d.   Mobilizing fat stores

I. Overview of the Circulatory System Components

A. Function. The circulatory system is a closed system of vessels that serves several functions, including:

1. **Delivery of nutrients and oxygen** to the body tissues

2. **Removal of waste products** from the tissues

3. **Maintenance of body temperature** via thermoregulation (see Chapter 16 of the Biology Review Notes)

4. **Transportation of blood cells**

5. **Delivery of hormones** from their site of production to their target tissues

B. Structures

1. The **heart** is a four-chamber organ that propels blood through the circulatory system (Figure 10-1).

   a. The heart tissue is comprised of **cardiac muscle cells,** which are interconnected by **intercalating disks.**

FIGURE 10-1.
Anatomy of the adult heart.

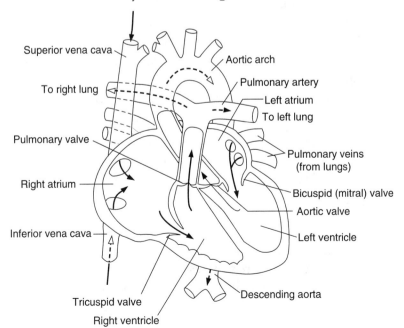

Superior vena cava
Aortic arch
To right lung
Pulmonary artery
Left atrium
To left lung
Pulmonary valve
Pulmonary veins (from lungs)
Right atrium
Bicuspid (mitral) valve
Aortic valve
Inferior vena cava
Left ventricle
Tricuspid valve
Right ventricle
Descending aorta

b. Blood enters the **atria** of the heart from the venous circulation and leaves the heart in **ventricles** via the arterial circulation.

c. **Valves** between the atrium–ventricle pair and ventricle–artery pair prevent the backflow of blood during contraction and drive the flow of blood in one direction.

2. The **conduction system** (Figure 10-2) is contained in the heart.

FIGURE 10-2.
Conduction system of the heart. (Reproduced with permission from Ville CA, Solomon EP, Davis PW: *Biology.* Philadelphia, Saunders College Publishing, 1985, p 749.)

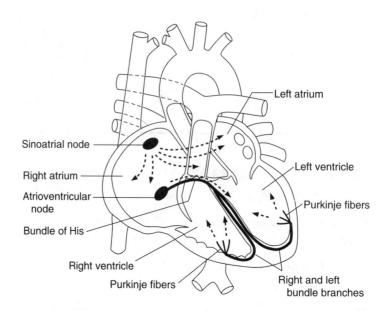

a. The **sinoatrial (SA) node** is a small group of cells found at the junction of the superior vena cava and the right atrium. The SA node is the **pacemaker of the heart;** it spontaneously depolarizes approximately 100 times every minute. **Depolarization causes atrial contraction.**

    (1) **Parasympathetic innervation** via the vagus nerve slows the heart rate to approximately 70 beats per minute in a resting state.

    (2) **Sympathetic innervation** accelerates the rate of depolarization.

b. The **atrioventricular (AV) node** is at the junction between the right atrium and the right ventricle. Atrial depolarization causes the AV node to depolarize.

c. The **bundle of His** carries the signal from the AV node through the interventricular septum.

d. The **left** and **right bundle branches** carry the impulse from the bundle of His to each ventricle, respectively.

e. **Purkinje fibers** transmit the impulse from the bundle branches into the tissue of the ventricles, which causes depolarization and, ultimately, ventricular contraction.

3. **Blood vessels** are composed of several layers of cells (Figure 10-3).

a. **Arteries** carry oxygenated blood away from the heart (except for the pulmonary artery, which carries deoxygenated blood). Arteries have **higher internal pressures** than veins. Arteries **do not contain valves,** but they do have thick layers of smooth muscle and connective tissue.

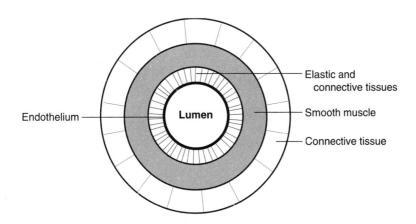

FIGURE 10-3.
Cross section of
a blood vessel.

b. **Veins** carry deoxygenated blood toward the heart (except for the pulmonary vein, which transports oxygenated blood). They have **lower internal pressures** than arteries. Veins **contain valves** that help to move blood against the force of gravity. They have a thick elastic layer and thin layers of smooth muscle and connective tissue. Veins **control blood pressure by controlling blood volume.**

c. **Capillaries** connect arterioles with venules and are the site of exchange between the circulation and the body tissues. **Capillary dynamics** describes the movement of fluid, nutrients, and waste products into and out of the capillary bed (Figure 10-4). More fluid leaves the capillary than returns to it.

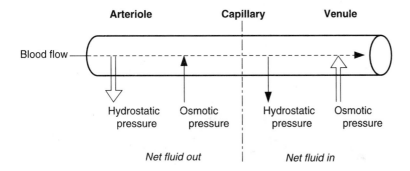

FIGURE 10-4.
Capillary dynamics. Note that the hydrostatic pressure is the dominant force acting on the arterial side of the capillary, whereas osmotic pressure is the dominant force acting on the venous side of the capillary. More net fluid exits than enters the capillary.

   (1) **Arterial side.** Blood entering the arterial side of the capillary has a high hydrostatic pressure that forces fluid out and a low osmotic pressure (caused by blood proteins) that attracts fluid (water). **Net movement is fluid out of the capillary.**

   (2) **Venous side.** On the venous side of the capillary, the osmotic pressure attracting water back into the capillary is greater than the hydrostatic pressure forcing fluid out of the capillary. **Net movement is fluid into the capillary.**

4. **Blood** is composed of plasma and cells.

  a. **Plasma** includes serum (blood fluid), platelets (cell fragments that assist in the clotting of blood), and proteins. Some of the more abundant proteins are albumin, immunoglobulins, fibrinogen, and blood-clotting enzymes.

  b. Types of **blood cells** are summarized in Table 10-1. White blood cells are discussed in Chapter 11 of the Biology Review Notes.

TABLE 10-1. Summary of blood cell types.

Cell Type	Other Name	Function	Appearance	Life Span
Red blood cell	Erythrocyte	Oxygen transport	Biconcave disks; no nucleus	120 days
Platelet	Thrombocyte	Initial blood clotting	Small, cytoplasmic fragments	10 days
White blood cell	Leukocyte	Immune function	Nucleated cells; depend on cell type	Variable

5. **Lymphatics** regulate the return of fluid to the circulation.

a. **Function.** Because more fluid leaves the capillary beds than returns, the body needs a means of returning the excess fluid to the circulatory system. This task is accomplished by the **lymphatic system.**

b. **Structures**

(1) The **lymphatics,** or **lymph vessels,** comprise a system of blind-ended channels that carry water, electrolytes, proteins, and waste material back to the bloodstream. Because lymph vessels contain valves but no muscle layer (Figure 10-5), they rely on the skeletal muscle in which they are embedded to propel fluid back toward the heart.

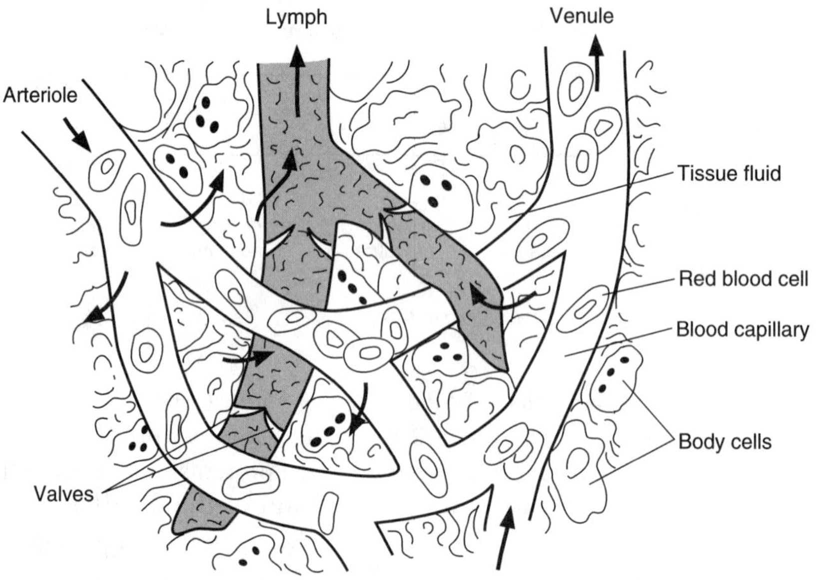

FIGURE 10-5.
Structure and relationship of lymph vessels. (Reproduced with permission from Ville CA, Solomon EP, Davis PW: *Biology.* Philadelphia, Saunders College Publishing, 1985, p 761.)

(2) The **lymph,** or fluid, is filtered by **lymph nodes** and **lymphatic tissues,** which aid the immune system in identifying foreign agents (see Chapter 11 of the Biology Review Notes).

c. **Anatomic divisions**

(1) **Central.** The sites of formation and maturation of white blood cells are the bone marrow and the thymus.

(2) **Peripheral.** The sites of initial sensitization of immune cells include the lymph nodes, tonsils, Peyer patches, and appendix.

(3) **Tertiary.** Solitary interepithelial lymphocytes are present.

II. Mechanisms of Circulation

A. Adult Circulation. Blood returns from the venous circulation and empties into the right atrium. Table 10-2 lists the structures that the blood passes through or passes by during circulation.

TABLE 10-2. Structures of adult blood circulation*.

Cardiac Circulation	Systemic Circulation	Pulmonary Circulation
Right atrium	Heart	Heart
Tricuspid valve	Aorta	Pulmonary artery
Right ventricle	Arteries	Lungs
Pulmonic valve	Capillaries	Pulmonary vein
Pulmonary artery	Veins	
Pulmonic circulation	Vena cavas	
Pulmonic vein		
Left atrium		
Mitral valve		
Left ventricle		
Aortic valve		
Aorta		

*Structures are listed in the order that they are involved in circulation.

B. Fetal Heart Circulation. The overall goal of the fetal circulation is to **deliver maternal nutrients and oxygen** to the left side of the fetal heart. Fetal circulation has several structures that are not found in adult circulation. Although blood cells are not exchanged between a mother and her fetus, nutrients, waste products, antibodies, such as immunoglobulin G (IgG), and blood gases are exchanged.

1. **Maternal circulation** flows from the systemic circulation to, in order, the placental artery, placental capillary bed, and placental vein.

2. **Fetal circulation to and from the placenta** flows from the umbilical arteries (deoxygenated blood) to the placenta, umbilical vein (oxygenated blood), ductus venosus, heart, systemic circulation, then back to the umbilical arteries.

3. **Structures in the fetal heart** include the following:

    a. **Ductus venosis.** Because oxygen and nutrients enter the fetal circulation through the umbilical vein, they must be transported directly to the left ventricle to maximize their delivery to the systemic circulation. The ductus venosis is a **connection between the umbilical vein and the inferior vena cava.** This duct allows substances to bypass the fetal liver.

    b. **Foramen ovale.** The **foramen ovale** is a **hole between the left and right atria** of the fetal heart. In the fetus, the lungs are not fully functioning because there is no gas exchange with the environment. The resistance of the collapsed lungs to blood flow in the fetus is high. Therefore, bypassing the pulmonary circulation is for delivering the bulk of the nutrients to the systemic circulation and for conserving energy.

    c. **Ductus arteriosus.** Because not all of the blood entering the right heart is transported through the foramen ovale, the ductus arteriosis assists in shunting blood that enters the right ventricle. The ductus arteriosus is a **connection between the pulmonary artery and the**

aorta. Again, this allows for direct delivery of nutrients into the systemic circulation by bypassing the fetal lungs.

4. **Fetal circulation in and around the heart** is as follows:

   a. Some blood entering the right atrium moves through the foramen ovale and into the left atrium. This bypasses the right ventricle and lungs. This blood is ultimately pumped into the aorta by the left ventricle.

   b. Some blood entering the right atrium moves into the right ventricle.

   c. Blood that enters the right ventricle is pumped into the pulmonary artery.

   d. From the pulmonary artery, most blood passes through the ductus arteriosus into the aorta.

III. Blood Pressure.

The atria are at a lower average pressure than the ventricles because the muscle walls of the atria are thinner and cannot generate as great a force of contraction. The left side of the heart is at a higher average pressure than the right side because the heart walls are thicker. The left side generates a greater force on contraction.

A. **Systolic blood pressure** is the pressure during heart contraction.

B. **Diastolic blood pressure** is the pressure during heart relaxation and filling.

The Immune System

11

I. Introduction. Many mechanisms enable the human body to respond to foreign substances. However, the same mechanisms that allow the body to resist bacterial infections, for example, can also cause tissue injury and disease under certain circumstances (e.g., autoimmunity). Therefore, **immunity** is defined as **a reaction to foreign agents** without implying a physiologic or pathologic outcome of this reaction. According to this definition, **foreign agents include microbes** (e.g., bacteria, viruses, fungi, parasites), **microbe-infected host cells, cancer cells,** and **macromolecules** (e.g., protein, polysaccharides).

II. Types of Immunity

A. **Natural immunity** (also called innate or native immunity) describes those defense mechanisms that are present before exposure to foreign agents. Natural immunity reactions are nonspecific, and defense mechanisms include the following:

1. **Physicochemical barriers**—skin and mucous membranes

2. **Molecules in the blood circulation**—complement

3. **Immune cells**—phagocytic cells (macrophages, neutrophils) and natural killer cells

4. **Soluble mediators**—cytokines (regulating substances) derived from immune cells

B. **Acquired immunity** is the stimulation or induction of other defense mechanisms by exposure to foreign substances (i.e., antigens). These reactions are specific for distinct molecules and increase in magnitude and effectiveness with each subsequent exposure to the eliciting stimulus.

1. The acquired, or specific, immune system has a **memory function** in which **reactive cells linger** after the stimulus has been eradicated so they can quickly respond to future encounters. This type of immunity also has the capacity to **amplify natural immunity protective mechanisms** and to **direct these mechanisms to the site of entry** of the antigen.

2. **Features of specific immunity** include:

    a. **Physicochemical barriers**—cutaneous and mucosal immune systems; antibodies in mucosal secretions

    b. **Molecules in the blood circulation**—antibodies

c. **Immune cells**—lymphocytes

d. **Soluble mediators**—lymphocyte-derived cytokines

3. **Types of specific immunity** include:

    a. **Active immunity**—an individual's specific immune reaction on exposure to antigen. A **lag period** is required for the immune system to become activated.

    b. **Passive immunity**—specific immunity conferred on an individual via the transfer of cells or serum from another immune person. Upon transfer, the immune responses are **immediately active.**

4. **Classes of specific immunity** include:

    a. **Humoral immunity**—passive immunity acquired via the transfer of plasma or serum. It is mediated by antibodies released by B cells.

    b. **Cell-mediated immunity**—passive immunity acquired via the transfer of lymphocytic cells.

III. Cells

A. **Lymphocytes** are the basic units of the immune system. They are derived from a **common precursor cell in the bone marrow.**

1. **T cells** are those lymphocytes that mature only after passage through the thymus. They have receptors on their cell surface that enable them to recognize antigens presented by major histocompatibility complexes. T cells regulate cell-mediated immunity. There are several important types of T cells.

    a. **Cytotoxic T cells** cause direct killing of cells that express foreign antigens on their cell surface. As a result, cytotoxic T cells play an important role in the elimination of viral-infected cells, cancer cells, and cells with an intracellular pathogen. Cytotoxic T cells have a $CD8^+$ surface marker.

    b. **Helper T cells** promote the activities of other cells through the **synthesis and secretion of cytokines,** which are soluble factors that bind to receptors on the surface of a target cell and initiate a physiologic change in that cell. Helper T cells have a $CD4^+$ surface marker.

    c. **Suppressor T cells** inhibit the activities of certain cells through cytokine mediators. Suppressor T cells have a $CD4^+$ surface marker.

2. **B cells** are involved in **humoral immunity,** which is a defense mechanism mediated by antibodies. **Antibodies** (Figure 11-1) are produced by mature B cells, known as **plasma cells,** in response to foreign antigens. Antibodies are made by a process of genetic recombination. A specific antibody is generated against each antigen.

    a. The **structure of antibodies** differs based on how many units the antibodies contain. The basic unit is shown in Figure 11-1. Immunoglobulin G (IgG) is a monomer and contains one basic unit. Immunoglobulin M (IgM) is a pentamer, and is made of five monomeric units linked together.

    b. There are **five classes of antibodies,** with each class containing specific antibodies. Each class of antibody has a somewhat different function. The classes are immunoglobulins (Ig) G, M, A, D, and E.

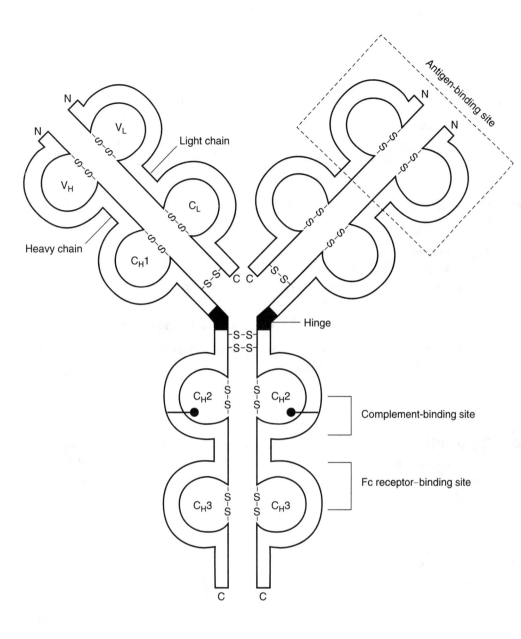

FIGURE 11-1.
Basic antibody structure. The structure shown is immunoglobulin G (IgG), which is a monomer.
V = variable region
C = constant region

Antigen-binding site

Light chain

Heavy chain

V_L

V_H

C_L

C_H1

Hinge

C_H2

C_H2

Complement-binding site

C_H3

C_H3

Fc receptor–binding site

●── Carbohydrate group

-S-S- Disulfide bond

(1) **IgG** is the major antibody in the bloodstream. It is usually the second antibody produced in an initial immune response. It crosses the placenta and, as a monomer, it has two antigen-binding sites.

(2) **IgM** is the primary antibody made in an immune response. As stated, it is a pentamer. Because it has a total of 10 antigen-binding sites, it is good for agglutinating bacteria.

(3) **IgA** is the primary antibody in secretions (e.g., saliva, breast milk). It is a dimer that has four antigen-binding sites.

(4) **IgE** is involved in allergic reactions and parasitic infections. It stimulates the release of histamine from mast cells and basophils. Structurally, it is a monomer.

(5) **IgD** helps B cells to recognize antigen. It is a membrane-bound monomer.

B. **Agranulocytes** are nongranular leukocytes. **Macrophages** are phagocytic agranulocytes that play a role in antigen presentation.

    1. **Phagocytosis.** Macrophages ingest bacteria, cell debris, and dead red blood cells. They scavenge for dead or damaged cells in the tissues.

    2. **Antigen presentation.** Macrophages have molecules on their surface called major histocompatibility complex molecules. These molecules present antigenic peptides on their cell surface so that T cells and B cells can recognize the antigen and initiate the appropriate response.

C. **Granulocytes** are multinucleated white blood cells that play a role in natural immune responses.

    1. **Neutrophils,** or polymorphonuclear cells, are phagocytic cells that are nonspecific in action because they do not involve a receptor-mediated event. They are effective in **phagocytosis of bacteria** nonspecifically.

    2. **Eosinophils** contain receptors for IgE on their cell surface. They participate in **defense against parasites** and in **allergic reactions.**

    3. **Basophils** generate **immediate hypersensitivity reactions** via their release of histamine when stimulated by IgE.

IV. Tissues

A. **Bone Marrow.** Blood cells, including those of the circulatory system, are produced in bone marrow. Some cells (e.g., B cells) complete maturation in the bone marrow; others require passage through other organs before gaining complete function (e.g., T cells must pass through the thymus). The cells of the bone marrow play a role in selecting the immune cells that react against self and subsequently destroying them.

B. **Spleen and Lymph Nodes** (Figure 11-2). Both the spleen and the lymph nodes are part of the lymphatic system (see Chapter 10 of the Biology Review Notes).

FIGURE 11-2.
Lymph node anatomy. Note that lymph ultimately returns to the bloodstream via the thoracic duct.

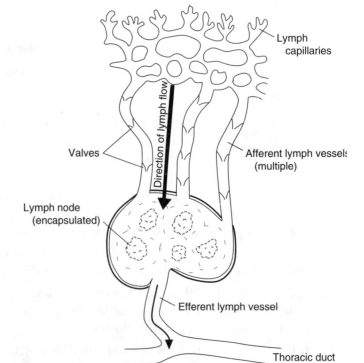

1. **Lymph nodes.** White blood cells segregate into specialized locations in the lymph nodes. As the lymph is filtered on its return to the circulatory system, foreign antigens are recognized by these immune cells, and an immune response is generated. This keeps bacteria from gaining access to the blood. Lymph nodes can be the site of cancer metastasis because they can be recognized as foreign.

2. **Spleen.** The spleen removes debris from circulating blood and clears defective red blood cells from the circulation. It also produces an immune response against foreign antigens.

12

The Digestive System

▓ I. Nutrition

A. **Introduction.** To meet energy requirements, organisms must ingest materials from the environment; these materials are usually present in the diet as polymers of simpler compounds. For the human body to use dietary components efficiently, it must first break down these complex polymers into their unit constituents. Larger substances are less readily absorbed by the intestinal epithelial cells. Furthermore, small subunits can be used more readily by the body to meet its own synthetic demands. The unit of measure for dietary energy is the **kilocalorie (kcal).**

B. **Nutrients**

   1. **Carbohydrates** yield 4 kcal of energy per gram and generally provide the greatest source of energy in the diet.

      a. Carbohydrates, or polysaccharides, are long chains of five- or six-carbon sugars called monosaccharides, which are the smallest functional units and cannot be further broken down.

         (1) **Monosaccharides** include glucose and fructose.
         (2) **Polysaccharides** include starch and glycogen.

      b. **Carbohydrate digestion** begins in the oral cavity with **salivary amylase** and is completed in the small intestine by exposure to **pancreatic amylase.** Intestinal epithelial cells absorb monosaccharides and disaccharides, which are further hydrolyzed into their monosaccharide subunits.

   2. **Fats** are lipids composed of the three-carbon molecule **glycerol** attached via phosphate linkages to **three fatty acids,** which contain long carbon polymer chains. When these carbon bonds are hydrolyzed, 9 kcal of energy are released per gram.

      a. **Saturated fatty acids** do not contain double bonds, whereas unsaturated molecules have either *cis* or *trans* double bonds.

      b. **Fat digestion** occurs when the hormone **cholecystokinin (CCK),** made in the lining of the duodenum, causes the release of **lipase** from the pancreas and **bile** from the gallbladder. These substances help emulsify the fat and form **micelles,** which are absorbed in the duodenum and jejunum.

3. **Proteins** are composed of chains of amino acids, which are the functional units. During proteolysis, 4 kcal of energy per gram are released from the hydrolysis of the peptide bonds.

   a. **Essential amino acids** must be consumed as part of the diet, whereas some other amino acids can be synthesized by the body.

   b. **Protein digestion** begins in the stomach by the action of **pepsin.** When the protein is transferred to the small intestine, CCK secretion is stimulated. This induces the release of **pancreatic proteolytic enzymes** (i.e., trypsin, chymotrypsin, elastase, numerous types of endopeptidase and exopeptidase). These enzymes complete protein digestion.

4. **Vitamins and minerals** are supplied to the body by the diet.

   a. **Vitamins** are organic molecules that aid in enzyme catalysis by acting as **coenzymes** [e.g., niacin is the coenzyme of nicotinamide adenine dinucleotide (NAD)]. They are either ingested or produced by bacteria within the gastrointestinal tract (e.g., vitamin K, vitamin B_{12}).

   b. **Minerals** are inorganic ions that can also aid in catalysis by acting as **prosthetic groups** (e.g., iron in the heme group of hemoglobin), in addition to playing roles in functions such as protein folding and electrochemical gradients.

II. Gastrointestinal Tract

A. Passage of Food

1. **Muscular control.** Food enters the body via the mouth and is eventually defecated through the anus (Figure 12-1).

   a. **Peristalsis,** which is a rhythmic, coordinated, wave-like movement of involuntary muscle contractions, propels ingested material unidirectionally through the digestive system.

   b. **Distention of a hollow organ** stimulates circular muscles to contract immediately behind the enlarged area. At the same time, the circular muscle in front of the enlarged area relaxes and the longitudinal muscle in between contracts, pushing the food bolus forward.

2. **Sphincters.** Sphincters are specialized rings of muscle that surround an orifice. The gastrointestinal tract is divided into compartments by several sphincters. Through contraction and relaxation, sphincters control the transition of food from one area to another.

   a. The **pyloric sphincter** governs the rate at which food enters the small intestine from the stomach.

   b. The **esophageal sphincters** prevent acidic stomach contents from moving back up into the esophagus.

   c. When there is **mechanical failure,** that is, when the esophageal or pyloric sphincters function abnormally, stomach acid can leak into the esophagus (heartburn) or the duodenum (ulcer formation).

3. **Secretions.** Enzymes assist in the digestion of nutrients. To make contact with the food, enzymes travel through ducts that empty into the gut lumen.

FIGURE 12-1.

The passage of food through the gut. On the *left*, a diagram of some of the major structures of the digestive tract is shown. On the *right*, the major structures of the digestive tract are listed in the order through which digesting food would pass.

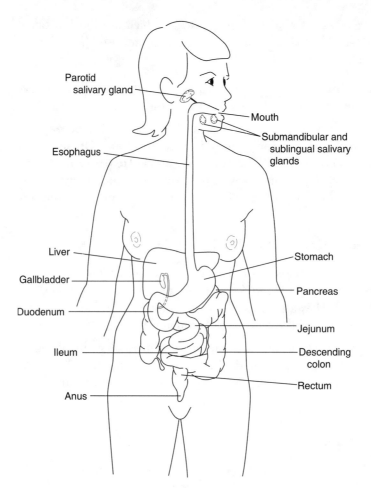

Mouth
Pharynx
Upper esophageal sphincter
Esophagus
Lower esophageal sphincter
Stomach
Pyloric sphincter
Duodenum
Jejunum
Ileum
Cecum
Ascending colon
Transverse colon
Descending colon
Sigmoid colon
Rectum
Anal sphincte
Anus

a. **Digestive enzymes are proteins.**

(1) Many digestive enzymes are released as **inactive precursors** called **zymogens,** or **preproenzymes** (Figure 12-2), which become active only when they reach the lumen of the gut.

(2) **Secretion of an inactive form** is thereby a means of **protection against self-digestion.**

(3) For example, **trypsin** is activated in the gut lumen only by stomach acid or by self-proteolysis by another trypsin molecule. Activated trypsin then goes on to activate the other digestive enzymes.

FIGURE 12-2.

The structure of zymogens.

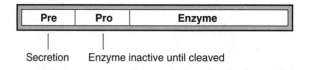

b. **The stimuli of gastrointestinal enzymes**.

B. Mouth and Pharynx. Food is taken into the mouth where it stimulates various sensations (e.g., taste, texture, odor, temperature). Digestion begins in the mouth and pharynx through two means.

1. **Mastication** is a mechanical manipulation that uses the teeth to break the food into smaller pieces.

2. Enzymatic breakdown occurs via the production of **saliva** by three pairs of salivary glands (i.e., parotid, submandibular, sublingual). Saliva acts to:

   a. Begin digestion of carbohydrates

   b. Lubricate food for easier passage into the esophagus

   c. Serve an antibacterial role through the action of **lysozymes**

C. Esophagus. The esophagus **transports the food** between the oral cavity and the stomach. The upper third of the esophagus is made of skeletal muscle, which is necessary for the voluntary action of swallowing. The middle third contains both skeletal and smooth muscle, and the lower third is smooth muscle. Smooth muscle, which undergoes involuntary movement, is under the control of the autonomic nervous system (see Chapter 8 of the Biology Review Notes). Smooth muscle lines the remaining gut wall of the gastrointestinal tract.

D. Stomach. The stomach stores, churns, and digests food. Digestion is accomplished through the **release of enzymes and acid.**

1. **Gastrin** is a hormone that is released early in the digestive process.

   a. **The release of gastrin from G cells is induced by:**

      (1) Stomach distention

      (2) Parasympathetic stimulation

      (3) Proteins in the stomach lumen

   b. **Gastrin stimulates:**

      (1) Stomach distention and motility (increased smooth muscle contraction and peristalsis)

      (2) The release of **pepsinogen,** which is converted to active **pepsin** by hydrochloric acid (HCl) and by pepsin proteins, from the chief cells

      (3) The secretion of HCl from parietal cells

2. To prevent damage to the stomach lining by acid, both **bicarbonate** (HCO_3^-) and **mucus** are produced, which, respectively, serve to neutralize the acid and to shield the stomach mucosa.

3. **Intrinsic factor** is a protein that binds to vitamin B_{12} and protects it from acid breakdown until it can be absorbed in the small intestine. Intrinsic factor is secreted by the parietal cells.

E. Small Intestine. Digestion is completed in the small intestine, and most of the absorption of nutrients occurs in the jejunum and the ileum.

1. To facilitate absorption, the lining of the intestine has numerous projections of gut mucosa (i.e., **villi**) and microscopic projections from the columnar epithelial cells (i.e., **microvilli**). Both of these modifications increase the surface area of the small intestine, assisting in both the absorption of nutrients and the secretion of mucus and enzymes.

2. The **duodenum** is the first region of the small intestine. It makes up approximately the first 12 inches of the human small intestine.

a. **Secretin** is a hormone whose release in the duodenum is stimulated by stomach acid. This hormone is produced by cells in the lining of the duodenum. Secretin has the following effects:

(1) Causes the pancreas to produce and secrete HCO_3^-

(2) Slows gastric motility and emptying

(3) Inhibits gastrin release

b. **CCK** is released in response to fatty acids and protein.

(1) **CCK stimulates the pancreas to release pancreatic enzymes:**

(a) **Trypsin** is released for protein digestion and activation of proenzymes.

(b) **Lipase** is released for fat digestion.

(c) **Amylase** is released for carbohydrate digestion.

(2) **CCK stimulates gallbladder contraction and emptying, which releases bile.** Bile is secreted by the liver, stored in the gallbladder, and released into the duodenum. Bile contains bile salts, cholesterol, and bilirubin (which is a product of hemoglobin degradation). Bile salts act like detergent to emulsify fats.

3. The **jejunum** is the upper two thirds of the small intestine. It releases enzymes (e.g., maltase, carboxypeptidase) and absorbs the majority of digesting nutrients.

4. The **ileum** is the lower one third of the small intestine. It completes nutrient absorption, and it reabsorbs bile acids for recycling.

F. **Colon.** The colon has several subdivisions, including the **cecum,** the **ascending colon,** the **transverse colon,** the **descending colon,** and the **sigmoid colon.** The colon serves several functions.

1. The colon **reabsorbs water and electrolytes** and thus has a role in osmoregulation.

2. The colon **forms and stores stool** for elimination from the body.

III. Accessory Organs (Figure 12-3)

FIGURE 12-3.
Anatomy of the upper gastrointestinal tract. (Reproduced with permission from Ville CA, Solomon EP, Davis PW: *Biology.* Philadelphia, Saunders College Publishing, 1985, p 703.)

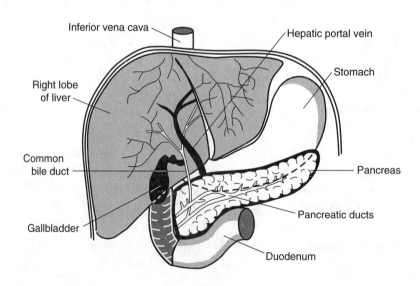

A. **Liver.** The liver is the most important metabolic organ. Functions of the liver are listed in Table 12-1.

TABLE 12-1. Functions of the liver.

Regulation of blood glucose via glycogen storage

Storage of essential vitamins

Interconversion of nutrients

Detoxification of drugs, including alcohol

Protective immunity via Kupffer cells (liver macrophages)

Destruction of RBCs (in addition to spleen)

Production and secretion of bile

Production of urea from ammonia (toxic), a byproduct of protein metabolism

Synthesis of plasma proteins (e.g., albumin, clotting proteins)

Manufacture of blood cells during embryogenesis

Release of HCO_3^-

Manufacture of lipoproteins for cholesterol transport

RBCs = red blood cells.

B. **Pancreas.** The pancreas serves both an endocrine function (see Chapter 9 of the Biology Review Notes) and an exocrine function. The exocrine pancreas is involved in digestion through its **production of pancreatic juice.** Pancreatic juice neutralizes stomach acid with bicarbonate ion, and it provides the enzymes necessary for the digestion of carbohydrates, fats, and proteins.

The Excretory System

I. The Role of the Excretory System in Body Homeostasis.

The ability to survive in osmotically unstable environments has been achieved by evolution of effective excretory systems. The simplest and smallest aquatic organisms use diffusion into the surrounding water to excrete metabolic wastes. Higher order animals, which have circulatory systems, have evolved kidneys through which blood passes and is filtered. **Kidney functions include:**

1. **Fluid and Electrolyte Balance**

2. **Control of Blood Pressure**

3. **Acid–base Balance**

4. **Stimulation of the Bone Marrow to Produce Red Blood Cells**

II. Mammalian Kidney Structure and Function

A. Gross Anatomy (Figure 13-1)

1. **Location.** The kidneys are paired organs lying behind the abdominal organs on each side of the body. They lie behind the peritoneum, against the ribs of the middle to lower back.

2. **Size.** The human kidney is approximately the size of a fist and accounts for less than 1% of total body weight.

3. **Blood flow and filtration.** The kidneys receive a massive blood flow—approximately 20% of the cardiac output. The kidneys filter plasma up to 125 ml/min, which approaches 170 L/day.

4. **Outer covering.** The kidney is covered with the renal capsule, which is a thin layer of connective tissue.

5. **Two functional regions produce urine:**

   a. The **cortex** is the outer functional layer.

   b. The **medulla** is the inner functional layer.

6. **Associated structures.** A **papilla** extends from the cortex into the medulla. The papilla funnels urine into the **renal pyramids,** which carry

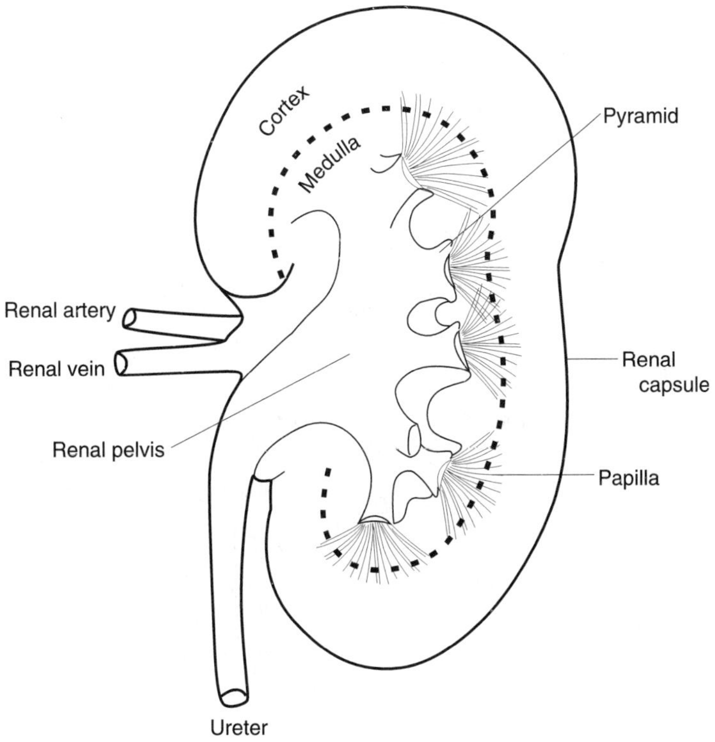

FIGURE 13-1.
The gross anatomy of
the human kidney.

urine to the **renal pelvis,** which is the hollow collecting chamber of
the kidney. The renal pelvis gives rise to the **ureters,** which are tubes
that carry urine to the **urinary bladder.** Urine leaves the bladder via the
urethra.

B. Microscopic Anatomy and Function

1. The **nephron is the functional unit of the kidney.** The human kidney con-
    tains more than 1,000,000 nephrons. The main purpose of the nephron is to al-
    low filtering of blood plasma, allowing resorption and secretion of key elec-
    trolytes and nutrients. The end product of this activity is the production of a
    concentrated urine.

2. To understand the function of the kidney, the **anatomy of the microcircula-
    tion** in the kidney must be known (Figure 13-2).

    a. **Toward the kidneys.** Blood enters the kidney from the **aorta** by the **re-
        nal artery.** The renal artery branches many times and gives rise to almost
        1,000,000 end branches known as **afferent arterioles.** The afferent arte-
        rioles lead to a complex capillary network called the **glomerulus.**

    b. **Away from the kidneys.** The **glomerular capillaries** are shaped like a
        ball of yarn, and they have pores that allow electrolytes and small mole-
        cules (i.e., molecules with molecular weights less than 200) to filter out of
        the blood. The blood that does not filter out of the glomerulus travels
        through the **efferent arterioles** to the **vasa recta vessels,** which reab-
        sorb water and solutes from the interstitial space. Blood eventually returns
        to the **renal vein** and the **vena cava.**

3. The **anatomy of the tubules** is also important in nephron function.

    a. The nephron begins at the **Bowman capsule,** which is a structure com-
        posed of a single cell layer that is adjacent to the glomerulus. **Blood fil-
        trate,** which filters out of the glomerulus, accumulates in the Bowman
        capsule.

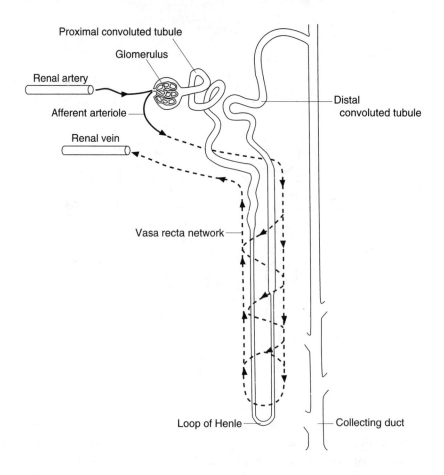

FIGURE 13-2.
The microscopic anatomy of the nephron. Note that the arrows show the direction of blood flow.

Proximal convoluted tubule

Glomerulus

Renal artery

Afferent arteriole

Renal vein

Distal convoluted tubule

Vasa recta network

Loop of Henle

Collecting duct

---

  b. From the capsule, the filtrate moves into the **proximal convoluted tubule.**

  c. From this tubule, the filtrate travels around a hairpin turn known as the **loop of Henle.**

  d. Filtrate then moves up a **thin ascending limb,** followed by a **thick ascending limb,** eventually reaching the **distal convoluted tubule.**

  e. The distal convoluted tubule empties directly into a **collecting duct,** which eventually drains into the **renal pelvis.**

C. Formation of Urine (Figure 13-3)

  1. Urine formation begins with the **ultrafiltration** of blood plasma and the accumulation of ultrafiltrate in the lumen of the Bowman capsule.

    a. Extensive filtration. Up to **25% of the water and solutes** flowing through the glomerulus is filtered into the Bowman space.

    b. Pressure difference. The driving force for filtration is the difference between hydrostatic pressure (blood pressure) and osmotic pressure in the glomerulus. The difference approaches **45 mm Hg.**

    c. Weight limitation. Because of the pore size of the glomerular capillaries, only particles with molecular weights less than several hundred can be filtered. Glucose, electrolytes, amino acids, and urea are filtered, whereas albumin, cells, and other large proteins are not filtered.

  2. Of the 170 L of plasma that are filtered per day, the **final urine volume** is only approximately 1.5 L. Thus, more than 99% of water and a large proportion of the electrolytes are reabsorbed.

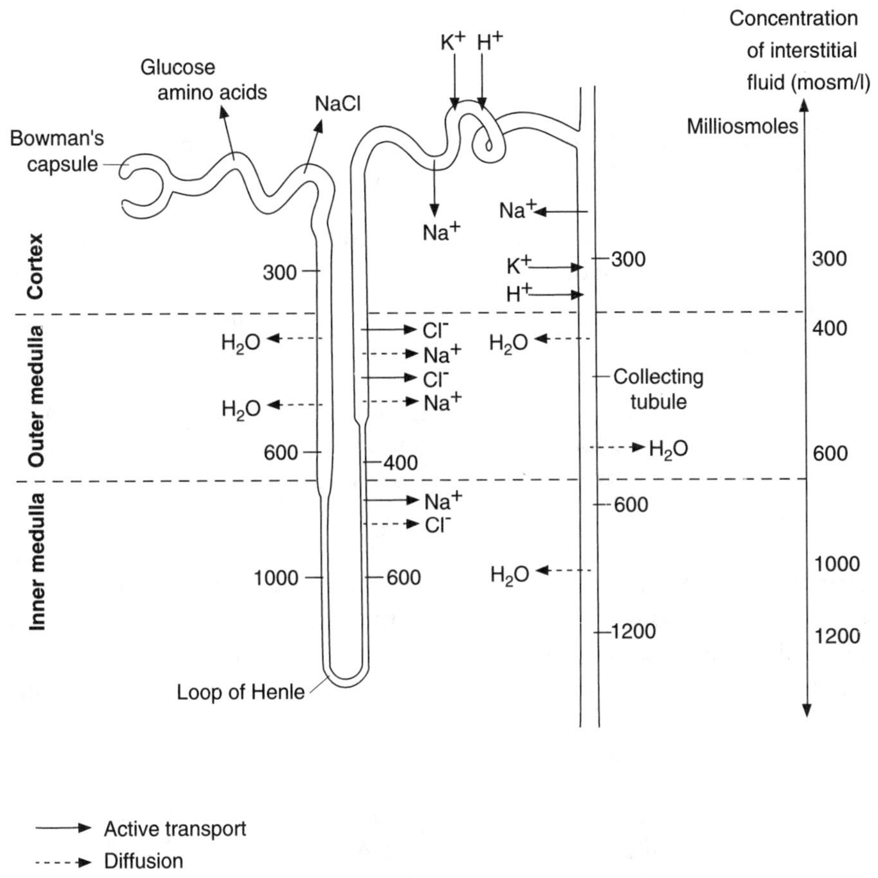

FIGURE 13-3.
The formation of urine.

→ Active transport

----→ Diffusion

3. Some substances appear in the urine in a concentration higher than in the blood. These substances are **selectively secreted** from the renal tubules into the urine.

4. From the Bowman capsule, the filtrate moves into the **descending limb of the loop of Henle.**

   a. The descending limb has very low permeability to sodium and chloride ions, and no active transport occurs there.

   b. This tubule is very permeable to water.

   c. A strong NaCl gradient exists in the interstitial space in this region.

5. The **thin ascending limb** is permeable to sodium and chloride ions, and some investigators believe that active transport of sodium ions occurs there.

6. The **thick ascending limb** shows almost no permeability to water and exhibits active transport of chloride ions from the lumen of the tubule into the interstitial space. Sodium ions passively follow.

7. The **distal convoluted tubule** is very active in transport.

   a. **Active transport of sodium ions** followed by the **passive movement of chloride ions** occurs there.

   b. Other distinct active transport proteins allow for a variety of other ions to be transported.

   (1) **Potassium–hydrogen ion cotransport** occurs. Potassium ions are excreted into the lumen from the tubule cell along with hydrogen ions. This cotransport provides a mechanism by which the body can excrete potassium ions and control its acid–base balance with hydrogen ions.

(2) The steroid hormone **aldosterone** plays a role in controlling the sodium ion and potassium–hydrogen ion transport in the distal tubule and in the collecting duct.

8. The **collecting duct** removes water from the hypotonic fluid entering the distal tubule and thereby produces hyperosmotic urine.

   a. **Antidiuretic hormone (ADH), or vasopressin,** must be present for the collecting duct to be permeable to water.

   b. In the **absence of ADH,** the duct is impermeable to water, and much water from the contents of the lumen is lost.

9. **Urine that leaves the collecting duct is concentrated** and contains the following: large amounts of nitrogenous waste (i.e., urea), less than 1% of the water and salts that were filtered, and secreted substances (e.g., drugs, toxins).

D. **Concentration Mechanism.** Although microscopically thin, the nephron is very long and spans from the cortex to the medulla of the kidney. Because the descending limb is water permeable but salts do not leave the tubule lumen, the osmolarity of urine increases as urine travels down the descending limb and is maximum at the loop of Henle. The loop of Henle is water impermeable, and salts stay in the tubule lumen.

1. As salts either leave the tubule passively or actively in the water-impermeable ascending limb, the urine osmolarity decreases. Finally, when urine passes down the collecting duct, it becomes **reconcentrated** because a tremendous amount of water leaves the urine (via ADH), concentrating the remaining solutes.

2. A **countercurrent feature** in the organization of the circulation of the nephron aids in maintaining the concentration gradient of the interstitium.

   a. The flow of urine in the tubules is opposite the flow of blood in the vasa recta (see Figure 13-2).

   b. Vasa recta blood flow begins at the thick ascending limb and flows around the loop of Henle to the thin descending limb.

   c. By selective resorption of salts and water, this countercurrent system aids in maintaining the concentration gradient of the interstitial fluid.

3. The **vasa recta vessels** form loop-like networks around each nephron.

   a. **Blood descends from the cortex** into the deeper portions of the medulla and forms the vasa recta networks.

   b. The **vasa recta then ascends toward the cortex.** Moving from the cortex to the medulla, blood in the vasa recta takes up salt and gives up water osmotically to balance the increasing osmotic load of the interstitial fluid.

   c. **As blood returns toward the cortex** from the medulla in the vasa recta network, the blood gives up salt and takes in water as it encounters an interstitial fluid of progressively lower osmolarity.

   d. The purpose of this system is to **maintain the concentration gradient of the interstitial fluid.** The vasa recta takes up salts and gives up water in the salty medulla, and it gives up salt and takes in water in the dilute cortex.

E. Hormonal Influences on the Nephron

1. **Aldosterone,** which is a steroid hormone produced in the adrenal cortex, acts on the distal convoluted tubule of the nephron.

   a. Aldosterone increases the active transport of **potassium ions** into the urine for **excretion** and of **sodium ions** from the urine into the cell for **reabsorption.**

   b. Aldosterone plays a major role in the **regulation of blood pressure** by controlling the level of sodium in the blood. Sodium retention in the body increases blood pressure by holding body water.

2. **ADH allows water reabsorption** from the collecting duct of the nephron.

   a. ADH is believed to **create pores** in the cells of the duct to allow massive water permeability and reabsorption.

   b. ADH is controlled by a **feedback regulation system.** Low blood pressure of high plasma osmolarity stimulates the hypothalamus to release ADH to the posterior pituitary gland.

   c. From the posterior pituitary, ADH is released into the bloodstream, where it reaches the target tissue in the nephron.

3. **The renin–angiotensin system** is another important hormonal system.

   a. The **juxtaglomerular apparatus** is a group of cells found where the afferent arteriole approximates the distal tubule (Figure 13-4).

   b. Stimulation by the **sympathetic nervous system** in times of low blood pressure, dehydration, or stress causes cells of the juxtaglomerular apparatus to release the enzyme **renin.**

   c. Renin enters the circulation, where it converts a serum protein that is made in the liver, **angiotensinogen,** to a decapeptide called **angiotensin I.**

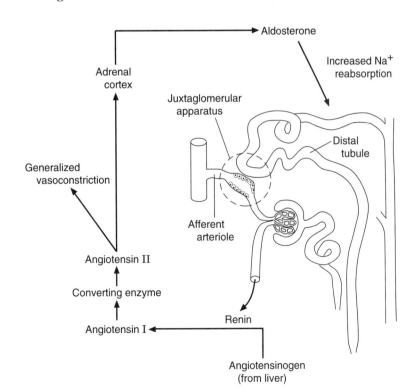

FIGURE 13-4.
The renin–angiotensin system.

d. Angiotensin I passes through the circulation. When it enters the lung, it encounters a converting enzyme, which removes two amino acids and leaves an eight-residue peptide, or **angiotensin II.** Angiotensin II has two important roles.

(1) Angiotensin II is a **strong vasoconstrictor,** thus it increases blood pressure.

(2) It also **stimulates secretion of aldosterone,** which retains sodium and thereby increases blood pressure.

The Muscles and the Skeletal System

I. Muscle System

A. Functions

1. **Controlled movement and posture.** Muscle cells, like neurons, can propagate action potentials. However, unlike neurons, muscle cells can also contract and generate force. This characteristic enables the body to control the movement of body parts and posture.

2. **Muscle pairs.** Muscles tend to contract in groups rather than in isolation. Because the force of a muscle contraction can generate a pull but not a push, muscles tend to be arranged in antagonistic pairs.

    a. **Flexors** bend parts of the body across joints, and **extensors** straighten them.

    b. **Abductors** move limbs away from the body's central axis, and **adductors** move them toward the central axis.

    c. **Levators** raise body parts, and **depressors** lower them.

    d. **Pronators** move parts of the body downward and backward, and **supinators** move them upward and forward.

    e. **Sphincters** close hollow body parts, and **dilators** enlarge them.

B. Structural Organization (Figure 14-1)

1. A **muscle fiber** is a single muscle cell. Muscle fibers are multinucleated, and they contain contractile filaments in their cytoplasm. Muscle fibers are arranged parallel to one another (see Figure 14-1). For a detailed description of muscle cell structure and the mechanism of muscle contraction, refer to Chapter 7 of the Biology Review Notes.

2. **Tendons** attach muscles to bones. The point of attachment that remains relatively fixed during contraction is called the **origin,** and the more mobile attachment site is termed the **insertion** (Figure 14-2).

C. Types of Muscle. There are three types of muscle: **skeletal, cardiac,** and **smooth** (Table 14-1).

FIGURE 14-1.
The structure of
skeletal muscle.

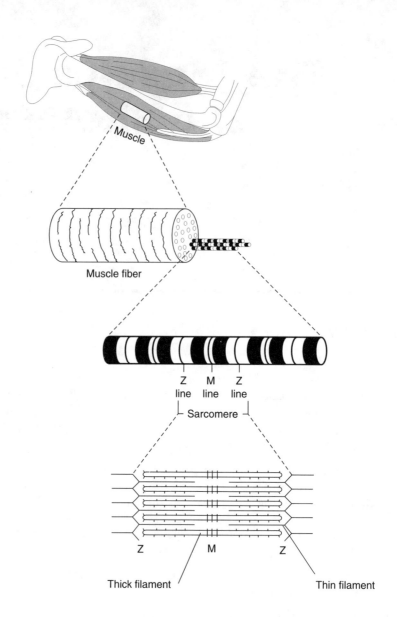

Muscle

Muscle fiber

Z
line　M
line　Z
line

Sarcomere

Z　M　Z

Thick filament　Thin filament

FIGURE 14-2.
Anatomy of the upper arm.

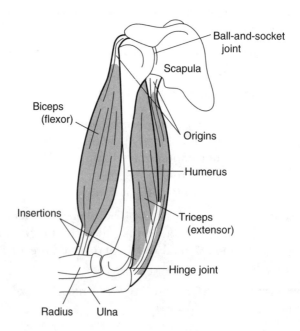

Ball-and-socket
joint

Scapula

Biceps
(flexor)

Origins

Humerus

Insertions

Triceps
(extensor)

Hinge joint

Radius　Ulna

TABLE 14-1. Comparison of muscle type-specific characteristics.

Characteristics	Skeletal	Cardiac	Smooth
Location	Attached to bones or cartilage via tendons	Heart tissue	Lining of hollow organs (e.g., gut, blood vessels)
Cell shape	Large, elongated, cylindrical, and blunt ends	Short, branching, and arranged end to end	Spindle shaped, flattened, and pointed ends
Number and location of nuclei	Multinucleated/peripheral	Multinucleated/central	One/central
Striations	Present	Present	Absent
Blood supply	Good	Rich	Fair
Control of contraction	Voluntary	Involuntary	Involuntary
Speed of contraction	Most rapid	Intermediate	Slowest
Ability to remain contracted	Least	Intermediate	Greatest

D. Nervous Control

1. **Muscles** are innervated by both **sensory and motor nerve fibers.** Motor innervation can be somatic or autonomic, depending on the type of muscle (see Chapter 8 of the Biology Review Notes).

2. **Transverse tubule** carries action potentials deep into the muscle tissue. Therefore, when an action potential from the nervous system causes depolarization of muscle fibers, the reaction of the muscle (i.e., contraction) can be better coordinated and synchronous because the depolarization is centrally located.

II. Skeletal System

A. Function. The human skeletal system is an **endoskeleton,** that is, it is internal, in contrast to the **exoskeleton** of insects, which is external. The function of the skeletal system is to:

1. **Support the structures** of the body

2. **Provide attachment sites** for muscle fibers

3. **Form blood cells**

4. **Store inorganic ions** (i.e., calcium, phosphorus)

5. **Protect internal organs** from injury

B. Structure

1. **Basic concepts** of the skeletal system are as follow:

   a. The human skeletal system is made up of both **cartilage** (see II D) and **bone.**

   b. A **joint** is the site where two or more bones join, or **articulate.**

   c. **Ligaments** attach bones to one another.

2. The **axial and appendicular skeletons** are the two subdivisions of the human skeletal system.

    a. The **axial skeleton** is made up of the bones that form the trunk and skull of the body. Its main function is to **protect internal organs.** The axial skeleton includes:

        (1) Vertebral column

        (2) Ribs and sternum

        (3) Fused bones of the skull

    b. The **appendicular skeleton provides support** for the appendages of the upper and lower extremities. Included in this subdivision are:

        (1) Bones of the shoulders and pelvis

        (2) Arms, wrists, hands

        (3) Legs, ankles, feet

3. **Several types of bones are based on shape.**

    a. **Long bones** include the femur, tibia, radius, and ulna.

    b. **Short bones** include the wrist and ankle bones.

    c. **Flat bones** include the cranial bones, sternum, and ribs.

    d. **Irregular bones** include the vertebrae.

4. There are several major **types of joints.**

    a. **Ball and socket joints** include the hip and shoulder joints, which give **many types of movement.**

    b. **Hinge joints** include the elbow and knee, which allow **motion in one plane only.**

    c. **Condylar joints** include the jaw joint, which allows **motion in two planes.**

    d. **Rotating joints** include the radius and ulna, which **only allow rotation.**

C. Bone

1. **Structure.** Bone is a specialized type of connective tissue (see Chapter 7 of the Biology Review Notes). Bone tissue is composed of cells that are embedded in a matrix of organic fibers and inorganic ions.

    a. **Cells**

        (1) **Osteoblasts** are cells in the active synthesis of bone matrix. They are stimulated by growth hormone.

        (2) **Osteocytes** are dormant osteoblasts that have surrounded themselves with matrix. They can be reactivated when a bone is injured.

        (3) **Osteoclasts** are multinucleated cells that remodel bone and release inorganic (i.e., calcium, phosphorus) and organic components. They are stimulated by parathyroid hormone.

b. Matrix

(1) Organic matrix includes collagen fibers (mostly type I) and glycoproteins.

(2) Inorganic matrix consists of ions, of which the most abundant form is calcium phosphate in a crystalline form called **hydroxyapatite**.

2. Types

a. Primary (immature) bone is the first bone formed in the fetus. It is also found during bone repair (i.e., it is temporary). Primary bone has irregular arrays of collagen and a low inorganic content.

b. Mature bone

(1) Spongy bone is found in the marrow space of long bones (Figure 14-3). Characteristics of the structure of spongy bone include the following:

(a) Interconnected trabeculae forming meshwork

(b) Bone marrow present in the spaces of the meshwork

(2) Compact bone is the hard, outer layer of bone (see Figure 14-3C). The structure of compact bone, which is solid and mature, is made up of numerous concentric units called **osteons** or **haversian systems.** Each osteon has central blood vessels and concentric rings of osteocytes embedded in a bone matrix.

FIGURE 14-3.
Bone anatomy. In **A),** note the periosteum, a fibrous outer layer over the bone. The compact bone is the outer layer of bone. The spongy bone is the inner layer. In **B),** the osteons (haversian systems), which are the small, functional units of mature bone, are shown. In **C),** the microstructure of an osteon is demonstrated. Note the lacunae containing osteocytes.

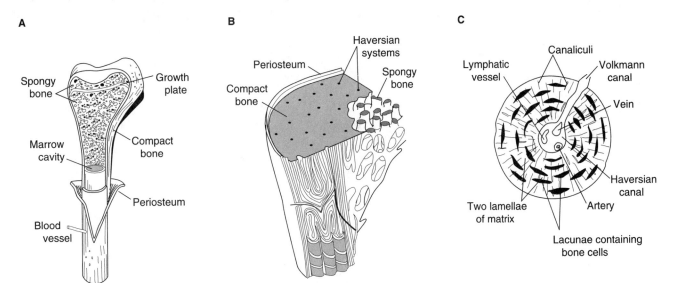

(a) Volkmann's canals carry blood vessels into the bone tissue from the outside.

(b) Haversian canals enclose blood vessels that bring nutrients to the osteon or haversian system.

(c) Lacunae are spaces in the bone matrix that contain the cell bodies of osteocytes.

(d) Canaliculi are networks of passageways between the lacunae that allow osteocytes to communicate and exchange nutrients.

3. **Bone formation**

    a. **Intramembranous bone** forms directly from connective tissue without a cartilage precursor. Examples include the bones of the skull.

    b. **Endochondral bone** forms from a cartilage precursor. The cartilage is reabsorbed and replaced by bone tissue. Examples include the long bones of the body (e.g., humerus, femur).

4. **Bone growth**

    a. Growth of the **periosteum** increases the **width** of bone. The periosteum is a fibrous layer of connective tissue that covers bone. It contains cells that can mature into osteoblasts or osteoclasts.

    b. Growth of the **epiphyseal plates** increases the **length** of bone. Epiphyseal plates (growth plates) are cartilaginous structures between the **diaphysis** (shaft) and **epiphysis** (end) of a bone. These structures function through puberty, then calcify and no longer function.

D. Cartilage. During embryogenesis, cartilage is the structure of support, although much of it is later replaced by bone tissue in the adult. Because cartilage is firm yet elastic, its support network is flexible. Cartilage does not contain blood vessels (therefore, diffusion provides nutrients), nor does it contain nerves or lymph vessels. Cartilage is found throughout the body, including the ears, nose, ribs, and joints.

1. **Hyaline cartilage** covers the ends of articulating bones to reduce friction.

2. **Chondrocytes,** or cartilage cells, secrete a hard, rubbery matrix and collagen fibers around themselves. Chondrocytes are the primary cells found in cartilage.

The Respiratory System ⒖

I. Function and Basic Anatomy of the Airways and Lungs

A. Function. Animals use oxygen and produce carbon dioxide during the process of cellular respiration. Organisms that are smaller than 0.5 mm in diameter can use diffusion alone for gas exchange. As organisms become larger, diffusion distances are increased and the ratio of surface area to volume is reduced. A circulatory system and respiratory system has evolved in larger animals to facilitate gas exchange.

B. Anatomy (Figure 15-1)

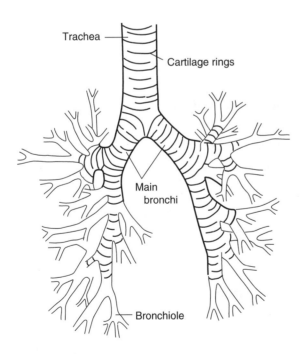

Trachea

Cartilage rings

Main bronchi

Bronchiole

FIGURE 15-1.
The airways of the lung.

1. **Structures of the airways** include the nose, mouth, pharynx, larynx, and trachea. Air enters the **nose** or **mouth** and moves into the **pharynx.** The pharynx is the upper throat and is located behind the nasal passages and behind the tongue. Air then moves into the **larynx,** the area of the

lower throat where the vocal cords are located. Air must pass between the two vocal cords to enter the **trachea.**

   a. The trachea is a rigid tube made of cartilaginous rings.

   b. The trachea is rigid to prevent collapse from the negative pressures generated during inspiration.

2. Regions of the airways

   a. The **main bronchi** are the two main branches of the trachea. There is a left and right main bronchus.

   b. **Bronchioles** are the smaller sets of branches created each time the main bronchus divides (which is more than 20 times). Most of the early branches have a cartilage-supported wall and are stiff. The later branches have smooth muscle in the wall, which allows for dilation or contraction.

   c. The **alveolus** is the smallest structure at the end of the branched network. Alveoli are lined with single cells and are spherical chambers where most gas exchange occurs (Figure 15-2). Gas exchange largely occurs across the cell membranes of the alveoli. There are more than 300 million alveoli in adult human lungs.

FIGURE 15-2.
The smallest components of the respiratory tree.

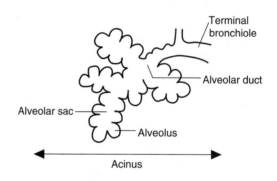

   d. **Alveolar sacs** rise from clusters of alveoli, and alveolar sacs communicate with one another via **alveolar ducts.**

   e. The **terminal bronchiole** carries the air to the alveolar network.

   f. An **acinus** is an alveolar network supplied by one terminal bronchiole.

3. Surfactant is a lipid material that lines alveoli. This substance decreases the surface tension of the spherical alveoli and reduces the likelihood of alveoli collapsing. Some premature infants have respiratory distress and alveolar collapse because they do not produce adequate amounts of surfactant.

II. Hemoglobin, Gas Exchange, and Respiratory Equations

A. Hemoglobin. Hemoglobin is a respiratory pigment that is the main oxygen carrier in the blood.

   1. Structure. Hemoglobin is a large molecule with a molecular weight of 68,000.

   a. Each molecule contains **four subunits,** and each subunit contains **a polypeptide chain** and **heme,** which is an iron-containing prosthetic group.

b. **Polypeptide chains** are either **alpha** or **beta.** Each hemoglobin molecule contains two alpha and two beta chains. Each chain has a heme moiety associated with it.

2. **Binding properties.** Each subunit can bind one molecule of oxygen. Thus, **one hemoglobin molecule can bind four oxygen molecules.** The binding of the first oxygen molecule makes the binding of the next oxygen molecule easier, which is referred to as **positive cooperativity.**

3. **Myoglobin versus hemoglobin. Myoglobin is a** storage pigment for oxygen located in muscle tissue. The major structural difference between myoglobin and hemoglobin is that myoglobin has only one subunit containing one heme group. Myoglobin can bind only one oxygen molecule, so it does not demonstrate positive cooperativity.

4. **Hemoglobin–myoglobin dissociation curves** (Figure 15-3). The dissociation curves show partial pressure of oxygen (PO_2) on the x-axis and the percentage of hemoglobin or myoglobin saturated with oxygen on the y-axis. Room air contains approximately 150 mm Hg of oxygen. Note that the curve for myoglobin is **hyperbolic,** whereas the curve for hemoglobin is **sigmoid.**

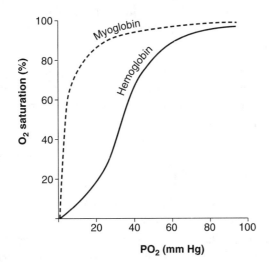

FIGURE 15-3.
The dissociation curves for hemoglobin and myoglobin.

a. **Myoglobin** has one heme group and binds only one oxygen molecule, so it quickly saturates with oxygen.

b. **Hemoglobin** is slower to take up its first oxygen molecule, and the binding of each subsequent oxygen molecule makes further binding easier (i.e., positive cooperativity), causing the upturn and sigmoid shape of the curve.

c. **Both curves flatten** as the pigments become fully oxygen bound.

5. **Factors affecting the dissociation curves.** The **oxygen affinity of hemoglobin** is labile. Affinity can be increased by decreasing temperature, basic blood pH, or low levels of diphosphoglycerate (DPG). This causes the hemoglobin–oxygen dissociation curve to shift to the left. Oxygen affinity of hemoglobin can be reduced by the following factors, which shift the curve to the right (Figure 15-4):

a. **Increases in temperature** make it more difficult to load hemoglobin with oxygen. Hemoglobin also gives up oxygen more easily at high temperatures. At high body temperatures, the rate of metabolism is higher, and the need for oxygen at the tissue level is greater.

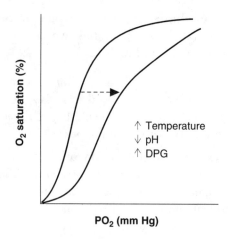

b. When **carbon dioxide concentration is increased,** carbon dioxide is converted to carbonic acid and **blood pH decreases.** A decrease in blood pH makes it more difficult to load hemoglobin with oxygen and makes oxygen unloading to the tissues easier. The effect of pH on hemoglobin–oxygen affinity is called the **Bohr effect.** The enhanced unloading of oxygen by hemoglobin is useful in periods of exercise, stress, or increased blood acidity.

c. **Increases in DPG.** Increases in the products of anaerobic metabolism decrease the affinity of hemoglobin for oxygen and increase the unloading of oxygen to the tissues. DPG is produced in anaerobic metabolism (glycolysis) and has a direct effect on hemoglobin. When anaerobic conditions exist, DPG levels rise, and oxygen is given up more easily by hemoglobin. This makes more oxygen available at the tissue level to provide for oxidative metabolism.

6. **Fetal hemoglobin.** The fetus has its own hemoglobin, and there must be a driving force for the diffusion of oxygen from the maternal side of the placenta to the fetal side. Fetal hemoglobin has a **higher oxygen affinity than adult hemoglobin;** this is what enhances oxygen transfer from mother to fetus. Therefore, the fetal hemoglobin–oxygen dissociation curve is to the left of the adult curve.

B. Gas Exchange

1. **Diffusion.** Oxygen must diffuse from the lumen of the alveolus to a red blood cell, and carbon dioxide must diffuse from the red blood cell or plasma to the alveolus.

2. **Layers.** Gases must diffuse through several layers (Figure 15-5). These layers are listed here in the order in which gas molecules encounter the structures:

   a. Fluid surface film of the alveolus (surfactant)

   b. Alveolar lining (membrane)

   c. Interstitial layer

   d. Capillary endothelial lining

   e. Blood plasma

   f. Wall of the red blood cell (membrane)

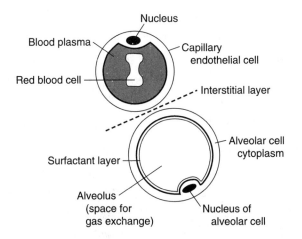

Nucleus

Blood plasma

Red blood cell

Capillary endothelial cell

Interstitial layer

Surfactant layer

Alveolar cell cytoplasm

Alveolus (space for gas exchange)

Nucleus of alveolar cell

FIGURE 15-5.

Schematic diagram showing the microscopic anatomy of gas exchange (in cross section).

C. Equations for Oxygen Loading and Unloading (Figure 15-6)

1. **Reactions at the red blood cells.** A series of important reactions occur at the red blood cell.

   a. **Hydrogen ion** plays an important role in oxygen loading and unloading. Hydrogen ion **binds to hemoglobin (Hb) to form HHb** (un-ionized hemoglobin). Hemoglobin is in the HHb form in the red blood cells that enter the lung (see Figure 15-6A). When a red blood cell approaches an alveolus, **oxygen** diffuses through the various layers to enter the red blood cell.

   b. **Oxygen** then moves to the HHb where it displaces the hydrogen ion from hemoglobin and **binds to hemoglobin itself, forming HbO$_2$**

FIGURE 15-6.

Equations showing oxygen loading and unloading at **A)** the red blood cell–alveolus interface and **B)** the red blood cell–tissue interface.

A

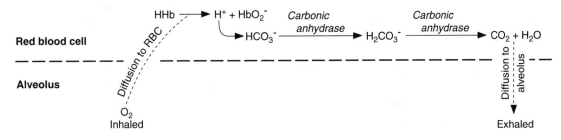

Red blood cell

Alveolus

HHb $\longrightarrow$ H$^+$ + HbO$_2^-$ — *Carbonic anhydrase* — *Carbonic anhydrase*

HCO$_3^-$ $\longrightarrow$ H$_2$CO$_3^-$ $\longrightarrow$ CO$_2$ + H$_2$O

Diffusion to RBC

O$_2$ Inhaled

Diffusion to alveolus

Exhaled

B

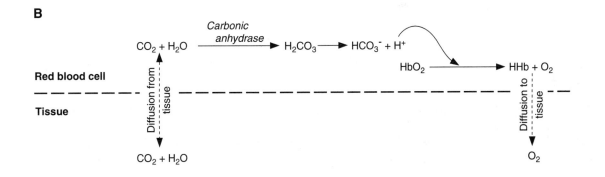

Red blood cell

Tissue

CO$_2$ + H$_2$O — *Carbonic anhydrase* $\longrightarrow$ H$_2$CO$_3$ $\longrightarrow$ HCO$_3^-$ + H$^+$

HbO$_2$ $\longrightarrow$ HHb + O$_2$

Diffusion from tissue

CO$_2$ + H$_2$O

Diffusion to tissue

O$_2$

     c.   The **displaced hydrogen ion binds to bicarbonate ion** in the cytoplasm of the red cell where **carbonic acid is formed (H_2CO_3).**

     d.   An enzyme called **carbonic anhydrase** then **converts carbonic acid to CO_2 and H_2O.** The carbon dioxide and water diffuse out of the red blood cell where they are expelled (i.e., exhaled).

  2.   **Reverse reactions at the tissues** (see Figure 15-6B)

     a. HbO_2 is the form of hemoglobin that carries oxygen to the tissues.

     b.   At the tissues, CO_2 and H_2O, products of oxidative metabolism, diffuse into the red cell. Carbonic anhydrase converts them to carbonic acid. Carbonic acid dissociates into hydrogen ion and bicarbonate ion.

     c.   The hydrogen ion displaces the oxygen from the HbO_2 and binds to Hb, forming HHb.

     d.   The bicarbonate ion stays in the red cell cytoplasm or diffuses out to the plasma.

     e.   The cycle repeats itself as HHb moves to the lungs to pick up more oxygen and to unload carbon dioxide and water.

III. Mechanics of Breathing

A. Inhalation and Exhalation

  1.   **Inhalation (inspiration)** requires energy and is an active process.

     a.   **Action.** During inhalation, the **diaphragm contracts** and pushes down on the liver and intestines. The intercostal muscles located between the ribs contract and move the rib cage upward and outward. The action is similar to that of a bellows.

     b.   **Function.** The function of the inspiratory muscles is to **increase the volume of the thorax.** As the volume of the thorax increases, the pressure within the airways of the lungs decreases with respect to the pressure outside the lungs.

  2.   The **pressure differential** brings air into the lungs. Air is not sucked into the airways; air is attracted into the airways by the pressure gradient created by increased thoracic volume.

  3.   **Exhalation (expiration)** is usually a passive process. (However, exhalation can be forceful when neck muscles are contracted and a different set of intercostal muscles are used.)

     a.   **Action.** The diaphragm relaxes and moves superiorly. The liver and intestines push back up on the base of the lungs. The intercostal muscles relax, and the rib cage moves down and in.

     b.   **Function.** The combination of muscle relaxation and recoiling of the lungs decreases the volume of the thorax, creating a higher pressure inside the airways than the pressure of air outside the body. Air moves down its pressure gradient and is exhaled.

B. Lung Spaces and Pressures

  1.   The **pleural space** of the thorax is shown in Figure 15-7. This space is filled with a small volume of pleural fluid, and there is a separate pleural lining for

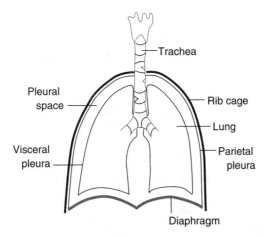

FIGURE 15-7.

Schematic diagram of the lung
linings and the pleural space.

each lung. The pleural space is the potential space between the following two
lung linings:

    a.   **Parietal pleura**—the lining on the inside of the rib cage

    b.   **Visceral pleura**—the lining directly on top of the lung

  2.   The lungs have a **continual elastic tendency** to collapse and pull away from
the chest wall. This is caused, in part, by the surface tension of the alveoli. The
elastic content of the lung also contributes to its recoil.

  3.   The **total recoil tendency** of the lungs can be measured by the amount of
negative pressure in the intrapleural space required to prevent collapse of
the lungs. This pressure is the **intrapleural pressure,** which is approximately −4 mm Hg. When the airways are open to atmospheric pressure, a
negative pressure of approximately −4 mm Hg is required to keep the lungs
expanded to normal size and to overcome the surface tension and elastic
fiber forces.

IV. Thermoregulation

A. Increases in Lung Ventilation Increase Heat Loss from the Respiratory System.

  1.   **When air is inhaled,** it is warmed and humidified.

  2.   **When air is exhaled,** it is cooled in the respiratory passages, conserving some
potentially lost heat. However, when the rate of ventilation increases, less time
is available to reabsorb heat energy.

B. Mammals and birds control heat loss via the respiratory system to regulate body temperature.
To increase heat loss, mammals breathe through
the mouth and hyperventilate. For example, a "panting" dog inhales through the nose
and exhales through the mouth. The exposed tongue encourages water evaporation
and, consequently, heat loss.

V. Protective Mechanisms Against Disease and Particulates

A.
The **upper respiratory tracts** are **lined with a ciliated mucosa,** which contains mucous cells.

1. **Mucus** is produced in the upper airways and is moved by cilia toward the mouth. The mucus is swallowed when it arrives in the throat.

2. The function of mucus is to **trap small particulate matter** such as dust, dirt, bacteria, and pollen.

B. The **nasal cavities** also trap particulates and are the first line of defense against particle inhalation.

1. **Nasal hairs and nasal mucus** trap many larger particles.

2. The small particles that travel down the bronchial tree may undergo **phagocytosis** by macrophages.

C. The lung is protected by the immune system; it has **resident macrophages** and a constant flow of **circulating immune cells** to protect it.

Skin

I. Structure of the Skin

A. The **epidermis,** which is derived from ectoderm, is made up of a **stratified squamous epithelium** that expresses intermediary filaments of keratin (see Chapter 7 of the Biology Review Notes). This epithelium includes several layers of cells, with the bottom layer attached to a basement membrane that divides the epidermis from the underlying dermis (see I B).

    1. As **dead cells** are removed from the skin's surface, they are **replaced by cells underneath.** The rate of cell replacement equals the rate of sloughing so that a constant epidermal thickness is maintained, although the overall thickness varies in different parts of the body.

    2. The **cells of the basal layer** just above the basement membrane **divide rapidly and continuously.** As the cells migrate up toward the body surface, they differentiate and begin to express the protein keratin. **Keratin** contributes to the mechanical strength and flexibility of the skin.

    3. Because the epidermis does not contain blood vessels, **the differentiating cells become nutrient deprived** and, therefore, less metabolically active. As the cells approach the surface of the skin, they lose their nuclei, die, and are shed by physical abrasion.

B. The **dermis** is the **connective tissue layer** between the epidermis and the hypodermis (see I C). Like other connective tissues (see Chapter 7 of the Biology Review Notes), the dermis is composed of collagen, reticulin, and elastic fibers. The fiber lattice acts as a scaffolding for the connection of the basement membrane as well as for skin-associated structures (e.g., hair, glands). Unlike the epidermis, the dermis has extensive capillary networks that nourish the dermis directly and the epidermis indirectly through the diffusion of nutrients and gases across the basement membrane. Many **skin-associated structures** are embedded in the dermis (Figure 16-1).

    1. Glands

        a. Sebaceous glands produce **sebum,** which is an oily substance that coats the exterior surface of the skin, slows the evaporation of water, and has antimicrobial effects. Sebum is secreted from ducts into the shaft of the hair follicle, thereby gaining access up through the epidermis to the surface of the skin.

FIGURE 16-1.

Microscopic structure of the skin. (Reproduced with permission from Ville CA, Solomon EP, Davis PW: *Biology*. Philadelphia, Saunders College Publishing, 1985, p 662.)

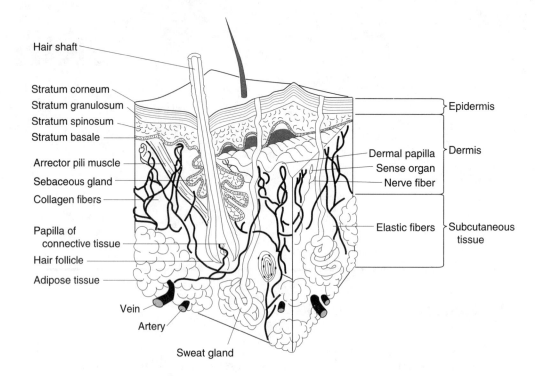

Hair shaft

Stratum corneum
Stratum granulosum
Stratum spinosum
Stratum basale

Arrector pili muscle
Sebaceous gland
Collagen fibers

Papilla of connective tissue
Hair follicle
Adipose tissue

Vein
Artery
Sweat gland

Epidermis
Dermal papilla
Sense organ
Nerve fiber
Dermis

Elastic fibers
Subcutaneous tissue

b. **Sweat glands** secrete metabolic waste products, salt and other ions, and water.

2. **Hair follicles** begin in the dermal layer and extend up through the epidermis from which they are originally derived. Hairs are closely associated with sebaceous glands as well as several sensory structures (see Chapter 8 of the Biology Review Notes). To make the hair stand up, the erector pili muscles contract, which pulls the hair shaft perpendicular to the surface of the skin.

C. **Hypodermis** is a layer of **subcutaneous tissue** below the dermis. In the hypodermis, **adipocytes,** or fat cells, are numerous. The adipocytes create a layer of subcutaneous fat that helps to insulate the body. Capillary networks tend to be sparse because adipocytes are less metabolically active than most cell types.

II. Function of the Skin

A. Homeostasis and Osmoregulation

1. **Homeostasis** is the tendency of organisms to **maintain an internal steady state,** despite changes in the external environment. In all organisms, a dynamic yet balanced internal state must be maintained. To accomplish this goal, metabolic processes must be monitored and constantly adjusted. These self-regulating control measures are exquisitely sensitive to small perturbations and are remarkably efficient in preventing excessive loss of time and energy.

2. **Osmoregulation** is the process that **maintains the water content of the body** in addition to **regulating** the concentration and distribution of the various ions.

    a. **Sweat glands.** Although the kidneys are the primary center for osmoregulation, the sweat glands in the skin excrete between 5% and 10% of the body's metabolic wastes, including salt and urea. Perspiration can vary from 0.5 L on a temperate day to 2–3 L on a hot day. The loss of both water volume and salt aids in the control of body osmolarity.

    b. **Protection against dehydration.** The skin plays another pivotal role in osmoregulation by protecting the body against dehydration. Human skin is impermeable to water and is, therefore, a barrier to water exchange with the environment. In other animals, such as amphibians, the skin is permeable to water, which allows those animals to osmoregulate directly with their environment.

B. **Thermoregulation.** The regulation of body temperature is an example of a homeostatic operation. Although some heat is dispelled through respiration, defecation, and urination, **90% of total heat loss is through the skin.**

    1. **When body temperature increases,** cells in the hypothalamus sense the increase and send out nerve impulses to compensate.

        a. **Increased sweat output.** Sympathetic neurons (see Chapter 8 of the Biology Review Notes) stimulate sweat glands to increase their output of sweat. The subsequent evaporation of the sweat from the surface of the skin helps to lower body temperature. Heat from the skin surface is dissipated by the conversion of sweat into water vapor.

        b. **Vasodilation.** Other nerve impulses travel to capillaries in the skin and cause them to vasodilate. This process increases the volume of blood being delivered to the surface of the skin so that more heat can radiate away.

    2. **When body temperature decreases,** the hypothalamus senses the heat loss.

        a. **Vasoconstriction.** The hypothalamus sends nerve impulses to induce vasoconstriction of skin capillaries, which reduces heat loss through radiation.

        b. **Muscle contraction (shivering).** In more extreme cases of heat loss, nerve impulses stimulate skeletal muscles to rapidly contract. The shivering generates heat without causing a great loss of energy because the amount of body movement is minimal.

C. **Physical protection.** The skin acts as a physical barrier between the body and the external environment. This physical separation serves several purposes.

    1. Entry of infectious agents is prevented.

    2. Damage from chemical toxins, extreme temperature fluctuation, and ultraviolet rays is reduced.

    3. The body is shielded from abrasive forces encountered during movement.

The Reproductive System

I. Male Reproductive System

A. Genitalia and Gonads. The male reproductive system is composed of the structures shown in Figure 17-1. The overall function of this system is to produce mature, active sperm and to deliver them outside the body.

FIGURE 17-1.

Male reproductive anatomy. (Reproduced with permission from Ville CA, Solomon EP, Davis PW: *Biology*. Philadelphia, Saunders College Publishing, 1985, p 934.)

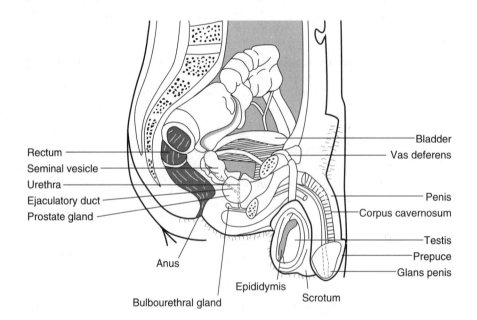

Rectum
Seminal vesicle
Urethra
Ejaculatory duct
Prostate gland
Anus
Bulbourethral gland
Epididymis
Scrotum
Bladder
Vas deferens
Penis
Corpus cavernosum
Testis
Prepuce
Glans penis

1. **Passage of sperm. Spermatogonium** are the male gametocytes (Figure 17-2).

   a. These progenitor cells arise in the **seminiferous tubules of the testes.**

   b. Spermatogonium are nourished by **Sertoli cells.** Development of spermatogonium takes several days, with the mature spermatozoa being concentrated and stored in the lower **epididymis** until ejaculation.

   c. Upon arousal, the penis becomes engorged with blood, and spermatozoa are propelled up into the **vas deferens** during ejaculation.

   d. From the vas deferens, the spermatozoa pass sequentially through the **urethra** and exit the body.

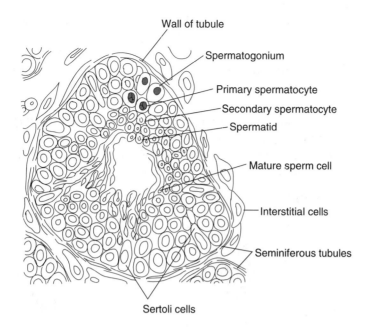

Wall of tubule
Spermatogonium
Primary spermatocyte
Secondary spermatocyte
Spermatid
Mature sperm cell
Interstitial cells
Seminiferous tubules
Sertoli cells

FIGURE 17-2.
Seminiferous epithelium. Note that the immature cells are spermatogonium, and they are on the periphery of the tubule. As cells undergo spermatogenesis and mature, they move toward the center of the tubule and become mature sperm cells. (Reproduced with permission from Ville CA, Solomon EP, Davis PW: *Biology.* Philadelphia, Saunders College Publishing, 1985, p 935.)

2. **Semen,** or ejaculate, contains **spermatozoa** and **seminal fluid.** One ejaculation produces 3–4 mL of semen and contains 300–500 million spermatozoa.

   a. The seminal fluid is **secreted by the male accessory sex glands,** of which there are three types.

      (1) The **prostate gland** is the largest seminal fluid–producing gland. There is one prostate gland.

      (2) The **seminal vesicles** are paired glands that secrete a component of semen.

      (3) The **bulbourethral (Cowper) glands** are paired, and they produce a mucoid secretion that is a component of semen.

   b. The fluid and its contents serve several purposes.

      (1) The **fluid** provides a vehicle for the **transport of the spermatozoa** out of the body.

      (2) **Fructose** in the fluid provides the spermatozoa with an energy source.

      (3) There may be **chemicals** in the fluid that protect the spermatozoa from the harsh environment of the uterus.

B. Spermatogenesis

1. **Gametogenesis.** Gametogenesis is the production of sex cells, or **gametes** (i.e., spermatozoa in men; ova in women).

   a. **Gametes** contain only one set of chromosomes (i.e., 23 chromosomes) and are **haploid.** (**Somatic cells** are **diploid;** they contain 23 pairs of chromosomes, or 46 chromosomes, with one member of each pair being contributed by each parent.)

   b. The **reduction in the number of chromosomes** occurs during **meiosis** (see Chapter 19 of the Biology Review Notes) as part of gametogenesis.

   c. When the egg and sperm unite **at fertilization, the diploid state is regained.**

2. **Spermatogenesis.** In all vertebrates, spermatogenesis takes place in the **testes.**

a. The **spermatogonia,** which are primitive, unspecialized germ cells, line the walls of the seminiferous tubules. Throughout embryonic development and before puberty, the spermatogonia divide mitotically to give rise to more spermatogonia. Only **after puberty** do the spermatogonia begin the process of spermatogenesis, which produces mature spermatozoa. Once spermatogenesis starts, it continues throughout a man's life.

b. The **steps of spermatogenesis** are shown in Figure 17-3.

FIGURE 17-3.
Spermatogenesis.

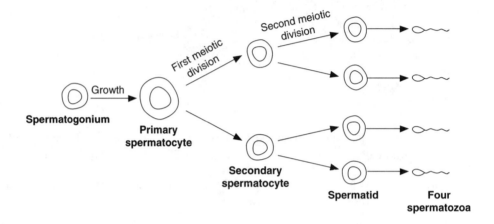

(1) The process begins with the growth of the spermatogonia into larger cells called **primary spermatocytes.**

(2) During meiosis I, the primary spermatocytes give rise to two **secondary spermatocytes,** each of which undergoes a second division, meiosis II, to yield four **spermatids.**

(3) All four spermatids mature into fertile **spermatozoa.**

3. **Hormonal control.** Spermatogenesis is regulated by secretions from the **anterior pituitary gland.**

a. **Luteinizing hormone (LH)** stimulates the **interstitial cells of Leydig** to produce **testosterone,** which then aids in the process of spermatogenesis.

b. Maintenance of spermatogenesis is assisted by **follicle-stimulating hormone (FSH)** and **growth hormone (GH).** For a summary of the male reproductive hormones, see Table 17-1 and Chapter 9 of the Biology Review Notes.

II. Female Reproductive System

A. Genitalia and Gonads. The structures of the female reproductive system are shown in Figure 17-4.

1. **The function of the female reproductive system is twofold:**

a. To produce fertile eggs or ova

b. To provide an environment capable of supporting embryonic development if an egg becomes fertilized

TABLE 17-1. Male reproductive hormones.

Endocrine Gland and Hormones	Site of Action	Activities Controlled
Anterior Pituitary		
Follicle-stimulating hormone (FSH)	Testes	Stimulates development of seminiferous tubules and maintenance of spermatogenesis
Luteinizing hormone (LH)	Testes	Stimulates interstitial cells of Leydig to release testosterone
Testes		
Testosterone	General	Before birth: development of primary sex organs and descent of testes into scrotum
		Puberty: growth spurt; development of reproductive structures; secondary sex characteristics (e.g., pubic and axillary hair, deep voice)
		Adult: maintenance of secondary sex characteristics; spermatogenesis

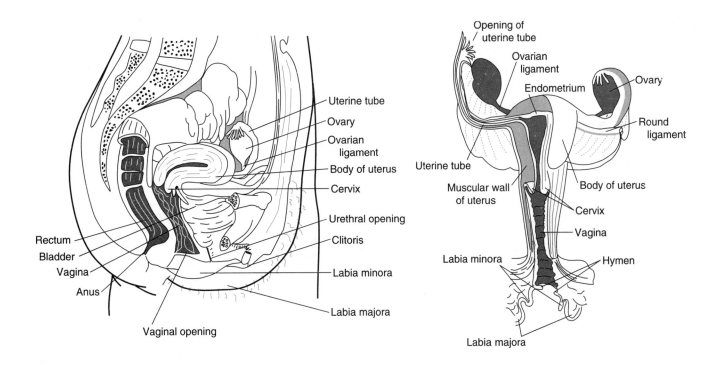

2. The **process of fertilization** is as follows: during intercourse, the man's penis is inserted into the woman's **vagina.** Upon ejaculation, spermatozoa travel up through the **cervix** into the **uterus** and ultimately reach the **fallopian tubes** or **oviducts.** In most pregnancies, fertilization takes place in the distal segment of the fallopian tube near the ovary.

B. Oogenesis. Table 17-2 compares oogenesis and spermatogenesis.

1. **Ova development**

   a. **Female embryos.** The **ova,** or eggs, begin development within the ovary from immature **oogonia** (Figure 17-5). Early in embryonic development, the oogonia divide mitotically to produce more oogonia, all of which are diploid. By the third month of embryonic development, the oogonia begin to develop into **primary oocytes** by starting

FIGURE 17-4.

Female reproductive anatomy. (Reproduced with permission from Ville CA, Solomon EP, Davis PW: *Biology*. Philadelphia, Saunders College Publishing, 1985, p 936.)

TABLE 17-2. Spermatogenesis versus Oogenesis.

	Spermatogenesis	Oogenesis
Meiosis	Continuous	Arrested in meiosis I until ovulation; meiosis II does not occur unless there is fertilization
Time frame	Throughout lifetime	Maximum number at birth
Meiotic products	Four fertile spermatozoa	One mature ovum and up to three nonviable polar bodies
Division of cytoplasm	Equal	Unequal (large ovum and small polar bodies)
Site of development	Entirely within testes	Meiosis I within ovary; meiosis II wherever fertilized
Hormones	FSH and GH: maturation of spermatozoa	FSH: stimulates follicle cells to produce estrogen
	LH: stimulation of Leydig cells to make testosterone	LH: stimulates corpus luteum to produce progesterone

FIGURE 17-5.
Oogenesis.

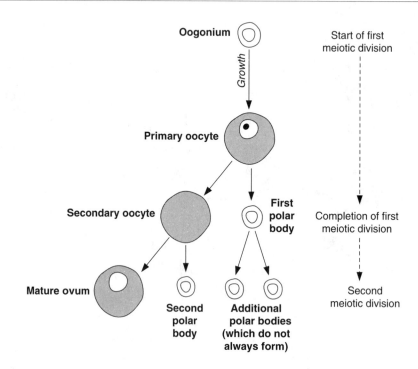

meiosis. However, meiosis is not completed; it is arrested in the prophase of meiosis I until ovulation.

b. **Menarche.** The beginning of ovulation at the onset of puberty is called **menarche.** A woman does not possess any fertile eggs until this time.

(1) At birth, a girl infant has approximately 400,000 primary oocytes, all of which are awaiting completion of meiosis I.

(2) Only a fraction of these primary oocytes survive until puberty, and even fewer (approximately 400) are ovulated.

c. **Ovulation.** The primary oocytes that are ovulated resume meiosis I, forming the **secondary oocyte** and the **first polar body.** At ovulation, the secondary oocyte is released from the ovary into the abdominal cavity and is then picked up by **fimbria** (cilia lining the oviduct), which draw the oocyte inside the oviduct.

d. **Fertilization.** Completion of meiosis II occurs only if the secondary oocyte becomes fertilized. The products of meiosis II are the mature **ovum** and the **second polar body.** By the time the ovum is mature, it is already fertilized and is technically a **diploid zygote.**

2. **Division of cytoplasm.** Unequal division of cytoplasm occurs during oogenesis. Most of the cytoplasm of an oogonia is ultimately transferred to only one of its meiotic products, the mature ovum. The remainder of the meiotic products, the polar bodies, contain almost nothing but a nucleus. This **unequal cytoplasmic division** ensures that the mature egg has enough cytoplasm and stored proteins to allow the zygote to begin development and to survive.

3. **Hormonal control.** The ovaries and the pituitary have a reciprocal effect on one another (Table 17-3). For a review of the endocrine glands, the hormones they produce, and the activities they control, see Chapter 9 of the Biology Review Notes.

TABLE 17-3. Female reproductive hormones.

Endocrine Gland and Hormones	Site of Action	Activities Controlled
Anterior Pituitary		
Follicle-stimulating hormone (FSH)	Ovary	Stimulates development of follicles; with LH, stimulates ovulation and secretion of estrogen
Luteinizing hormone (LH)	Ovary	Stimulates ovulation and development of corpus luteum (including progesterone release)
Prolactin	Breast	Milk production
Ovary		
Estrogens	General	Puberty: growth spurt; development of secondary sex characteristics (e.g., pubic and axillary hair, breast development)
		Adult: maintenance of secondary sex characteristics; oogenesis
	Reproductive structures	Monthly preparation of endometrium; makes cervical mucus more alkaline and thinner
Progesterone	Uterus	Maintains endometrium for pregnancy
	Breasts	Stimulates development of mammary glands

a. During oogenesis, cells surrounding the developing ovum **assist in the maturation process** and form a spherical structure called a **follicle.**

  (1) The follicle continues to grow under the influence of **FSH** released from the anterior pituitary gland. In addition, FSH **stimulates the cells of the follicle to produce estrogen.**

  (2) As **estrogen levels increase,** the follicles begin to inhibit the further release of FSH.

b. **Ovulation** is achieved with the aid of **LH.** After ovulation, the cells of the follicle are transformed into a structure called the **corpus luteum.** LH stimulates the corpus luteum to **produce progesterone.**

C. **Menstrual Cycle.** The menstrual cycle is approximately 28 days. It occurs from menarche to menopause, and it can be divided into four phases (Figure 17-6).

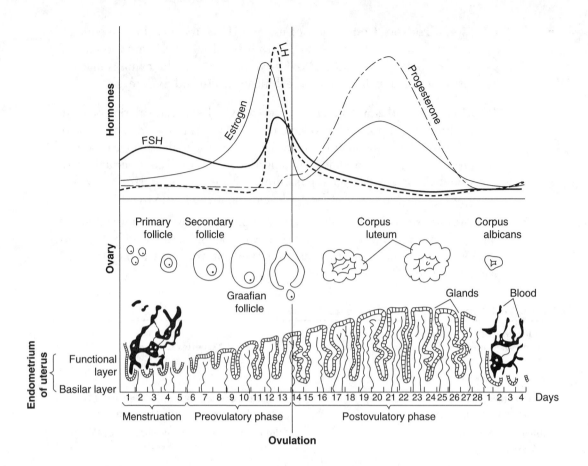

FIGURE 17-6.

The menstrual cycle. (Reproduced with permission from Ville CA, Solomon EP, Davis PW: *Biology*. Philadelphia, Saunders College Publishing, 1985, p 939.)

1. **First phase: menstruation (days 1–5).** Maintenance of the uterine lining depends on the continued presence of progesterone. Initially, the progesterone is produced by the corpus luteum under the stimulation of LH. However, the life span of the corpus luteum is approximately 10 days, and if implantation of a fertilized egg does not occur, the corpus luteum regresses. This event coincides with a decrease in progesterone concentration, which induces the lining of the uterus to slough and causes the characteristic bleeding.

2. **Second phase: follicular, or preovulatory, phase (days 6–13).** A maturing oocyte is surrounded by a growing mass of follicular cells that release estrogen in response to FSH stimulation. The estrogen helps to prepare the uterine lining for fertilization. Normally, FSH and LH are suppressed by high levels of estrogen and progesterone. However, during menstruation, both of these hormones are abruptly withdrawn, removing the negative feedback inhibition and causing a rise in FSH and LH at the beginning of the follicular phase. As the follicular cells begin to produce estrogen, the negative feedback is reestablished, causing a decline in FSH and LH levels toward the end of the follicular phase.

3. **Third phase: ovulation (day 14).** The small, abrupt rise in estrogen near the end of the follicular phase causes a surge in FSH and LH release. High plasma concentrations of estrogen appear either to suspend negative feedback or to induce a positive feedback on FSH and LH. Regardless of the mechanism, this FSH/LH surge causes the release of the developing oocyte from the follicle, which is the process of ovulation.

4. **Fourth phase: luteal, or postovulatory, phase (days 15–28).** Once the oocyte is released from the developing follicle, the remaining follicular cells are transformed into the corpus luteum under the influence of LH. The corpus luteum then begins production of progesterone and estrogen, also with the help of LH.

    a. **Progesterone** continues preparation of the uterus for fertilization. It promotes mammary gland development and, in conjunction with estrogen, prohibits additional ovulation by reestablishing negative feedback on FSH and LH.

    b. The second peak of **estrogen** results from estrogen production both by the corpus luteum and by the maturing uterine lining. Under the influence of estrogen and progesterone, the uterine lining continues to proliferate, developing new blood vessels and glands. If fertilization does not occur, the corpus luteum regresses, and the cycle repeats.

D. Pregnancy

1. **Placenta**

    a. **Structure.** On approximately day 7 of embryonic development, the **embryo begins to implant** into the endometrial lining of the uterus. At this time, the placenta is formed from both fetal (developing trophoblast and chorionic villi) and maternal (endometrium) tissues.

    b. **Functions**

        (1) Stimulation of the placenta by estrogen and progesterone promotes **vascularization, glandular development, secretory activity, accumulation of fluid, and endometrial proliferation.**

        (2) The placenta is the **organ of exchange between the fetus and the mother.** The placenta provides:

            (a) Nutrients and oxygen to the fetus

            (b) Removal of waste products from the fetal circulation

            (c) An endocrine organ for the production of estrogen, progesterone, and human chorionic gonadotropin (hCG)

2. **Human chorionic gonadotropin.** hCG plays a key role in pregnancy because it maintains the corpus luteum beyond its normal 10-day life span. As a result, progesterone production continues, preventing sloughing of the endometrium and subsequent ovulation, both of which would be detrimental to the developing fetus. By approximately the second month of pregnancy, the placenta is able to produce progesterone in sufficient quantities so that a positive feedback loop is established, ensuring proper maintenance of the placenta throughout gestation. Excess hCG is excreted in the mother's urine and is the basis for most pregnancy tests.

3. **Fetal membranes.** There are four membranes that surround the fetus. However, only two of the membranes contribute to fetal structures. They are the yolk sac and the allantois (Figure 17-7).

    a. The **amnion** is the closest membrane to the fetus. It creates a fluid-filled cavity (i.e., the amnionic cavity) around the developing embryo. The fluid is derived from the maternal circulation and from fetal excretory products. The amnionic cavity serves several functions:

        (1) Absorbs shocks

        (2) Allows fetal movement and growth

        (3) Prevents adhesion of the amnion to the fetus

        (4) Regulates temperature

        (5) Protects the fetus during birth

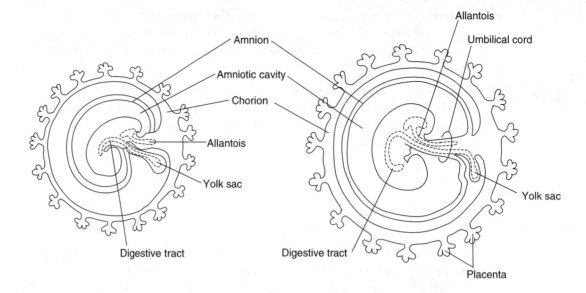

FIGURE 17-7.
Structure of the fetal membranes. (Reproduced with permission from Ville CA, Solomon EP, Davis PW: *Biology.* Philadelphia, Saunders College Publishing, 1985, p 965.)

b. The **chorion** is the fetal contribution to the placenta.

c. The **yolk sac** connects to the umbilical cord within the chorionic cavity. Functions include:

(1) Initial blood cell development

(2) Formation of the germ cells

(3) Nutrient transfer before formation of a functional placenta

(4) Provision of endodermal derivatives of the gastrointestinal tract and respiratory system

d. The **allantois** contributes to the following:

(1) Blood cell formation

(2) Connection between the bladder and umbilical cord

(3) Umbilical artery and vein formation

Development

18

I. Human Embryology

A. **Fertilization,** which is the **union of a spermatozoon and an ovum,** marks the beginning of human embryonic development.

    1. **Functions.** Fertilization serves three functions:

        a. Restores the diploid state when the haploid nuclei of the sperm and ovum unite

        b. Determines the sex of the offspring, which is determined by the sex chromosome carried by the sperm cell

        c. Initiates development

    2. **Capacitation and the acrosome reaction**

        a. **Capacitation.** Upon entry into the female reproductive tract, spermatozoa are not fully capable of fertilization. The spermatozoa must first undergo capacitation, which is a process that **strips the coat of glycoprotein** molecules off the surface of the spermatozoa. (The glycoproteins adsorb to the spermatozoa during maturation in the epididymis.) These molecules are removed by the proteolytic enzymes and high ionic strength of the estrogen-primed uterus.

        b. **Acrosome reaction.** After capacitation, spermatozoa are capable of activation via the acrosome reaction.

            (1) The acrosome is the **cap-like structure** at the head end of the sperm.

            (2) During the acrosome reaction, this cap breaks down, releasing enzymes (e.g., hyaluronidase) that **degrade the cells of the corona radiata** and help the spermatozoon to penetrate the oocyte (Figure 18-1).

            (3) It is important that activation occurs in close proximity to the oocyte because once spermatozoa are activated, their viability is greatly reduced.

    3. **Fusion of membranes and pronuclei**

        a. **Fusion.** Once a spermatozoon has penetrated the corona radiata, it comes into contact with the **zona pellucida,** which is a protective membrane

FIGURE 18-1.

Phases of oocyte penetration.

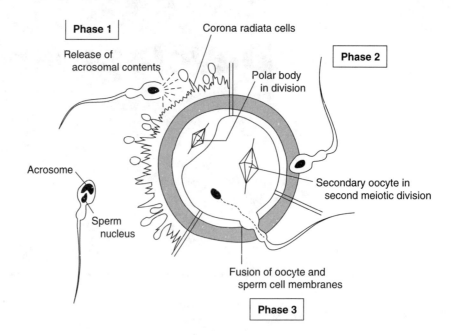

Phase 1

Release of
acrosomal contents

Corona radiata cells

Phase 2

Polar body
in division

Acrosome

Sperm
nucleus

Secondary oocyte in
second meiotic division

Fusion of oocyte and
sperm cell membranes

Phase 3

that surrounds the oocyte and stimulates the zona reaction. After passing through the zona pellucida, **the plasma membrane of the spermatozoon fuses with that of the oocyte** (see Figure 18-1).

b. **Male and female pronuclei.** Fusion stimulates the completion of meiosis II (see Chapter 17 of the Biology Review Notes) and allows for entry and formation of the **male pronucleus** in the cytoplasm of the newly formed zygote (Figure 18-2). When the male pronucleus and **female pronucleus** come into contact, their nuclear membranes break down, their chromosomes intermingle, and a diploid nucleus is established. This completes the process of fertilization.

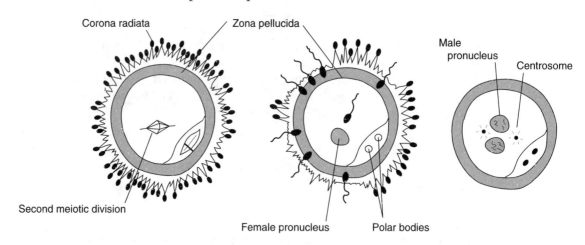

Corona radiata

Zona pellucida

Male
pronucleus

Centrosome

Second meiotic division

Female pronucleus

Polar bodies

FIGURE 18-2.

Formation of male and
female pronuclei.

4. **Advantages of large numbers of spermatozoa.** Movement of spermatozoa is undirected, so large numbers help to ensure that a few come into contact with the oocyte. The acidic pH of the uterus and phagocytic degradation greatly decrease the number of spermatozoa. Multiple spermatozoa can work together in a coordinated fashion to break through the corona radiata.

5. **Barriers to polyspermy.** Fusion of one oocyte with one spermatozoon results in creation of a genetic diploid state. However, if multiple spermatozoa entered the oocyte, polyploidy could arise. Polyspermy results in excess chromosomes and is incompatible with life. There are several barriers to multiple spermatozoa entry.

a. **Negative charge.** Spermatozoon penetration stimulates **hyperpolarization of the membrane of the zygote.** This enhanced negative charge repels further binding of spermatozoa.

b. **Cortical reaction.** Hyperpolarization mobilizes calcium, the displacement of which results in **fusion of cortical granules** in the cytoplasm of the zygote with the plasma membrane.

c. **Zona reaction.** The cortical reaction **releases enzymes that modify the zona pellucida,** which impairs subsequent spermatozoa penetration. Strongly acidic glycoproteins are released along with the modifying enzymes. These proteins polymerize on the surface of the zona pellucida and form a protective coat around the zygote.

B. **Cleavage** is a rapid series of mitotic divisions. Upon fertilization, there is a dramatic increase in the metabolic rate, oxygen consumption, and protein synthesis of the zygote, all of which prepare the zygote for cleavage. During cleavage, the embryo migrates down the fallopian tube.

1. Cleavage **increases the number of cells** comprising the embryo but without any protoplasmic growth because each interphase period is too brief to allow the cells to grow. Hence, with each division, the **cells become progressively smaller.** The small size of the cells enables them to move about with ease, partitioning the zygote into distinct regions in preparation for future developmental events.

2. The zygote is called a **morula** when it reaches the 16-cell stage. This state is reached as the embryo enters the uterus. At this time, the zona pellucida is fully dissolved.

   a. The morula consists of a group of centrally located cells, the **inner cell mass,** which gives rise to the embryo proper.

   b. The morula contains a surrounding outer cell layer, the **outer cell mass,** which later forms the **trophoblast.** The trophoblast is the fetal contribution to the placenta (see Chapter 17 of the Biology Review Notes).

C. **Blastulation** occurs when fluid begins to accumulate between the inner and outer cell masses, creating an internal cavity called the **blastocoele,** or **blastocyst cavity** (Figure 18-3A).

FIGURE 18-3.
Blastocyst formation.

A

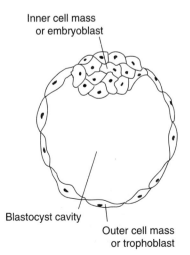

Inner cell mass or embryoblast

Blastocyst cavity

Outer cell mass or trophoblast

B

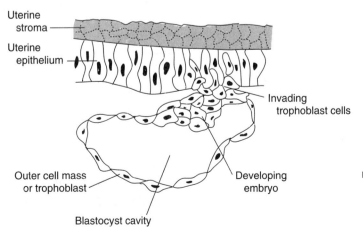

Uterine stroma

Uterine epithelium

Invading trophoblast cells

Outer cell mass or trophoblast

Developing embryo

Blastocyst cavity

1. The **embryoblast** is the inner cell mass that polarizes to one end of the embryo.

2. At this time, the developing zygote as a whole is referred to as **the blastocyst,** and implantation begins.

3. The cells of the trophoblast invade the endothelial layer of the uterus, establishing the initial connections of the placenta (see Figure 18-3B).

D. **Gastrulation** occurs during the third week of embryonic development and creates a **trilaminar disk** composed of the three germ layers: **endoderm, mesoderm, and ectoderm.**

1. Before gastrulation, cells of the embryoblast migrate to form two parallel planes of cells—the **hypoblast** and the **epiblast** (Figure 18-4). When the **bilaminar disk** is formed, the amnionic cavity and the primitive yolk sac are formed coordinately (see Chapter 17 of the Biology Review Notes).

FIGURE 18-4.
The bilaminar disk.

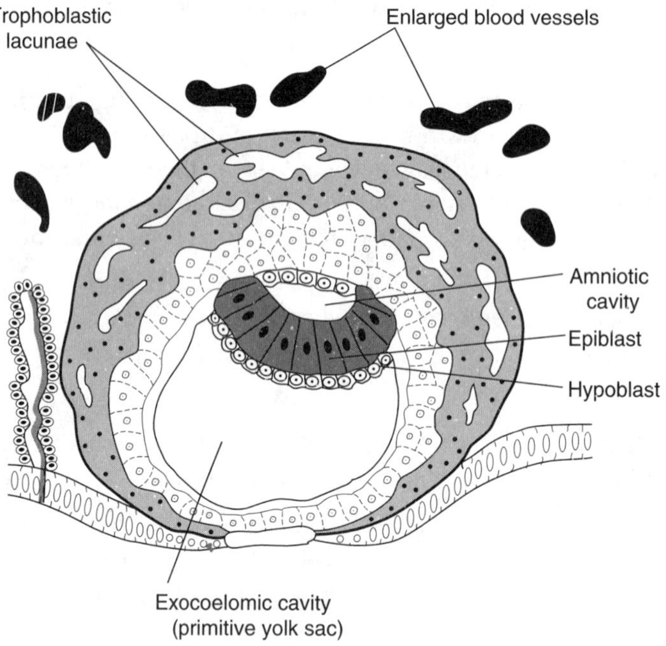

Trophoblastic lacunae

Enlarged blood vessels

Amniotic cavity

Epiblast

Hypoblast

Exocoelomic cavity
(primitive yolk sac)

2. Gastrulation begins with an **invagination of the epiblast** along its superior surface, which produces the **primitive streak** (Figure 18-5).

FIGURE 18-5.
Formation of the trilaminar disk.

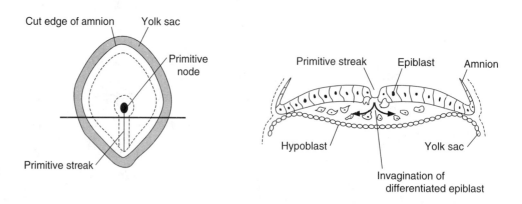

Cut edge of amnion   Yolk sac

Primitive node

Primitive streak

Primitive streak   Epiblast   Amnion

Hypoblast   Yolk sac

Invagination of differentiated epiblast

a. **Invagination.** As the epiblast invaginates, some of its cells differentiate and then migrate between the hypoblast and the epiblast.

b. **Formation of the trilaminar disk.** Some of these differentiated cells displace the hypoblast to form the embryonic endoderm, and others come to lie between the newly formed endoderm and the epiblast to form the embryonic mesoderm. The remaining undifferentiated epiblast is referred to as the ectoderm, and the trilaminar disk is completed.

    c.   **Differentiation.** The three germ layers of the trilaminar disk eventually give rise to the anatomic features of the body (Table 18-1).

TABLE 18-1. Germ layer derivatives.

Endoderm	Mesoderm	Ectoderm
Linings of internal organs and ducts (respiratory, gastrointestinal, urinary, eustachian tube, tympanic cavity)	Cartilage and bone	Central and peripheral nervous system
	Muscle (skeletal, cardiac, smooth)	Epidermis and associated structures (e.g., hair, nails)
	Dermis and connective tissue	
	Blood cells	Cornea and lens of eye
Parenchyma of:		
Liver	Cardiovascular, excretory, reproductive, and lymphatic systems	Inner ear
Tonsil		
Thyroid	Organs:	Tooth enamel
Thymus	Adrenal cortex	Nasal olfactory epithelium
Pancreas	Gonads and their ducts	Mammary and pituitary glands
Parathyroid	Spleen	Adrenal medulla
	Kidneys	

E.   **Neurulation** refers to neural plate formation and the development of a neural tube. The **brain and spinal cord**, which arise from these embryonic structures, are among the first organs to develop.

    1.   The **notochord.** During the second week of embryonic development, mesodermal cells differentiate and form a **cylindrical rod along the length of the embryo** (the notochord). This serves as a flexible skeletal axis for all chordates. In vertebrates, the notochord is later replaced by a bony vertebral column, and its remnants become part of the intervertebral disks.

    2.   The **neural plate.** Cells of the notochord secrete factors that induce the overlying ectoderm to thicken and form the neural plate (Figure 18-6). The neural plate invaginates to become the **neural groove** and ultimately the **neural tube,** which later forms the brain and the spinal cord.

A

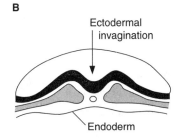

B

C

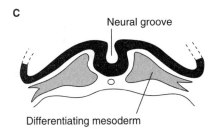

D

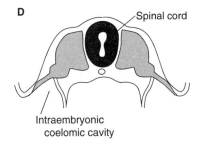

FIGURE 18-6.
Neural tube formation.

II. Developmental Mechanisms.
Embryonic development is a highly complex sequence of events that must be exquisitely orchestrated. A high degree of communication must take place between cells to allow for tissue, organ, and system development. Some general developmental concepts are discussed in the following paragraphs.

A. **Differentiation** is the process by which immature cells or tissues develop into mature cells or tissues with specialized functions. Differentiation is accompanied by specific protein expression and cytoskeletal modifications so that structures are created that assist the functions required of the specialized, mature cells.

B. **Determination** is the process that occurs as cells undergo development and their destiny becomes progressively more restricted. For example, a single-cell zygote has the potential to develop into any type of specialized eukaryotic cell (Figure 18-7). As the three germ layers are formed, the destiny of a cell within a given layer becomes limited, although many possibilities are still possible. The cell continues to differentiate until a single pathway of differentiation is chosen.

FIGURE 18-7.
The process of determination.

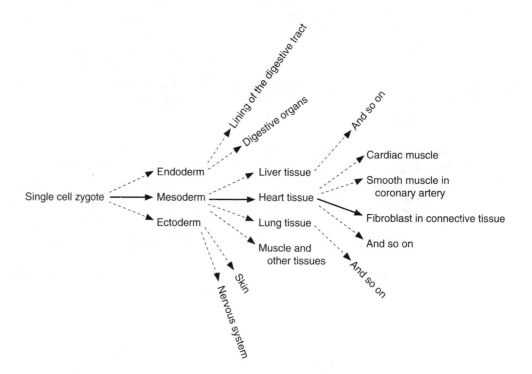

C. **Induction** is the process by which a chemical mediator released from one part of the embryo causes a specific morphogenic effect in another part by inducing a particular developmental pathway. For instance, the dermis of the skin, which is derived from the mesoderm, releases a substance that causes the overlying ectoderm to differentiate into epidermis. As a consequence of simultaneous induction of neighboring cells, tissues and ultimately organs can be formed.

Genetics

19

I. Introduction

A. Basic Definitions

1. **Genetics** is the study of the heritable information in organisms.

2. A **gene** is a unit of genetic information encoded in DNA (see Chapter 4 of the Biology Review Notes).

   a. The **genotype** of an organism is its genetic makeup, including the information in all its genes. The **potential** characteristics or traits of an organism are encoded in its genotype.

   b. The **phenotype** of an organism is its actual or **expressed** traits. A specific phenotype results from the expression of specific genes.

3. Genes are carried on **chromosomes,** which are discrete structures made up of DNA and associated histone proteins. The position of a gene on a chromosome is called its **locus.**

4. A **diploid** cell contains two sets of chromosomes, one set inherited from each parent. Each chromosome is paired with another chromosome. The two chromosomes of a pair are called **homologous chromosomes** or **homologs.**

   a. Homologous chromosomes carry genes for the same traits at corresponding loci. Therefore, homologs are functionally similar. However, homologs do not necessarily contain identical genetic information.

   b. If N is the number of functionally different chromosomes, then diploid cells have $2N$ chromosomes. Each species has a characteristic diploid number of chromosomes: **Humans have 46** ($2N = 46$), dogs have 78, fruit flies have 8.

   c. Homologs look alike in the **karyotype** of an organism, which is a stained preparation of all the chromosomes. In a karyotype, the different types of chromosomes can be distinguished by size, centromere location, and pattern of dark and light bands.

5. The **somatic cells** are the diploid cells that make up an organism. All the somatic cells in an organism have the same genotype.

B. Sexual Reproduction (Figure 19-1). **Gametes (germ cells)** are produced by diploid organisms. A germ cell, which is **haploid,** has half of the diploid number of

chromosomes. **Human germ cells have 23 chromosomes** ($2N = 46$; $1N = 23$), which is one of each type of chromosome.

FIGURE 19-1.

Sexual reproduction.

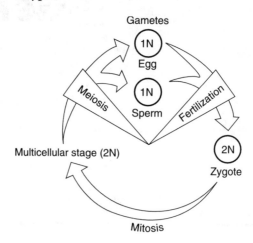

1. The **germ line** of an organism includes the gametes and the cells that give rise to them. In the germ line, new gametes are produced through a special cell division called **meiosis.**

2. In sexual reproduction, **each parent contributes one set of homologs to the offspring.** Sexual reproduction results in unique combinations of genetic information in each offspring.

    a. In **fertilization,** the father's gamete (spermatozoon) fuses with the mother's gamete (egg) to produce the diploid **zygote** or fertilized egg.

    b. The zygote grows by **mitotic divisions.**

II. Mendel and the Principles of Heredity

A. **Mendelian Inheritance.** Gregor Mendel first proposed many of the fundamental principles of genetics. In the late nineteenth century, he recognized the existence of units of heritable information for the observable traits of organisms. This was the first concept of the gene.

1. Mendel studied the **inheritance of traits in pea plants.** In a single plant, each trait occurs in either of two forms, for example, yellow or green seeds, round or wrinkled seeds, short or tall stems. The following abbreviations are used in Mendelian genetics.

    a. **P—parental generation.** Each parental strain is pure breeding, meaning that it produces offspring with only one of the alternative forms of a trait.

    b. **F1—first offspring (filial) generation.** These plants are crossed with each other to produce the F2 generation.

    c. **F2—second offspring generation.** These plants are produced by crossing two F1 plants.

2. **Mendel's method** was to cross two pure-breeding strains with contrasting forms of a trait (Figure 19-2).

3. **Mendel's conclusions** include the following.

    a. The information for a trait (pod color) is a discrete, heritable factor (gene).

    b. Genes come in pairs, called **alleles.** Alleles are the different forms of a gene for a particular trait.

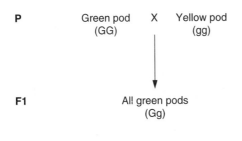

P	Green pod (GG)	X	Yellow pod (gg)

F1 All green pods
(Gg)

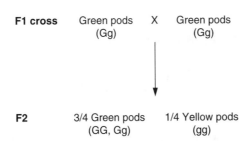

F1 cross	Green pods (Gg)	X	Green pods (Gg)

F2 3/4 Green pods 1/4 Yellow pods
(GG, Gg) (gg)

    c.   In the diploid organism, a **dominant allele** of a gene may mask the phenotypic expression of the **recessive allele.** For the pod color gene, G is the dominant allele (green); g is the recessive allele (yellow).

        (1) The pure-breeding **P-generation plants are homozygous** for their alleles: GG (green) and gg (yellow).

        (2) All the **F1 plants are hybrids,** or organisms carrying both alleles of a particular gene. The F1 plants are **heterozygous** for the two alleles. Although Gg is the F1 genotype, only the dominant allele G shows in the phenotype (green).

    d.   The two alleles segregate when a hybrid produces gametes. This **segregation** occurs randomly, so that half of the gametes receive the G allele, and half receive the g allele. This is **Mendel's first law—the law of random segregation.**

    e.   The F1 cross described above is called a **monohybrid cross** (one trait is segregating). In fertilization, each F1 parent contributes a gamete containing either G or g to the offspring. Which gametes are combined is determined by a random event.

    4.   The **F2 genotypes can be predicted** using the **Punnett square method** (Table 19-1). The alleles contributed by the spermatozoon and egg are placed along the top and left side, respectively. The F2 offspring resulting from each fertilization event are placed inside the squares.

TABLE 19-1. Prediction of F2 phenotypes using a Punnett square; monohybrid cross.

		F1 Spermatozoa	
		½ G	**½ g**
F1 Eggs	**½ G**	¼ GG	¼ Gg
	½ g	¼ gG	¼ gg

F1: Gg (green) × Gg
F2 genotypes: ¼ GG, ²⁄₄ Gg, ¼ gg (1:2:1)
F2 phenotypes: ³⁄₄ green, ¼ yellow (3:1)

5. The **genotype** of the phenotypic green plant **can be determined by a test-cross.**

    a. If the genotype is GG, all the progeny will be Gg (green).

    b. If the genotype is Gg, half the progeny will be Gg (green) and half will be gg (yellow).

6. Segregation and fertilization are both random events. Therefore, the **rules of probability** can be used to predict genotypes or phenotypes in mendelian crosses.

    a. The **multiplication rule** states that the probability that two events will both happen equals the product of the probabilities that each independent event will happen. For example, in the F1 cross (Gg × Gg), the probability that an F2 plant will have yellow pods can be determined as follows:

        (1) A plant with yellow pods (gg) must receive a g allele from both the egg and the spermatozoon. The probability of g in the egg = $\frac{1}{2}$. The probability of g in the spermatozoon = $\frac{1}{2}$.

        (2) The probability of g in the egg and in the spermatozoon is the product of the probabilities of each: $\frac{1}{2} \times \frac{1}{2} = \frac{1}{4}$. Therefore, 25% of the F2 plants should have yellow pods.

    b. The **addition rule** states that the probability that either of two events will happen is predicted by adding the probabilities of the alternate events. For example, in the F1 cross, the probability that an F2 plant is Gg can be determined as follows:

        (1) The probability of G from the egg and g from the spermatozoon = $\frac{1}{2} \times \frac{1}{2} = \frac{1}{4}$.

        (2) The probability of g from the egg and G from the spermatozoon = $\frac{1}{2} \times \frac{1}{2} = \frac{1}{4}$.

        (3) The probability of either of these events happening is the sum of the probabilities of each: $\frac{1}{4} + \frac{1}{4} = \frac{1}{2}$. Therefore, 50% of the F2 plants should be Gg.

B. Independent Assortment. Mendel's second law is the **law of independent assortment.** This law states that the genes for different traits are inherited (assorted) independently from each other. Mendel performed a **dihybrid cross** in which two different traits segregated (Figure 19-3).

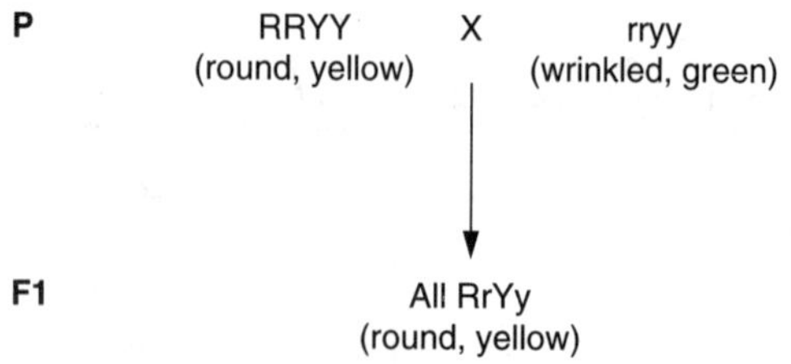

FIGURE 19-3.
Mendel's dihybrid cross in which two different traits (i.e., color and shape) are segregating. Y = yellow; y = green; R = round; r = wrinkled.

P	RRYY	X	rryy
	(round, yellow)		(wrinkled, green)

                    ↓

F1   All RrYy
               (round, yellow)

1. The phenotypes of the F2 progeny fit the Punnett square for independent inheritance of the genes for seed color and shape (Table 19-2).

2. As in the monohybrid cross, each of the traits exhibits a 3:1 phenotypic ratio (i.e., 12 round:4 wrinkled).

TABLE 19.2. Prediction of F2 phenotypes in a dihybrid cross.

		F1 Spermatozoa			
		RY	**Ry**	**rY**	**ry**
	RY	RRYY	RRYy	RrYY	RrYy
F1 Eggs	**Ry**	RRYy	RRyy	RrYy	Rryy
	rY	rRYY	rRYy	rrYY	rrYy
	ry	rRyY	rRyy	rryY	rryy

F2 phenotypes: $^9/_{16}$ round yellow, $^3/_{16}$ round green, $^3/_{16}$ wrinkled yellow, $^1/_{16}$ wrinkled green (9:3:3:1)

III. Population Genetics

A. Population genetics is concerned with the relative **frequencies of dominant and recessive alleles** in a population of interbreeding organisms.

1. The **gene pool** is the sum of all the genotypes in a population at any given time.

2. A population is in **genetic equilibrium** when the gene pool remains constant from one generation to the next. Genetic equilibrium occurs only under the following "ideal" conditions:

    a. Mating is completely random.

    b. The population is very large.

    c. There is no net change in the gene pool caused by mutations.

    d. The population is isolated (i.e., there is no migration in or out).

    e. All genotypes have equal reproductive success.

B. The **Hardy-Weinberg principle** states that, under conditions of genetic equilibrium, the frequencies of alleles in a gene pool remain constant from generation to generation. The frequency of an allele in a population determines the proportion of gametes that will contain that allele. The random probability of combinations of alleles results in predictable genotype frequencies in the offspring.

1. **Hardy-Weinberg equation.** The **genotype frequencies in a gene pool** can be calculated if the allele frequencies are known, and vice versa.

    a. For the two alleles A and a, let p represent the frequency of the dominant allele A, and let q represent the frequency of the recessive allele a.

    b. The **sum of the allele frequencies** must equal 100% of the genes for that locus in the population: $p + q = 100\%$, or $p + q = 1$. If the frequency of one allele is known, the other can be derived by these equations: $1 - p = q$ or $1 - q = p$.

    c. The **frequencies of the genotypes** in the offspring can be predicted from the allele frequencies and from the probability of each combination of alleles.

        (1) The combination of two gametes containing the same allele occurs with a probability of:

            (a) $p \times p = p^2$, for the homozygous dominant genotype (AA)

            (b) $q \times q = q^2$, for the homozygous recessive genotype (aa)

(2) The combination of gametes containing different alleles occurs with the probability of: $(p \times q) + (p \times q) = 2pq$, because the heterozygote (Aa) can be formed in either of two ways.

d. The **sum of the genotype frequencies must equal 100% (or 1):**

(1) $p^2 + 2pq + q^2 = 1$

(2) AA + Aa + aa = 1

e. The **allele frequencies** in this generation **can be determined from the genotype frequencies.**

(1) All the gametes from the homozygous AA and half the gametes from the heterozygous Aa will contain the p allele. Therefore, $p =$ frequency AA + $\frac{1}{2}$ frequency Aa.

(2) Likewi.se, $q =$ frequency aa + $\frac{1}{2}$ frequency Aa

2. **A Hardy-Weinberg problem**

a. It is given that $p =$ the frequency of allele A = 0.7, and $q =$ the frequency of allele a = 0.3.

b. From the equation $p^2 + 2pq + q^2 = 1$, the **genotype frequencies** in the next generation are as follows:

(1) AA = $0.7 \times 0.7 = 0.49$, or 49%.

(2) aa = $0.3 \times 0.3 = 0.09$, or 9%.

(3) Aa = $2(0.7 \times 0.3) = 0.42$, or 42%

c. The **allele frequencies** in this population are as follows:

(1) A = $0.49 + \frac{1}{2}(0.42) = 0.7$

(2) a = $0.09 + \frac{1}{2}(0.42) = 0.3$

d. Because the allele frequencies remained constant, this population is said to be in **Hardy-Weinberg equilibrium.**

3. **Application.** The Hardy-Weinberg equation applies to **nonevolving populations.** If the gene pool of a population is changing, then the actual frequencies in the population will not fit those predicted by the equation.

IV. Meiosis

A. The **process of meiosis** (Figure 19-4). A diploid (2N) organism produces haploid (1N) gametes through meiosis, which is a special division that **reduces the chromosome number by half.** Meiosis is necessary for fusion of two gametes to produce a zygote with a diploid number of chromosomes.

1. Meiosis involves **two sequential divisions**—meiosis I and meiosis II. The entire process results in four different haploid daughter cells, which form the gametes (Table 19-3).

2. **Meiosis I** is the reductional division in which the chromosome number is halved. In meiosis I, homologous chromosomes are paired, then separated.

a. **Prophase I.** The first phase takes approximately 90% of the time for meiosis.

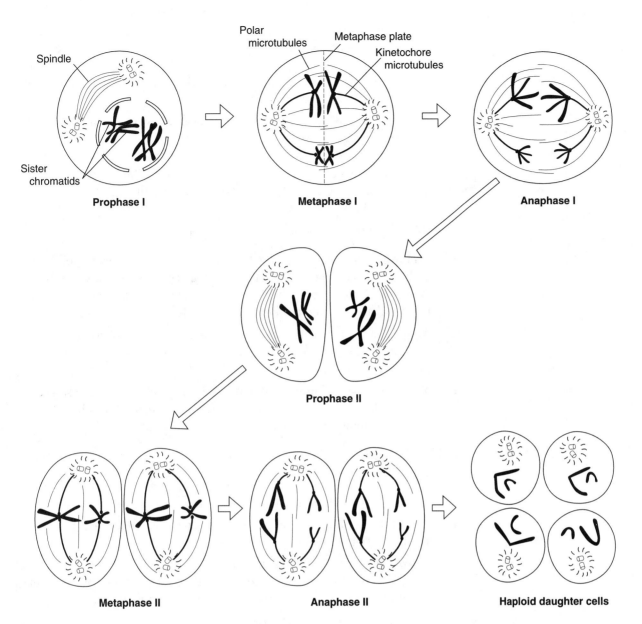

FIGURE 19-4.
The process of meiosis.

TABLE 19-3. Summary of meiosis.

Stage	Event
Interphase I	Chromosome replication; sister chromatids attach at centromere
Prophase I	Synapsis of homologous pairs, crossing over at chiasmata; spindle forms
Metaphase I	Homologous pairs line up at metaphase plate, with centromeres attached to microtubule fibers from opposite poles
Anaphase I	Homologous pairs of chromosomes separate and move toward opposite poles; centromeres do not split
Metaphase II	Individual chromosomes, consisting of two chromatids, line up at metaphase plate
Anaphase II	Centromeres split; sister chromatids separate and move toward opposite poles

(1) Homologous chromosomes pair through a process called **synapsis.** The genes on one homolog line up side-by-side with the same genes on the other homolog. A complex of proteins forms between the paired chromosomes. Four **chromatids,** the two sisters of each homolog, are involved at this stage.

(2) The paired homologs undergo **crossing over** at several sites. In this process, chromatids break, and homologous segments are exchanged between the paired chromosomes. The visible structures formed by crossovers are called **chiasmata.** Chromosome pairs are physically held together by their chiasmata through the next stage of meiosis.

(3) The **meiotic spindle** also develops during prophase I.

    b. **Metaphase I.** At this stage, the homologous pairs of chromosomes line up at the metaphase plate. The sister chromatids of each chromosome are attached to the same pole. The paired homologs are attached to opposite poles and are oriented randomly.

    c. **Anaphase I.** The crossovers are resolved. The homologs move, centomeres first, toward opposite poles. (The sister chromatids of each chromosome remain together.)

    d. **Telophase I–cytokinesis–interphase II.** The cell divides into two cells, each of which contains a haploid chromosome number. Interphase II is of very short duration, and no DNA replication occurs.

3. **Meiosis II** is called the equational division. In meiosis II, sister chromatids are separated from each other (as in mitosis).

    a. During **prophase II,** the spindle develops.

    b. In **metaphase II,** the chromosomes line up on the metaphase plate, with sister chromatids facing opposite poles.

    c. In **anaphase II–telophase II,** the sister chromatids are separated and move as individual chromosomes toward the poles. Four daughter cells are produced, each with a haploid number of chromosomes.

B. Comparison of Meiosis I and Mitosis (Table 19-4). Mitosis produces two daughter cells that are genetically identical to the parent cell and to each other. Meiosis produces four haploid daughter cells that differ genetically from the parent cell and from each other.

TABLE 19-4. Comparison of events in meiosis I and mitosis.

	Meiosis I	Mitosis
Prophase	Homologs synapse (pair) and cross over	No synapsis; no crossing over
Metaphase	Paired homologs line up on plate	Individual chromosomes line up on plate
Anaphase	Centromeres remain intact; homologs separate	Centromeres divide; sister chromatids separate

C. The Role of Meiosis in Genetic Variability. Meiosis and fertilization involve chromosome sorting and recombining, resulting in new combinations of genes in the offspring. The genes in a population are reshuffled with each successive generation.

1. In meiosis I, the homologs orient randomly at the equator. This results in a **random segregation** to one pole or the other and an equal probability for either homolog to be present in a particular gamete.

    a. Each of the homologous pairs (23 in humans) assorts independently of the others. This means that **a human gamete has a possibility of 2^{23}, or 8 million, different chromosome assortments.**

    b. **Crossing over** also provides variation by exchanging homologous segments that carry different information (alleles).

2. **Fertilization** is random, meaning that the 8 million possible eggs can combine with any of the 8 million possible spermatozoa to give **70 trillion diploid combinations.**

V. Mutations

A. Mutations are changes in the genetic material of an organism. Mutations that affect gene function can result in a new phenotype. These are heritable changes, and they are a continuing source of variability in populations.

1. **Some mutations involve a change in the number of chromosomes.** Such changes result from an abnormal meiotic event called **nondisjunction.** In this process, a homologous pair of chromosomes fails to separate during anaphase I or II. This results in one gamete having both copies of the chromosome, and the other gamete having none.

    a. **Aneuploidy,** which is an abnormal chromosome number, occurs when a gamete created by nondisjunction (a gamete receives two of the same type of chromosome or no copy) gets fertilized. Aneuploidy is transmitted to all cells by mitosis, and usually results in miscarriage of a fetus.

    b. **Polyploidy** occurs when there are too many chromosomes in a gamete. For example, a nondisjunction that produces an extra copy of chromosome 21 (trisomy 21) results in a fetus with Down syndrome.

2. **Most mutations result in changes in DNA sequence.**

    a. Mutations can be large, involving large regions of DNA. Large mutations may alter chromosome structure and, therefore, be detected as an **abnormal karyotype.**

    b. Mutations can be as small as a single nucleotide change in the DNA. Such changes are called **point mutations.**

B. Mechanisms of Chromosome Alterations (Figure 19-5)

1. **Breaks in a chromosome** can cause a loss or gain of DNA information.

    a. A **deletion** is the loss of DNA sequences. A deletion within a gene almost always negatively affects the phenotype.

    b. A **duplication** is the presence of an extra copy of a sequence on the same chromosome.

2. Chromosome breaks are often accompanied by **rearrangements of DNA sequences.**

    a. An **inversion** is when a sequence reattaches in the reverse orientation.

    b. A **translocation** involves the joining of DNA from one chromosome onto another chromosome.

FIGURE 19-5.

Mechanisms of chromo-
some alterations.

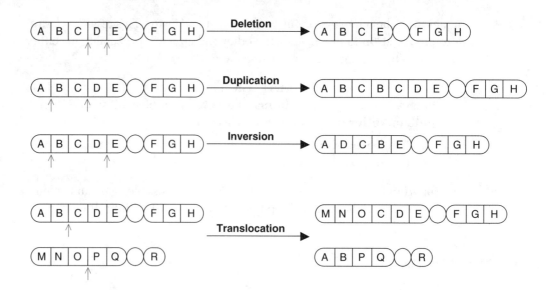

c. **Amplification** refers to the production of many extra copies of a sequence. Amplified DNA may be found in the chromosome or on extra-
chromosomal elements.

d. When a chromosome is rearranged, the expression of genes near the
breakpoints may be influenced by new neighboring sequences. This phenomenon is called **position effect.**

C. Effects of Mutations on Proteins

1. A **reading frame shift** is when a mutation changes the codon sequence in the
DNA. This results in a new sequence of amino acids past the point of the mutation.

2. A **missense mutation** results in the substitution of one amino acid for another.

3. A **nonsense mutation** creates a new stop codon, resulting in premature termination of a polypeptide chain.

4. **Silent mutations** have no detectable effect on phenotype.

   a. A mutant codon may code for the same amino acid as the normal codon
   (i.e., redundant codons).

   b. A mutation may occur between genes or in an **intron.**

   c. A mutation may alter a protein with a nonessential or redundant function.

VI. Sex Linkage

A. Sex Determination.
Sex is a genetically determined trait. In humans, males and
females have 22 homologous pairs of chromosomes, or **autosomes.**

1. **Sex chromosomes** are the twenty-third pair of chromosomes.

   a. **Females** have two X chromosomes (**XX**).

   b. **Males** have one X and one Y chromosome (**XY**).

2. Even though the **X and Y chromosomes** pair during meiosis I, they **are not
homologous.** The Y is small and carries few genes; the X is large and carries
many essential genes.

3. In humans, male is the **heterogametic sex;** that is, it is the sex that produces two different kinds of gametes and determines the sex of the offspring

(Table 19-5). Maleness in humans is determined by a specific area on the Y chromosome called the **testes-determining factor.** However, mechanisms of sex determination vary in different organisms. In bees, for example, unfertilized eggs (haploid) become males, while fertilized eggs (diploid) become females.

TABLE 19-5. Determination of maleness in humans.

Spermatozoa

		X	Y
	X	XX	XY
Eggs			
	X	XX	XY

The ratio of female to male offspring is 1:1.

B. Sex-linked Genes

1. Sex-linked genes are genes on the X chromosome. These genes have special **patterns of inheritance** because of the different sex chromosomes in males and females.

   a. Sons receive the X chromosome only from their mothers and the Y chromosome only from their fathers. All daughters, but no sons, receive their father's X chromosome.

   b. **Males only have one X chromosome.** Therefore, any sex-linked recessive gene (received from the mother) is expressed in the male phenotype.

   c. **Females have two X chromosomes** and need two copies of a recessive gene to show the phenotype.

   d. **More males than females have recessive, sex-linked disorders,** such as color blindness, hemophilia, and Duchenne muscular dystrophy.

2. **Males and females both have two copies of the autosomal genes.** However, females have two copies of sex-linked genes and males only have one.

   a. **Cells in female mammals compensate** for this inequality by **inactivating one of the X chromosomes** during embryogenesis, leaving only one active copy of the sex-linked genes.

   b. The inactive X chromosome contracts into a dense body called a **Barr body.**

   c. **Inactivation of X chromosomes is random** in each cell. For heterozygous sex-linked alleles, therefore, each allele is active in about one half of the female's cells.

VII. Pedigree Analysis

A. **Pedigrees** show a **family's history** for the inheritance of a particular trait. Pedigrees are used to analyze the segregation of inherited disorders in humans.

   1. In determining a pedigree, **males are symbolized as squares and females as circles.** Horizontal lines represent mating partners, and vertical lines connect offspring to their parents.

   2. **Genotypes** are shown next to the symbols. An individual with the disorder is shown by a solid or crossed square or circle.

B. To determine the **inheritance pattern** in humans, whether the inherited disorder is dominant or recessive, the number of unafflicted individuals is compared with the number of afflicted individuals in the pedigree.

1. **Recessively inherited disorders** are indicated by a 3:1 ratio of unafflicted to afflicted family members (Figure 19-6). Genotypes are determined by assessing family members above and below the afflicted individual in the pedigree; parents and offspring must be heterozygous.

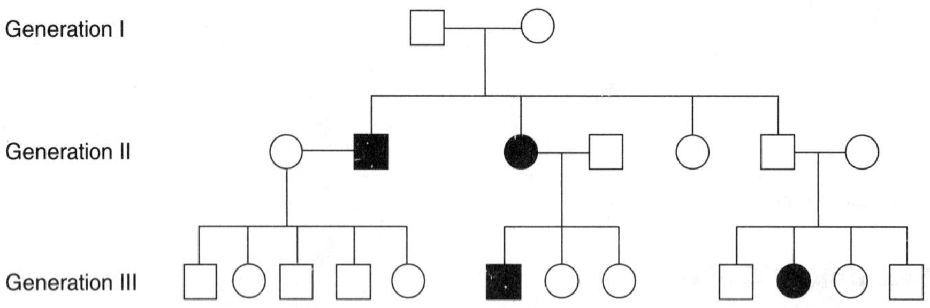

FIGURE 19-6.
A pedigree demonstrating a recessively inherited disorder.

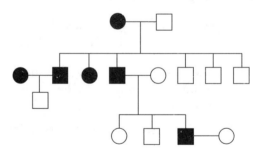

a. **Recessive disorders often skip generations** because the heterozygotic family members, or **carriers**, are phenotypically normal.

b. When **two carriers mate,** each offspring has a **1 in 4 chance of being homozygotic** and having the disorder. Each offspring has a 3 in 4 chance of being normal (2 of 3 of these offspring are carriers themselves).

c. Examples of recessively inherited disorders include phenylketonuria, cystic fibrosis, Tay-Sachs disease, and sickle-cell anemia.

2. **Dominantly inherited disorders** are indicated by a 1:1 ratio in a family (Figure 19-7). A single copy of the dominant gene is sufficient to significantly affect phenotype. Dominant traits **do not usually skip generations.**

FIGURE 19-7.
A pedigree demonstrating a dominantly inherited disorder.

a. Family members who are **heterozygotic for lethal dominant traits do not usually reproduce,** so these genes are less common than lethal recessive genes in a population.

b. The exception is **late-acting dominant lethal genes,** which show up later in life, after an individual has reproduced. Each offspring has a 1 in 2 chance of receiving the dominant gene. Examples include Huntington chorea and Alzheimer disease.

3. A **sex-linked recessive trait affects more males than females** (Figure 19-8). Such traits are passed from a normal carrier female to all of her sons, who are afflicted. The trait is then passed from the afflicted sons to all of their daughters, who are carriers.

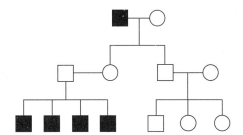

FIGURE 19-8.
A pedigree demonstrating the inheritance of a sex-linked recessive disorder.

VIII. Gene Mapping

A. Genetic Linkage

1. **Linked genes** are genes that are located on the same chromosome. Linked genes are an **exception to Mendel's law of independent assortment.**

    a. Genes that are adjacent to each other on the chromosome are inherited as a unit (i.e., they go through meiosis and fertilization together). Such genes do not assort independently.

    b. Most of the offspring have the parental genotype at closely linked loci.

2. Genes on the same chromosome but some distance apart can be separated by **crossing over** during meiosis. A crossover can result in exchange of information between paired homologous chromosomes (Figure 19-9).

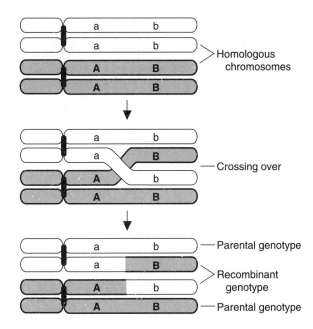

FIGURE 19-9.
The process of crossing over.

    a. If the homologs carry different alleles of the exchanged genes, the result is a **new combination of alleles** on the chromosome. This recombination event results in a **recombinant chromosome.**

    b. The **frequency of recombination** between two genes reflects the frequency of crossing over, which is proportional to the distance between the genes.

    c. Recombination events result in production of recombinant offspring.

B. Mapping Genes

1. **Gene mapping** can be performed when recombination frequencies are used to assign a gene to a particular chromosome and to a region of the chromosome. Recombination frequencies can also be used to determine the distance between linked genes.

2. The following is an example of mapping the genes for body color and wing shape in *Drosophila*.

   a. The **dihybrid testcross** is shown in Figure 19-10.

FIGURE 19-10.

A dihybrid testcross used to map the genes for body color and wing shape in *Drosophila*. The recombination frequency of 1% is 1 map unit. Therefore, this testcross demonstrates that the genes b and vg are 22 map units apart.

P	b^+b, vg^+vg (grey body, normal wings)	X	bb, vgvg (black body, vestigial wings)

F1	Grey, normal: 400 Black, vestigial: 380 Parentals: 780 flies (>50%)	Black, normal: 120 Grey, vestigial: 100 Recombinants: 220 flies

Recombination frequency between b and vg = 220 recombinants/1000 total offspring = 22%

   (1) A recombination frequency of 1% is defined as **1 map unit** on a chromosome.

   (2) Therefore, b and vg are 22 map units apart.

   b. The greater the distance between two genes on the chromosome, the greater the chances of a crossover between them, and the greater the recombination frequency.

20

Evolution

I. Natural Selection

A. Charles Darwin. In the 1850s, Charles Darwin published *On the Origin of Species by Means of Natural Selection.* In this book, Darwin presented evidence that species present today evolved from ancestral species. Darwin also proposed a mechanism for evolution that he called **natural selection.**

1. The **theory of natural selection** in based on the following three major concepts:

    a. In any population, **more individuals are produced each generation than can be supported by the environment.** This leads to competition for the limited natural resources and survival of only a fraction of individuals each generation.

    b. The likelihood of survival is not random but depends in part on the fitness of an individual, or **survival of the fittest. Fitness** refers to the inherited traits that make an individual suited to the surrounding environment.

    c. **Individuals who are better suited to their environment are likely to leave more offspring than less fit individuals.** This **differential reproduction** among individuals of a population leads to the gradual accumulation of favorable traits in the population. The gene pool changes over time as the population adapts to its environment.

2. There are **three major modes of natural selection.**

    a. **Stabilizing selection** involves selection of more intermediate rather than extreme phenotypes. This type of selection reduces variability in a population and is seen in relatively stable environments.

    b. **Directional selection** involves selection of a particular phenotypic trait during a time of environmental change.

    c. **Diversifying selection** involves selection of the extreme phenotypes in a population.

B. Nonadaptive Mechanisms of Population Change

1. **Genetic drift** is a chance change in the gene pool of a population. Genetic drift is likely to occur only in very small populations.

    a. The **bottleneck effect** is one type of genetic drift in which a random event, such as a disaster, drastically reduces the size of a population.

b. The **founder effect** occurs when a small group of individuals from a parent population colonizes a new area and starts a new population.

2. **Gene flow** involves the migration of individuals between populations.

3. **Nonrandom mating** (inbreeding) is usually based on proximity.

II. The Concept of Species

A. Definition. A species is a **group of individuals with the potential to interbreed** in nature. This mating produces viable, fertile offspring.

B. Reproductive Isolation. Individuals of different species are said to be reproductively isolated. The different mechanisms of isolation include the following:

1. **Geographic barriers** between species

2. **Temporal isolation** because species mate at different times

3. **Physiologic isolation** because of mechanical incompatibility between individuals of different species

4. **Ecological and environmental isolation** because species inhabit different niches

C. Speciation. Speciation is the formation of one or more new species from a previously existing species.

1. There are **two main modes of speciation.**

   a. In **phyletic speciation (anagenesis),** an ancestral species evolves over time into a new species.

   b. In **divergent speciation (cladogenesis),** an ancestral species splits, forming more than one new species over time.

2. There are **three major mechanisms of speciation** based on biogeographical criteria.

   a. In **allopatric speciation,** a geographic barrier isolates two populations, which then evolve independently.

   b. **Sympatric speciation** occurs because a genetic change in a subgroup of a population causes it to become reproductively isolated from the rest of the population. Thus, the gene pool is divided without geographic separation.

   c. **Parapatric speciation** involves the gradual divergence among members of a population to form different species. Parapatric speciation also does not require geographic separation.

III. The Origin of Life

A. Chemical Evolution. Earth is approximately 4 billion years old. The first living organisms are proposed to have arisen by a gradual process of chemical evolution. This process is thought to have involved four stages.

1. **Abiotic (nonliving) synthesis.** First, organic compounds were synthesized from inorganic precursors available in the atmosphere and seas of the primitive

Earth (e.g., water, methane, ammonia, hydrogen gas). This process of abiotic (nonliving) synthesis led to the accumulation of small organic compounds.

2. **Formation of organic polymers.** Organic compounds were joined together to form organic polymers.

3. **Formation of protobionts.** Organic molecules aggregated together to form droplets called protobionts. It is thought that protobionts had some of the properties of living cells, such as metabolism, excitability, and a distinct internal environment.

4. **Evolution.** The evolution of heredity began with the origin of genetic information.

B. **Earliest Fossil.** According to the fossil record, the earliest organisms were prokaryotic cells that arose about 3 billion years ago.

C. **Classification.** All organisms are grouped into five **kingdoms** (Figure 20-1). Organisms within the same taxonomic categories are related by their evolutionary history (phylogeny).

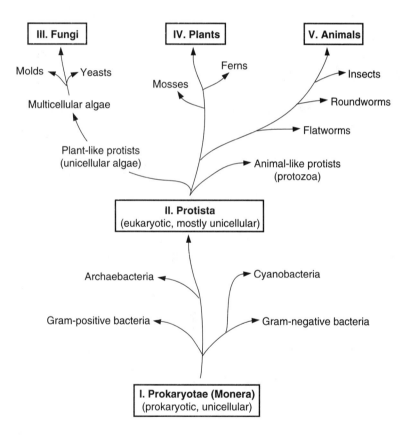

FIGURE 20-1.
The five kingdoms used in taxonomic categorization.

IV. Comparative Anatomy. Anatomic similarities between organisms in the same taxonomic group provide evidence for evolution from a common ancestor.

A. **Homology** is similarity due to common ancestry. An example of homologous structures are the forelegs, wings, flippers, and arms of chordates. Although evolved for different functions, all of these structures are built from similar skeletal elements.

1. Closely related organisms that look different in adults go through **similar stages in their embryonic development.** For example, all vertebrates go

through similar embryonic stages, including a stage in which they have gill slits. These develop into gills in fish and into various other structures in different vertebrates.

2. The idea that embryonic development is a replay of an organism's evolutionary history is referred to as **"ontogeny recapitulates phylogeny."**

B. **Analogy** is similarity between species that are not evolutionarily related. Analogous structures may evolve independently because of some common selective advantage. This type of evolution is called **convergent evolution.** For example, the wings of insects and birds have evolved independently. Although they are both used for flying, they are built from entirely different structures.

Biology

PRACTICE TESTS

Time: 45 minutes

Directions: This test contains as many biology passages as you may encounter on the real MCAT. There are also several independent multiple-choice questions at the end of this test. The time allotted approximates the time allowed on a real MCAT to solve the given number of questions. Choose one best answer for each question.

Passage I (Questions 1–7)

The auditory system depends on several energy forms for the production of auditory signals that are relayed to the brain. Sound entering the auditory canal sets up movement of the eardrum, or tympanic membrane. This movement is transmitted to the middle ear ossicles—the malleus, the incus, and the stapes. A connection between the middle ear and pharynx, called the eustachian tube, allows pressure between the middle ear and upper airways to be equilibrated. The footplate of the stapes inserts into the oval window of the cochlea. By moving into and out of the fluid contained in the cochlea, the stapes footplate sets up motion in the cochlear fluid. Because fluid is noncompressible, pressure changes and stimulation of the basilar membrane occur. This membrane contains stereocilia, which detect motion of the cochlear fluid and, in turn, fire action potentials in response to cochlear fluid movement. Neurons in the eighth cranial nerve (CN VIII) carry the action potentials to the auditory region of the cerebral cortex after passing through the auditory regions of the midbrain and thalamus.

When the middle ear becomes infected, the tympanic membrane becomes red, thickened, and painful. The middle ear cavity often becomes filled with fluid and may fill with pus. If the infection is ignored, permanent scarring of the eardrum may occur, and eardrum perforation may ensue. Perforations of the eardrum often become permanent, and they greatly interfere with the patient's hearing ability.

Recently, a new drug known as FGF was tested in guinea pigs to determine if eardrum perforations could heal more rapidly in the presence of FGF. Fifty female guinea pigs underwent placement of eardrum perforations in both ears surgically, while under anesthesia. Twenty animals underwent placement of a 1-mm perforation in each ear, whereas thirty animals had a 2-mm perforation placed in each ear. Gelfoam, a sterile spongy material, was saturated with either phosphate buffered saline (PBS) or liquid FGF. The saturated gelfoam containing either PBS of FGF was placed in direct contact with the eardrum perforations immediately after the perforations were performed. PBS was placed in contact with the left eardrum of all animals, and FGF was placed in contact with the right eardrum of all animals.

The wounds were inspected at 3 days, 5 days, and 8 days following the placement of either PBS of FGF. The figure below shows the percentage of eardrum wound closures after treatment with gelfoam-PBS and gelfoam-FGF.

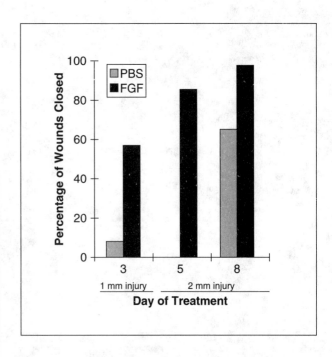

Figure 1. Percentage of eardrum wound closures after treatment with gelfoam-PBS and gelfoam-FGF.

1. Based on the passage, which statement best describes the energy transfers that occur when sound interacts with the middle and inner ear?

   A. Sound energy is converted from mechanical to electrical.
   B. Sound energy is converted from chemical to mechanical.
   C. Sound energy is converted from mechanical to chemical.
   D. Sound energy is converted from electrical to mechanical.

2. The mucosal cells lining the eardrum can best be described as:

   A. epithelial.
   B. connective.
   C. contractile.
   D. neurosecretory.

3. Which of the following served as controls in the experiments?

   I. Gelfoam-PBS
   II. Gelfoam-FGF
   III. Left ear perforation
   IV. Right ear perforation

   A. II only
   B. I and III only
   C. II and IV only
   D. I and IV only

4. Based on Figure 1 in the passage, which of the following statements regarding eardrum healing is best supported by the information presented?

   A. FGF speeds the healing of 2-mm injuries at 5 days post-injury.
   B. FGF speeds the healing of eardrum perforations of 1-mm injuries at 8 days post-injury.
   C. FGF speeds the healing of 2-mm injuries at 8 days post-injury.
   D. FGF speeds the healing of eardrum perforations of 1-mm injuries at 3 days post-injury.

5. Which of the following lacks a control group?

   A. Animals with a 1-mm injury, 3 days post-injury
   B. Animals with a 2-mm injury, 5 days post-injury
   C. Animals with a 1-mm injury, 5 days post-injury
   D. Animals with a 2-mm injury, 8 days post-injury

6. Which of the following statements is least supported from the information presented?

   A. FGF leads to faster healing of experimental eardrum perforations in the first several days post-injury.
   B. FGF decreases the percentage of animals whose experimental eardrum perforations are not closed at 3 days post-injury.
   C. FGF decreases the area of perforation remaining at 3 days.
   D. FGF may have less effect on the speed of eardrum perforation healing at periods of 8 days post-injury compared to 3 days post-injury.

7. FGF has been shown to increase the rate of cell division and replication in eardrum. FGF is best described as a drug that induces:

   A. mitogenesis.
   B. carcinogenesis.
   C. transformation.
   D. transduction.

Passage II (Questions 8–15)

Recently, researchers have discovered that a mutation of chromosome 10 in humans causes Crouzon's disease, which is associated with facial and skull deformities in children. This finding was made by an in-depth study of a family that was afflicted with Crouzon's disease. Through mapping studies of family members, the chromosome containing the mutation was identified.

Crouzon's disease was originally named after a French neurologist, Dr. Pierre Crouzon, who first described the group of deformities associated with this syndrome in 1912. Within several years of his landmark paper describing the condition, scientists discovered that transmission was through a predictable genetic route. Crouzon noted that 50% of offspring inherited the condition if either parent had the condition.

Recent studies have shown that the mutation of chromosome 10 affects a region that codes for growth factor receptors. Growth factors are small peptides that are produced by various cells in the body, including fibroblasts and osteoblasts. When growth factor substances are released by body tissues, they may bind to cell surface receptors in other regions of the body. These receptors, when bound by growth factors, initiate a kinase mechanism internally in the cell. The kinase system produces an intracellular response leading to increased cell division and growth.

When researchers identified the sequence that was affected by the mutation, they discovered that it coded for the fibroblast growth factor receptor 2. They found that in patients with Crouzon's disease, fibroblast growth factor receptors are produced but do not function normally. In addition, recent studies have shown that the cranial sutures from the skulls of children with Crouzon's disease contain abnormally low levels of fibroblast growth factor receptor 2.

Fibroblast growth factor is produced by a variety of cells to increase mitotic activity and collagen synthesis of fibroblasts, ultimately leading to connective tissue growth. It binds specifically to its cell surface protein receptor.

In a series of experiments, a researcher studied children who had Crouzon's disease and stenosis (fusion) of cranial skull sutures. The researcher also studied children who did not have Crouzon's disease, and were otherwise normal, but had isolated (nonsyndromic) stenosis of cranial sutures. The data from experiments comparing the counts of cells expressing fibroblastic growth factor receptor 2 are given in the table below.

TABLE I. Counts of cells expressing fibroblastic growth factor receptor 2 in sutures of children with Crouzon's disease and nonsyndromic cranial stenosis.

Suture Type	Cell Counts (cells/mm²)*
Crouzon's disease, stenosis	11.4 ± 5.6
Crouzon's disease, no stenosis	24.8 ± 4.2
Nonsyndromic, stenosis	39.3 ± 7.6
Nonsyndromic, no stenosis	44.4 ± 8.1

*Values represent mean +/− standard deviation.

8. Which of the following best describes the mutation associated with Crouzon's syndrome?

   A. Gene mutation
   B. Chromosome mutation
   C. Allele mutation
   D. Nonsense mutation

9. What is the most likely mode of inheritance for Crouzon's disease?

   A. Sex-linked recessive
   B. Autosomal dominant
   C. Random mutation
   D. Autosomal recessive

10. What is the most likely reason that the growth factor receptor of Crouzon's patients is nonfunctional?

   A. The receptors are no longer cell surface receptors.
   B. The receptors are down-regulated.
   C. The receptors bind other growth factors.
   D. The receptors have a different three-dimensional conformation.

11. Which of the following reactions are occurring intracellularly in response to growth factor receptor binding?

   A. Oxygenation
   B. Phosphorylation
   C. Reduction
   D. Oxidation

12. Based on information presented in the passage, which of the following tissues would *least likely* utilize growth factors to mediate growth?

   A. Bone tissue
   B. Connective tissue
   C. Glandular tissues
   D. Skin

13. In laboratory experiments in an animal model system, a substance that is known to noncompetitively inhibit the fibroblast growth factor receptor is injected into developing embryos. Which of the following findings would be expected?

   A. Abnormal growth of the embryos based on the inability of growth factors to bind receptors
   B. Abnormal growth of the embryos based on inhibition of growth factors
   C. Normal growth of the embryos, because binding of growth factors will be unaffected
   D. Normal growth of the embryos, because an excess of growth factors are present

14. Based on the data, which one of the following statements is most accurate?

   A. Crouzon's disease correlates with cranial stenosis.
   B. Crouzon's disease correlates with nonsyndromic stenosis and low levels of fibroblast growth factor receptor 2.
   C. Crouzon's disease correlates with fibroblast growth factor levels and the degree of cranial stenosis in children.
   D. Crouzon's disease correlates with low levels of fibroblast growth factor receptor 2.

15. Which cells are most likely involved in the cranial stenosis described in this passage?

   I. Osteoclasts
   II. Fibroblasts
   III. Osteoblasts

   A. I only
   B. II only
   C. I and III only
   D. II and III only

498

Passage III (Questions 16–22)

Skin grafts are thin slices of skin that contain both dermis and epidermis. These grafts may be taken from an anesthetized donor with a special surgical instrument that allows the harvesting of very thin skin grafts. There are two basic types of skin grafts—full-thickness grafts and partial-thickness grafts. Full-thickness grafts contain the full thickness of dermis and all of the epidermis. The partial-thickness grafts contain all the epidermis and only the upper portions of the dermis.

The advantage of the partial-thickness skin graft over the full-thickness skin graft is that the split graft has a higher survival rate overall when transferred from a donor area to a recipient area of the same animal or person. However, the split graft has a higher rate of contraction or shrinkage after transfer from donor to recipient area. The full-thickness graft is more durable and generally maintains a better appearance than split grafts.

Skin grafts must be placed on a vascularized bed of tissue, such as a raw wound surface. The graft survives for several days until capillaries from the recipient site can grow into the graft and vascularize it. By day 4 or 5 after skin graft placement on a recipient site, the graft becomes stable and adequately vascularized. If blood vessels do not enter the graft within 72 hours, the graft usually dies. In addition, grafts may not survive if they are sheared or damaged during healing, or if they are immunologically rejected because of incompatibility of donor and recipient.

A series of experiments were conducted with laboratory animals and skin grafts. The experiments are described below:

Experiment 1

A split-thickness skin graft was taken from the belly of a mouse donor and placed on the hind leg of a rabbit recipient.

Experiment 2

A full-thickness graft was then taken from the back of a rabbit and placed on a rat belly recipient site.

Experiment 3

A split-thickness graft was taken from the belly of a rat donor and placed on the neck region of a mouse recipient.

The data table below describes graft status 3, 5, and 7 days after the above skin graft transfers were performed. Grafts were examined, and those that were viable were shown as (+). The grafts that did not survive at the time of examination were shown as (−).

TABLE 2. Skin graft status after transfer.

Experiment #	Days After Graft Transfer	Graft Viability
1	3	+
2	3	+
3	3	+
1	5	+
2	5	−
3	5	−
1	7	+
2	7	−
3	7	−

+ = viable; − = nonviable.

16. Which of the following might be found in a full-thickness skin graft but not in a split-thickness graft?

   A. Epidermal cells
   B. Keratin
   C. Pigment cells
   D. Sweat glands

17. Which cellular elements of skin are most likely responsible for the shrinkage of split-thickness grafts?

   A. Fibroblasts
   B. Epidermal cells
   C. Endothelial cells
   D. Nerve cells

18. Analysis of the split-thickness experimental data presented in the passage suggests that:

   A. rat-to-mouse transfers show delayed graft rejection.
   B. rabbit-to-mouse transfers are more susceptible to early rejection.
   C. mouse-to-rabbit transfers show delayed graft rejection.
   D. mouse-to-rat transfers are more susceptible to early rejection.

19. According to the data in the passage, how do split-thickness grafts survive compared with full-thickness grafts in the rabbit-to-rat transfer?

   A. Full-thickness grafts survive longer.
   B. Split-thickness grafts survive longer.
   C. There is no difference in graft survival between these graft types.
   D. There is not enough information to determine graft survival.

499

20. According to the data presented, how does skin graft survival vary according to graft type?

    A. Split-thickness grafts survive longer.
    B. Full-thickness grafts survive longer.
    C. Split-thickness grafts survive longer only on rabbit donors.
    D. More data is needed to draw any conclusions based on graft type.

21. If a split-thickness skin graft from a normally hair-bearing area of skin is transferred to a hairless area of the same animal, which of the following would be true?

    A. The animal will grow hair at the recipient site.
    B. The animal will not grow hair at the recipient site because differentiation will not occur.
    C. Induction will occur such that the dermis of the recipient site will influence the donor graft not to grow hair.
    D. Hair growth will depend on whether the graft has enough dermal thickness to include hair follicles.

22. What is the most likely mechanism by which a skin graft survives the first 48 hours after transfer?

    A. Capillary ingrowth
    B. Aerobic metabolism
    C. Diffusion of nutrients into the graft
    D. Lymphatic vessels

Passage IV (Questions 23–28)

Dietary fat is hydrolyzed in the gut to form fatty acids, glycerides, and cholesterol. Following absorption and resynthesis to triglycerides by mucosal cells of the small intestine, fats are secreted into the intestinal lymphatics as chylomicrons, and they enter the bloodstream via the thoracic duct. In the liver, processing of chylomicrons occurs.

Fatty acids and cholesterol are the major lipids requiring transport in the plasma. Because both are insoluble in water, fatty acids and cholesterol require transport in hydrophilic complexes, collectively referred to as lipoproteins. There are several types of lipoproteins, with low-density lipoproteins (LDL) constituting a major lipoprotein carrying cholesterol in the bloodstream. High-density lipoprotein (HDL) also carries cholesterol in the serum. However, LDL tends to deliver cholesterol to cells of the body from the serum, whereas HDL carries excess cholesterol from cells of the body back to LDL and the liver.

Familial hypercholesterolemia (FH) is a relatively common autosomal dominant disorder characterized by an increased plasma concentration of LDL. Patients with this condition may be homozygous or heterozygous. Patients with a homozygous form of the disease have a more severe set of symptoms.

Primary hypertriglceridemia (PH) is a disease that results in the accumulation of triglycerides in tissues of the body. It is transmitted by an autosomal recessive route. This condition is caused by a deficiency in the enzyme lipoprotein lipase.

23. Which of the following would be most likely associated with the homozygous form of FH?

    A. Elevated levels of triglycerides in the blood
    B. Elevated levels of lipoprotein lipase
    C. Deposition of cholesterol in body tissues
    D. Elevation of HDL as a compensatory mechanism

24. Which of the following strategies would *least likely* decrease the severity of FH in afflicted patients?

    A. Provision of a drug that decreases LDL levels directly
    B. Provision of a drug that decreases the synthesis of cholesterol in the liver and increases the synthesis of HDL
    C. Provision of a drug that interferes with the mechanism of cholesterol binding to HDL and chylomicrons
    D. Decreasing the dietary intake of cholesterol

25. The vessels that transport lipids through the intestine following absorption are known as:

    A. lacteals.
    B. thoracic ducts.
    C. capillary beds.
    D. lymph nodes.

26. Which statement best describes the relationships presented in the passage?

    A. There is a cycle in which LDL delivers cholesterol to extrahepatic cells, whereas cholesterol is returned to LDL from extrahepatic cells via HDL.
    B. Mechanisms exist that transport HDL-bound cholesterol from the liver to the tissues of the body to prevent overaccumulation of cholesterol in the liver.
    C. HDL and LDL mediate the transport of cholesterol from the intestine to the circulation via chylomicrons.
    D. Chylomicrons require lipoproteins such as LDL and HDL to provide a polar surface that allows transport in the plasma.

27. A male patient is found to have a lipid-related disease. By interviewing the patient, it is discovered that his parents were not affected by a lipid-related disease. However, his maternal grandmother did show evidence of a lipid-related disease, and she died from complications of it. Based on this evidence, one may expect which of the following statements to be true?

A. The patient may have FH.
B. The patient may have PH.
C. The patient may have FH or PH.
D. The patient has neither FH nor PH.

28. Consider that FH is determined by alleles on a single locus of a human chromosome. If a child has a severe form of FH with grossly elevated levels of serum cholesterol, and the parents of this child have mild forms of the disease, which of the following best explains this phenomenon?

A. Complete dominance of FH
B. Incomplete dominance of FH
C. Codominance of FH
D. Incomplete penetrance of FH

Passage V (Questions 29–34)

Extensive surgical procedures frequently involve significant blood losses. Depending on the overall health of a patient, surgical blood losses can increase the risk of complications to the patient's health. Large blood losses have been linked to higher rates of postoperative heart attack, stroke, and bleeding problems. Recently, researchers have evaluated the effect of isovolemic hemodilution (IHD) in extensive surgical procedures.

IHD is defined as the reduction of the percentage of red blood cells in the blood by withdrawal of red blood cells and simultaneous replacement with cell-free substitutes. The procedure is performed in several steps. First, the patient has a volume of blood removed prior to surgery. Second, the same volume of blood that is removed prior to surgery is replaced with liquid albumin or other viscous fluid. The theory behind IHD is to dilute the patient's blood before surgery, so that the blood losses that occur during surgery are of a more dilute blood. In the third and final step, which is performed once bleeding stops after completion of surgery, the blood that was initially removed is given back to the patient as an auto-transfusion. The IHD procedure may be useful because it decreases the risk of transmitting viruses, such as the human immunodeficiency virus (HIV), because the patient's own blood is the only blood source.

To evaluate the effect of IHD in patients undergoing extensive surgery, measurements of heart rate (HR) in beats per minute, systolic blood pressure (SBP) in mm Hg, percent of blood volume comprised of red blood cells (PCV%), and arteriovenous oxygen content difference (AVOC) were measured. By definition, AVOC is the percentage difference in oxygen content between the arterial and venous blood. The data is shown in the table below:

TABLE 3. Data showing effect of isovolemic hemodilution (IHD) on patients undergoing extensive surgery.

Measurement	Pre-IHD	Post-IHD	Post Auto-Transfusion
Heart rate (HR)	87	98	87
Systolic blood pressure (SBP)	120	102	126
PCV%	40	32	36
AVOC	31	30	30

PCV% = Percent of blood volume that is red blood cells; AVOC = arteriovenous oxygen content difference.

29. Which of the following would be expected as a result of IHD?

A. An increase in SBP
B. An increase in AVOC difference
C. An increase in HR
D. An increase in the PCV%

30. A physiologic response to the first step of the IHD procedure would be expected to produce:

A. vasoconstriction of capillary beds
B. changes in pulmonary function
C. increased urine production
D. vasodilation and bronchodilation

31. Immediately following the first step of the IHD procedure, but prior to the second step, a blood sample is drawn from the patient. The blood sample is assayed for the presence of hormones normally released from the pituitary gland. Which of the following would be expected to be elevated?

A. Melanocyte-stimulating hormone (MSH)
B. Thyroid-stimulating hormone (TSH)
C. Antidiuretic hormone (ADH)
D. Follicle-stimulating hormone (FSH)

32. When comparing the pre-IHD and post auto-transfusion stages, the IHD procedure is *least likely* to:

A. maintain blood pressure.
B. maintain AVOC.
C. maintain heart rate.
D. maintain PCV%.

33. Which one of the following glands would most likely be activated by the IHD procedure?

   A. Thyroid
   B. Adrenal
   C. Parathyroid
   D. Thymus

34. If AVOC values of a patient in the post-IHD stage (step 2) increase to 40, then it is likely that:

   A. there is decreased oxygen extraction by body tissues.
   B. there are increased oxygen levels in the arterial blood.
   C. there is increased oxygen extraction by body tissues.
   D. there are decreased oxygen levels in the arterial blood.

Questions 35–40 are NOT based on a descriptive passage.

35. Several genetic diseases are caused by variations in the number of chromosomes possessed by a zygote. Aneuploidy results when the normal chromosome complement of a cell is increased or decreased by one or more chromosomes. The process that best accounts for aneuploidy is:

   A. random mutation.
   B. translocation.
   C. crossing over.
   D. nondisjunction.

36. During starvation, fat stores and lean body mass both decrease. Associated with the prolonged starvation is the onset of tissue swelling or edema. The onset of edema is most likely attributed to:

   A. decreased serum albumin.
   B. increased hydrostatic pressure of the blood.
   C. increased oncotic pressure of the blood.
   D. decreased activity of the heart.

37. The pineal gland in animals has been studied extensively. Studies in hamsters and other animals have shown that the pineal gland is sensitive to the amount of light seen by the eyes each day. The main role of the pineal gland is believed to be:

   A. controlling of seasonal fertility or sex drive.
   B. regulating sleep cycles.
   C. mediating feeding cycles.
   D. regulating fat storage.

38. Glucose is labeled with radioactive carbon 14 and added to a culture of liver cells. Insulin is then added to the culture. Assuming that the glucose is metabolized as an energy source, the radioactive carbon would be least expected to be associated with which liver cell structure?

   A. Cell surface receptors
   B. Cytoplasm
   C. Mitochondria
   D. Nucleus

39. A collection of frog eggs are stored in a glass vial containing pond water. The eggs are fertilized by the addition of sperm. Two days later, a drug known to be an inhibitor of endodermal tissues is added to the vial. If the eggs are able to develop into tadpoles, one might expect abnormalities in which one of the following systems?

   A. Digestive system
   B. Nervous system
   C. Skeletal system
   D. Circulatory system

40. Which one of the following processes does NOT occur in intracellular organelles?

   A. Oxidative phosphorylation
   B. Protein glycosylation
   C. Electron transport
   D. Glycolysis

Answers and Explanations to Biology Practice Test I

1. **A**   The basic mechanism of hearing is reviewed in the first passage. Eardrum movement is a form of mechanical energy, which is transmitted to the cochlear fluid. The conversion of movement of cochlear fluid (mechanical energy) to action potentials (electrical energy) in the cochlea then occurs. Chemical energy conversions do not enter this process.

2. **A**   Choice A is correct because the eardrum is lined with skin similar to that in the ear canal. Connective tissue cells (choice B) are not found as lining cells. They are found in the deeper layers of tissues or are associated with organs. Contractile cells are found in muscle tissues. Therefore, choice C is not correct because the eardrum is moved by sound energy and is a passive structure. Neurosecretory cells (choice D) are neuronal-like cells that have a secretory function.

3. **B**   A control is a standard that allows a researcher to test an experimental manipulation against an object, subject, or group. To see if gelfoam-FGF has any effect on healing, it must be compared with a similar manipulation. By placing saline (PBS) on gelfoam and applying it to the opposite ear, one can see if healing is affected by FGF. The possible effect of gelfoam application to the eardrum is removed from consideration by the use of gelfoam-PBS as a control. In addition, the placement of a left-eardrum perforation experimentally also acts as a control for the right-eardrum perforation. Many students confuse experimental groups with control groups. The experimental procedure is one that is done to evaluate a permutation. The control is what the experimental procedure is compared against.

4. **D**   This question can be answered by evaluating Figure 1. At 3 days, there is a significant difference between the percentage of wounds closed comparing FGF and PBS groups. At 8 days, there is less of a difference, which makes statement D a better choice than statement C. The question asks for the best-supported statement, which does not mean that only one statement is correct. On the MCAT, it is common to see several correct statements following an MCAT question. Choice A is incorrect because there is no control group for comparison. Choice B is incorrect because 1-mm injuries were evaluated only at 3 days; there was no 8-day evaluation.

5. **B**   This question can be answered by looking at Figure 1. The 2-mm injury group at 5 days post-injury has no PBS group acting as a control.

6. **C**   The statement that is least supported is the correct answer, so each of the statements need to be read carefully. Choice A is a correct statement. Choice B is indirectly supported by the data in the passage. Look at Figure 1 at 3 days post-injury. By increasing the percentage of wounds closed, FGF is decreasing the percentage of wounds that do not close. Choice D is a reasonable and correct inference from Figure 1. Choice C is the answer to this question because there is no data in the passage that allows evaluation of the area of perforations.

7. **A**   Mitogenic substances cause cell division. Carcinogenesis, the development of malignancy, is not discussed or implied in the passage. Transformation and transduction are means by which bacteria exchange genetic material.

8. **A**   The passage states that Crouzon's disease is associated with a sequence that coded for a specific protein (fibroblastic growth factor receptor 2). Although a chromosome is ultimately affected by the mutation, the actual mutation occurs at the level of the gene. Thus, choice B is eliminated. Always use the process of elimination to determine the best answer. Choice C is not the best answer because allele mutation is not a valid term. An allele is a form of a gene and does not imply a mutation. A nonsense mutation is a specific type of mutation that does not give rise to a protein.

9. **B**   In the second paragraph of the passage, it is stated that 50% of offspring inherit the condition from either parent. Autosomal dominant inheritance would produce 50% afflicted offspring if one parent had the condition. Because either parent can pass the condition to offspring, the inheritance is not sex-linked (choice A). And, because it appears that there is no carrier state, recessive processes (choice D) are unlikely. Choice C is unlikely because a random mutation at the level of the same gene would have to occur each generation.

10. **D**   This question asks why the receptors are nonfunctional, not about the quantity of receptors. Choice A is not reasonable because there is no information in the passage to suggest that the receptor location changes. Choice B could explain why there may be fewer receptors, but does not deal with receptor function. Choice C is tricky. It suggests that receptors may be nonfunctional because they bind other growth factors. It is not a wrong statement, but before selecting a choice, choice D should be evaluated. Choice D gives a clear mechanism as to why the receptors may be nonfunctional. Choice C provides more of a sequelae and less of a mechanism for receptor nonfunction; therefore, choice D is the best answer.

11. **B**   The passage states that a kinase system is associated with the receptor. Kinase reactions involve phosphorylation of cellular proteins.

12. **C**   The question asks which tissue is least likely to utilize growth factors. The passage states that fibroblasts and osteoblasts produce these growth factors. The process of elimination can be used to find the least likely target tissue of the growth factors. Bone tissue is a likely target because osteoblasts produce growth factors. Similarly, connective tissue and skin are likely targets because they contain large numbers of fibroblasts. The only tissue that does not seem to go with the others is the glandular tissues.

13. **A**   A noncompetitive inhibitor binds to the receptor at a location away from its primary binding or active site, and interferes with the function of the primary binding site, making it difficult for growth factors to bind to receptors. Because the passage implies that growth factors are important for cellular growth, one would expect abnormal embryo growth when a substance that noncompetitively inhibits the fibroblast growth receptor (and interferes with the function of the primary binding site) is injected into developing embryos.

14. **D**   This question tests for overconclusion or misunderstanding of the conclusions reached in the passage. The process of elimination should be used. Choice A is incorrect because Table 1 shows that subjects can have cranial stenosis without having Crouzon's disease. Choice B incorrectly implies that Crouzon's disease correlates with otherwise normal children with an isolated stenosis. Choice C is incorrect because Crouzon's disease correlates with receptor levels not growth factor levels. This choice also incorrectly states that there is a correlation with the degree of stenosis. The degree of stenosis is not stated in the passage. Choice D is a correct statement and is the best choice by default.

15. **D**   The passage states that both fibroblasts and osteoblasts produce growth factors. In addition, one should know that osteoblasts lead to bone formation, and fi-

broblasts lead to connective tissue formation. Both osteoblasts and fibroblasts are involved in normal bone growth, and they most likely play a role in abnormal bone growth such as that described in cranial stenosis. Osteoclasts are bone-resorbing cells, and they lead to bone destruction. Their role in cranial stenosis is unlikely.

16. **D** The passage mentions that a split-thickness graft contains part but not all of the dermis. The dermis contains sweat glands, sebaceous glands (oil-producing glands), blood vessels, and nerve endings. The epidermis contains epidermal cells and keratin. Pigment cells can usually be found between the epidermis and the dermal layers.

17. **A** This question tests the understanding of the basic cells found in the body. Epidermal cells are found on the surface of the skin, whereas endothelial cells line internal body structures (e.g., blood vessels). Simple nerve cells do not have a shrinkage potential. Fibroblasts secrete collagen and elastin proteins, which may contribute to contraction of a graft. In addition, fibroblasts may become associated with other cells that have some contractile properties.

18. **C** When reading the listed experiments in the passage, you should outline in the margin which animal tissues were transplanted and where they were transplanted. This process greatly speeds analysis of data. In addition, evaluate Table 2 carefully. Note that experiments 1 and 3 present split-graft data. Experiment 2 refers to full-thickness grafts. Evaluating Table 2, notice that for both experiments 1 and 3, grafts are nonviable at either 5 or 7 days. Use the process of elimination to reject choices that do not make sense. Choice A is incorrect because rat-to-mouse transfers are nonviable at 5 days. Choices B and D are incorrect because the experiments do not describe rabbit-to-mouse or mouse-to-rat transfers. Choice C is correct because Table 2 shows that mouse-to-rabbit transfers are still viable at 7 days.

19. **D** The passage implies that split-thickness grafts have a higher survival rate than full-thickness grafts. However, the question does not ask about generalities; it asks about graft survival in a particular experiment (i.e., rabbit-to-rat transfer). The rabbit-to-rat transfer is performed in experiment 2 and involves only full-thickness grafts. There is no data allowing us to see how split-thickness grafts survive.

20. **D** This question tests for overgeneralizations in evaluating passages and data. The question asks about skin-graft survival based on data. The passage states that split-thickness grafts have a higher survival rate but does not provide information about immunologic rejection or compatibility. Neither the passage nor Table 2 supplies data that allows a generalization to be made about the immunologic survival of split-thickness or full-thickness grafts.

21. **D** Hair follicles are found in the dermis. If the split-thickness graft contains enough dermis to include the follicles, hair will grow. This question deals with fully differentiated, mature tissues. Processes such as induction, differentiation, and determination occur during development. Thus, choices B and C are incorrect. Choice A is not as good as choice D because you do not know if the split-thickness graft contains enough dermis to include hair follicles.

22. **C** The passage states that vascularization of the graft occurs during the first several days after placement on a raw surface. The passage does not explain how the graft survives during the time in which capillaries are growing. The process of elimination (and common sense) are used to find the best answer. Choice A is incorrect because capillaries grow during the first several days, and they cannot vascularize the graft for a couple of days. Choice B is incorrect because there is not a good supply of oxygen to the graft. Furthermore, anaerobic metabolism is more likely to keep the graft viable. Lymphatic vessels drain tissue fluid from a region of the body and do not provide nourishment. Choice C, or the diffusion of nutrients, is the best choice.

23. **C** The passage discusses the role of low-density lipoproteins (LDL) in the body and states that LDL delivers cholesterol to cells of the body. With a homozygous form of familial hypercholesterolemia (FH), the patient has two copies of the genetic trait and more severe symptoms. Choice A is incorrect because it describes what is expected with the primary hypertriglyceridemia (PH) disease. A low level of lipoprotein lipase is associated with PH, and there is no evidence in the passage that indicates a relationship with FH. Choice D is incorrect because the passage does not support the statement that elevation of high-density lipoprotein (HDL) is a compensatory mechanism. Also, this idea is counter to what is expected with homozygous FH. Elevated levels of LDL not HDL would be expected. Choice C is the best choice because with elevated levels of LDL, large amounts of cholesterol would circulate. A correct inference is that this could lead to deposition of cholesterol in body tissues.

24. **C** To answer this question correctly, identify the choice that would not lower low-density lipoprotein (LDL) or serum cholesterol. Choice A lowers LDL directly and should decrease the severity of familial hypercholesterolemia (FH) disease. Choice B should decrease the level of cholesterol in the blood and increase the transport of cholesterol from the body tissues to the liver. These are both helpful to patients with FH. Decreasing cholesterol intake should also help patients. Choice C is the answer because the drug would interfere with the ability of high-density lipoprotein (HDL) to transport cholesterol away from body tissues.

25. **A** Fat is absorbed in the form of chylomicrons into the lacteals of the small intestine. It is propelled along with lymph fluid to the thoracic duct, where it empties into the large veins of the neck. Capillaries are not involved in this process. Lymph nodes act as filters and centers for immune cells in the body. Although lymph nodes can be found in the intestine, they are not vessels that transport lipids through the intestine.

26. **A** Choice A is implied by the passage in the second paragraph. Choices B and C are incorrect statements and are contraindicated by paragraph two of the passage. Choice D is a nonsense choice that sounds correct but uses the terms described in the passage incorrectly. Chylomicrons, low-density lipoprotein (LDL), and high-density lipoprotein (HDL) are separate entities.

27. **B** The question specifically states that the patient's parents did not have the condition but a grandparent did. This is the key to answering this question. The disease cannot be an autosomal dominant inherited disease like familial hypercholesterolemia (FH) because a parent of the patient would have had the disease. The disease could be a recessively transmitted disease, with a grandparent having the disease and the child of the grandparent (the patient's parent) being a carrier of the disease. If this were the case, both of the patient's parents must have been carriers.

28. **C** If both parents had mild forms of the disease, they were heterozygous. The child is homozygous and has a worse form of the disease than either parent. Codominant allelic interaction occurs when each gene makes an equally strong contribution to the phenotype. Therefore, the child has a more severe form of the disease because the child has two copies of the gene. Incomplete dominance falls between codominance and complete dominance: the phenotype of a heterozygote (Aa) is intermediate between the phenotypes of homozygous (AA) and (aa). An example is the cross of red flowers with white flowers making pink flowers. Incomplete penetrance means that a phenotype is not always expressed or fully expressed. For example, there are diseases in which an individual possesses the gene for a severe disease but may never show any evidence of the disease. Others with the same gene may show a mild form of the disease or may die from the disease.

29. **C** While reading the passage about isovolemic hemodilution (IHD), think about the basic physiology of the procedure. When the patient is bled, the blood pressure should fall, and the heart rate should rise as a compensatory mechanism. The percentage of red blood cells in the blood volume (PCV%) would be expected to decrease because there is a loss of red blood cells. IHD causes a rise in the heart rate. The other choices are incorrect, based on an inspection of the post-IHD column of Table 3.

30. **A** The first step of the isovolemic hemodilution (IHD) procedure is explained in the passage. It involves the removal of blood from the patient, which causes stimulation of vasoconstriction of peripheral capillary beds to maintain the blood pressure. Stimulation of the sympathetic nervous system would also be expected. There is no evidence that pulmonary function would change. Decreased urine production is expected in times of blood volume loss because of the increased release of antidiuretic hormone by the posterior pituitary gland.

31. **C** During dehydration or blood volume loss, the posterior pituitary gland releases antidiuretic hormone (ADH). ADH acts to increase reabsorption of water in the collecting ducts of the kidney nephrons.

32. **D** Table 3 needs to be carefully evaluated to answer this question. Compare the pre-isovolemic hemodilution (IHD) column with the post auto-transfusion column. Note that systolic blood pressure (SBP), heart rate (HR), and arteriovenous oxygen content difference (AVOC) are stable. Only the percentage of red blood cells in the blood volume (PCV%) decreases.

33. **B** The adrenal gland is activated during periods of stress. The adrenal cortex produces cortisol, which is a steroid hormone that helps the body deal with stress. The adrenal medulla also releases epinephrine, norepinephrine, and amine hormones, which increase heart rate and blood pressure acutely. The thyroid gland produces thyroid hormone and calcitonin. Thyroid hormone increases the metabolic rate, and calcitonin decreases serum calcium. The parathyroid glands produce parathyroid hormone, which increases serum calcium. The thymus gland is the maturation center for T lymphocytes.

34. **A** This question tests the understanding of a basic definition in the passage and tests if the basic principles can be applied. Arteriovenous oxygen content difference (AVOC) describes the percent difference in oxygen content between the arterial and venous blood. If the body tissues do not extract oxygen well from the arterial blood, the venous blood will have a high oxygen content, and the AVOC will decrease. If oxygen is extracted well from the arterial blood, the venous blood oxygen content will be low, and the AVOC will increase. The AVOC provides no information about the oxygen content of the arterial blood. Information is given only about the oxygen content difference between arterial and venous blood.

35. **D** Nondisjunction at meiosis can cause homologous chromosomes to fail to disjoin at the first meiotic division, which causes two of the resulting gametes to carry a double dose of the chromosome. The other two gametes lack the chromosome entirely.

36. **A** With protein starvation, serum albumin levels fall. Because albumin is the dominant serum protein, a low albumin level gives rise to low serum oncotic pressure. This leads to less fluid reabsorption in the capillary beds and tissue fluid accumulation. The tissue fluid leads to edema.

37. **A** The pineal gland has been linked to seasonal fertility in animals. It is believed that the duration of daily sunlight stimulates centers in the brain to respond to seasonal changes and to mating times. In humans and higher animals, the pineal gland is postulated to have a role in the sex drive.

38. **D** The labeled glucose binds to cell-surface receptors, which require insulin to bring glucose into the cell. Glucose may be metabolized in the cytoplasm by gly-

colytic enzymes. Labeled carbon molecules may also be found in the mitochondria undergoing Krebs cycle. It is less likely that the radioactive label would be found in the nucleus.

39. **A** The lining of the digestive system develops from endoderm. The nervous system develops from ectoderm, and the circulatory and skeletal systems develop from mesoderm.

40. **D** Glycolysis occurs in the cytoplasm. Oxidative phosphorylation and electron transport occur in mitochondria. Protein glycosylation occurs in the Golgi apparatus.

Time: 45 minutes

Directions: This test contains as many biology passages as you may encounter on the real MCAT. There are also several independent multiple-choice questions at the end of this test. The time allotted approximates the time allowed on a real MCAT to solve the given number of questions. Choose one best answer for each question.

Passage I (Questions 1–7)

An essential role of biologic membranes is to allow movement of all compounds necessary for normal cell function to cross the barrier selectively. These compounds include a vast array of sugars, amino acids, steroids, fatty acids, anions, and cations. These substances must enter and exit in a coordinated and balanced manner for the cell to function normally. Disturbances of these balances can often cause serious problems.

Mediated transport can be active, passive, or coupled. A few metabolites of low molecular weight are presumed to move or diffuse across the membrane freely. The rate of flow is directly proportional to the concentration gradient across the membrane. The simple facilitated diffusion is called passive transport. Net transport can occur only by diffusion. The kinetics mimic simple Michaelis-Menten enzyme kinetics; that is, the system can be saturated and both K_m and V_{max} values can be obtained.

Active transport occurs against a concentration gradient. This process must be driven by some energy-yielding reaction. Coupled transport is transport of two different solutes that may occur in the same direction (symport) or in the opposite direction (antiport). The active transport process requires energy, is coupled to energy-yielding reactions, and is directional.

Two sets of experiments were performed by different researchers evaluating transport systems.

Experiment 1

A previously unknown species of deep water fish is discovered on an expedition. Experiments are performed to measure the rate of transport of glucose and ethylene glycol from the exterior to the interior of the blood cells from this deep water fish. The following data is obtained (Figure 1).

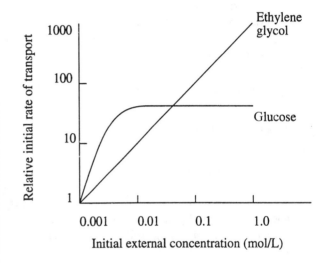

Figure 1.

Experiment 2

Researchers studying antibiotics at a pharmaceutical company discover two new peptide antibiotics (antibiotic A and antibiotic B) that promote cation transport. Two artificial membrane systems, each containing one of the antibiotics, are prepared. The initial rate of potassium ion transport as a function of temperature is obtained and is shown in Figure 2.

509

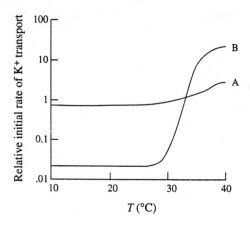

Figure 2.

1. Which one of the following compounds will most readily diffuse through a typical membrane at pH 7 without a transport protein?

   A. $CH_3(CH_2)_3$—OH

   B. CH_3—$\overset{\overset{\displaystyle O}{\|}}{C}$—$NH_2$

   C. H_3N—CH—$\overset{\overset{\displaystyle O}{\|}}{C}$—$NH_2$
                  $\underset{\displaystyle OH}{|}$

   D. HO—$(CH_2)_3$—OH

2. Glucose is more polar than ethylene glycol. The spontaneous diffusion of glucose through cell membranes compared with ethylene glycol would be expected to be:

   A. faster.
   B. slower.
   C. the same.
   D. undeterminable.

3. The most likely explanation for the difference in the two curves in Figure 1 is:

   I. glucose is more polar and cannot diffuse linearly.
   II. ethylene glycol has a specific carrier.
   III. glucose has a specific carrier.

   A. I and III only
   B. I and II only
   C. III only
   D. II only

4. Comment on the following statement using data presented in experiment 2:

   One class of peptide antibiotic promotes ion transport and is lipid soluble. It is cyclic, and it can bind ions and diffuse with them across the membrane. Antibiotic A is a member of this class.

   A. According to the data, this statement is most likely true.
   B. This statement is most likely contradicted by the data.
   C. The data does not relate to this statement.
   D. More data is needed giving transport rates for temperatures greater than 40°C.

5. Based on the data shown in Figure 2, which one of the following statements regarding antibiotic B is true?

   A. It forms an ion channel in the membrane.
   B. It is a cation carrier and diffuses across the membrane.
   C. Both A and B are likely true.
   D. Neither A nor B are likely true.

6. In animal cells, the active uptake of many different solutes is coupled to the passive transport of sodium ions. If 10 solutes are transported per sodium ion, and the internal concentration of sodium is maintained at 0.01 of the external concentration, what ratio of internal-to-external concentration will be maintained for each of the 10 solutes?

   A. 1:1
   B. 1:10
   C. 1:100
   D. 1:1000

7. Consider the data presented in experiment 1. A drug that is a known blocker of active transport in all blood cells is added to the extracellular fluid prior to the initiation of the experiments. Which one of the following would be expected?

   A. The plot for ethylene glycol would most likely plateau.
   B. Glucose transport would most likely cease.
   C. Ethylene glycol transport would likely cease.
   D. Glucose transport would likely become linear.

Passage II (Questions 8–14)

The polymerase chain reaction (PCR) is an in vitro method used to amplify specific DNA segments. In PCR, DNA strands are separated by heat denaturation, and DNA primers are annealed to the 3′ ends at the region of interest. DNA polymerase catalyzes the extension of the complementary strand. At this point in the process, the quantity of genetic material is doubled, and the cycle can be repeated.

PCR in combination with reverse transcriptase can be used to amplify viral RNA. Reverse transcriptase (an enzyme present only in certain viruses) uses an RNA template to synthesize complementary DNA (cDNA), which is then used in PCR.

Recently, detection of human immunodeficiency virus (HIV) RNA from blood cells has been made possible through the use of PCR and reverse transcriptase. The presence of viral RNA indicates expression of the infectious virus.

The following table summarizes the results of a study using patients who tested positive for HIV infection. The diagnosis was based on a serologic assay for antibodies to HIV.

TABLE I. Summary of study using HIV-positive patients.

Subject Number	Drugs	Symptoms*	Viral RNA Detection Using PCR**
I	None	++	+
2	None	++	+
3	None	+	−
4	AZT	+	+
5	AZT	+++	+
6	AZT	−	−
7	None	−	−
8	None	+++	+
9	AZT	++	+
10	AZT	+	−

*Symptoms: +++, ++, +, and − denote severe, moderate, low, and no symptoms associated with AIDS, respectively.
**Polymerase chain reaction (PCR) results: + denotes HIV RNA expression; − denotes no expression.
AZT = azidothymidine.

8. Which one of the following is needed for the PCR to occur?

   A. Helicase
   B. DNA ligase
   C. Nucleotides
   D. RNA

9. Which of the following statements regarding the process of PCR is true?

   A. Polymerization of the complimentary strand is in the 3′-to-5′ direction.
   B. Reverse transcriptase is present in most eukaryotic cells.
   C. A primer is necessary for DNA polymerase to initiate synthesis of complementary DNA.
   D. A primer is necessary for RNA polymerase to initiate synthesis of complementary RNA.

10. Reverse transcriptase uses the following viral RNA template:

    5′ AUCAGGUUAGAC 3′

    Which one of the following sequences represents the viral cDNA formed?

    A. 5′ GTCTAACCTGAT 3′
    B. 5′ TAGTCCAATGTG 3′
    C. 5′ UAGUCCAAUGUG 3′
    D. 5′ GUCUAACCUGAU 3′

11. If the cDNA formed in question 10 is to be used in PCR, which of the following nucleotide sequences could be used as the DNA primer?

    A. 5′ CACATT 3′
    B. 5′ CAGATT 3′
    C. 5′ ATCAGG 3′
    D. 5′ GGACTA 3′

12. The viral cDNA inserts into a host cell chromosome. The genetic material of the virus and the host cell is then transcribed and translated. Which step occurs in the cytoplasm?

    A. Binding the ribosome to the messenger RNA (mRNA)
    B. Cleaving of introns
    C. Adding adenine residues at the 3′ end of mRNA
    D. Adding a 5′ methyl cap

13. Which one of the following statements is true based on the data presented in Table 1?

    A. Patients 1, 2, and 8 all have moderate symptoms.
    B. The blood serum of patients 5, 6, and 7 contains antibodies specific for HIV.
    C. Patients 5, 6, and 7 all express the infectious virus.
    D. The azidothymidine (AZT) treatment of patient 6 is most likely responsible for the absence of symptoms associated with AIDS.

14. Results from the study indicate:

    A. Treatment with AZT correlates with a decrease in symptoms associated with AIDS.
    B. Treatment with AZT significantly decreases RNA expression of HIV.
    C. Patients without AZT treatment had significantly fewer symptoms associated with AIDS.
    D. Testing positive for RNA expression of HIV correlates with an increase in symptoms associated with AIDS.

5 I I

Passage III (Questions 15–22)

The cardiovascular physiology of a fetus is quite different from that of an adult. These differences arise from the fact that the fetus receives oxygenated blood from the placenta rather than the lungs. The fetal umbilical vein is analogous to the adult pulmonary vein in that both are responsible for delivering oxygenated blood to the heart. The fetal heart then pumps the blood to the rest of the fetal body through the systemic circulatory system.

The differences between the fetus and adult also manifest in the type of hemoglobin that is carried in red blood cells. If you were to plot both adult and fetal hemoglobin on an oxygen dissociation curve, the fetal hemoglobin curve would be to the left of the adult hemoglobin curve.

The majority of fetal blood is shunted away from the lungs, providing only the flow needed for development. Two structures, the foramen ovale and the ductus arteriosus, allow blood flow to bypass the fetal lungs. Blood flows directly from the right atrium to the left atrium through the foramen ovale. The ductus arteriosus provides a pathway for blood from the pulmonary artery to the aorta.

At birth, the umbilical cord is cut, making the infant depend on its own respiratory system. Lung expansion and the presence of oxygen causes pulmonary vasodilation. During the first couple of days, the ductus arteriosus constricts, and the foramen ovale functionally closes, which results in increased blood flow to the lungs. The infant's cardiovascular system rapidly becomes like that of an adult.

15. In the fetal cardiovascular system, which structure listed below contains the most oxygenated blood?

   A. The right atrium
   B. The left atrium
   C. The umbilical artery
   D. The umbilical vein

16. In the adult cardiovascular system, which structure listed below contains the most oxygenated blood?

   A. The left atrium
   B. The pulmonary artery
   C. The right atrium
   D. The superior vena cava

17. In the adult cardiovascular system, which structure listed below contains the most pressure?

   A. The pulmonary artery
   B. The aorta
   C. The pulmonary vein
   D. The right ventricle

18. If the foramen ovale failed to close after birth, which one of the following actions is most likely to occur?

   A. Pressure in the pulmonary circulation would drop.
   B. Blood would be shunted from the left atrium to the right atrium.
   C. Systemic blood flow would increase.
   D. Systemic venous pressure would increase.

19. If the ductus arteriosus failed to close after birth, which of the statements below would be FALSE?

   A. Pressure in the pulmonary artery would increase.
   B. Oxygenated blood would be shunted to the lungs.
   C. Pressure in the left ventricle would increase.
   D. Blood would be shunted from the aorta to the pulmonary artery.

20. Which of the following substances listed below cannot diffuse between the maternal and fetal circulatory systems?

   A. A virus
   B. Antibodies
   C. Alcohol
   D. Platelets

21. If the ductus arteriosus fails to close, which of the following can be expected to occur?

   A. The lungs would compensate for decreased oxygen content by using mechanisms such as releasing angiotensin-converting enzyme (ACE).
   B. The ductus venosus would take over some of the function of the ductus arteriosus.
   C. Low oxygen content in the blood would be expected, and an increased respiratory rate would be of little value in increasing blood oxygen levels.
   D. Special fetal blood vessels, such as the ductus venosus and foramen ovale, would decrease the amount of blood shunted around the lungs and minimize low blood oxygen levels.

22. Which of the following is/are true regarding the fetal circulatory system?

    I.   Fetal hemoglobin has a lower affinity for oxygen than adult hemoglobin.

    II.   The resistance to bloodflow in the fetal lungs is high because the fetal lungs are filled with fluid.

    III. The umbilical artery carries deoxygenated blood

    A.   I only
    B.   I and II only
    C.   II and III only
    D.   I and III only

Passage IV (Questions 23–29)

The visceral pleura is a tissue-paper thin membrane that lies against the outer surface of the lung and follows the external contour of the lung. The parietal pleura lines the inner aspect of the chest wall. The pleural space is defined as the potential space between these pleura, and it contains approximately 30 ml of fluid.

The elastic recoil of the lung pulls the visceral pleura inward, and the recoil of the lung pulls the parietal pleura outward. The net pressure in the pleural space at the end of passive exhalation is lower than atmospheric pressure. In the pleural space, fluid flows from the parietal surface into the pleural space, with subsequent reabsorption by the capillaries of the visceral pleura. This system is well balanced and ordinarily prevents the collection of excess pleural fluid. Through this mechanism, the pleural fluid is exchanged at the rate of 35% to 70% per hour in healthy people. However, when a disease process involves the pleura, the rate of pleural fluid production dramatically increases. This is because inflammation increases the capillary permeability of the pleura and increases the movement of fluid from the pleural membrane capillary beds into the pleural space.

The forces that control the volume of fluid in the pleural space are governed by the Starling equation. The hydrostatic pressure in the capillaries of the visceral pleura is much lower (i.e., only 16 cm H_2O) than the hydrostatic pressure in the capillaries of the parietal pleura (i.e., 35 cm H_2O). The oncotic pressure in both the visceral and parietal pleurae blood vessels is approximately 29 cm H_2O. When abnormalities in the hydrostatic and oncotic pressure, capillary permeability, or lymphatic drainage systems occur, pleural fluid collections form. Pleural inflammation, owing to infectious or noninfectious causes, leads to a high protein-containing pleural fluid collection in the pleural space. Alterations in the systemic and pulmonary venous pressures or heart failure can also increase fluid collections in the pleural space.

A malignant effusion is a clinical entity in which cancer cells invade the pleural space from a nearby malignant tumor or develop from within the pleural space itself, causing a large fluid collection in the pleural space. The cancer cells cause inflammation and interfere with the resorption of pleural fluid. Breast, lung, and ovarian cancers are well known to spread to the pleural space. Mesothelioma is a type of cancer that develops from cells within the pleural space and is associated with asbestos exposure.

23. Which of the following membrane(s) must have net movement of fluid out from the membrane surface into the pleural space?

    A.   Visceral pleura
    B.   Parietal pleura
    C.   Both the visceral and parietal pleura
    D.   Neither the visceral nor the parietal pleura

24. The significantly lower hydrostatic pressure affecting the visceral pleura is best explained by the fact that:

    A.   the visceral pleura is supplied by the low-pressure pulmonary circulation, whereas the parietal pleura is supplied by the high-pressure systemic circulation.
    B.   the visceral pleura is a very thin membrane, whereas the parietal pleura is a much more substantial membrane that requires higher perfusion pressures to provide good bloodflow.
    C.   the plasma oncotic pressure exerts a selectively greater effect on the visceral pleura.
    D.   the albumin concentration in plasma is relatively lower in the parietal pleura.

25. The pressure gradient favoring the movement of fluid into the pleural space from the parietal pleura is:

    A.   35 cm H_2O.
    B.   29 cm H_2O.
    C.   6 cm H_2O.
    D.   64 cm H_2O.

26. If the hydrostatic pressure in the visceral pleural capillaries increased by 50%, the net pressure gradient would be associated with:

    I.   a change in the direction of net fluid flow.
    II.   no change in the direction of net fluid flow.
    III. a net pressure gradient of 5 cm H_2O.

    A.   I only
    B.   II only
    C.   I and II only
    D.   II and III only

27. Based on the information in the passage, the volume of pleural fluid exchanged per day at the upper limit would best be approximated as:

    A. 0.5 l.
    B. 1 l.
    C. 2 l.
    D. 4 l.

28. Which of the following mechanisms are not consistent with the formation of malignant effusions?

    A. Increased capillary perfusion pressure
    B. Lymphatic obstruction
    C. Increased capillary permeability
    D. Venous obstruction

29. Which of the following is most likely to cause the formation of a pleural effusion?

    A. Increased resorption of pleural fluid
    B. A low serum albumin concentration
    C. A decrease in the venous pressure within the pulmonary veins
    D. An improvement of cardiac function in a patient with heart failure

Passage V (Questions 30–35)

A biologist studies three populations of mice. The three populations were named A, B, and C. Field observations of the mice were made, and the geographic boundaries of the living area for each mouse population were noted. In addition, the mating behavior of the mice were studied. Mouse populations A and B were found to nonselectively mate with one another, and they produced viable offspring.

Because of a difference in the appearance of the mouse populations with respect to hair color and hair length, a genetic analysis of each mouse population was made. A genetic difference noted between mice in populations A, B, and C was in the coding for hair length. Mice populations A and B were also found to carry a dominant form of the gene (Y) that codes for long hair. Both populations A and B also carried the recessive form of the gene (y), which was found to code for short hair. Finally, the frequency of short-haired mice in populations A and B was determined to be 81%.

Field observations of the geographic boundaries for populations A, B, and C were as follows:

Observation 1

Populations A and B were found to have overlapping geographic boundaries.

Observation 2

Populations A and C had geographically isolated populations.

Observation 3

Populations B and C had geographically isolated populations.

For populations A and B of mice, assume random intermating, viable offspring production, no intermating, and no immigration or emigration.

30. Mice populations A and B do NOT demonstrate which of the following?

    A. Speciation
    B. Competition
    C. Selective mating
    D. Two of the above

31. Mice populations A and C do not tend to mate with one another and do not produce viable offspring. The most likely explanation for these observations is:

    A. natural selection.
    B. emigration.
    C. genetic drift.
    D. geographic isolation.

32. If all the mice carrying gene Y went on a foraging expedition and were eaten by predators, which of the following best describes the effect this would have on the population gene frequencies?

    A. Natural selection
    B. Emigration
    C. Speciation
    D. Genetic drift

33. The frequency of heterozygous long-haired mice in populations A and B is:

    A. 1%.
    B. 9%.
    C. 18%.
    D. 81%.

34. What fraction of long-haired mice in populations A and B do not carry a gene for short hair?

    A. 1/81
    B. 1/9
    C. 1/18
    D. 1/19

35. Which of the following is the best description of the principle on which gene frequency calculations for the mouse populations are based? (Assume conditions of genetic equilibrium.)

   A. The gametes predict the allele frequencies expected.
   B. All genotypes in an ideal population show a variety of reproductive successes to provide variation within the population.
   C. Mutations occur randomly only, and they are not factored into allelic frequency calculations.
   D. The frequencies of alleles in the gene pool remain constant from generation to generation.

Questions 36–40 are NOT based on a descriptive passage.

36. Menstruation is prevented by increased levels of which one of the following hormones?

   A. Oxytocin
   B. Luteinizing hormone
   C. Estrogen
   D. Progesterone

37. During inspiration, which of the following processes occurs?

   A. The rib cage is depressed.
   B. The diaphragm moves inferiorly.
   C. Intrapulmonic pressure is positive with respect to atmospheric pressure.
   D. Intrapleural pressure is positive.

38. Which pair of the following pairs do NOT match?

   A. Cornea/ectoderm
   B. Kidney/endoderm
   C. Heart/mesoderm
   D. Thymus/endoderm

39. Which of the following is NOT a gastrointestinal hormone?

   A. Pepsin
   B. Cholecystokinin
   C. Secretin
   D. Gastrin

40. How do meiosis I and mitosis differ in anaphase?

   A. In meiosis I, homologs synapse and crossover; in mitosis, there is synapsis and no crossing over.
   B. In meiosis I, paired homologs line up on the plate; in mitosis, centromeres divide, and sister chromatids separate.
   C. In meiosis I, centromeres remain intact, and homologs separate; in mitosis, centromeres divide, and sister chromatids separate.
   D. In meiosis I, centromeres divide, and sister chromatids separate; in mitosis, centromeres remain intact, and homologs separate.

Answers and Explanations to Biology Practice Test 2

1. **A** The passage mentions that movement of molecules across membranes is important, but it does not specifically state which chemical groups are best at moving across membranes. However, the answer can be predicted based on general principles. Recall that nonpolar molecules are better for diffusing through lipid membranes. Look carefully at each of the structures shown among the choices, and note that all of the choices have some element of polarity. However, choice A is the least polar of the choices.

2. **B** The spontaneous diffusion of glucose through cell membranes is slower than ethylene glycol because glucose is more polar than ethylene glycol.

3. **C** Notice that the transport of glucose can be saturated, and the transport of ethylene glycol cannot be saturated. This suggests that a carrier exists for glucose that can be saturated and shows a maximum velocity of transport. Generally speaking, all membrane carriers have the ability to be saturated and have some element of specificity. Thus, statement III is correct. Statement I is incorrect because the presence or absence of polarity does not cause the ability to be saturated in transport. Statement II is unsupported, because the ability to be saturated is not seen in the data presented.

4. **B** To answer this difficult question, start by looking at the data for antibiotic A given in Figure 2. Note that the rate of potassium transport is affected little by increasing temperature. Generally speaking, as the temperature increases, membrane fluidity increases. If the antibiotic described in this question crossed the membrane and diffused with bound ions, one would expect it to be very sensitive to temperature and to have a rate of transport that rises markedly with increasing temperature. Antibiotic A is not affected by temperature to any great extent, and it is most likely not part of this class.

5. **B** Antibiotic B is temperature dependent, showing little transport activity at low temperatures and high transport activity at biologic temperatures. Choice A is most likely incorrect, because ion channels would be present at all temperatures. They are stable membrane elements and are not very temperature dependent. Choice B is correct, because with higher temperatures, membrane fluidity increases, and diffusion rates greatly increase.

6. **C** Because the transport of each solute is independent of the others, the ratio depends only on the sodium concentration gradient. Therefore, the ratio of sodium internal to sodium external is 0.01 to 1, or 1 to 100.

7. **B** The drug that is incubated with the extracellular solution prior to beginning experiment 1 will block active transport proteins. Look at Figure 1 and note that ethylene glycol cannot be saturated. It is most likely able to passively diffuse across the membrane without a carrier. However, glucose can be saturated and is carrier dependent. Glucose requires active transport to enter cells. Therefore, if the active transport of glucose is blocked, glucose transport will cease.

8. **C** Nucleotides are needed for DNA polymerase to synthesize the complementary strand of DNA. Helicase works to unravel double stranded DNA but, in the polymerase chain reaction (PCR), the DNA is denatured by heat. In PCR, a DNA primer is used rather than a RNA primer.

9. **C** Polymerization of the complementary strand is in the 5′ to 3′ direction. Thus, choice A is incorrect. Choice B is incorrect based on information given in the passage. Viruses bring reverse transcriptase into cells, but eukaryotic cells do not have their own reverse transcriptase. Choice D is incorrect, because an RNA primer is needed for DNA synthesis.

10. **A** If the RNA template is 5′ AUCAGGUUAGAC 3′, the complementary DNA (cDNA) formed is 3′ TAGTCCAATCTG 5′. Remember that the strands should be antiparallel with respect to the 5′/3′ orientation.

11. **C** The complementary DNA (cDNA) formed from question 10 was 3′ TAGTC-CAATCTG 5′. Therefore, the DNA primer for PCR is 5′ ATCAGG 3′. Recall the statement in the passage that the DNA primer is annealed to the 3′ end of the DNA to be polymerized.

12. **A** Ribosomes binding to messenger RNA (mRNA) is a part of translation, which occurs in the cytoplasm. The cleavage of introns and the addition of a 5′-methyl cap and a polyadenylated 3′ tail are posttranscriptional modifications that occur in the nucleus.

13. **B** This question can be answered by looking carefully at Table 1. Choice B is true because as stated in the passage, all patients in the study tested positive in serologic assays for antibodies to HIV. Choice A is incorrect, because patient 8 had severe symptoms. Choice C is incorrect because patient 6 does not demonstrate RNA expression of HIV. Choice D lacks convincing support.

14. **D** Based on the data presented in this passage, treatment with or without azidothymidine (AZT) did not correlate with the severity of symptoms or with the presence of viral RNA. Thus, choices A, B, and C are eliminated.

15. **D** This question was based on information recall. As stated in the passage, the umbilical vein carries blood directly from the placenta, where the fetal blood is oxygenated. Thus, the umbilical vein is closest to the site of oxygenation. The umbilical artery carries deoxygenated blood to the placenta, and contains the least oxygenated blood.

16. **A** As stated in the first paragraph of the passage, the pulmonary veins carry oxygenated blood from the lungs to the heart (left atrium).

17. **B** The blood vessel with the most pressure is the vessel closest to the outflow of blood from the heart to the systemic circulation. Because the aorta is the vessel accepting blood from the left ventricle, it contains the blood under the most pressure (at least 100 mm Hg). Right ventricular pressure (approximately 40 mm Hg) is much lower than aortic pressure, which makes sense conceptually. The right ventricle must pump blood through the resistance of only the pulmonary circulation, which has much lower resistance than the systemic circulation.

18. **B** In the fetus, blood-flow through the foramen ovale travels from right to left. In the adult, the pressure on the left side of the heart is much higher than on the right side. As a result, blood flows from left to right through any defect between the right and left sides of the heart.

19. **C** In the fetus, blood-flow through the ductus arteriosus goes from the pulmonary artery to the aorta. In the adult, or after birth, the blood pressure is much higher in the aorta than in the pulmonary artery. As a result, oxygenated blood from the aorta would shunt back to the lungs through the remaining ductus arteriosus. The pressure in the aorta would be transmitted to the pulmonary circulation. Choices A, B, and D are all true.

20. **D** Platelets and red blood cells theoretically do not leave the maternal circulation to exchange with the fetus. Chemicals such as alcohol and drugs, electrolytes,

glucose, amino acids, immunoglobulin G (IgG) antibodies, and viral particles are among the substances that are exchanged across the placenta.

21. **C** The ductus venosus is a vessel that bypasses the fetal liver and carries blood from the umbilical vein to the inferior vena cava. It has no direct relation to the ductus arteriosus. Choices B and D can be eliminated. Choice A is incorrect because angiotensin-converting enzyme (ACE) is involved in the renin–angiotensin system and has no relation to oxygenation. ACE is found in lung tissue and aids in the conversion of angiotensin I to angiotensin II. Choice C is the best answer because the shunting caused by a patent ductus arteriosus overwhelms the lungs with blood, decreasing the ability to effectively oxygenate blood. As might be imagined, increasing the respiratory rate does not help, because the problem is one of circulation rather than ventilation.

22. **C** Statement I is false because fetal hemoglobin has a higher affinity for oxygen than adult hemoglobin. This is what "drives" the diffusion of oxygen across the placenta. Statement II is true. At the time of birth, fluid is rapidly emptied from the lungs, and breathing of air begins. Fluid within the lungs of the fetus creates a high pulmonary vascular resistance, which promotes bloodflow through the foramen ovale and ductus arteriosus rather than through the pulmonary vasculature. Statement III is true.

PASSAGE IV

23. **B** The parietal pleura has a net outward pressure of 6 cm H_2O (35 − 29). The visceral pleura has a net inward pressure of 13 cm H_2O [oncotic pressure (29 cm H_2O) − hydrostatic pressure (16 cm H_2O)]. Inward pressure indicates an absorptive function.

24. **A** Choice A seems plausible. The pulmonary circulation has a lower pressure than the systemic circulation. Choice B does not seem plausible. Although the visceral pleura may be very thin, both pleural linings are thin. One would not expect thin membranes to require much perfusion pressure. Choices C and D are very unlikely because there is no reason why the oncotic pressure of albumin concentration would be higher in one pleural lining.

25. **C** The pressure gradient equals the hydrostatic pressure minus the oncotic pressure. As provided in the passage, 35 cm H_2O − 29 cm H_2O = 6 cm H_2O.

26. **D** Statements II and III are correct. The new pressure calculation is 29 − (16 + 8) = 5 cm H_2O. The net pressure would still be inward, which indicates an absorptive function.

27. **A** If 30 ml of pleural fluid is exchanged at a maximum of 70% per hour, then 21 ml is exchanged per hour. Per day, this would represent (24 hours) (21 ml/hour) ≅ 500 ml.

28. **A** The passage states that in malignant effusions, cancer cells interfere with the resorption of pleural fluid. Choices B and D provide mechanisms by which there may be less resorption of pleural fluid. Thus, they can be eliminated. Choice C is consistent with increased inflammation, so it can be eliminated as a choice. Choice A is the best answer.

29. **B** Increased resorption of pleural fluid would tend to decrease the chances of forming an effusion. An increase in venous pressures may help form an effusion, but a decrease would not make an effusion likely. Heart failure may lead to an effusion, but an improvement in cardiac function in such a patient would make an effusion less likely. A low serum albumin concentration decreases oncotic pressures. Hydrostatic pressures do not decline however, and pleural effusions form.

PASSAGE V

30. **D** Statements A and C are correct. The passage mentioned that viable offspring were produced. This implies that they were from the same species. In addition, the passage also pointed out the nonselectivity of mating. Competition is not discussed in the passage.

31. **D** Because mouse populations A and C are not able to mate and produce viable offspring, they must be distinct species. The diagram suggests geographic isolation, which is one of the most important factors leading to speciation.

32. **D** Genetic drift implies that the genetic constitution of a population is dramatically affected by a random event, such as the loss of a gene through catastrophe. For example, consider a population of 10 people, only one of which has a gene for red hair. Great changes in the gene pool of this population would be expected if the one person with red hair died without reproducing.

33. **C** The Hardy-Weinberg equations can be used to solve this problem. The frequency of the recessive condition is given as 81%. Remember that the Hardy-Weinberg equations are: $p^2 + 2pq + q^2 = 1$, and $p + q = 1$. Thus, $y^2 = 0.81$, and $y = 0.9$. Since $p + q = 1$, and $y = 0.9$, Y must equal 0.1. The heterozygous frequency is the $2pq$ term, and it is equivalent to $(2)(0.1)(0.9) = 0.18$.

34. **D** The percent of long-haired mice who do not carry a gene for short hair is $Y^2 = (0.1)^2 = 0.01$, or 1%. Thus, the fraction of all long-haired mice who do not carry a gene for short hair is the percent of long-haired mice who do not carry a gene for short hair divided by the percent of all long-haired mice. Thus, $1\% \div (1\% + 18\%) = 1/19$.

35. **D** Choices A and B are incorrect statements. In a Hardy-Weinberg population, there should not be a variety of reproductive successes. Although choice C may be a true statement, it does not answer the question being asked. The Hardy-Weinberg principle states that, under conditions of genetic equilibrium, the frequencies of alleles in a gene pool remain constant from generation to generation.

36. **D** This question tests the understanding of the menstrual cycle and its key associated hormones. Remember that oxytocin stimulates contraction of the smooth muscle in the uterus and breast tissue. Luteinizing hormone causes ovulation. Estrogen has many effects, but it is especially important in causing endometrial growth. Progesterone causes final endometrial growth and prevents menstruation after fertilization (under the influence of human chorionic gonadotropin). Progesterone is the main ingredient of birth control pills.

37. **B** During inspiration, the diaphragm contracts and moves inferiorly (pushing against the liver and intestines). The rib cage expands, and both the intrapulmonic pressure and intrapleural pressure are negative.

38. **B** The kidney develops from mesoderm. The other paired structures (i.e., cornea/ectoderm, heart/mesoderm, thymus/endoderm) are all correct.

39. **A** All of the substances given as choices (i.e., pepsin, cholecystokinin, secretin, and gastrin) are involved in digestion. However, pepsin is an enzyme. It forms from pepsinogen, which is a zymogen enzyme released into the stomach and activated to pepsin by hydrochloric acid. The other choices are all important hormones in the digestive process.

40. **C** Choice A describes the differences between meiosis I and mitosis in prophase. Choice B describes the differences between these two processes in metaphase. Choice D has the description reversed. Therefore, the best answer is choice C, which states: in meiosis I, centromeres divide and sister chromatids separate; in mitosis, centromeres remain intact, and homologs separate.

Time: 45 minutes

Directions: This test contains as many biology passages as you may encounter on the real MCAT. The time allotted approximates the time allowed on a real MCAT to solve the given number of questions. Choose one best answer for each question.

Passage I (Questions 1–8)

An investigator isolates three strains of bacteria from the blood of an ill patient. The bacteria are named strains A, B, and C. Each bacterial strain is grown in vitro in nutrient-rich growth media. A number of tests are performed on each strain, including tests for Gram stain and appearance, for metabolism of the organism, for the ability to ferment lactate, for the presence of coagulase, and for the ability to lyse red blood cells. The results of each of these tests for each strain are listed in Table 1.

TABLE 1. Results of tests performed on strains A, B, and C.

Strain	Gram Stain	Lactate Fermentation	Coagulase	Hemolysis
A	–	+	–	+
B	+	+	–	+
C	+	+	+	+

+ = positive; – = negative.

Coagulase is an extracellular product of some staphylococci that exists in several antigenically different forms, each of which is able to induce antibody formation and has the unique characteristic of clotting various mammalian plasmas. Coagulase does not react directly with fibrinogen but forms a thrombin-like substance by reacting with a coagulase-reacting factor of plasma. Hemolysins are peptide substances produced by some types of staphylococci that lyse red blood cells. Bacteria can use nutrients released by lysed red blood cells to grow and multiply their number.

Catalase is an enzyme not possessed by strain C but retained by strains A and B. Catalase detoxifies substances that may otherwise harm the cell, and it has an oxidative function in destroying hydrogen peroxide.

Figure 1 below shows the effect of addition of substance X to a nutrient medium of growing strain-A bacteria. The substance is added to the media at the time at which "X" is marked on the graph.

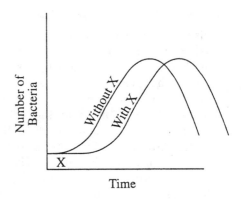

Figure 1.

1. Which strain would be LEAST sensitive to a substance that inhibited cell wall synthesis?

   A. Strain A
   B. Strain B
   C. Strain C
   D. All strains would be equally sensitive.

2. The strain that is susceptible to cell-wall inhibiting antibiotics and possesses the ability to grow in a hydrogen peroxide and blood-containing nutrient medium is most likely:

   A. strain B only.
   B. strain A or C only.
   C. strain B or C only.
   D. none of the strains.

3. Based on the information in the passage, a reasonable suggestion is that Figure 1 most likely shows strain A being exposed to a substance that:

   A. inhibits cell wall synthesis.
   B. slows protein synthesis.
   C. slows nuclear chromosome formation.
   D. inhibits aerobic metabolism.

4. Coagulase acts most like which endogenous substance?

   A. Thrombin
   B. Prothrombin
   C. Fibrin
   D. Fibrinogen

5. Strain C bacteria are grown in a nutrient medium and are lysed by a chemical agent. An extract of these lysed bacteria is injected into a rabbit. Two weeks later, a blood sample is taken from the rabbit. A second sample of living strain C bacteria growing in a nutrient medium is then exposed to this blood sample. Which of the following would be expected from this second sample of strain C bacteria?

   A. An ability to coagulate plasma
   B. An ability to grow in hydrogen peroxide
   C. Both A and B
   D. Neither A nor B

6. Which strain(s) have anaerobic potential?

   A. Strain A only
   B. Strains A and B
   C. Strains B and C
   D. Strains A, B, and C

7. Which strain is most likely to inhabit the colon and to be least sensitive to an antibiotic affecting the synthesis of bacterial cell walls?

   A. Strain A
   B. Strain B
   C. Strain C
   D. None of the above

8. An investigator grows strain C in culture medium and adds a small amount of antibiotic X to the medium. He notes an initial decrease in the number of viable bacteria; however, within 24 hours, the surviving bacteria have reexpanded the colony. The investigator then adds antibiotic Y to the colony, followed by antibiotic Z. The bacterial counts initially decline, yet the colony ultimately survives and reproduces. Which terms given below accurately describe the phenomenon described?

   I. Antibody mediated
   II. Mutation acquired
   III. Plasmid mediated

   A. II only
   B. III only
   C. I and III only
   D. II and III only

Passage II (Questions 9–16)

Septic shock is the most common cause of death in intensive care units in this country. Septic shock usually results when bacteria release synthesized products (exotoxins) or bacterial-surface components (endotoxins) into the bloodstream of infected patients. This results in a high temperature, a decrease in the vascular resistance of the blood vessels, a generalized bloodflow maldistribution, and a normal or increased cardiac output. The ventricular myocardium (cardiac muscle) becomes depressed in contractility and dilated in shape. There is an expansion in the volume of the ventricles. Normal or high cardiac outputs are maintained by high heart rates.

Data describing the left ventricular dynamics associated with the acute and recovery phases of septic shock are given in Table 2 below. Left ventricular end-diastolic volume (LVEDV) is defined as the volume of blood in the left ventricle at the end of diastole. Recall that diastole is the period of ventricular filling. Left ventricular end-systolic volume (LVESV) is the volume of blood in the left ventricle at the end of systole (ventricular contraction). Stroke volume (SV) is the volume of blood ejected with each heartbeat, and the ejection fraction (EF) is the fraction of blood in the left ventricle ejected with each heartbeat.

TABLE 2. Phases of septic shock.

Phase	LVEDV	LVESV
Acute	200 ml	150 ml
Recovery	100 ml	50 ml

LVEDV = left ventricular end-diastolic volume; *LVESV* = left ventricular end-systolic volume.

A study was performed in which 33 survivors of septic shock were compared to 21 nonsurvivors on the basis of mean left ventricular ejection fraction, end-diastolic left ventricular volume index (EDVI; ml blood per square meter of body surface area), and the time in septic shock. The data from this study is given in Table 3.

TABLE 3. Ejection fraction (EF) and end-diastolic volume index (EDVI) based on time while in septic shock.

	Time (days)	EDVI (ml/m²)	EF (%)
Survivors	1	40	40
	2–5	38	42
	6–14	55	55
Nonsurvivors	1	48	44
	2–5	44	43
	6–14	—	—

9. Based on the data given in the passage, the ratio of stroke volumes between the acute and recovery phases of septic shock is:

    A. 1:1.
    B. 1:2.
    C. 2:1.
    D. 3:1.

10. Which one of the following substances is most likely to induce septic shock?

    A. Bacterial cell walls
    B. Bacterial nuclei
    C. Membrane-bound organelles
    D. High vascular resistance

11. The ejection fraction determined from data in the acute phase of septic shock is closest to which one of the following values?

    A. 10%
    B. 25%
    C. 40%
    D. 50%

12. Which of the following best describes the high cardiac outputs associated with septic shock?

    A. Increased vascular resistance
    B. Tachycardia
    C. Increased contractility
    D. Ventricular constriction

13. A muscle biopsy of left ventricular myocardium in a septic shock patient would probably show:

    A. thinned smooth muscle.
    B. thinned smooth muscle with intercalated disks.
    C. thickened striated muscle.
    D. thinned striated muscle with intercalated disks.

14. A decrease in vascular resistance associated with a normal cardiac output in a septic shock patient is associated with a blood pressure described as:

    A. hypotensive.
    B. normotensive.
    C. hypertensive.
    D. none of the above.

15. Based on the data collected in the study, if the mean body surface area of the survivors is 2.5 m², the mean ejection fraction and EDV at day 1 for these patients are approximately:

    A. 0.40 and 40 ml, respectively.
    B. 0.40 and 100 ml, respectively.
    C. 0.44 and 44 ml, respectively.
    D. 0.44 and 110 ml, respectively.

16. As the EDVI increases in the normal heart, one would expect a change in the overlap and crosslinking of which proteins in cardiac muscle?

    A. Actin and myosin
    B. Troponin and tropomyosin
    C. Actin and troponin
    D. Myosin and tropomyosin

Passage III (Questions 17–24)

Antibacterial drugs can be described as bacteriostatic or bacteriocidal. Bacteriostatic drugs have the property of inhibiting bacterial multiplication. For these drugs, bacterial multiplication resumes when the agent is removed. Bactericidal drugs have the property of killing bacteria. With these antibacterial drugs, bacterial action is irreversible. The affected organisms can no longer reproduce, even when the agent is removed from contact with the bacteria.

Antibacterial drugs have many possible modes of action, including protein synthesis inhibition, protein denaturation, cell-membrane inhibition, disruption of cell membranes, formation of oxidizing agents in bacterial cells, or chemical antagonism. Each of these modes of action have been exploited by researchers looking for new antibacterial substances to control bacterial induced illnesses.

Figure 2 below is a plot that shows the effects of drug X on a given small population of bacteria. The plot gives the relationship between drug X concentration and the time required to kill 50% of the bacterial population.

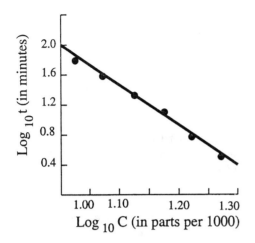

Figure 2.

17. Two important antibiotics, clindamycin and penicillin, are known inhibitors of cell-wall formation and cross-linking. These antibiotics most likely interfere with:

 A. capsule formation.
 B. pili function.
 C. flagella function.
 D. peptidoglycan.

18. Which of the following is NOT true about the antibacterial actions depicted by the plot?

 A. The plot demonstrates bacteriostatic activity.
 B. The plot suggests that as the concentration of drug X increases, the time required to kill 50% of the bacteria in the population decreases.
 C. The plot demonstrates bacteriocidal activity.
 D. None of the above are false.

19. Ten minutes after adding drug X to the suspension of bacteria, the number of surviving bacteria is:

 A. approximately 100.
 B. approximately 1000.
 C. approximately 10,000.
 D. undeterminable from the given information.

20. If 1 hour and 40 minutes are required to kill 50% of the bacterial population, based on the data presented in the passage, the concentration of drug X should be:

 A. 1 part per 100 parts.
 B. 1 part per 10 parts.
 C. 10 parts per 1 part.
 D. 100 parts per 1 part.

21. What concentration of drug X is required to kill all of the bacteria in the population in 100 minutes?

 A. Between 0 and 10 parts per thousand
 B. Between 10 and 100 parts per thousand
 C. Between 100 and 1000 parts per thousand
 D. There is not enough information to determine the concentration.

22. Which of the following observations is most consistent with an antibacterial drug that interfered with protein synthesis?

 A. Bacterial endoplasmic reticulum was disrupted.
 B. Glycosylation of proteins in the Golgi apparatus of bacterial cells was disrupted.
 C. Posttranslational modification was altered.
 D. Bacterial ribosomes were disrupted.

23. Which of the following is the least likely action of drug X on bacterial cells?

 A. Lysis of nuclear membranes
 B. Oxidation of DNA
 C. Inhibition and lysis of the cell wall
 D. Inhibition of protein synthesis

24. If drug X acts to inhibit the reproduction of the bacteria in the population, it most likely inhibits:

 A. mitosis.
 B. meiosis.
 C. binary fission.
 D. budding.

Passage IV (Questions 25–32)

The ventilator is a machine utilized extensively in hospitals to mechanically assist the respiration of patients. The ventilator attaches to an endotracheal tube that either passes through the nose or the oropharynx into the trachea of a patient. Through the endotracheal tube, the ventilator delivers breaths to the patient. The ventilator has settings that allow the clinician to vary the fraction of oxygen delivered (F_iO_2), volume delivered to the patient per breath (tidal volume), number of breaths delivered automatically to the patient per minute (IMV), and the amount of positive pressure maintained in the airways at the end of expiration (PEEP). The term "minute ventilation" describes the volume of gas delivered to a patient per minute.

Overbreathing occurs when a patient on a ventilator breathes spontaneously at a rate higher than the IMV. The ventilator allows patients to breathe as fast as they wish; however, it ensures that the patient receives a minimum number of breaths per minute.

The clinician can follow the ventilatory status of a patient by monitoring blood gas values. A sample of arterial blood is withdrawn from a patient and is analyzed. A blood gas analysis provides the blood pH (normal = 7.40), partial pressure of oxygen (P_{O_2}; normal = 100 mm Hg), partial pressure of carbon dioxide (P_{CO_2}; normal = 40 mm Hg), and bicarbonate concentration in blood ([HCO_3^-]; normal = 24 mEq/dl). These values are expressed by a notation that lists blood pH first, followed by P_{O_2}, P_{CO_2}, and bicarbonate concentration.

Consider the following clinical situation. A patient is connected to a ventilator with settings as follows: IMV = 8, F_iO_2 = 50%, tidal volume = 750 ml, and PEEP = 5 cm H_2O. Blood pH = 7.36, P_{O_2} = 70 mm Hg, P_{CO_2} = 46, and bicarbonate concentration = 20 mEq/dl. The notation for this blood gas is 7.36/70/46/20.

25. Which of the following does not affect minute ventilation?

    A. IMV
    B. Tidal volume
    C. F_iO_2
    D. Overbreathing

26. PEEP is likely to have which effect in the lungs of a ventilated patient?

    A. It increases lung expansion during inhalation.
    B. It aids in oxygen delivery to the tissues.
    C. It decreases surface tension in small bronchioles.
    D. It holds alveoli open during exhalation.

27. Which of the following are functions of the lungs?

    I. Acid–base regulation
    II. Participation in the renin–angiotensin system
    III. Storage and breakdown of erythrocytes

    A. I only
    B. I and II only
    C. II and III only
    D. I, II, and III

28. Raising which of the following would tend to increase P_{O_2} without affecting P_{CO_2}?

    A. Tidal volume
    B. IMV
    C. F_iO_2
    D. None of the above

29. A patient who is breathing with the aid of a ventilator develops a fever. The body temperature of the patient rises significantly. What effect does this have on the lungs and tissues?

    A. It leads to a lower affinity of oxygen for hemoglobin.
    B. It leads to an increase in blood pH.
    C. It leads to a decrease in tissue unloading to the tissues.
    D. It leads to a higher affinity of oxygen for either hemoglobin or myoglobin.

30. A ventilated patient who has severe acidosis of the blood with a pH of less than 7.30, could be helped by which of the following maneuvers?

    I. Increasing the IMV rate
    II. Administering intravenous bicarbonate
    III. Increasing the F_iO_2

    A. I only
    B. I and II only
    C. II and III only
    D. I, II, and III

31. Consider the clinical situation given in the passage. Increasing the F_iO_2 to 70% without changing the other settings is most likely consistent with which blood gas notation?

    A. 7.46/85/40/22
    B. 7.30/85/50/18
    C. 7.36/85/40/22
    D. 7.36/85/46/20

32. The organ most responsible for the compensatory retention and excretion of bicarbonate in response to altered pH is the:

    A. liver.
    B. kidney.
    C. spleen.
    D. lung.

Passage V (Questions 33–40)

Hormones are substances secreted by many tissue types, including endocrine glands, portions of the brain, and the gastrointestinal tract. The term "hormone" comes from a Greek word that can be translated as "to excite." Although hormones are viewed as primarily excitatory in nature, they also have many important inhibitory functions. It is also well known that inhibitory pathways are important in regulating hormone synthesis and release.

524

Hormones consist of various classes of molecules, including steroids, peptides, glycopeptides, iodine-containing compounds, and others. Most hormones are released into the bloodstream and are carried throughout the body, where they regulate various processes, such as the synthesis and degradation of chemicals and the utilization of energy. Some hormones, especially the steroid hormones, bind to nuclear receptors and act to modify the transcription of proteins. However, peptide and glycopeptide hormones bind to cell-surface receptors and act to modify cell activities in the cytoplasm.

The rate of secretion of a particular hormone varies under different conditions. In some cases, the resting rate is modified by specific stimuli. For example, the hormone insulin increases in the bloodstream in response to an increased serum glucose concentration. In other cases, hormone release is cyclic. The hypothalamus and pituitary gland release several hormones on a cyclic basis.

The control of hormone release is very important. Two basic hormonal control mechanisms exist—negative feedback and positive feedback. In negative feedback, an increased concentration of a secreted hormone can inhibit the stimulus to synthesize or secrete that hormone. Positive feedback systems are also important, but they are associated with potential instability of the organism. Positive feedback systems are found less often in mammalian hormonal control systems.

33. The passage best supports which of the following statements regarding hormones?

   A. Positive feedback is unstable and is used only in cases of severe stress.
   B. All hormones tend to have an excitatory function in addition to intermittent inhibitory functions.
   C. Hormones are the main regulators of metabolic homeostasis.
   D. Hormone secretion is strictly controlled.

34. Which of the following hormones is not released by the anterior pituitary gland?

   A. Adrenocorticotropic hormone
   B. Thyroid-stimulating hormone
   C. Oxytocin
   D. Growth hormone

35. Using molecular biology techniques, the DNA-binding domain of the cortisol receptor is removed and replaced by the DNA-binding domain of the estrogen receptor. The hybrid receptor is placed into cells lacking endogenous receptors. Which of the following statements regarding cortisol and estrogen is true?

   A. Estrogen inhibits transcription of genes that normally respond to cortisol.
   B. Cortisol stimulates transcription of genes that normally respond to cortisol.
   C. Estrogen stimulates transcription of genes that normally respond to cortisol.
   D. Cortisol inhibits transcription of genes that normally respond to estrogen.

36. Which of the following hormones does not act on the nucleus?

   A. Estrogen
   B. Follicle-stimulating hormone
   C. Thyroid hormone
   D. Aldosterone

37. The thyroid gland is an important regulator of various metabolic processes. Certain diseases act to counteract normal thyroid function. For example, in patients with Grave's disease, a high concentration of antibodies are made by the body that act as agonists. These antibodies tend to bind the thyroid-stimulating hormone (TSH) receptor in the thyroid gland. A correct expectation would be that:

   A. there would be elevated TSH levels in the bloodstream.
   B. there would be a decrease in thyroid hormone levels in the bloodstream.
   C. there would be increased synthesis of TSH in the anterior pituitary gland.
   D. there would be elevated thyroid hormone levels in the bloodstream.

38. The effects of a drug that acts to decrease the levels of an important hormone in the bloodstream is best counteracted by which of the following processes?

   A. Negative feedback
   B. Positive feedback
   C. Mutation
   D. Transduction

39. Which of the following endocrine glands produce hormones of distinctly different chemical classes?

    A.   The ovary
    B.   The anterior pituitary gland
    C.   The parathyroid gland
    D.   The adrenal gland

40. Which of the following hormones is *least likely* to utilize a plasma membrane-associated second messenger mechanism?

    A.   Amine hormones
    B.   Peptide hormones
    C.   Steroid hormones
    D.   Glycopeptide hormones

Answers and Explanations to Biology Practice Test 3

1. **A**   Table 1 indicates that strain A has a negative Gram stain. Strains B and C have positive Gram stains. Gram-negative bacteria have thin cell walls. However, the survival of Gram-negative bacteria is less dependent on having a cell wall than that of the Gram-positive bacteria. This is because Gram-negative bacteria inhabit protected areas such as the gastrointestinal tract. Gram-positive bacteria inhabit the skin, mouth, and other areas of trauma and desiccation. Therefore, Gram-positive bacteria are most susceptible to cell wall inhibitory substances, such as some antibiotics. Gram-negative bacteria (strain A) are least susceptible to inhibited cell wall synthesis.

2. **A**   Table 1 and the information in the passage should be carefully evaluated. Gram-positive bacteria are susceptible to cell wall–inhibiting antibiotics, so strains B and C are the choices to consider further. The passage clearly states that strain C does not have catalase. Thus, it is known that strain C probably does not grow in a hydrogen peroxide-containing environment. Therefore, strain B is correct.

3. **B**   Strain A is a Gram-negative organism and is not susceptible to cell wall–inhibiting antibiotics. Thus, choice A should be eliminated. There are no nuclear chromosomes in bacteria, so choice C should be eliminated. In bacteria, anaerobic metabolism easily replaces the energy demands when aerobic metabolism is shut down, thus, choice D is not the best choice. Choice B (slows protein synthesis) is the best answer.

4. **B**   The passage implies that coagulase behaves like the precursors of thrombin (prothrombin). Note that the passage states that coagulase reacts with a factor in plasma to become a thrombin-like substance.

5. **D**   One would expect that the rabbit formed antibodies in serum against coagulase. Coagulase and other bacterial proteins are released into the supernatant injected into the rabbit when the bacteria were lysed. Thus, when a sample of the rabbit serum is inoculated into a medium containing strain C bacteria, inactivation of the bacterial coagulase by antibodies is expected. In addition, strain C bacteria do not contain catalase and cannot grow in hydrogen peroxide–containing media.

6. **D**   Because all of the strains have the ability to ferment lactate (lactic acid), they all possess the ability to utilize anaerobic metabolism.

7. **A**   The explanation to this question is similar to that for question 2. Gram-negative bacteria prefer protected sites, especially the gastrointestinal tract. In addition, as discussed earlier, they are less sensitive to substances affecting cell wall synthesis.

8. **B**   Adding antibiotic to a colony selects out those bacteria possessing resistance to that antibiotic. Frequently, antibiotics kill all exposed bacteria. In this problem, however, information is given stating that addition of numerous antibiotics fail to kill all bacteria. These bacteria are highly resistant to antibiotics, and acquire this resistance by plasmids. Plasmids are small, circular molecules of double-

stranding DNA that occur naturally in both bacteria and yeast. Plasmids replicate as independent units as the host cell proliferates. They also carry resistance genes to specific antibiotics from one group of bacteria to another.

PASSAGE II	9. **A**	The passage states that the stroke volume is the volume of blood ejected with each heartbeat. The left ventricular end diastolic volume (LVEDV) is the blood in the left ventricle at the end of ventricular filling. The left ventricular end systolic volume (LVESV) is the volume at the end of ventricular contraction. The difference between these volumes is the stroke volume. The stroke volumes of each of the acute and recovery phases is 50 ml, and thus, the ratio is 1:1.
	10. **A**	This is an information recall question. The passage states that bacterial surface components (endotoxins) are a cause of septic shock. Only choice A describes a component of the bacterial cell surface.
	11. **B**	The data in Table 2 shows that the volume in the ventricle at the end of ventricular filling is 200 ml. A total of 50 ml is ejected. Therefore, 50/200 = 25%.
	12. **B**	The passage states that septic shock is associated with decreased contractility, ventricular dilatation, and decreased resistance of the blood vessels. Thus, choices A, C, and D can be eliminated. Choice B is supported by a statement at the end of the first paragraph, which says that high outputs are maintained by high heart rates.
	13. **D**	This question tests understanding of the basic structure of muscle. The heart contains striated muscle, which has intercalated disks. This muscle is known as cardiac muscle. Smooth muscle is found in hollow, slowly contracting organs such as the intestine, stomach, and bladder. The status of the thickness of the heart muscle can be determined from the passage, which states that there is an expansion in ventricular volume. This suggests dilatation and thinning.
	14. **A**	Blood pressure is generated when output from the heart is driven against a resistance of the vasculature. If the vascular resistance is low and the cardiac output is not elevated, blood pressure will fall.
	15. **B**	The mean ejection fraction for survivors (40%) is given in the first horizontal line in Table 3. The end diastolic volume (EDV) is given in the table indirectly as the end diastolic volume index (EDVI). Notice that the only difference between the EDV and EDVI is that the EDVI is measured per square meter. The EDV is calculated by multiplying the surface area by the EDVI. Thus, $(40 \text{ ml/m}^2)(2.5 \text{ m}^2) = 100$ ml.
	16. **A**	This question tests the understanding of the important proteins in muscle tissue. Recall that the sarcomere contains thin filaments (actin), and thick filaments (myosin). There are additional proteins associated with actin, namely troponin and tropomyosin. For details, review Chapter 7 of the Biology Review Notes.
PASSAGE III	17. **D**	Remember that peptidoglycan is the important component of bacterial cell walls. Some bacteria have a capsule exterior to the cell wall. The capsule functions to protect bacteria from attackers, prevent dehydration, and allow attachment to surfaces. Pili are short, thin extensions from bacterial cells. These are useful for attachment to surfaces.
	18. **A**	The plot (Figure 2) shows that the concentration of drug X correlates with the time necessary to kill 50% of the bacterial population. This plot shows killing activity, not bacteriostatic activity. Thus, choice A is a false statement, so it correctly answers the question being asked. Choices B and C are true statements and should be eliminated.
	19. **D**	There is no information provided in the passage to allow this calculation to be performed. Data relating the numbers of bacteria surviving versus time (after adding drug X) is necessary.
	20. **A**	One hour and 40 minutes equals 100 minutes. The plot gives time as a log base 10 value. The log base 10 of 100 equals 2. Looking at the plot for 2 minutes, there is a

corresponding value of log C approximately equal to 1.00. This means that C is about 10. Because the units are given in parts per thousand, 10/1000 equals 1:100.

21. **D** The plot (Figure 2) only gives data on the concentration of drug X and time to kill 50% of the bacteria. There is no data given to predict how long it will take to kill all of the bacteria.

22. **D** This question tests the understanding of how bacterial cells synthesize proteins. Bacteria do not contain membrane-bound organelles. Thus, choices A and B are incorrect. Choice C is unlikely because posttranslational modification occurs after protein synthesis. In addition, it is more important in eukaryotic cells. Therefore, choice D (disruption of bacterial ribosomes) is the best answer.

23. **A** Choice A is incorrect because bacteria do not have nuclear membranes. The other choices are plausible.

24. **C** Bacteria reproduce (divide) by binary fission. Fungi use budding, and eukaryotes may use mitosis, meiosis, or both. Therefore, a drug that inhibits bacterial reproduction must inhibit binary fission.

---

25. **C** The passage defines minute ventilation as the volume of gas delivered per minute. The intermittent mandatory ventilation (IMV), tidal volume, and any additional breathing (overbreathing) would effect overall volume. However, the fraction of oxygen in inspired gas (F_iO_2) would have no effect on minute ventilation.

26. **D** It is stated that value of PEEP is associated with airway-positive pressure at the end of expiration. Thus, choices A, B, and C are not supported by any information given in the passage. Choice D relates to expiration, and it is a reasonable explanation for how PEEP works in the lung.

27. **B** The lungs play an important role in acid–base balance. The lungs adjust mainly the acute changes in acid–base status, whereas the kidney adjusts chronic acid–base imbalances. The lungs also produce angiotensin-converting enzyme (ACE), which speeds the conversion of angiotensin I to angiotensin II. Thus, the lungs have a role in the renin–angiotensin system. The storage and breakdown of erythrocytes (i.e., red blood cells) is the function of the spleen.

28. **C** The P_{CO_2} is the partial pressure of carbon dioxide gas. The way to eliminate carbon dioxide is to increase the rate of exhalation (through ventilation). Ventilation is effective in reducing carbon dioxide levels in the blood, whereas hypoventilation increases carbon dioxide levels. Thus, both the tidal volume and intermittent mandatory ventilation (IMV) affect ventilation overall and play a role in affecting CO_2. The F_iO_2 would not affect ventilation or P_{CO_2}.

29. **A** This question tests understanding of the Bohr effect. An increase in body temperature, a decrease in pH, or an increase in the anaerobic products of metabolism (e.g., diphosphoglycerate) will shift the oxygen–hemoglobin dissociation curve to the right. This shift implies a lower affinity of oxygen for hemoglobin. This has useful consequences because it makes it easier for hemoglobin to unload oxygen to the tissues. At higher temperatures, metabolic rates tend to increase and there are greater tissue requirements for oxygen.

30. **B** The goal of this question is to find techniques to correct the acidosis (low pH). Test each statement to see if each maneuver increases pH. Increasing the intermittent mandatory volume (IMV) rate would decrease P_{CO_2} and lead to a lower level of carbonic acid, which would increase pH. Administering bicarbonate would also increase pH by neutralizing acid. Increasing the fraction of oxygen in the ventilated air would have no effect on pH.

31. **D** This question tests the understanding of the concepts and notation introduced in the passage. Increasing the oxygen concentration alone increases oxygen content in the blood. It does not affect carbon dioxide exchange or blood pH. Thus, a choice that has an unchanged pH and an unchanged carbon dioxide partial pressure would be correct. This makes choice D the best.

32. **B** The kidney attempts to correct blood pH induced by other organs of the body by retaining or excreting bicarbonate. The liver and spleen are not important organs in acid–base regulation.

33. **D**   Choice A is partially supported, but issues of stress are not discussed in the passage. Choice B is not supported by the passage and is an incorrect statement. Choice C is not discussed in the passage. Hormones do play a role in metabolic regulation, but so do enzymes and allosteric modulators. For example, glucose can act as a positive allosteric modulator and stimulate phosphofructokinase, which is the key controlling enzyme in glycolysis. Overall, choice D is best supported by the passage.

34. **C**   Oxytocin is produced in the hypothalamus and is released by the posterior pituitary gland. Adrenocorticotropic hormone, thyroid-stimulating hormone, and growth hormone are released by the anterior pituitary gland.

35. **D**   This question tests the understanding of hormone sites and actions. The DNA-binding domain is the part of the receptor that interacts with the DNA. The hormone-binding domain binds the hormone. In this case, the estrogen DNA-binding domain is placed on a cortisol receptor. When cortisol binds, it is the estrogen genes that are affected. This can give rise to inhibition of transcription of genes that normally respond to estrogen.

36. **B**   The steroid hormones and iodine-containing hormones (e.g., thyroid hormone) tend to diffuse into cells, bind receptors, and act on the nucleus. Choices A and D are steroid hormones. Choice C is an iodinated hormone. Only follicle-stimulating hormone (FSH) is not a steroid or an iodinated hormone. FSH is a glycopeptide, which binds a cell-surface receptor.

37. **D**   The antibodies described in this question bind to the thyroid-stimulating hormone (TSH) receptor and act as agonists. Recall that agonists stimulate the receptor. Increased stimulation of the TSH receptors in the thyroid gland would lead to excess thyroid hormone production. One can also expect that the excess thyroid hormone production would cause thyroid hormone to feedback to the hypothalamic-pituitary axis and decrease TSH production. This is an example of negative feedback.

38. **B**   A drug that decreases an important hormone in the bloodstream would be naturally counteracted by hormonal control mechanisms. Positive feedback control could allow the decreased level of the important hormone to positively feedback and stimulate further synthesis of the hormone. Mutation is a random event and would not necessarily counteract decreased hormonal levels. Transduction is a genetic process in bacteria.

39. **D**   The adrenal gland has two distinct regions—the adrenal cortex and the adrenal medulla. The adrenal cortex produces steroid hormones (e.g., cortisol, aldosterone, androgens), whereas the adrenal medulla produces amine hormones (e.g., epinephrine, norepinephrine). The ovary, the anterior pituitary gland, and the parathyroid gland generally produce one distinct chemical class of hormone.

40. **C**   The steroid hormones bind intracellular receptors and act on the nucleus. They do not utilize cell membrane–associated second messengers. Choices A, B and D (i.e., amine hormones, peptide hormones, glycopeptide hormones) all use a second messenger [e.g., cyclic adenosine monophosphate (cAMP)] system.

Organic Chemistry

REVIEW NOTES

General Concepts

$\textcircled{\text{\small I}}$

HIGH-YIELD TOPICS

I. Basic Introduction

II. Electronegativity and Bond Formation

III. Acid–Base Theory

IV. Energy and Kinetics

I. Basic Introduction

Success in the organic chemistry sections of the MCAT requires a thorough knowledge and understanding of the basics. These review notes show you an assortment of reactions that give a general overview of organic chemistry. **Do not memorize reactions!** Instead, familiarize yourself with how and why the reactions occur. Use the principles and concepts presented in the Organic Chemistry Review Notes and subsequent practice tests to gain an understanding of the types of processes that molecules undergo as they try to attain more favorable energy states. The key is to understand trends and principles.

The appendix to the Organic Chemistry Review Notes provides a summary of the rules for nomenclature in organic chemistry. As you review each functional group, be sure to flip back to this appendix to review the nomenclature for that group.

What are the basics?

1. Atoms are mostly fluffy electron clouds (atomic orbitals). What differentiates them is the number of electrons in the outer shell and how far away this shell is from the nucleus. These outer shell electrons determine physical properties and reactivity.

2. Molecules are formed when two atoms join their atomic orbitals to form a larger electron cloud (molecular orbital, MO). The sharing of electrons in an MO constitutes a covalent bond. Electrons can move within an MO and they gather around the more electronegative atom of the bond. This focus of electrons in particular regions of a molecule affects the physical properties and chemical reactivities of the molecules.

3. In most cases, bonds form between species that are electron deficient (**electrophiles**) and those that are electron rich (**nucleophiles**). Thus, it is important to be able to recognize which types of atoms and molecules are nucleophiles and which are electrophiles.

4. When analyzing chemical reactions, remember that a reaction is a collision between two molecules. Organic reactions (e.g., bonds breaking and forming) occur because they involve energy-releasing processes or because enough energy is applied to force the reaction. In general, everything strives toward lower energy.

5. Lower energy species are more stable and less reactive, whereas higher energy species are less stable and more reactive.

II. Electronegativity and Bond Formation

A. Importance of Electronegativity and Valence Electrons in Bond Formation

A great way to remember the electronegativity order of key elements, going from the highest electronegativity to the lowest, is to learn the expression: **FONClBrISCH: pronounced "fawn-cul-brish."** This expression will help you to remember that the key elements (fluorine, oxygen, nitrogen, chlorine, bromine, iodine, sulfur, carbon, and hydrogen) descend predictably in electronegativity strength compared to one another. **Electronegativity is defined as the ability of an atom to attract electrons.**

From this order, recognize that **electronegativity increases as you move to the right on the periodic table.** Halogens (group VII), with seven valence electrons, need only one more electron to attain the energetically favorable complete outer shell octet. Thus, they have a relatively high affinity for electrons. After gaining one electron, group VI elements still need another electron to reach a complete octet; thus their affinity for an electron is not as great as the halogens. Group V atoms have an even lower affinity for an electron.

Electronegativity decreases as you move down the periodic table. Coincidentally, the atomic radii of the elements increase greatly. An electron added to the outer shell of a relatively large atom such as iodine does not feel as strong a nuclear charge (because of **shielding** by the electrons in energy levels below) as an electron added to fluorine. Also, the outer-shell electrons of a large atom such as iodine are not held as tightly as those of smaller atoms because of their greater distance from the positively charged nucleus.

As you move to the left of the periodic table, the elements are increasingly willing to give up electrons. By releasing a few electrons, the next lower energy level that contains a full octet becomes the shell. For example, in group IA, Na^+ is Na, which has given up one electron to expose a full outer shell of electrons.

All atoms not in this list have electronegativities lower than hydrogen. All members of FONClBrISCH (except H) are on the right side of the periodic table. They need to gain three or fewer electrons to obtain a complete octet of electrons in their outer shell.

The number of valence electrons determines how many bonds are formed. Halogens (group VII) have seven electrons in their outer shell and generally form one bond to establish a complete octet. Atoms in group VI (oxygen) have six valence electrons, so they generally form two bonds to complete an octet. Nitrogen and other group V elements form three bonds to complete their octet. Carbon, one column to the left on the periodic table, has four valence electrons and forms four bonds.

B. Types of Bonds

1. **Ionic Bonds**

   Ionic bonds occur between two atoms of different electronegativities. The electronegative atom takes an electron from another atom that possesses a low ionization potential (willing to give up an electron to obtain a completely filled outer shell of electrons).

SECT. III
ORGANIC
CHEMISTRY
REVIEW
NOTES

533

Typical ionic bonds involve halogens and metals (e.g., NaCl, KI). **These bonds are strong.** Furthermore, crystal lattices form, involving a highly ordered system with extensive intermolecular bonding. The intermolecular bonds give these compounds high melting and boiling points. To solvate these molecules, the intermolecular interactions of the solid must be replaced by interactions with solvent. In other words, polar solvents must be used to solvate these highly polar molecules. Ionic bonds can also occur between charged clusters of atoms ($NH_4^+ OH^-$, $NH_4^+CH_3COO^-$, and so on).

2. **Covalent Bonds**

Covalent bonds involve the sharing of electrons, but it is not a "give and take" relationship as with ionic bonds. They occur in diatomic molecules, such as O_2 or Cl_2, and between atoms with similar electronegativity. Polar covalent bonds involve atoms that have different electronegative strength but not to the point where an ionic bond forms. The movement of electrons toward the more electronegative atom results in a partial positive charge on one end of the bond (lower electronegativity end) and a partial negative charge on the other end (higher electronegative end).

3. **Hydrogen Bonds (H-bonds)**

Hydrogen bonds are relatively weak intermolecular interactions in which a slightly acidic (partially + or δ^+) hydrogen forms a weak dipole interaction with a neighboring basic (partially − or δ^-) atom. Look for hydrogen atoms attached to N, O, and F. These atoms tend to be good donors of hydrogen toward H-bonds. Good acceptors are electronegative atoms with lone pair electrons, such as O, N, and F. Hydrogen bonds account for many physical properties of compounds in organic chemistry.

C. Atomic, Molecular, and Hybrid Orbitals

1. **General Ideas**

The **atomic orbitals (AO)** are theoretic regions around the nucleus where the probability of finding an electron is high. Each energy level contains its own AO.

The **covalent bond** involves a sharing of electrons. **This bond between two atoms is an overlap of two atomic orbitals.** The overlap of two AO forms two molecular orbitals (MO)—one bonding MO (lower energy) and one antibonding MO (higher energy). Electrons fill the lower energy bonding MO first, and then they fill the higher energy antibonding MO. **If the number of electrons in the bonding orbitals is the same as that in the antibonding orbitals, no bond will form between the two atoms.**

The **hybridization** of AO involves a mixing of AO on an atom to create a hybrid AO. These new AO allow for greater overlap when forming MO, leading to a stronger (lower energy) bond. The hybridization determines the shape of the molecule.

2. **Atomic Orbitals**

Atomic orbitals describe a cloud in which electrons of a particular energy level are likely to be found about the nucleus of an atom. These orbitals have specific shapes, depending on their energy.

For organic chemistry, it is important to know the following:

s orbital: Spherically symmetric about the nucleus
p orbital: Dumbbell shaped with nucleus at the center

With the exception of the first energy level, which contains only the s orbital, each principal energy level has one s orbital and three p orbitals, arranged 90° from each other (Figure 1-1). Each orbital can hold two electrons. Remember from the overview of atomic orbitals in the General Chemistry Review Notes that the filling order is: $1s^2$, $2s^2$, $2p^6$, $3s^2$, $3p^6$, $4s^2$, $3d^{10}$, $4p^6$, $5s^2$, $5p^6$, and so on, filled from lowest to highest energy.

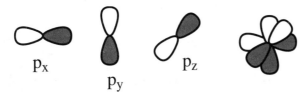

p_x

p_y

p_z

FIGURE 1-1.
The arrangement of the p orbitals.

3. **Molecular Orbitals**

Molecular orbitals (MO), one bonding and one antibonding, are created when atomic orbitals from two atoms combine and form a single electron cloud. The two electrons in this MO are shared by the contributing atoms. Each MO can hold two electrons. Two simple examples follow.

   This diagrammatic method is an easy way to conceptualize simple molecules. Such diagrams become exponentially more difficult as more electrons and atoms are added to the picture, but they give you an idea of what to think about as you draw a line on the paper to designate a bond.

   Remember that bonds form because it is energetically favorable for the atoms to be bonded rather than unbound. In Figures 1-2 and 1-3, note that the energy of the 1σ MO is lower than that of the 1s AO. Thus, the electrons of H_2 are in a lower energy state than they would be individually. Conversely, electrons occupying the He 1s AO are lower in energy than the electrons in the $1\sigma*$ MO and they prefer to stay that way. Thus, He is not a diatomic gas. **Often when you break a bond and form another in an organic reaction, you are removing the electrons from a higher energy MO and placing them into a lower energy MO.**

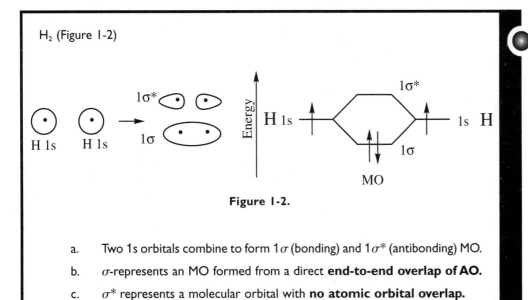

H_2 (Figure 1-2)

Figure 1-2.

EXAMPLE 1-1

FIGURE 1-2.
Molecular orbital diagram for H_2.

   a.   Two 1s orbitals combine to form 1σ (bonding) and $1\sigma*$ (antibonding) MO.

   b. σ-represents an MO formed from a direct **end-to-end overlap of AO.**

   c. $\sigma*$ represents a molecular orbital with **no atomic orbital overlap.**

   d.   Two electrons (one from each H) fill the 1σ MO, and a bond forms.

SECT. III
ORGANIC
CHEMISTRY
REVIEW
NOTES

535

FIGURE 1-3.
Molecular orbital diagram for He₂.

He₂ (Figure 1-3)

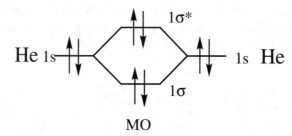

Figure 1-3.

a. Four electrons (two from each He) fill the 1σ and $1\sigma^*$ MO.

b. Because both the higher energy $1\sigma^*$ MO and the 1σ MO are occupied, a bond does not form between two He atoms. This type of orbital filling occurs for all noble gases and is the reason why they do not exist as diatomic species. It is energetically preferable for electrons to remain in the lower energy AO. A bond will form only when electrons fill more "bonding" MO than antibonding MO.

4. **Hybrid Orbitals**

Hybridized atomic orbitals are created when atomic orbitals on an atom mix together. Carbon contains four electrons in its valence shell ($2s^2$, $2p^2$). The s and p orbitals can be mixed to form the sp^3, sp^2, or sp hybrid orbitals. The types of hybrids and the formation of double and triple bonds are shown in Figures 1-4 to 1-8.

a. sp^3 (Figure 1-4)

FIGURE 1-4.
The sp³ hybrid. The solid arrow, out of the plane of the paper; the dashed arrow, into the plane of the paper.

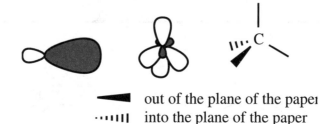

◄──── out of the plane of the paper
·····IIII into the plane of the paper

The sp^3 hybrid orbitals can be thought of as one s and three p orbitals mixing to form four sp^3 orbitals. In Figure 1-4, a single sp^3 hybrid orbital is shown at left and the orientation of all four of the sp^3 hybrids and their geometry are shown at right.

The four sp^3 hybrids, each containing one electron, can form four σ (direct overlap) bonds. The hybrid orbitals are arranged **tetrahedrally** about the nucleus to maximize the distance between the electrons in the four σ-bonds. Thus, the bonds of an sp^3 hybridized carbon have a bond angle $\approx 109.5°$. These orbitals are longer than s orbitals and more ovoid than p orbitals. Their shape permits a greater overlap volume with AO of other atoms when forming MO. Larger overlap results in lower energy and more stable MO.

b. sp² (Figure 1-5)

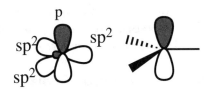

FIGURE 1-5.
The sp² hybrid.

One s and two p orbitals mix to form three sp² orbitals, leaving one unhybridized p orbital. The three sp² orbitals are arranged on the same plane (120° apart) and are perpendicular to the axis of the p orbital. Each of the sp² orbitals is equal in energy and contains one electron. The unhybridized p orbital is slightly higher in energy and also contains one electron.

The sp² orbitals can form a σ-bond (direct end-to-end overlap of AO) and the **p orbital can form a π-bond with a properly aligned p orbital, resulting in a double bond** (Figure 1-6). π-bonds, unlike σ-bonds, are sideways overlaps of p orbitals. The overlap is not as great as with end-to-end overlaps, which occur for σ-bonds. Thus, the π-MO is higher in energy compared with the σ-MO of a double bond. In a σ-bond, the electrons are found mainly between the two nuclei. For a π-bond, the electrons are mostly found above and below the bond and are more accessible for electrophilic species.

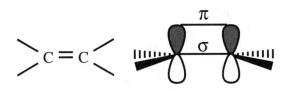

FIGURE 1-6.
The double bond.

c. sp (Figure 1-7)

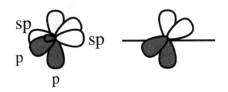

FIGURE 1-7.
The sp hybrid.

One s and one p orbital mix to form two sp orbitals, leaving two unhybridized p orbitals. The two sp orbitals are arranged 180° apart and are perpendicular to the p orbitals (which are perpendicular to each other). For **carbon,** each of the two hybridized orbitals and the two unhybridized p orbitals contains one electron.

The sp orbitals can each form a σ-bond and the two p orbitals can form π-bonds with two properly aligned p orbitals, resulting in a triple bond (Figure 1-8). Think of the π-electrons surrounding the two nuclei in a barrel-shaped cloud of electrons.

FIGURE 1-8.
The triple bond.

SECT. III
ORGANIC
CHEMISTRY
REVIEW
NOTES

537

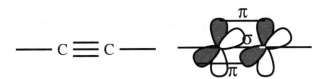

Note: Atoms connected with just σ-bonds can be rotated about the bond. Those atoms connected by σ- and π-bonds, however, require more energy, because to rotate about a double bond, the π-bond must be broken. Thus, compounds with multiple bonds are more rigid than those with just single bonds.

D. Hybridization, Molecular Shape, and Polarity

The type of hybridization determines the shape of the molecule, which in turn determines the polarity of the molecule. **Hybridization occurs with atoms other than carbon,** for example, **nitrogen** (sp^3 in ammonia–NH_3) and **oxygen** (sp^3 in water and ethers). **Boron** is sp^2 hybridized, with an electron in each hybridized orbital and an empty p orbital. The resulting trigonal planar shape of boron results from the hybridized orbitals and the empty p orbital(s) (Figure 1-9).

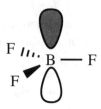

FIGURE 1-9.

The sp^2 hybridization of BF_3.

1. Polarity

Recall that polar covalent bonds are dipoles consisting of an electron-rich region and an electron-deficient region. The net polarity of a molecule is the vector sum of its component dipoles. **Dipole moments** measure the polarity of molecules as a whole. Figures 1-10 and 1-11 show different types of hybridized molecules with or without dipoles. Note that the net dipole moment is derived by the vector sum of the bond moments of the molecules. Thus, CCl_4 and CO_2 have no net dipole moment, whereas the other molecules have a net dipole moment.

FIGURE 1-10.

Examples of sp^3 hybridized molecules with or without dipoles (CCl_4, CH_2Cl_2, and H_2O).

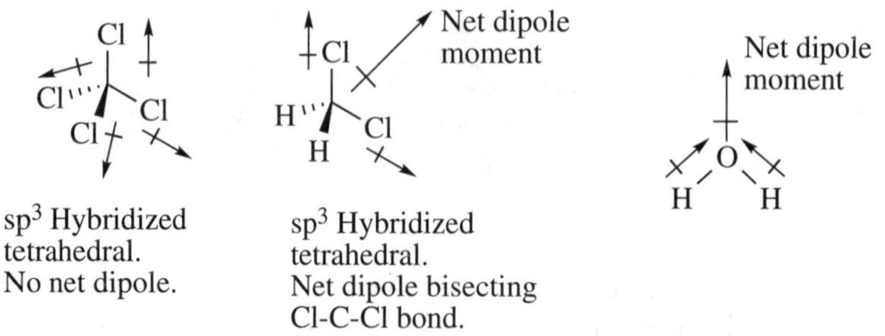

sp^3 Hybridized
tetrahedral.
No net dipole.

sp^3 Hybridized
tetrahedral.
Net dipole bisecting
Cl-C-Cl bond.

Net dipole
moment

FIGURE 1-11.

Examples of sp^2 and sp hybridized molecules with or without dipoles (acetone, CO_2).

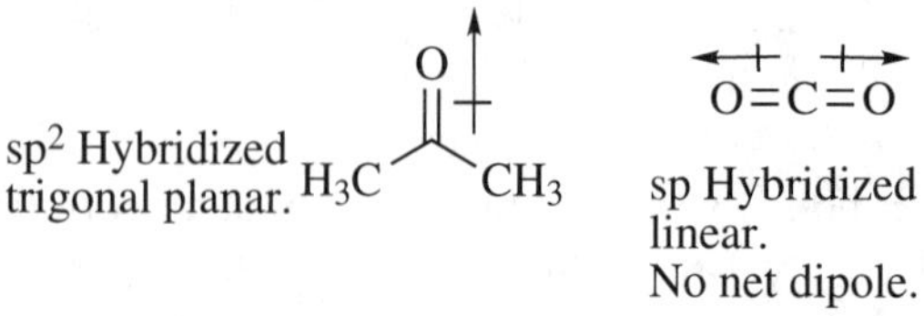

sp^2 Hybridized
trigonal planar.

sp Hybridized
linear.
No net dipole.

Why is polarity important? The net polarity of a molecule affects the interactions of that molecule with other molecules (of its own kind or different ones). Such physical properties as melting point, boiling point, density, and solubility are affected by the degree of intermolecular interaction.

2. Solubility and Solvation

The phrase "like dissolves like" means that only polar solvents can solvate polar compounds. Solvation involves breaking intermolecular interactions of the solute and replacing them with interactions of the solute with the solvent. Nonpolar solvents cannot interact with polar solutes and are thus unable to dissolve polar compounds. Nonpolar solids or liquids do not dissolve in polar solvents. The new interactions between the nonpolar solute and the polar solvent are not strong enough to replace the dipole-dipole interactions stabilizing the solvent molecules (e.g., oil–nonpolar and H_2O do not mix). Nonpolar compounds, however, dissolve in nonpolar solvents because nonpolar solvents do not have the strong intermolecular interactions that hold molecules together.

E. Resonance Forms and Delocalization

A problem associated with Lewis structures (see General Chemistry Review Notes) is that they tend to position electrons in a single location (in a bond between two atoms). Two or more equivalent Lewis structures that differ only in the position of the electrons are referred to as resonance structures, or forms. An example of these forms is shown in Figure 1-12.

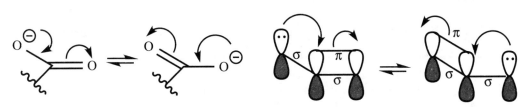 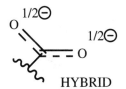

FIGURE 1-12.
Resonance forms and resonance hybrid for carboxylate. *Arrows represent movement of two electrons.*

The **resonance hybrid** is a structure that takes into account the individual resonance forms of a compound and is **more stable** than any of the individual resonance forms that contribute to its formation. Resonance structures are therefore contributors to the overall resonance hybrid of a molecule. **The more stable a particular resonance form, the more it contributes to the overall resonance hybrid.** This fact indicates that electrons in a π-bond are not always located between the two atoms of the original bond. Rather, they are spread out or **delocalized,** which enhances stability. Note: Only π-bonded electrons or free electrons in a p orbital can delocalize in a molecule.

Neutral species are also stabilized through resonance delocalization of electrons. Benzene is highly stabilized because of multiple resonance forms; two resonance structures and the resonance hybrid are shown in Figure 1-13. Note that the **resonance hybrid for benzene suggests a single π-molecular orbital spread over the six atoms of the ring.**

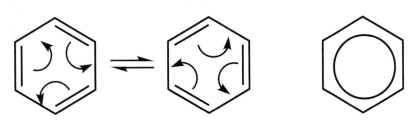

FIGURE 1-13.
Resonance structures and resonance hybrid for benzene.

When drawing resonance forms of a molecule, remember to:

1. Move only the electrons. The positions of the atoms must be preserved.

2. Maintain proper Lewis structures (no five-bonded carbons, etc.).

3. Conserve the charge and the number of unpaired electrons.

SECT. III
ORGANIC
CHEMISTRY
REVIEW
NOTES

539

Figure 1-14 illustrates how to move electrons to generate a resonance structure.

FIGURE 1-14.
Electron movements associated with resonance structures.

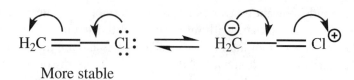

More stable

To estimate the relative stability of resonance structures, look at the overall **viability** of the forms. In general, **forms with more covalent bonds are more stable.** Resonance forms in which charges are located on atoms that stabilize them (e.g., negative charges on electronegative atoms) are also more stable. Finally, forms with complete octets and fewer charges are also more stable.

III. Acid–Base Theory

A. General Ideas

1. Brønsted-Lowry Definition of Acids and Bases

A Brønsted-Lowry acid is any molecule or ion that can donate a proton.

A Brønsted-Lowry base is any molecule or ion that can accept a proton.

Consider the dissociation of HCl in water:

$$HCl + H_2O \rightleftharpoons H_3O^+ + Cl^-$$

Acid 1   Base 2   Acid 2   Base 1

Using the Brønsted-Lowry (BL) definitions, note that this reaction includes two acids, HCl and hydronium ion, and two bases, water and chloride ion. All BL acid–base reactions involve two conjugate acid–base pairs in equilibrium. In evaluating this reaction, note that HCl acts as a BL acid by donating a proton to water. The water molecule acts as a BL base by accepting the proton. The hydronium ion can act as a proton donor to the chloride ion, and thus act as a BL acid. The chloride ion can act as a base by accepting a proton from the hydronium ion. Remember that these reactions are in equilibrium. Note also how each BL acid becomes a conjugate base and vice versa.

2. Lewis Definition of Acids and Bases

A Lewis acid is any species that can accept an electron pair.

A Lewis base is any species that can donate an electron pair.

A Lewis acid–base reaction creates a **coordinate covalent bond** in the reaction product. The Lewis system is useful for classifying reactions that occur in solvents other than water or in the complete absence of a solvent. In the Lewis system, all cations are acids and all anions are bases.

Consider the compound BF_3 (see Figure 1-9). The boron atom shares six electrons with the three fluorine atoms and has a vacant 2p orbital that can accept a pair of electrons. Thus, BF_3 can act as a Lewis acid and accept a pair of electrons from a Lewis base. Ammonia (NH_3) is a great example of a Lewis base. The lone pair of electrons on the nitrogen of ammonia can be donated to a suitable Lewis acid, such as BF_3, to create a coordinate covalent bond.

B. The Dissociation Equilibrium

According to Brønsted, acids are compounds that donate protons (protonate bases). To donate protons, the equilibrium must shift to the right. Look at the following dissociation equation:

$$HA + H_2O \rightleftharpoons H_3O^+ + A^-$$

$$K_a = [H_3O^+][A^-]/[HA] = (\text{products/reactants}) \text{ or } (\text{dissociated/protonated})$$

If the equilibrium shifts to the right, the K_a should increase. In other words, strong acids are characterized by large K_a (small pK_a) values. It follows then that weak acids are characterized by small K_a (large pK_a) values.

C. Acidity Trends

The more stable the conjugate base (A^-), the stronger the acid (HA). If A^- is unstable (more reactive and basic), the dissociation equilibrium will shift to the left, resulting in a weaker acid.

D. How to Stabilize the Conjugate Base (A^-)

1. **Increase Electronegativity**

   Increasing the electronegativity of A^- increases acidity. More electronegative conjugate bases can better hold on to the extra electron after the proton is released from the acid.

   $$\underline{HF} > H_2\underline{O} > \underline{N}H_3 > \underline{C}H_4 \text{ (stronger to weaker acid)}$$
   $$pK_a \quad 3.2 \qquad 16 \qquad 38 \qquad 48$$

   Another way of thinking is that the H–F bond is more polarized than the C–H bond because of the higher electronegativity difference. Thus, it is easier for H–F to lose an H^+.

2. **Spread Out the Charge**

   a. Spread Over a Large Volume

      This factor overrides the electronegativity trend. A charge in a small volume will be more unstable because of the repulsion from nearby electrons. The resulting reactive conjugate base is more likely to shift the dissociation equilibrium to the left.

      $$HI > HBr > HCl > HF \text{ (stronger to weaker acid)}$$
      $$pK_a \quad -10 \quad -9 \qquad -7 \qquad 3$$

      Iodine (I) is the least electronegative halogen, but the anion I^- is the largest, and it can disperse the negative charge over a large volume (compared with F^-), making it less apt to reverse the deprotonation reaction. Remember: **Spread the charge; increase stability.**

   b. Resonance Effect

      Conjugate bases with multiple resonance forms are more stable than those without and, thus, the acids are stronger. The conjugate base of acetic acid has greater charge delocalization (see carboxylate delocalization, Figure 1-12) than the conjugate of methanol (CH_3O^-),

SECT. III
ORGANIC
CHEMISTRY
REVIEW
NOTES

541

resulting in a more stable A⁻ for acetic acid. Again, spreading the charge stabilizes A⁻.

$$CH_3COOH > CH_3OH$$
$$pK_a \quad 4.7 \qquad 16$$

c.   Resonance Combined with Inductive Effects

In fluoroethane (CH_3CH_2F), the presence of the electronegative (electron attracting) fluorine places a partial positive charge (δ^+) on the CH_2 to which it is bound. This carbon, in turn, pulls electron density toward itself from the C–C bond, which places a δ^+ on the carbon of the CH_3 group. This action is called the inductive effect. The effect decreases with increasing distance from the electronegative substituent.

The inductive effect often increases acidity. Consider acetic acid.

$$Cl{-}CH_2{-}COOH > CH_3COOH$$
$$pK_a \quad 2.86 \qquad\qquad 4.76$$

Why does adding the chloride atom increase the acidity (decrease pK_a) of acetic acid? When an electronegative atom is placed near the functional acid group of acetic acid, the electronegativity of Cl polarizes the C–Cl bond and, through inductive effects, further polarizes the O–H bond, making the proton more δ^+. This action weakens the O–H bond and the proton is released more easily.

The inductive effect can also be thought of as stabilizing the conjugate base by helping to spread out the negative charge (Cl pulls electron density toward itself).

E.   A Few Last Words

Weaker acids have stronger conjugate bases. This statement makes sense, because weaker acids have less stable (more reactive or stronger) conjugate bases (A⁻).

If HA and A⁻ represent a conjugate acid–base pair, then K_a of HA = $[H_3O^+][A^-]/[HA]$ and K_b of A⁻ = $[HA][OH^-]/[A^-]$. Thus, $K_a^{HA}K_b^{A^-} = [H_3O^+][OH^-] = K_w$, a constant. This formula is a general truism for any **conjugate pair** and quantifies the dissymmetric relationship between the relative strengths of the acid and its conjugate base (i.e., **the stronger the acid, the weaker the conjugate base**).

Reactions of acids with bases: HA + B $\rightleftharpoons$ BH⁺ + A⁻

The equilibrium will favor the side with the weaker acid–base pair. Strong bases are needed to deprotonate weak acids, and strong acids are needed to protonate weak bases. In the preceding example, B must want the proton more than A⁻. The weaker an acid HA, the stronger a base A⁻. Thus, B must be a strong base to hold on to the proton from a weak acid.

The **Henderson-Hasselbalch equation:** pH = pK_a + log [A⁻]/[HA], states that when the pH of a solution is equal to the pK_a of a dissolved acid, half of the acid will be protonated and the other half will be deprotonated. (See also Chapter 10.)

IV. Energy and Kinetics

Reactions sometimes occur spontaneously (in organic chemistry, bonds break and form) because the products are more stable than the reactants. In other cases, even though the products are energetically more stable, the application of energy is still needed because of the initial energy barrier that must be surpassed to move the reaction forward. We use the energy versus reaction coordinate to depict (in two dimensions) the energy of a species as it goes from one form to another. Remember that a species that is lower in energy is more stable and less reactive. **(The energy referred to is the Gibbs' free energy, G.)**

A. Enthalpy

The change in enthalpy of a reaction ($\Delta H°$, in which ° denotes standard conditions, 1 atm for a gas, 1 M for solution) measures the difference in the relative enthalpies (heat content or potential energy) of the reactants and products. The reactions are as follows:

Exothermic if $\Delta H° < 0$, indicating that heat is liberated during the course of the reaction.

Endothermic: $\Delta H° > 0$, indicating that heat is absorbed during the course of the reaction.

The energy diagrams in Figure 1-15 show the two processes; it is assumed that ΔG and ΔH have the same sign. Note that for each process, reactants pass through a transition state, have an associated activation energy, and form products.

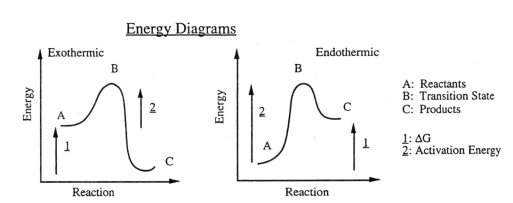

Energy Diagrams

A: Reactants
B: Transition State
C: Products

1: ΔG
2: Activation Energy

FIGURE 1-15.
Exothermic and endothermic reactions.

B. Activation Energy

The **activation energy** barrier must be surpassed for a reaction to occur. The height of this barrier determines the rate at which the reaction occurs. Enough energy must be available to push a reaction forward to the **transition state** (point B of the energy diagrams). The transition state, where bonds are being partially formed and/or broken, represents an intermediate between reactants and products. Once the reaction reaches this point, it can roll either way (forward or back) depending on the conditions and the equilibrium. **Catalysts** accelerate a reaction by decreasing the energy difference between the starting material and the transition state, thus decreasing the activation energy.

C. Gibbs' Free Energy: $\Delta G°$ Standard Free Energy Change

The standard free energy change ($\Delta G°$) measures the driving force or the push of a reaction. When $\Delta G° < 0$, the reaction is considered spontaneous. The more negative the $\Delta G°$ of a reaction, the greater the tendency of the reaction to go forward. Spontaneous reactions have higher initial free energies and the products have lower free energies.

The following equation: $\Delta G° = \Delta H° - T\Delta S°$, in which $\Delta S°$ is the change in entropy or randomness, indicates that free energy depends on three factors; enthalpy, entropy, and temperature.

SECT. III
ORGANIC
CHEMISTRY
REVIEW
NOTES

543

To understand how you push a reaction forward, look at the preceding equation and each of the factors. Exothermic reactions ($\Delta H° < 0$), or reactions that increase entropy (producing products in a more random phase), tend to make ΔG more negative. In addition, increasing the temperature of a reaction increases the magnitude of the $T\Delta S°$ term and makes it easier to surpass the activation energy barrier. Both of these effects help to push the reaction forward and result in a more negative ΔG.

Consider another relationship:

$$\Delta G° = -RT \ln K_{eq}$$

in which K_{eq} = [products]/[reactants]. This relationship quantifies the relationship between $\Delta G°$ and the size of the equilibrium constant. This information is important. You should be able to predict that the larger the negative value of $\Delta G°$, the larger the K_{eq}. If product molecules predominate at the reaction equilibrium, then K_{eq} is high. This favorable formation of product is then reflected in a low $\Delta G°$.

D. Reaction Order

The order of a reaction describes how the concentration of the reactants affects the rate of the reaction. For the reaction: $mA + nB \rightarrow$ product, rate = $k[A]^m[B]^n$ (k is the rate constant). **The order of the reaction = m + n.** Become familiar with the following types of reactions.

Zero Order: The rate of the reaction is constant and independent of the reactant concentration. An example is an enzyme-catalyzed reaction that is under conditions of substrate saturation (enough substrate so that the enzyme is working as hard as possible).

First Order: The rate depends on the concentration of one of the reactants.

Second Order: The rate depends on the concentration of two of the reactants. The reactants can be the same molecule (A + A $\rightarrow$ product) or two different molecules. Most reactions that you will encounter are first or second order.

Alkanes and Their Chemistry, Stereochemistry, and Reaction Mechanisms

I. Alkanes	
II. Stereochemistry	**HIGH-YIELD TOPICS**
III. Free Radical Reactions	
IV. Nucleophilic Substitution and Elimination	

I. Alkanes

A. Empiric Formula

Alkanes are carbon compounds consisting of single bonds (s) between each carbon. They have the general formula: C_nH_{2n+2}. Alkanes are described as saturated because the carbons of the alkane are bound to as many hydrogens as possible. A review of the naming of alkanes is provided in the Appendix to this section.

When n > 3, it is possible for several molecules to have the same atoms but different connections. These compounds are **structural isomers** of one another. In Figure 2-1, note that the structural isomers butane and 2-methylpropane have a general formula of C_4H_{10} but different connectivity. **Structural isomers generally differ also in their physical properties** (e.g., boiling and melting points, solubilities, and densities) and their spectroscopic properties [e.g., nuclear magnetic resonance (NMR) and infrared (IR) spectroscopy].

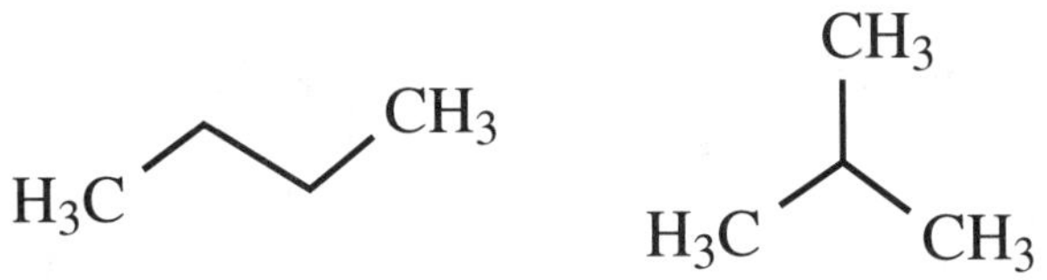

FIGURE 2-1.
Two structural isomers.

B. Physical Properties

The state of alkanes at room temperature is as follows:

n = 1–4: gases

n = 5–17: liquids

n > 18: solids

SECT. III
ORGANIC
CHEMISTRY
REVIEW
NOTES

545

Alkanes are **highly nonpolar** and insoluble with water. They are effective solvents for nonpolar compounds. Polar compounds cannot be dissolved in alkanes.

The melting points and boiling points of these compounds are relatively low. As the carbon chain length increases, the melting and boiling points increase because of the increase in the **van der Waals** intermolecular interactions. These interactions are caused by the transient dipoles that form as electrons move in their orbitals within a molecule. These dipoles can induce dipoles to form in other molecules, and weak dipole–dipole attractive interactions occur between these molecules. Remember that melting and boiling points are directly related to intermolecular interactions.

With increased branching, boiling point decreases because of fewer and weaker van der Waals interactions. The branches act like arms to increase intermolecular distances, thus decreasing the strength of van der Waals interactions.

Melting point is trickier. In many cases, melting temperature is higher because branching enhances symmetry, which in turn enhances the ability of the molecules to form crystal lattices. As an example, cycloalkanes have high melting points because of their high degree of symmetry.

Combustion of alkanes involves the complete oxidation of the alkane to form CO_2 and H_2O. These processes are exothermic. **More heat is released from a longer carbon chain** because of the larger numbers of C, H, and O atoms in the molecule. **Between isometric forms, the one that releases more energy is the less stable isomer.**

C. Conformation

Remember that the atoms about a single bond are free to rotate. **Rotational isomers are also known as conformers and are generated by rotating substituents about single bonds.** Figure 2-2 shows the rotational isomers for butane. You can generate these isomers by looking down the long axis of a molecule and seeing how the substituents are positioned with respect to one another. Realize that for a given alkane, certain rotational isomers are more energetically favorable than others.

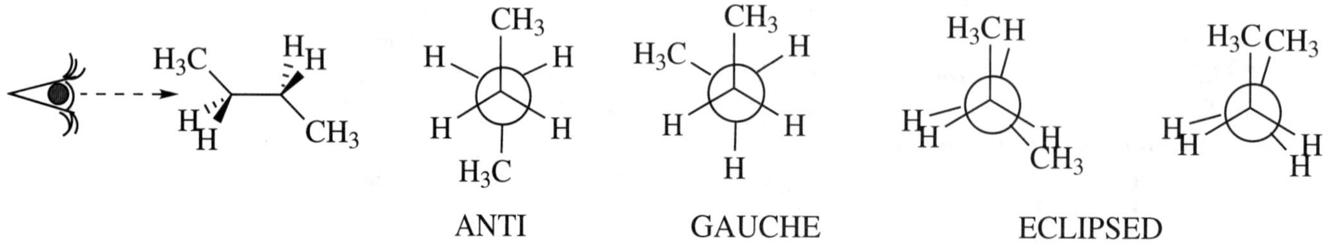

ANTI   GAUCHE   ECLIPSED

FIGURE 2-2.
Rotational isomers of butane.

Of the different rotational isomers possible, the basic forms—**anti, gauche,** and **eclipsed**—are shown in Figure 2-2. The anti and gauche forms are known as **staggered** conformations, because the bonds emanating from the two carbons into the plane of the paper do not overlap as they do in the eclipsed conformer.

The stability of conformers is dictated by two factors: steric interactions and eclipsing strain. Steric interactions occur when the atoms get too close and "bump" into one another. Eclipsing strain occurs when the bonds and substituents overlap.

Moving from left to right in Figure 2-2, the forms are shown from lowest to highest energy. It is important to realize that the percentage of time a molecule spends in each conformation is directly related to the energy of the conformation; i.e.,

CHAP. 2
ALKANES AND
THEIR CHEMISTRY,
STEREOCHEMISTRY,
AND REACTION
MECHANISMS

546

the highest energy conformations are the least populated. The eclipsed form (far right) is the least stable and the highest in energy because of the proximity of the methyl groups and the fact that it is an eclipsed conformation. The anti form is the most stable because of the large separation between the methyl groups in a staggered conformation. The eclipsed forms are less stable than any staggered form given the overlap of the bonds and the substituents.

D. Cycloalkanes

Ring strain is caused by the geometry of the ring and the fact that sp^3 carbons normally assume an angle of $109.5°$. The more this angle deviates from this value, the greater the ring strain. Ring strain is measured by examining the energy released per CH_2- group on combustion. Cyclopropane has the greatest and cyclohexane has the least energy released per CH_2 group. Thus, the three-membered ring of cyclopropane is highly strained and cyclohexane has no ring strain.

Cyclohexane is unique because it is possible to have all of the carbons perfectly tetrahedral and all of the bonds staggered. This conformation is called the **chair.** In the chair conformation in Figure 2-3, note that there are two different orientations for substituents to attach: axial (along the vertical axis) and equatorial (along the belt line of the ring). Cyclohexane can also be in a **boat** form, but this conformation is less stable because of repulsive flagpole interactions.

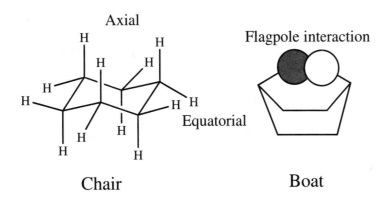

Chair

Boat

FIGURE 2-3.
Chair and boat forms of cyclohexane. The circles in the boat form represent substituents.

The concept of **ring flip** is illustrated in Figure 2-4. The form of the chair at left contains two groups that are close to one another. The repulsive interactions between groups lead to ring flips, which spread bulky groups to equatorial and more distant locations. In Figure 2-4, 1,3-diaxial interactions are the cause for the placement of larger substituents in the **equatorial** (around the equator) positions instead of the **axial** positions (vertical axis). This action occurs as a result of flips in the ring. These flips occur constantly and are in equilibrium based on their relative energies. Thus, the form with the larger substituent in the equatorial position would have the highest concentration.

FIGURE 2-4.
Ring flip.

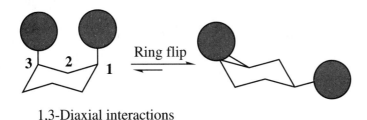

1,3-Diaxial interactions

SECT. III
ORGANIC
CHEMISTRY
REVIEW
NOTES

547

II. Stereochemistry

A. Importance

Many reactions occur **stereospecifically** (give different products depending on the stereochemistry of the substrate) or **stereoselectively** (yield one stereoisomer more than another). Thus, it is important to be able to name, classify, and identify stereoisomers. **An important example involves thalidomide,** the drug used in the 1960s to alleviate morning sickness. Two stereoisomers were coadministered; one provided the intended relief while the other was later found to cause severe birth defects.

B. Terms and Definitions

Become familiar with the following terms:

Stereoisomers: Isomers that have identical connectivity but different spatial configurations; two types are **enantiomers** and **diastereomers.**

> **Enantiomers:** Stereoisomers that are nonsuperimposable mirror images of each other

> **Diastereomers:** Stereoisomers that are not enantiomers

Asymmetric carbon: An sp^3 carbon with four different substituents, often referred to as a **chiral carbon.** Stereoisomers are formed by changing the orientation of the substituents of the chiral carbon.

Optically active compounds: Compounds that rotate plane-polarized light are optically active (chiral). Compounds designated "l" rotate the plane of the polarized light counterclockwise. Compounds designated "d" rotate the plane of the polarized light clockwise.

> As a **general rule of thumb:** If you can draw an internal mirror plane through a molecule (drawing the plane down the center of an atom is allowed), the molecule is **not** optically active and is **achiral.**

C. Enantiomers

An example of enantiomers on your body is your hands: they are mirror images and you cannot superimpose them. In organic chemistry, if a compound contains a single chiral carbon, its enantiomer can be drawn by switching any two substituents on the chiral carbon. The compounds then become nonsuperimposable on one another.

1. **Absolute Stereochemistry**

   R and S are used to identify and label chiral carbon. The assignment of R or S is determined by the priority of the substituents on the chiral carbon. Priorities are determined by the following process:

   - Look at the atom attached to the carbon. Rank by atomic number.

   - If there is a tie, go to the next atom and rank by atomic number.

   - Look for a point of difference such as a branch point. If there still is a tie, go to the next atom. Keep going until there is a higher ranking atom. An example is shown in Figure 2-5.

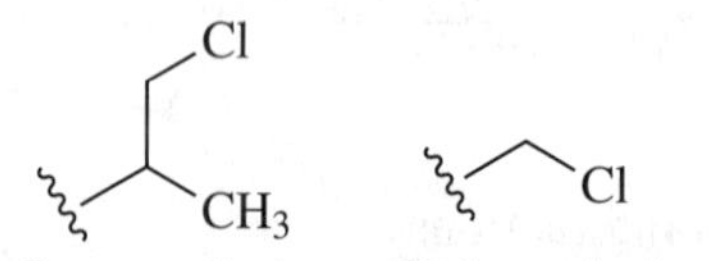

FIGURE 2-5.
Assigning priority for a branch point.

Lower priority   Higher priority

- Look for multiple bonds. Caution: they are counted as if they were the same number of singly bonded atoms; i.e., a CH–CH₂ double bond counts as four carbons and three hydrogens. See the examples in Figure 2-6.

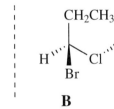

$$\begin{array}{l} \xi - \underset{H}{C} = CH_2 \\ \downarrow \\ C H \\ \xi - \underset{H}{C} \rule{0.5cm}{0.4pt} H \\ C \end{array}$$

$$\begin{array}{l} \xi - \underset{H}{C} = O \\ \downarrow \\ O \\ \xi - \underset{H}{C} - O \\ C \end{array}$$

$$\begin{array}{l} \xi - C \equiv CH \\ \downarrow \\ C C \\ \xi - \underset{CC}{C} \rule{0.3cm}{0.4pt} H \end{array}$$

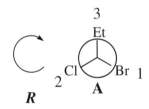

Higher priority   Lower priority

FIGURE 2-6.
Priority assignments for multiple bonds.

- Remember to look for rankings according to atomic weight and **not** the total weight of the substituent group.

a. **Steering Wheel Approach**

Place the lowest priority substituent (often hydrogen) into an imaginary steering column. Look straight at the wheel and see if the other three ranked substituents go high-to-low priority clockwise (*R*) or counterclockwise (*S*). Recognize that if a chiral center is assigned *R*, its mirror image is *S*.

Figure 2-7 shows a chiral molecule and its enantiomer. The geometry of the enantiomers (at left) reveals that they are nonsuperimposable mirror images of each other. When using the steering wheel approach to assign priority of substituents, compound A shows an *R* conformation and compound B shows an *S* conformation.

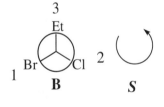

A   **B**   *R*   **A**   **B**   *S*

FIGURE 2-7.
Assigning *R* and *S* absolute stereochemistry to two enantiomers, A and B, using the steering wheel approach.

b. **Fischer Projections**

Fischer projections can also be helpful in assigning absolute stereochemistry. Think of the substituents along the horizontal bonds as a bow tie. To assign *R* or *S*, rank the substituents as described previously. Put the lowest priority group at the top by rotating the entire projection by **180°** (rotations by 90° or 270° result in the representation of the other enantiomer), or hold one atom and rotate the other three atoms.

In Figure 2-8, the Br is held and the other three positions are rotated to place the lowest priority H at the top. With this action, you are just spinning the chiral carbon about one of the bonds. Assign the compound by examining the orientation of the groups from high priority to low priority (*R*-clockwise, *S*-counterclockwise).

FIGURE 2-8.
Using Fischer projections to assign absolute stereochemistry.

$$\begin{array}{c} Cl \\ H \rule[0.5ex]{0.3cm}{0.4pt}\!\!\mid\!\!\rule[0.5ex]{0.3cm}{0.4pt} Br \\ Et \end{array}$$
Bow tie

$$\begin{array}{c} Cl \\ H \rule[0.5ex]{0.3cm}{0.4pt}\!\!\oplus\!\!\rule[0.5ex]{0.3cm}{0.4pt} Br \quad \textbf{hold} \\ Et \end{array}$$
Fischer

$\longrightarrow$

$$\begin{array}{c} H \\ Et \rule[0.5ex]{0.3cm}{0.4pt}\!\!+\!\!\rule[0.5ex]{0.3cm}{0.4pt} Br \\ {}_{3} Cl {}_{1} \\ {}_{2} \quad \textbf{\textit{R}} \end{array}$$

$$\begin{array}{c} H \\ Br \rule[0.5ex]{0.3cm}{0.4pt}\!\!+\!\!\rule[0.5ex]{0.3cm}{0.4pt} Et \\ {}_{1} Cl {}_{3} \\ {}_{2} \quad \textbf{\textit{S}} \end{array}$$

549

2. **Physical Properties**

Enantiomers are **optically active.** One enantiomer rotates plane-polarized light in one direction and the other rotates it in an equal but opposite direction. **All other physical (e.g., melting and boiling points, and solubilities) and spectroscopic (e.g., NMR and IR) properties of enantiomers are identical.** Thus, enantiomers are hard to separate, purify, and characterize.

3. **Racemic Mixture**

A racemic mixture is a solution with an equal concentration of two enantiomers. The solution will not rotate plane polarized light; it is rotated in one direction by one enantiomer and rotated to an equal degree in the opposite direction by the other enantiomer.

D. Diastereomers

1. **Stereochemistry**

Diastereomers, defined as stereoisomers that are not enantiomers, are compounds with two or more asymmetric centers.

Remember: For n-chiral centers in a molecule, there are 2^n possible stereoisomers.

Study Figure 2-9. Note that some compounds are nonsuperimposable mirror images and others are not. Be sure you understand which pairs are enantiomers and which are diastereomers. (Answers are provided in the legend.)

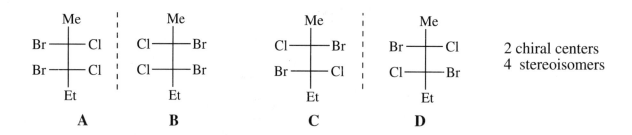

2 chiral centers
4 stereoisomers

FIGURE 2-9.
Enantiomers and diastereomers. Compounds A through D each have 2 chiral centers and 2^2, or 4, stereoisomers. (A,B) and (C,D) are pairs of enantiomers. (A,C), (A,D), (B,C), and (B,D) are pairs of diastereomers.

2. **Physical Properties**

Diastereomers have **different** melting and boiling points, solubilities, and spectroscopic properties. Thus, diastereomers can be isolated, purified, and characterized. Diastereomers also have different, but not opposite, optical activities.

E. Meso Compounds

A meso compound has asymmetric centers and an internal mirror plane of symmetry. Meso compounds are not optically active and do not possess enantiomers. Try to draw a line of symmetry through a compound to see if it is a meso compound. Compounds A and B in Figure 2-9 are both meso compounds.

Figure 2-10 illustrates two sets of compounds with ***R*** and ***S*** configurations. Compound **A** is a meso compound because you can draw a mirror plane down the middle of the molecule. **B** is a mirror image of **A** and is also a meso compound. Notice that both **A** and **B** are superimposable. Compounds **A** and **B** are identical because they just flip onto one another. Compounds **C** and **D** are not meso compounds; they are enantiomers. (**C,A**) and (**D,A**) are pairs of diastereomers.

CHAP. 2
ALKANES AND
THEIR CHEMISTRY,
STEREOCHEMISTRY,
AND REACTION
MECHANISMS

550

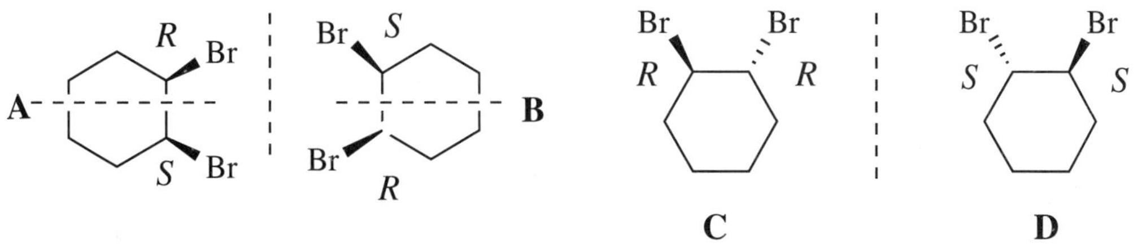

FIGURE 2-10.
Examples of meso compounds, enantiomers, and diastereomers.

III. Free Radical Halogenation of Alkanes

A. The Basics

Free radical halogenation of alkanes involves initiation (formation of halogen radical), propagation (chain reaction resulting in product and halogen radical), and termination steps (two radicals coming together to form a bond). Once the initial radical is formed, the rest goes on by itself. Lower energy radicals are more selective (Br• is the most selective radical), which means that lower energy halogen radicals preferentially remove hydrogens that form lower energy (more stable) alkyl radicals.

B. Types of Bond Cleavage

Heterolytic cleavage involves the breaking of a bond such that both electrons from the bond are taken by one of the atoms.

$$\text{Example: } H_2O \rightarrow H^+ + OH^-$$

Homolytic cleavage involves the breaking of a bond such that one electron goes to one side and the other goes to the other side. Unlike heterolytic cleavage, the products are not charged. The radicals that are formed are reactive because they are electron deficient and want a full outer shell.

$$\text{Example: } HO\text{–}OH \text{ (hydrogen peroxide } H_2O_2) \rightarrow HO\bullet + \bullet OH$$

C. Reaction Sequence

The steps of free radical reactions are detailed in Figure 2-11 and as follows.

Initiation: The halogen radicals are formed by reacting with light or heat. This step is highly endothermic and ends at point A on the energy graph in Figure 2-11.

Propagation: The halogen radical then pulls off a proton from the alkane (homolytic cleavage) to form HX and the alkyl radical. The alkyl radical then splits up another X_2 molecule and the propagation steps go on until one of the starting materials runs out or the radicals are consumed by termination steps.

Note that points **A** to **C** on the graph involve formation of the alkyl radical. This step is highly endothermic and requires energy input to overcome the activation energy barrier. After **C** is formed, the formation of the alkyl halide and the halogen radical (**C to E**) is highly exothermic, with a relatively small activation energy barrier from points **C** to **D**.

Termination: Combination of any two radicals creates a nonradical species and propagation steps stop. This step is best depicted at point **E**. Termination steps generally are energetically favorable.

SECT. III
ORGANIC
CHEMISTRY
REVIEW
NOTES

551

Initiation $\quad X_2 \xrightarrow[\text{or } \Delta]{hv} \quad X\text{-}X \longrightarrow 2 X^\bullet$

Propagation $\quad X^\bullet \quad H\text{-}H_2C\text{-}R \longrightarrow R\text{-}\overset{\bullet}{C}H_2 + HX$

$\quad\quad\quad\quad\quad R\text{-}\overset{\bullet}{C}H_2 \quad X\text{-}X \longrightarrow R\text{-}CXH_2 + X^\bullet$

Termination $\quad 2\ R\text{-}\overset{\bullet}{C}H_2 \longrightarrow RCH_2CH_2R$

$\quad\quad\quad\quad\quad R\text{-}\overset{\bullet}{C}H_2 + X^\bullet \longrightarrow R\text{-}CXH_2$

$\quad\quad\quad\quad\quad 2\ X^\bullet \longrightarrow X_2$

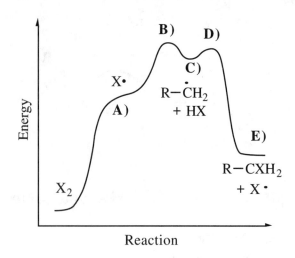

FIGURE 2-11.

Free radical halogenation: the reactions and energy diagram. *Single-headed arrows* identify single electron movements.

D. Energy and Stability of Radicals

Many questions can be answered by understanding stability concepts. Remember from the review of acids and bases in Chapter 1 that spreading the charge increases stability. Radicals are electron deficient and so the attachment of electron-donating substituents, like carbons, leads to greater stabilization (**inductive effect, spreading the charge**). In Figure 2-12, the stability of radicals is ranked high to low. Note that **radicals are stabilized by delocalization and resonance.**

FIGURE 2-12.
Stability of radicals.

Radicals can be stabilized by **delocalization.** For alkyl radicals, the p orbital of the radical can line up with an σ C–H bond to give the resonance forms shown in Figure 2-13. If R is an alkyl group, several more of these types of resonance forms can be drawn. **Thus, the more substituted alkyl radicals are more stable.** Furthermore, the alkyl groups can be considered electron-donating substituents that can stabilize the electron-deficient radical. **In all cases, stability is enhanced by spreading the electrons.**

FIGURE 2-13.
Resonance forms contributing to the stability of radicals.

For the halides (high to low reactivity), F• > Cl• > Br•. I• is unreactive. This order relates to the fact that F is highly electronegative and is willing to form a bond. F• is high enough in energy to pull off any proton to form any alkyl radical (primary to benzyl). Br•, on the other hand, is lower in energy and is thus **more selective** of which H atom it pulls off. Given a choice, the Br• species pulls off the H atom that leads to the most stable alkyl radical because it is the easiest H atom to remove. Halogenation and analogous radical reactions are successful only with Cl• or Br•. Unfortunately, F• is too reactive and I• is not reactive enough for these reactions.

E. Stereochemical Aspects

If the alkane is a pure enantiomer, the resulting product will be a mixture of two enantiomers. Halogen attack can occur from either the top or bottom face to give two different products. Thus, racemization occurs. Figure 2-14 illustrates the production of two enantiomers from free radical reaction.

CHAP. 2
ALKANES AND
THEIR CHEMISTRY,
STEREOCHEMISTRY,
AND REACTION
MECHANISMS

552

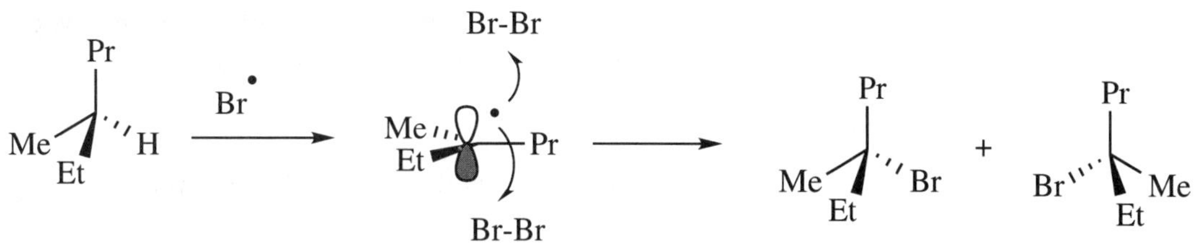

FIGURE 2-14.
Enantiomers produced from free radical reaction. Do not memorize this process; just understand that it occurs.

IV. Nucleophilic Substitution and Elimination

To understand these critically important mechanisms fully, you must know why they occur, how they occur, and what products they produce.

A. General Ideas

Reactions often occur (bonds break and new ones form) between a molecule that is electron rich (δ^-) and one that is electron deficient (δ^+). Such is the case in radical halogenation, because radicals are the electron-deficient species, as well as with nucleophilic substitutions and eliminations.

Substitutions and eliminations involve the reaction between an electrophile (electron-deficient species) and a nucleophile (electron-rich species). **Eliminations result in alkenes and substitutions result in alkanes with different substituents.** Note also that electron-rich and electron-deficient species exist, because of the formation of dipoles caused by differences in electronegativity. The types of substitutions and eliminations can be distinguished by mechanism and product distribution.

The substitutions are commonly known as S_N1 and S_N2 reactions. The eliminations are commonly known as E1 and E2. **Substitution and elimination reactions compete in many instances.** The conditions of the reaction and compounds involved favor one type of reaction over another.

B. S_N1

An S_N1 reaction involves two steps and is a **unimolecular reaction** (first-order reaction, see Chapter 1 of the Organic Chemistry Review Notes). The **first step** involves the **dissociation of the leaving group (electron-accepting species) from the substrate, resulting in a carbocation.** The carbocation is considered an intermediate. **Intermediates** are characterized as high-energy valleys in the energy diagram that either go forward to create product or degrade back to starting materials. The **second step** involves the **attack of the carbocation by a nucleophile from either face of the sp² hybridized carbocation.**

In Figure 2-15, the first step of the S_N1 reaction involves the formation of the carbocation intermediate. The second step involves the nucleophilic attack of the carbocation, leading to a substituted product. Note that the nucleophile can attack from either face. The energy graph (Figure 2-15, at right) shows the formation of the carbocation intermediate (C+).

FIGURE 2-15.
S_N1 reaction mechanism. Note the two steps, the ability of the nucleophile to attack from either face, and the energy diagram depicting the reaction.

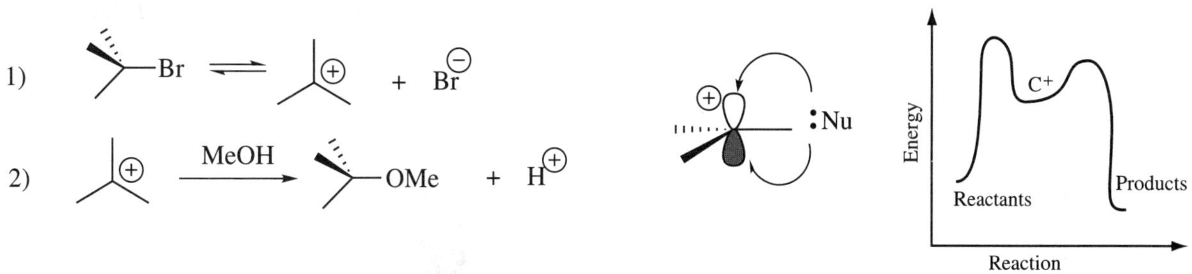

1. Rate-Determining Step

The step with the highest activation energy determines the rate of the reaction. In this process, the formation of the carbocation is the rate-determining step.

553

Because the formation of a more stable carbocation requires less energy, the stability of the carbocation directly affects the rate of the reaction.

2. **Carbocation Stability**

Carbocation stability (Figure 2-16) parallels radical stability (see preceding section III) and for similar reasons.

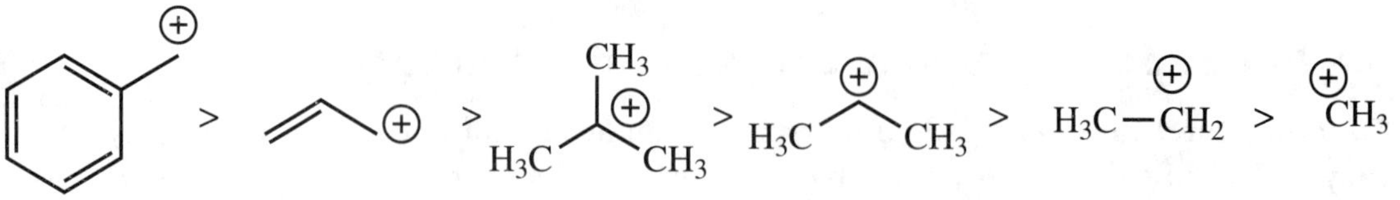

FIGURE 2-16.
Carbocation stability.

Increased substitution results in more groups that can donate electrons (electron induction) to stabilize the carbocation (remember: spread out the charge; increase stability). The benzyl and the allyl are especially stable because of **delocalization** of the positive charge via resonance.

3. **Carbocation Rearrangement**

Figure 2-17 shows that carbocations can migrate through shifts to form a more stable carbocation.

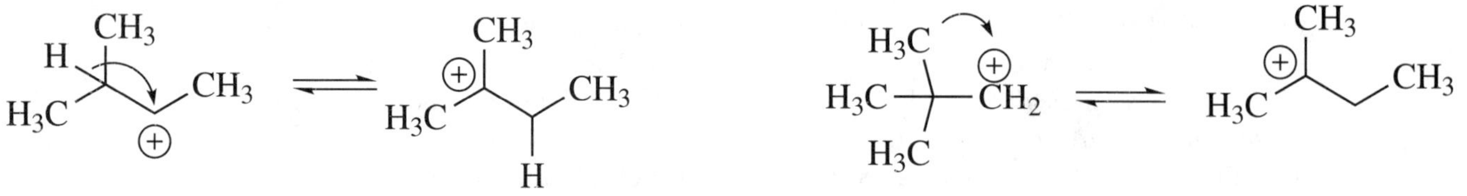

FIGURE 2-17.
Carbocation rearrangement to form the most stable carbocation.

4. **First-Order Rate**

Rate of the reaction depends only on the concentration of the substrate. The strength and concentration of the nucleophile are not as important, because nucleophilic attack is **not** the rate-limiting step.

5. **Stereochemical Considerations**

If you start with an optically pure material (only one enantiomer present), the result will be a mixture of stereoisomers. This change occurs because the carbocation is sp² hybridized and can be attacked by the nucleophile from either face, resulting in two different stereoisomers.

C. S_N2

S_N2 is a **one-step, bimolecular** (second-order, see Chapter 1 of the Organic Chemistry Review Notes) reaction. Refer to Figure 2-18 and follow the steps of the reaction closely.

The nucleophile approaches the electrophile along the line of the electrophile-leaving group bond, the dipole formed by the electronegative-leaving group having

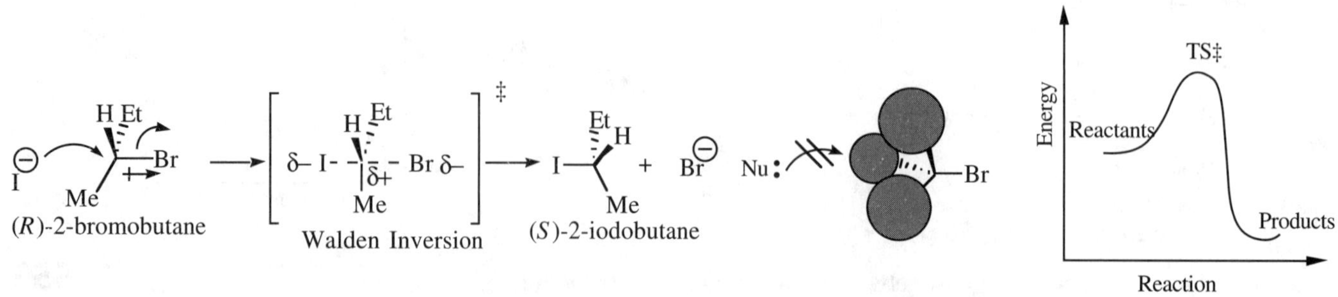

FIGURE 2-18.
S_N2 reaction mechanism. Note the single step, transition state, geometry of the nucleophilic attack, and the energy diagram depicting the reaction.

made the carbon of the bond δ^+. The nucleophile attacks as the leaving group leaves. This action correlates with the transition state (TS) shown on the energy graph in Figure 2-18. During this stage, the electrophile is flattened out like an umbrella in the wind. The new bond between the nucleophile and the electrophile is formed and the electrophile-leaving group bond is broken. Because the reaction is one-step, there is **no rate-determining step.**

1. **Steric Considerations**

   If the electrophile has too much steric bulk (large alkanes or branched alkanes), the reaction will occur slowly or not at all. The same holds true for bulky nucleophiles.

2. **Stereochemical Considerations**

   An inversion of stereochemistry follows the nucleophilic attack. Optical activity is maintained, although the product will have a different optical rotational value.

3. **Second-Order Rate**

   Unlike S_N1, the **rate depends on the concentration of both the electrophile and the nucleophile.**

D. S_N1 and S_N2: Differences and Preferences

Consider the following to predict which substitution mechanisms are favored.

1. **Electrophile**

   Both reactions prefer strong electrophiles. In terms of substitution, however, opposite trends are at work. S_N2- **prefers less substituted electrophiles (primary or secondary carbons)** so the attacking nucleophile can approach the electrophile. Tertiary electrophiles will not undergo S_N2.
   S_N1- **prefers more substituted electrophiles (Tertiary > Secondary > Primary)** because of the stability of the carbocations that are formed after dissociation of the leaving group.

2. **Nucleophile**

   Both reactions work well with good nucleophiles, but **the S_N2 reaction is more dependent on the strength of the nucleophile.** Remember that the rate-determining step of the S_N1 reaction is the formation of the carbocation, which is independent of the nucleophile.

   What makes a good nucleophile?

   a. **Good nucleophiles are generally good bases.** Do not think that all strong bases are good nucleophiles. The only possible generalization is that for a group of nucleophiles in which the attacking atom is the same, the stronger base is the better nucleophile.

   b. **Charged nucleophiles are always more powerful than their uncharged counterparts.**

   c. **The halogens are good nucleophiles because of their ability to polarize (fluffiness).** The electron cloud around the nucleus is large and the outer electrons are shielded from the positive charge of the nucleus. This situation makes it easy for larger atoms to donate electrons to electrophiles.

SECT. III
ORGANIC
CHEMISTRY
REVIEW
NOTES

555

Good examples of nucleophiles are as follows:

- Conjugate bases of weak acids: ^-CN, RO^-, HO^-, RS^-, among others

- Halogens: I^-, Br^-, Cl^-

- Neutral molecules with lone pairs: RNH_2, ROH, H_2O, RSH

- Carbon nucleophiles: R_2CuLi

3. **Leaving Group**

Both S_N2 and S_N1 reactions prefer good leaving groups. **For the S_N1 reaction, a better leaving group lowers the activation energy of the rate-determining step.**

What makes a good leaving group?

Good leaving groups are conjugate bases of strong acids (i.e., weak bases). A good leaving group can stabilize the extra electron it gains from dissociation from the carbon. Thus, groups such as I^-, Br^-, are good leaving groups.

^-OH is considered a poor leaving group (strong base), but H_2O is considered a good leaving group (weak base). Figure 2-19 demonstrates how you can improve a leaving group by modifying it. In this example, the poor leaving group, the hydroxyl, is protonated to make it a weaker base and a better leaving group. This reaction then proceeds via an S_N1 mechanism. Thus, protonation can allow for displacement of OH via an **S_N1-type reaction.** S_N2 does not work by this method.

FIGURE 2-19.

Improving a leaving group by protonation, allowing an S_N1 reaction.

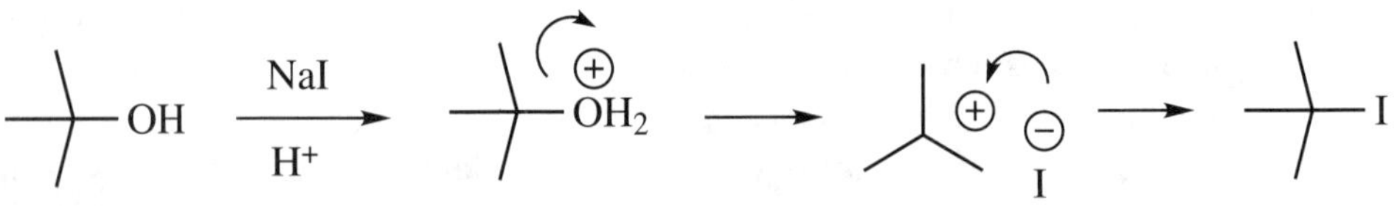

4. **Stereochemical Implications**

If the starting material of an S_N2 reaction is chiral, the product will be chiral **with inversion of stereochemistry.** For S_N1, the product will be a racemic mixture because of the formation of the carbocation and nucleophilic attack occurring in two different directions.

5. **Solvent Effects**

Both reactions favor polar solvents. For **S_N2, aprotic solvents** (no protons that can be involved in hydrogen bonding) are favored. For **S_N1, protic solvents** (good donors of protons for H-bonds), such as alcohols, are favored because of their ability to stabilize the anion and cation products of the rate-limiting step of the reaction.

6. **Mechanisms**

A summary of mechanisms for the substitution reactions follows.

- S_N1 goes through a mechanism that involves an **intermediate,** whereas S_N2 goes through a single step with a transition state.

- The rate of the S_N1 is **dependent on substrate concentration** but not on nucleophile concentration or strength.

CHAP. 2
ALKANES AND
THEIR CHEMISTRY,
STEREOCHEMISTRY,
AND REACTION
MECHANISMS

556

- The **rate** of the S_N2 reaction is **dependent on both substrate and nucleophile** concentration and strength.

- The **products** of S_N1 reactions can be the result of **carbocation rearrangements.** These rearrangements do not occur for S_N2.

E. E1

Like S_N1, E1 is also a **two-step, unimolecular** reaction. Refer to the example in Figure 2-20.

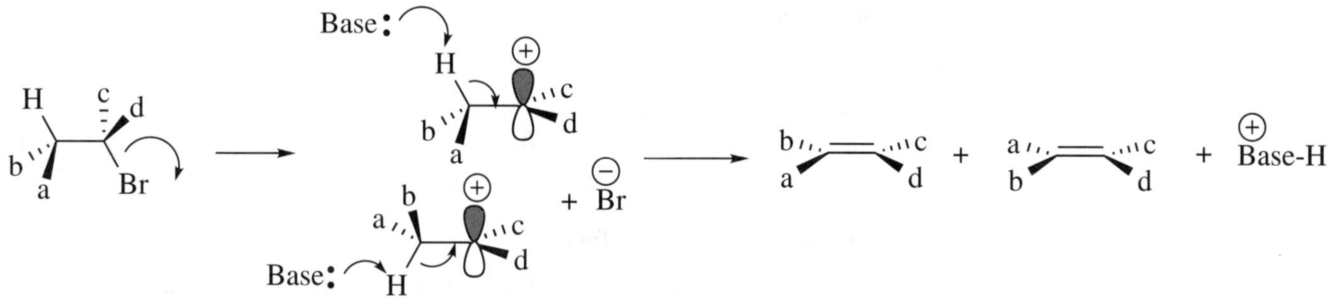

The first step involves the dissociation of the leaving group from the substrate, resulting in a carbocation intermediate (just like S_N1). The second step involves the removal of a proton by a base and the formation of a double bond. The energy diagram for this process is analogous to the S_N1 energy diagram. **The rate-determining step is again the carbocation formation.**

FIGURE 2-20.
E1 mechanism. Note the two steps and carbocation formation.

1. Rearrangements

Like the S_N1, the carbocations can rearrange to a more stable carbocation.

2. Alkene Stability

On elimination, several different double-bonded molecules can result. The more stable double bond will form preferentially. In most cases, **the product with the increased number of substituents on the double bond (higher substitution) is favored.** This arrangement increases stability. In addition, the **trans isomer is more stable than the cis form** because of eclipsing strain. (See the Appendix for a review of *cis/trans* designations.)

Figure 2-21 shows which alkene products are most stable in E1 reactions (listed from high to low stability).

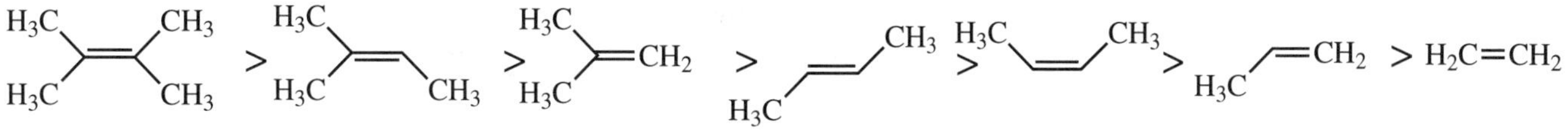

3. Rate

Like S_N1, the rate of E1 is dependent on the concentration of the substrate and independent of the concentration or strength of the base. **In general, E1 is outcompeted by S_N1 and is not used as an elimination reaction.**

FIGURE 2-21.
Alkene stability in E1 reactions.

F. E2

Like S_N2, E2 is a **single-step, bimolecular** reaction. Refer to the example in Figure 2-22.

SECT. III
ORGANIC
CHEMISTRY
REVIEW
NOTES

557

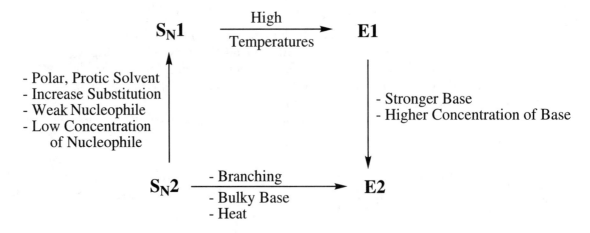

FIGURE 2-22.
E2 mechanism. Note the transition state and double-bond formation.

The base deprotonates the substrate when the proton is **antiperiplanar** to the leaving group. In this orientation, the proton is on the positive end of the dipole of the molecule. Electrons move from the broken C–H bond to the C–C bond to form a double bond as the leaving group departs. The energy diagram resembles the diagram for the S_N2 reaction.

1. **Rate**

   The rate of the E2 reaction depends on the concentration of the substrate and base along with the strength of the base (stronger bases are more effective). By increasing the steric bulk of the base, fewer S_N2 side reactions occur.

2. **Stereochemical Considerations**

   Given the nature of the antiperiplanar orientation of the substrate, specific products can be expected. E1 gives a mixture of products, but in E2, **rearrangement does not occur.** Remember that E2 is a one-step reaction.

   Key point: E2 is a more effective elimination reaction than E1.

G. Take-Home Points to Understand

1. **Summary Chart**

   The chart in Figure 2-23 sums up the reactions discussed in this chapter and the conditions favoring the reaction types. Note that you can control the reaction path by controlling the conditions of the reaction.

$$S_N1 \xrightarrow[\text{Temperatures}]{\text{High}} E1$$

- Polar, Protic Solvent
- Increase Substitution
- Weak Nucleophile
- Low Concentration of Nucleophile

- Stronger Base
- Higher Concentration of Base

$$S_N2 \xrightarrow[\text{- Heat}]{\substack{\text{- Branching} \\ \text{- Bulky Base}}} E2$$

FIGURE 2-23.
Summary chart of reaction types.

CHAP. 2
ALKANES AND
THEIR CHEMISTRY,
STEREOCHEMISTRY,
AND REACTION
MECHANISMS

2. **More General Rules**

   a. Primary alkyl halides undergo S_N2 or E2, depending on the base.

   b. Secondary alkyl halides undergo S_N2 with weak bases, E2 with strong bases, and S_N1 when protic solvents are used.

   c. Tertiary alkyl halides undergo S_N1 with no S_N2. E1 also occurs, but is more of an annoying side reaction that ruins yield. E2 is the only observed reaction with a strong base.

Alkenes and Alkynes

Alkenes

and Alkynes

I. **General Information**

II. **Key Reactions**

HIGH-YIELD TOPICS

I. General Information

A. Empiric Formula

Alkenes are hydrocarbons that possess a double bond between adjacent carbon atoms in the hydrocarbon backbone. The double bond acts as the dominant functional group of the molecule. **For alkenes, the general formula is: C_nH_{2n}.** (See the review of nomenclature for alkenes and alkynes in the Appendix.)

Alkynes are hydrocarbons that possess a triple bond between adjacent carbon atoms in the hydrocarbon backbone. The triple bond is the dominant functional group. **For alkynes, the general formula is: C_nH_{2n-2}.**

B. Structure and Physical Properties

Like alkanes, the **melting and boiling points of alkenes and alkynes increase with chain length.** Unlike alkanes, **no free rotation** occurs about the double bond (alkene) or triple bond (alkyne) because of the presence of the π-bonds. The carbon–carbon double bond is shorter and stronger than a carbon–carbon single bond owing to the π-interaction and increased s-character of the σ-bond. Similarly, a carbon–carbon triple bond is stronger and shorter than a carbon–carbon double bond.

The stability of the multiple bond increases with substitution. For double bonds, *cis* **is less stable than** *trans* because of eclipsing interactions of the substituents. The carbons of multiple bonds are slightly more electronegative than sp^3 carbons. The triple-bonded carbon is slightly more electronegative than the double-bonded carbon.

C. Types of Reactions

Most reactions of alkenes and alkynes take advantage of the accessible electrons in the π-bond. The three basic types are as follows:

1. **Electrophilic attack.** The π-bond provides a source of electrons for electrophiles to attack. These reactions go through a carbocation intermediate or an intermediate with a partial positively charged carbon.

SECT. III
ORGANIC
CHEMISTRY
REVIEW
NOTES

559

2. **Reductions** can occur that convert the multiple bond to a more saturated bond.

3. **Oxidations** (or additions of oxygen) can occur.

II. Key Reactions

A. Electrophilic Attack

Multiple bonds are characterized as electron-rich species with relatively accessible electrons in the π-bond(s). Given the nature of the π-bond, with its sideways overlap, the electron can be donated to form new s-bonds.

1. Addition of Hydrogen Halides (HX Attack)

This reaction, in which an alkene is converted by HCl, HBr, or HI into the corresponding alkyl halide, is a good example of an electrophilic attack (Figure 3-1). The π-electrons from the double bond attack the polarized HX molecule and form a bond with the hydrogen, creating a carbocation at the more substituted carbon. The anion can then attack the carbocation from either the top or bottom face, leading to the nucleophile attached to the more substituted position. Figure 3-1 demonstrates that even with only one starting material, two products are formed because of the nonselective attack of the carbocation by the nucleophile.

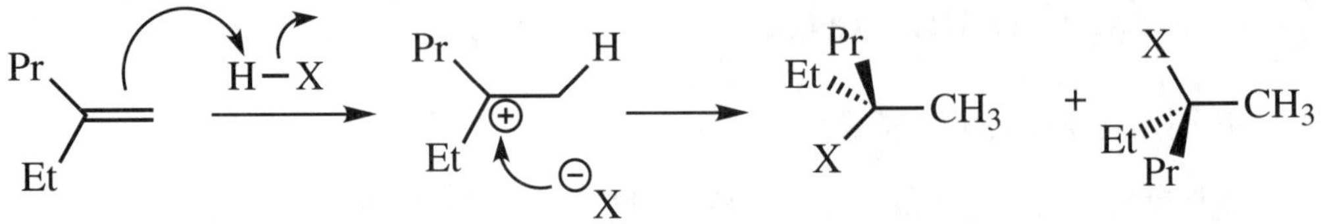

FIGURE 3-1.

Electrophilic attack with a carbocation intermediate.

It is important to know **Markovnikov's rule: in the addition of an acid to the carbon–carbon double bond of an alkene, the hydrogen of the acid attaches itself to the carbon that already holds the greater number of hydrogens.** With some rewording, Markovnikov's rule states that **electrophilic addition to a carbon–carbon double bond involves the intermediate formation of the more stable carbocation.**

Markovnikov's rule occurs because the breaking of a double bond occurs more easily in the direction that forms a more stable carbocation intermediate. Thus, the initial electrophilic attack forms the more substituted (stable) carbocation.

FIGURE 3-2.

Two examples of the addition of halogen reaction. Mechanisms look complicated on first glance, but are shown for understanding, not memorization.

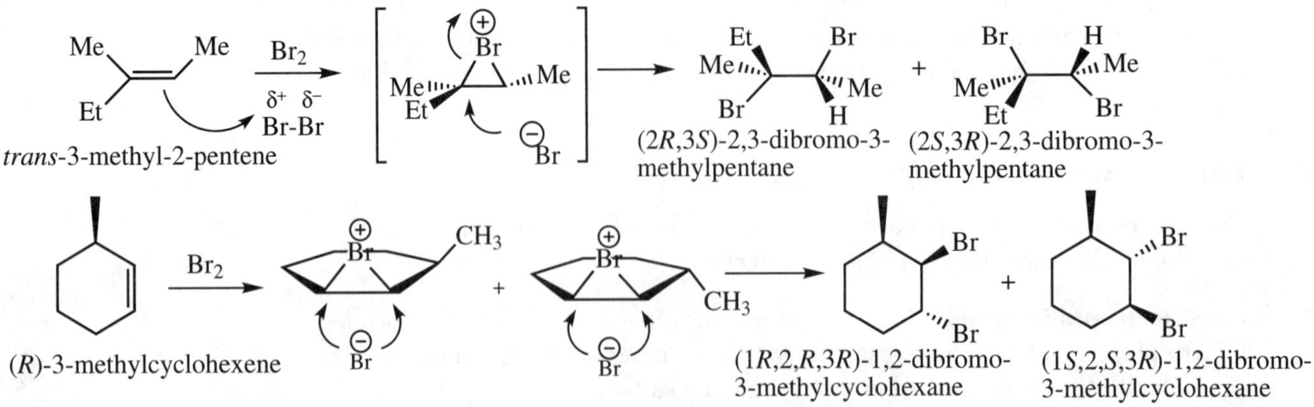

2. Addition of Halogens

This reaction is another example of electrophilic attack. Figure 3-2 shows the mechanisms for the addition of halogens across a double bond.

These reactions begin when electrons from the double bond attack the positive end of the halogen dipole. A three-membered ring forms, as is shown in Figure 3-2. Both carbons are highly δ^+ (partially positive) because of the electron-deficient, positively charged halogen of the ring. The nucleophile attacks this intermediate from the opposite side of the ring (owing to steric hindrance). Furthermore, the attack occurs at the more substituted carbon, because it can better stabilize the partial positive charge. Thus, **Markovnikov's rule is observed.**

A similar mechanism occurs for alkynes (Figure 3-3). The three-membered ring in this case is highly strained and is thus **higher in energy,** i.e., has a high energy activation barrier. In most cases, high energy activation barriers are surpassed by heating.

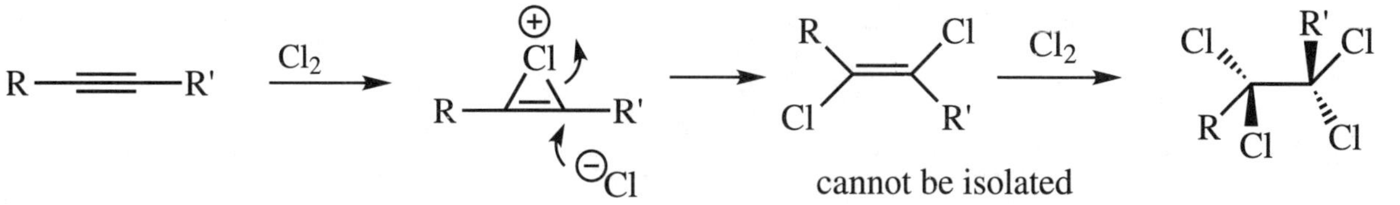

FIGURE 3-3.

Addition of halogens across a triple bond. Mechanism shown for understanding, not memorization.

cannot be isolated

B. Anti-Markovnikov Reactions

These important reactions result in the nucleophile attaching to the lesser substituted carbon.

1. **Radical Halogenation**

   This reaction is important because an anti-Markovnikov product is formed (Figure 3-4). Using a **peroxide** to initiate the reaction, the electron-deficient bromine radical attacks the double bond, leaving the more stable and substituted radical. The more stable radical is formed by the addition of the bromine radical to the lesser substituted site. The reaction propagates as another bromine radical is formed and continues until the reaction terminates or the starting material is consumed. This process results in **an anti-Markovnikov addition of bromine to the alkene.** Even so, note that the trend of going through the more stable (lower energy) intermediate is preserved.

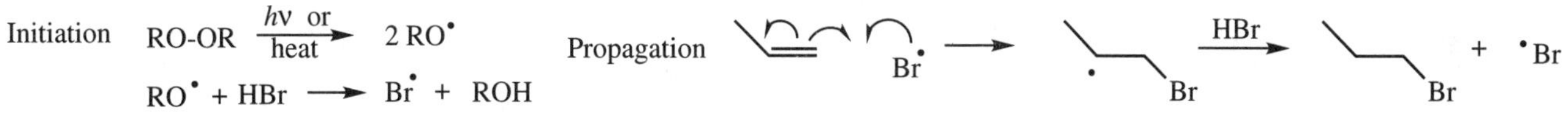

FIGURE 3-4.

Radical halogenation, an example of an anti-Markovnikov reaction.

2. **Hydroboration**

   In this reaction (Figure 3-5), the electron-deficient boron attacks the double bond at the less substituted site, leaving the partial positive charge on the other more substituted carbon. A hydrogen is then delivered to this site and oxidation using hydrogen peroxide removes the boron and replaces it with a hydroxy. Thus, this hydroboration represents an anti-Markovnikov addition of OH. Again, note the trend of going through the more stable (lower energy) intermediate.

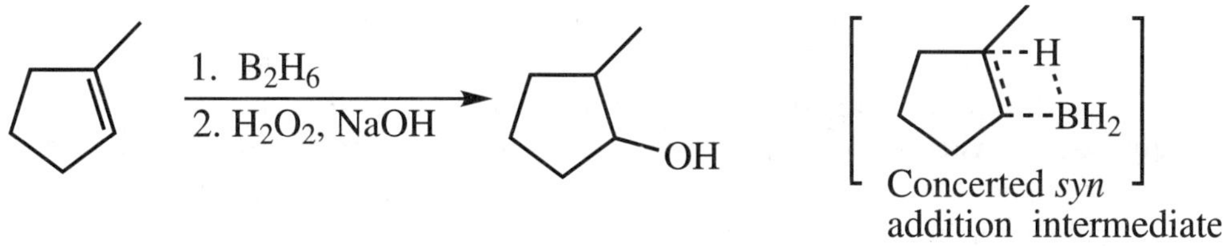

FIGURE 3-5.

Hydroboration reaction, an example of anti-Markovnikov addition.

Concerted *syn* addition intermediate

SECT. III
ORGANIC
CHEMISTRY
REVIEW
NOTES

561

C. Hydration of Multiple Bonds

Water adds to the more reactive alkenes in the presence of acids to yield alcohols. This addition follows Markovnikov's rule. A hydrogen atom from water adds to the carbon of the double bond that contains more hydrogens. The $-OH$ group from water adds to the carbon of the double bond containing fewer hydrogens. This reaction will hydrate both double and triple bonds in the presence of dilute acid. In both cases, the reaction starts with the electrophilic attack of the proton, resulting in the most substituted carbocation.

Figure 3-6 shows the hydration reaction for both double and triple bonds. For the double bond, the carbocation is attacked by water and Markovnikov addition is observed. For alkynes, the carbocation is attacked by water and keto–enol tautomerism occurs. (See Chapter 6 of the Organic Chemistry Review Notes for a review of keto–enol tautomerism.)

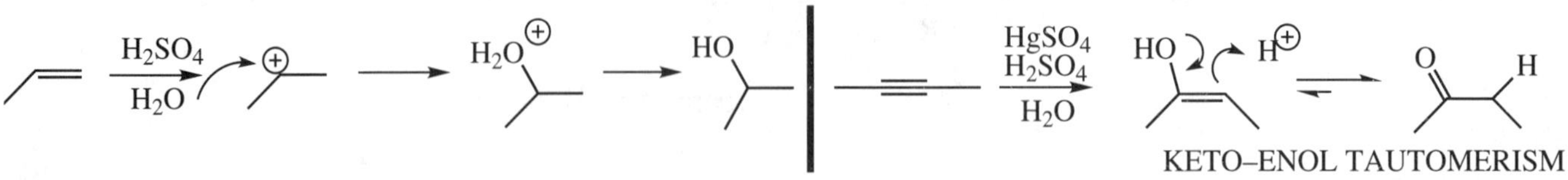

KETO–ENOL TAUTOMERISM

FIGURE 3-6.
Hydration reactions for double bonds (left) and triple bonds (right).

D. Oxidations

To identify oxidizing agents, look for multiple oxygens in the agents themselves; $KMnO_4$ and OsO_4 are good examples. The multiple bonds are oxidized by the addition of oxygen to the bonds.

Treatment with **$KMnO_4$ or OsO_4** creates *cis* (same side) diols (Figure 3-7). If the starting material is optically active, two products form (diastereomers) because of the two different *cis* additions that could occur.

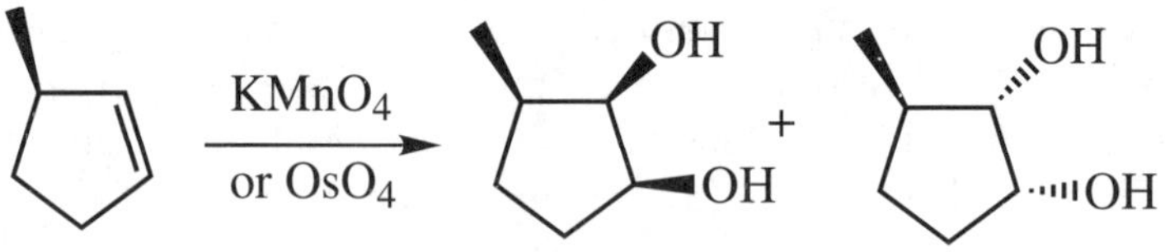

FIGURE 3-7.
Oxidation by $KMnO_4$ or OsO_4.

Ozonolysis (Figure 3-8) splits up the double bond and puts carbonyls in its place. This reaction is easy to recognize because of the products. Be aware that the starting materials can be linear or cyclic. Also, depending on the substitution of the double bond, an aldehyde or a ketone will result.

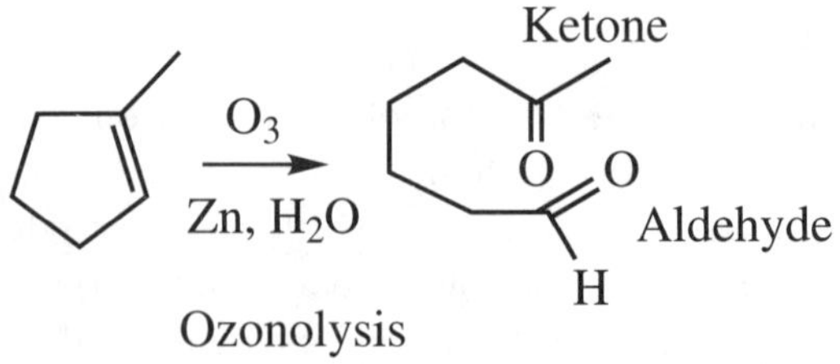

FIGURE 3-8.
Ozonolysis reaction.

Ozonolysis

E. Reductions

In organic chemistry, the word **reduction** generally refers to the addition of hydrogen. In the case of multiple bonds, it means that the bonds become more saturated.

Catalytic hydrogenation of multiple bonds results in a *cis* addition of hydrogen. As shown in Figure 3-9, the location of hydrogen addition can be deduced experimentally by the addition of deuterium instead of hydrogen. It is then possible to follow the reduction process and see where the hydrogen adds.

Figure 3-10 shows the mechanism by which a metal catalyst helps reduction reactions. Presumably, the hydrogen binds to the metal catalyst and the reaction is controlled such that the substrate is attacked on only one face.

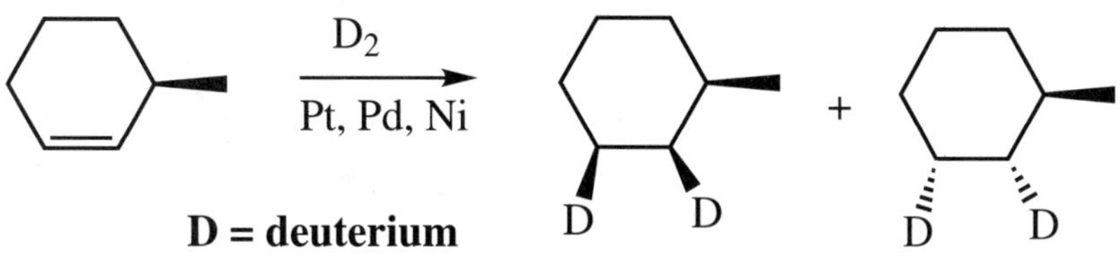

FIGURE 3-9.
Reduction of a double bond. Use of deuterium.

Catalytic hydrogenation can be used to reduce alkynes as well as alkenes. The difficult part is stopping the reduction of the triple bond before complete reduction occurs. Special care is needed when reducing a triple bond to a double bond to ensure that over-reduction does not occur. Otherwise, triple bonds are reduced to the carbon–carbon single-bonded alkane.

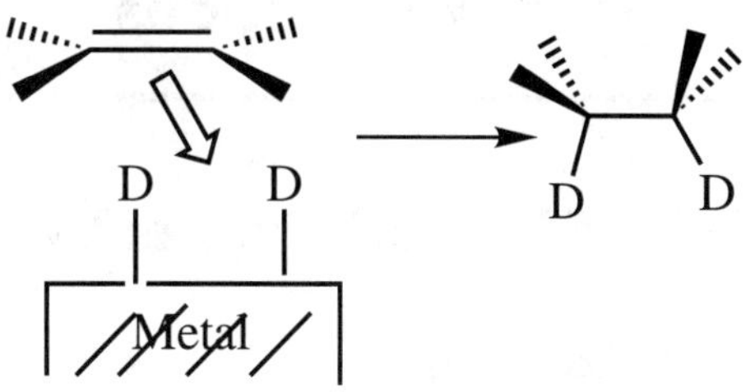

FIGURE 3-10.
How a catalyst aids in the reduction of the double bond.

F. Formation of Alkynes

This concept is straightforward. Recall that alkenes are formed by the elimination of hydrogen and a leaving group. To form a triple bond (alkyne), the same step is carried out twice through an E2 mechanism (Figure 3-11).

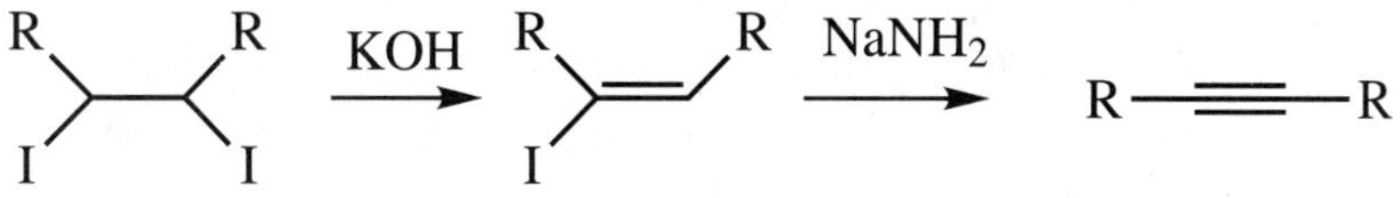

FIGURE 3-11.
Formation of alkynes.

SECT. III
ORGANIC
CHEMISTRY
REVIEW
NOTES

563

Benzene

Benzene

HIGH-YIELD TOPICS	**I.** Structure and Physical Properties
	II. Key Reactions

I. Structure and Physical Properties

A. Stability Through Resonance

Conjugation refers to molecules with p orbitals next to π-bonds or an extended series of overlapping p orbitals. These conjugated structures are more stable than their unconjugated counterparts because **resonance** allows for electron **delocalization.** Thus, these compounds release less energy on combustion when compared with their unconjugated counterparts.

Recall that the allylic and benzylic radicals and carbocations are highly stabilized owing to resonance. This factor determines the outcome of the reactions in which these compounds are intermediates.

Structurally, in order for these compounds to form conjugated structures, they must be able to line up all of their p orbitals. Thus, conformationally, these compounds favor a planar geometry. 1,3-butadiene is a good example of a compound with planar geometry (Figure 4-1).

FIGURE 4-1.
Arrangements of 1, 3-butadiene. Note the structure (left), the p orbitals for the molecule (center), and a representation of the molecular orbitals (right).

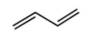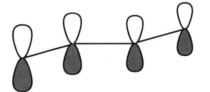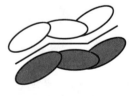

Once the four p orbitals for 1,3-butadiene line up, they can form molecular orbitals over the four atoms in the chain. Each p orbital contains one electron, and these four electrons fill the lower energy bonding molecular orbitals to capacity. This situation is energetically favorable, and is like the filling of an outer electron shell for an atom. Thus, the molecule is highly stabilized.

Benzene has a similar molecular orbital picture (Figure 4-2). Benzene is a planar six-membered ring with six p orbitals. These p orbitals come together to form molecular orbitals over all six atoms. The p orbital electrons fill the lower energy bonding molecular orbitals to capacity, creating an energetically favorable situation that makes benzene highly stabilized. Think of benzene as a flat carbon ring with a π-electron cloud above and below the ring (see Figure 4-2).

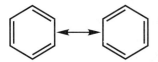 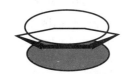 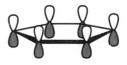

B. Aromaticity

Aromatic compounds usually have double bonds, are stable, and generally are found as five-, six-, or seven-membered rings. Theoretically, aromatic compounds are thought to have cyclic clouds of delocalized π-electrons above and below the plane of the molecule.

How can you be sure that a compound is aromatic?

A compound is considered aromatic if it has ($4n + 2$) π-electrons ($n = 0$, 1, 2, etc.) and is in a cyclic form. In addition, each member of that cyclic compound must be associated with at least one sp² hybridized atom. Thus, you can determine whether or not a particular compound is aromatic by calculating the number of its π-electrons and seeing if that value is predicted by the formula: 2, 6, 10, etc.

Benzene is an aromatic compound and contains six π-electrons. Many compounds, however, which do not look exactly like benzene, are aromatic. Study the compounds in Figure 4-3 to determine whether or not each compound is aromatic. Use the formula provided. Each double bond represents two π-electrons. Unpaired electrons are also counted directly. Sum all of the π-electrons associated with the double bonds and unbound electrons. If the sum is compatible with a value predicted by the formula, the compound is aromatic.

  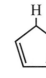 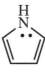 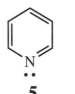 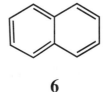

1　　　**2**　　　**3**　　　**4**　　　**5**　　　**6**

Compound 1 observes the rules for aromaticity. It has 2 π-electrons associated with the double bond. If $n = 0$, the formula could yield the integer 2. Thus, the compound is aromatic.

Compound 2 has a negative charge (2 π-electrons) associated with it. These electrons occupy a p orbital and are delocalized within the ring. Compound 2 is aromatic because it has a total of 6 π-electrons associated with it. The formula can give a value of 6 if $n = 1$.

Compound 3 is not aromatic because this structure has 4 π-electrons, and the formula cannot give a value of 4. The conjugate base of structure 3 is structure 2 (compound 2).

Compound 4 is aromatic. The lone pair on nitrogen lines up with the π-bonds of the ring and the system becomes aromatic. If $n = 1$, the formula predicts 6 electrons, because 4 π-electrons are associated with the 2 double bonds and there are 2 unpaired electrons.

Compound 5 is aromatic only if there is no donation of the lone pair into the ring. If the lone pair is considered in this structure, there would not be aromaticity.

Compound 6 is aromatic because of conjugation through the cyclic system and 10 π-electrons. Note that if $n = 2$, the formula predicts 10 π-electrons.

FIGURE 4-2.

Benzene: resonance structures (left), resonance hybrid (center), and π-electron cloud above and below the ring (right).

FIGURE 4-3.

Various aromatic and non-aromatic compounds. (See text for details.)

SECT. III
ORGANIC
CHEMISTRY
REVIEW
NOTES

565

II. Key Reactions

A. Electrophilic Aromatic Additions

Like alkenes and alkanes, the benzene ring is electron rich and the π-orbital electrons are accessible to electrophiles. Various electrophiles can add to benzene rings but they are strongly electrophilic and follow the same general reaction as shown in Figure 4-4. The electrophile is attacked by the ring and a resonance-stabilized carbocation forms. This intermediate is quickly deprotonated to re-establish aromaticity. An electrophilic aromatic addition product is formed.

FIGURE 4-4.

Mechanism of electrophilic aromatic addition.

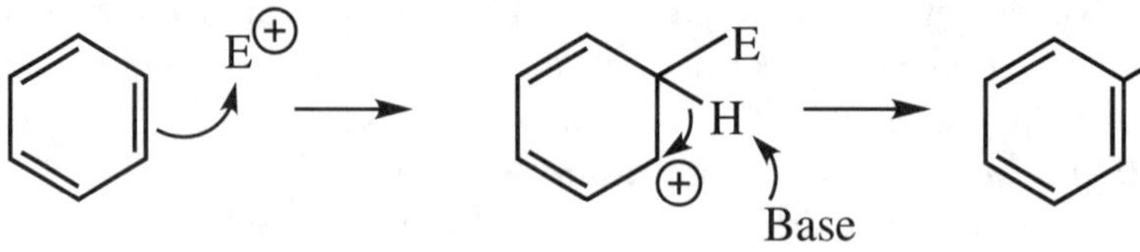

Figure 4-5 depicts a particular example of electrophilic aromatic addition: the **Friedel Crafts Acylation reaction.** In this reaction, the $AlCl_3$ functions as the Lewis acid that polarizes the carbonyl (more than it is normally), and makes the carbon highly electrophilic. Remember that Lewis acids are good electron acceptors. The $AlCl_3$ pulls electrons from the Cl of the acid chloride, which weakens the C–Cl bond. Electrophilic addition results in the aromatic ketone.

FIGURE 4-5.

Electrophilic addition: the Friedel Crafts Acylation reaction. Do not memorize this reaction, but follow and understand it.

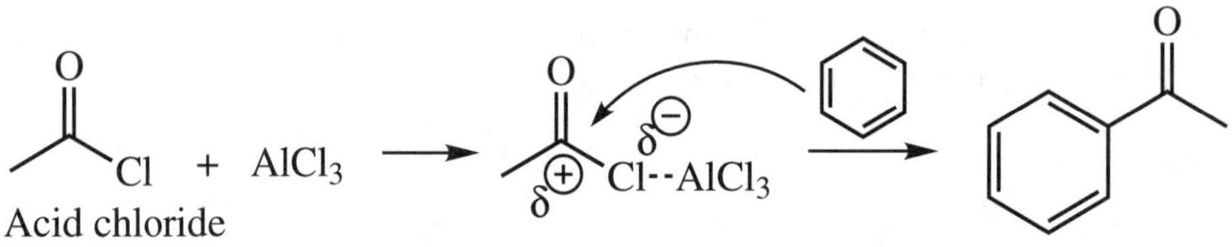

Other groups can add to the ring to give addition products. The **major reactions** are **bromination, nitration,** and **alkylation.**

The take-home message is that several different electrophilic aromatic additions can occur. Several examples are shown in Figure 4-6. Memorizing individual mechanisms is not necessary because all of these reactions are similar. Halogenation can occur as the diatomic halogen is polarized by the Lewis acid (in this case, $FeBr_3$). Nitration (adding an NO_2 group to the ring) can also occur. Chloroethane can be placed on a ring via Friedel Crafts alkylation. The Lewis acid activates the electrophile in a manner similar to the acylation described previously.

FIGURE 4-6.

Examples of various electrophilic aromatic additions.

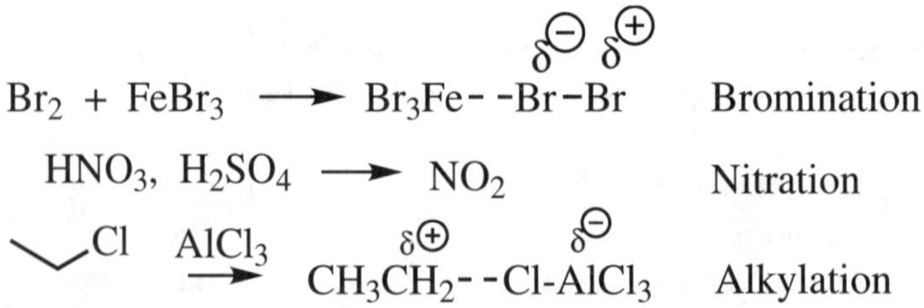

B. Substituent Effects

Whether a substituent takes electron density out of or donates electron density to the aromatic ring plays a large role in the physical characteristics and reactivity of the benzene ring. Remember that aromatic rings have fluffy electrons clouds above and below the plane of the ring, and it is the electrons that are susceptible to attack by an electrophile. If an electron-withdrawing group is placed on the ring, the relatively nonpolar benzene becomes polar because of the shift in the electron cloud toward the electronegative substituent. This change then alters the physical properties of the compound (e.g., melting and boiling points).

How is electrophilic addition affected if a group is already attached to the ring?

Any group attached to a benzene ring affects the **reactivity** of the ring and determines the **orientation** of substitution. **When an electrophilic reagent attacks an aromatic ring, it is the group already attached to the ring that determines where and how readily the attack occurs.**

1. **Activators and Deactivators**

   A group that makes the ring more reactive than benzene is an **activating group.** A group that makes the ring less reactive than benzene is a **deactivating group.**

   a. **Determination of Orientation**

      A group on a ring directs incoming substituents into an **ortho, para,** or **meta** position on the ring with respect to the initial group. For example, the −OH group of phenol directs an incoming substituent to an ortho or para position on the ring with respect to the −OH group. A nitro group on a benzene ring would direct incoming substituents to a meta position on the ring with respect to the nitro group.

   b. **Activators**

      Groups that are strong activators are ortho/para directors; i.e., electrophilic additions take place at the ortho and para positions (relative to the activator). For the most part, this orientation is attributable to the electron-releasing capability of the strongly activating substituents (amine groups and hydroxyl groups are good examples).

      In Figure 4-7, the amino group is a strong activator and ortho/para director. The amino group directs to the ortho/para position because from these positions, the lone pairs on the nitrogen donate electrons into the ring to help stabilize the carbocation intermediate. This situation would not occur if substitution were at the meta position.

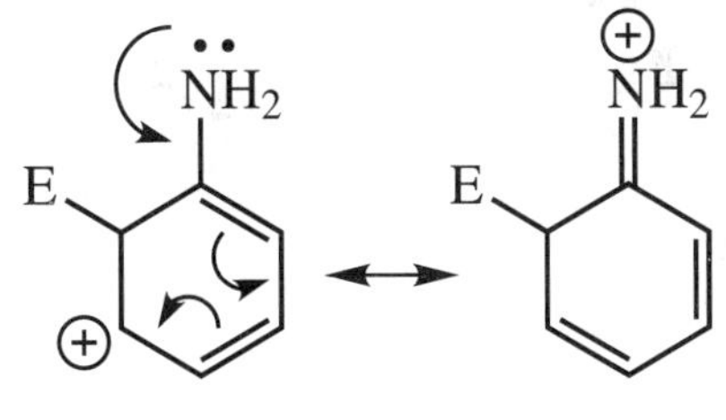

ortho E attack

FIGURE 4-7.
Activators: ortho/para directors. An example of how adding in the ortho position stabilizes the carbocation intermediate.

   c. **Deactivators**

      Deactivating substituents often direct to the meta position; halogens are an exception. Common deactivators and meta directors (Figure 4-8) include the nitro group, −CN group, −COOH group, and −SO₃H group. These substituents have δ⁺ atoms attached directly to the ring and tend to draw electron density out of the ring, thus deactivating

SECT. III
ORGANIC
CHEMISTRY
REVIEW
NOTES

567

the ring toward electrophilic attack. Electrophilic addition can still occur, although when it does, these groups direct the incoming electrophile to the position meta to the substituent. Only after meta attack does the highly unstable intermediate **not** occur.

FIGURE 4-8.
Deactivators: meta directors.

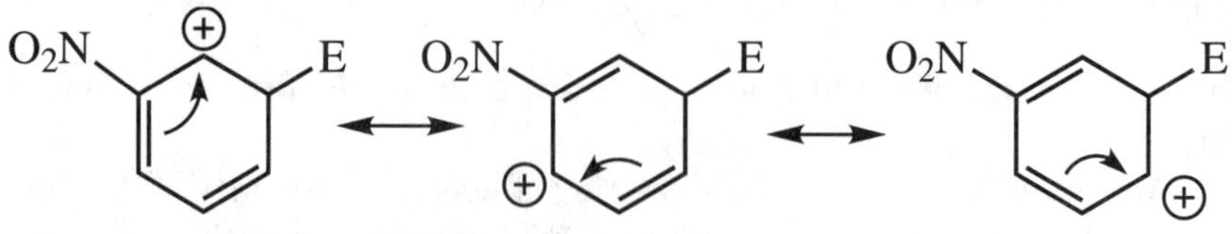

Meta attack

d. **Halogens**

Halogens are **deactivators** because of their electronegativity. They pull electron density out of the ring. Because of the presence of lone pairs, however, they are **also ortho/para directors.**

2. **Summary**

Activating: *ortho/para directors*	$-NH_2$, $-NHR$, $-OH$
Moderate activators: *ortho/para directors*	$-OCH_3$
Weak activators: *ortho/para directors*	$-C_6H_5$, $-CH_3$
Deactivating: *meta directors*	$-NO_2$, $-CH$, $-COOH$, $-SO_3$, $-CHO$
Deactivating: *ortho/para directors*	$-F$, $-Cl$, $-Br$, $-I$

If there is more than one substituent on the ring, refer to the following priority order (high to low) to decide where the electrophile will substitute:

o, p **activators** > *o, p* **deactivators (halogens)** > *m* **deactivators**

Figure 4-9 shows the o, p activating effects of the $-OH$ group overriding the meta deactivating effects of the nitro group. Thus, Br adds ortho and para to the $-OH$ group.

FIGURE 4-9.
Example of priority assignment for deciding where electrophile will substitute on multisubstituted ring.

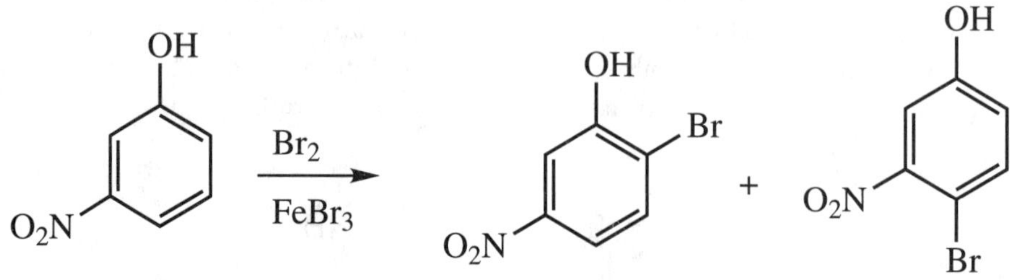

Alcohols and Ethers

5

I. Key Points
II. Physical Properties
III. Reactions
IV. Phenols

HIGH-YIELD TOPICS

I. Key Points

Alcohols and ethers contain an sp³ hybridized oxygen that is electronegative and has two lone pairs of electrons. Alcohols and ethers differ in that **alcohols have a hydrogen bound to oxygen, whereas ethers have an alkyl group bound to oxygen.** This structural dissimilarity accounts for the noticeable difference in the chemistry between the compounds. (See the review of nomenclature for these compounds in the Appendix.)

II. Physical Properties

A. Structure

Because alcohols and ethers contain an sp³ hybridized oxygen as the main functional group, the shape of the C–O–C bond is **bent,** with an angle of less than 109.5°. This configuration results from the repulsion of the lone pair of electrons of the oxygen (just like water). The electronegativity of the oxygen polarizes the compound, thus making alcohols and ethers good solvents for polar organic compounds. Ethers are less reactive than alcohols because of the lack of the hydrogen on the oxygen.

B. Melting and Boiling Points

Alcohols can form intermolecular hydrogen bonds. Figure 5-1 shows the hydrogen bonding that can occur between two alcohol molecules. Note that the hydrogen of one molecule forms a hydrogen bond with the oxygen of another molecule. **Ethers cannot form intermolecular hydrogen bonds,** because they have no hydrogen bound to oxygen. Thus, **alcohols have higher melting and boiling points than similar ethers.** The boiling point of ethers is similar to that of alkanes of comparable molecular weight.

FIGURE 5-1.

Hydrogen bonding of alcohols.

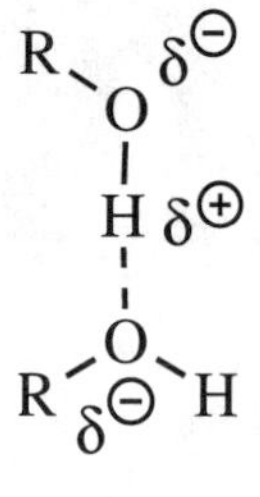

An increase in chain length raises the melting and boiling points for both alcohols and ethers, owing to an increase in the van der Waals interactions between molecules. Increased branching is associated with a decrease in van der Waals interactions, and a lowering of melting and boiling points.

Both short-chain alcohols and ethers can hydrogen bond with water, allowing them to mix in water. This ability indicates that the intermolecular interactions of water molecules can be replaced by interactions of the water with the alcohol or the ether. The water solubility of both alcohols and ethers decreases, however, with an increase in chain length. As the carbon chain length increases, the hydrophobic nature of these molecules increases.

III. Reactions

Alcohols and ethers often undergo reactions in the presence of acids in which the oxygen becomes protonated. The positive charge is then reacted with a base or nucleophile.

A. Reactions with Acids: Dehydration and Nucleophilic Attack

1. Alcohols

Treatment of alcohols with strong acids results in the displacement or elimination of the –OH group. Recall that –OH is a poor leaving group. Figure 5-2 illustrates the **substitution and elimination** reactions of alcohols. In step I, the oxygen donates a lone pair of electrons (Lewis base) and becomes protonated. In step II, water leaves to form a **carbocation;** this is the rate-limiting step. Finally, in step III, the carbocation is attacked by a nucleophile via an S_N1-type reaction or is eliminated by an E1 reaction.

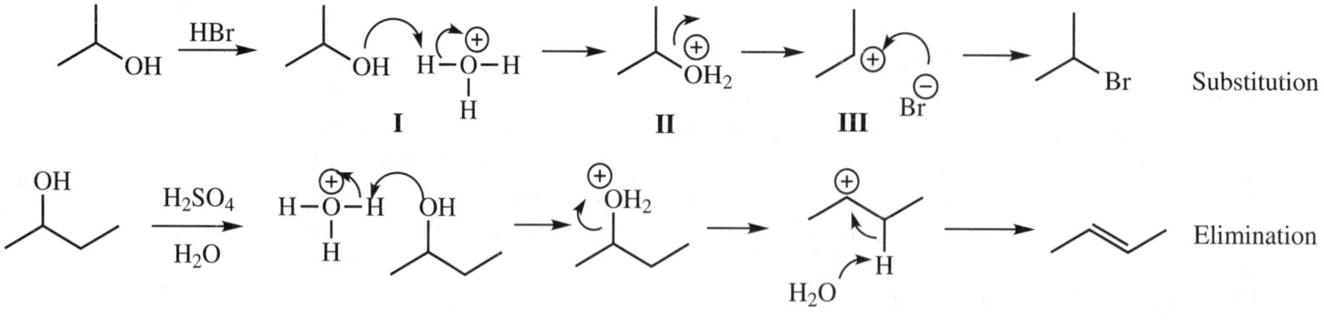

FIGURE 5-2.

Substitution and elimination reactions of alcohols.

Elimination occurs when the conjugate base of the acid is not a good nucleophile (as in the case of H_2SO_4). The carbocation formation occurs mainly with secondary and tertiary alcohols. Because of the nature of the reaction, rearrangements to form the more stable carbocation occur and result in a mixture of products. For primary alcohols, after protonation, water is displaced by a nucleophile in an S_N2-type reaction.

The S_N2-type reaction is also involved in the treatment of alcohols with PBr_3 or $SOCl_2$. These reactions result in the formation of alkyl bromides or chlorides, respectively (Figure 5-3). The O–P or O–S bond forms, putting a positive charge on the oxygen. Cl^- or Br^- acts as the nucleophile and displaces the species, resulting in the formation of the alkyl halide.

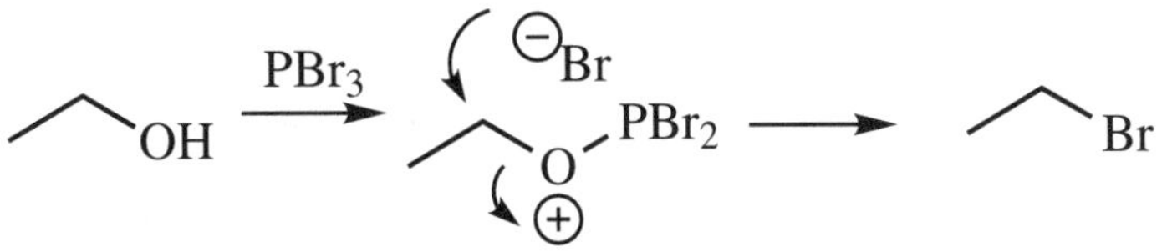

FIGURE 5-3.
Formation of alkyl halides by reaction of alcohols with PBr_3 or $SOCl_2$.

2. **Ethers**

Similar reactions with acids occur with ethers by an S_N2 process. These reactions result in cleavage of the ethers (Figure 5-4). The acid protonates the oxygen, and this species is attacked by the conjugate base of the acid. In the example in Figure 5-4, the size of the nucleophile and bulk of the electrophile cause the nucleophile to attack the primary electrophilic carbon instead of the more crowded carbon on the right. This reaction is an **anti-Markovnikov** addition of iodine.

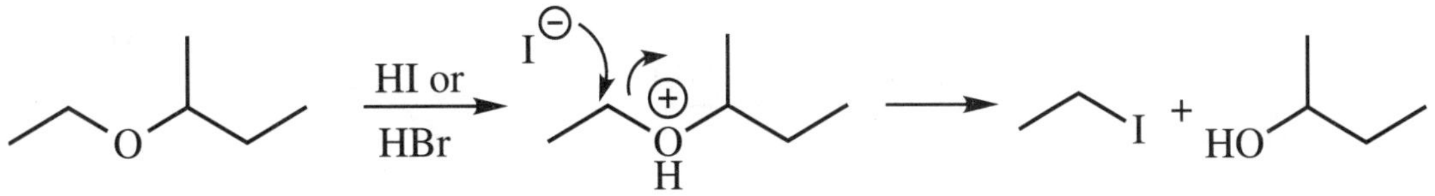

B. Alcohols as Nucleophiles

FIGURE 5-4.
Cleavage of ethers by acid.

The C–O bonds of alcohols are polarized because of the electronegativity of O. This polarization results in a δ^- at the oxygen, making it a decent nucleophile. **Alcohols can be used as solvent/nucleophiles for S_N1 reactions as a result of their polar protic nature.** (See examples of these reactions in Chapter 6 of the Organic Chemistry Review Notes.)

C. Ether Formation

A popular way to synthesize an ether is to react an alcohol with a strong base. The resulting alkoxide is a highly nucleophilic species that reacts with primary alkyl halides and produces an ether by an S_N2 mechanism. This reaction is known as the **Williamson ether synthesis** (Figure 5-5).

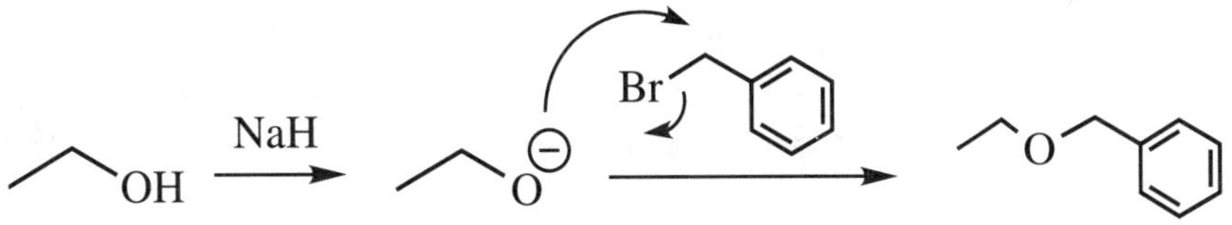

FIGURE 5-5.
Williamson ether synthesis (synthesis of an ether from an alcohol).

D. Epoxides

Epoxides are three-membered oxygen-containing rings that are highly strained owing to the acuteness of bond angles. They are susceptible to nucleophilic attack because of the electronegativity of oxygen that causes polarization of the C–O bond.

SECT. III
ORGANIC
CHEMISTRY
REVIEW
NOTES

571

Figure 5-6 demonstrates how epoxides are formed and how they may act as intermediates in reactions. In this reaction, a six-membered ring containing one double bond (halohydrin) is treated with base. An epoxide is formed (shown in lower left structure of Figure 5-6). Note that the epoxide is in the form of a **cis ring**. In this example, two enantiomers are formed, because the nucleophile can attack either carbon of the epoxide.

FIGURE 5-6.

Reaction involving an epoxide. The epoxide is shown at the lower left of the figure.

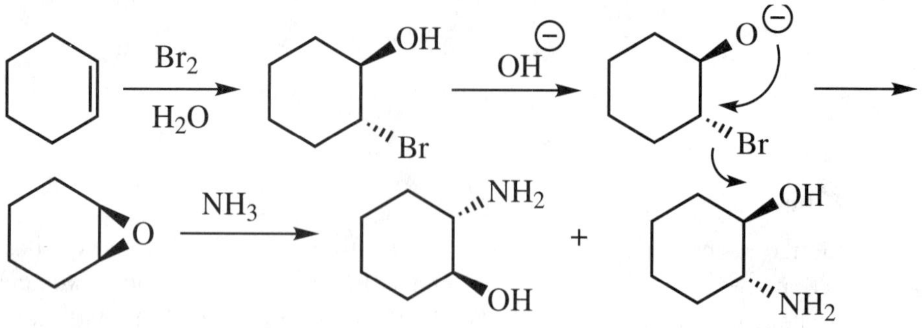

E. Oxidation of Alcohols

Chromium reagents, such as CrO_3, convert alcohols to carbonyl compounds. Secondary alcohols are oxidized to ketones (Figure 5-7).

FIGURE 5-7.

Oxidation of a secondary alcohol to a ketone.

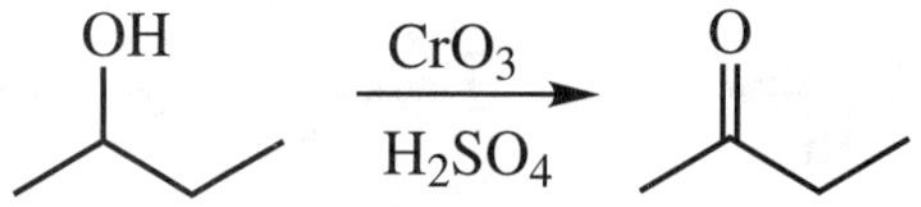

Primary alcohols are converted to aldehydes and then to carboxylic acids (Figure 5-8). A special reagent, known as pyridinium chlorochromate (PCC), allows the isolation of the aldehyde that results from oxidation of the primary alcohol without over-oxidation to the carboxylic acid.

FIGURE 5-8.

Oxidation of a primary alcohol to an aldehyde and ultimately to a carboxylic acid. Structure of the reagent pyridinium chlorochromate (PCC) is also shown.

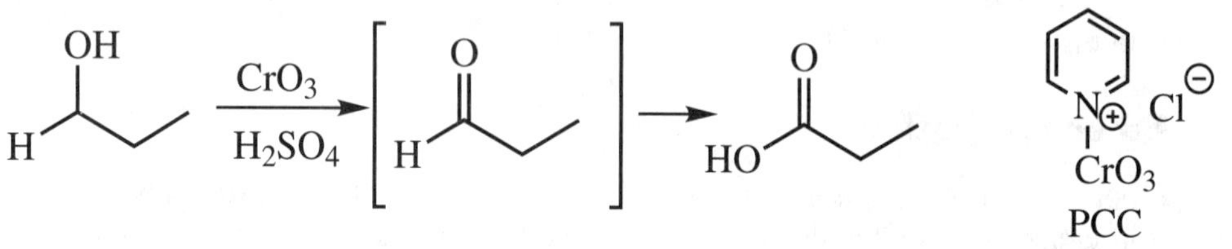

F. Formation of Alcohols and Ethers by Reduction

Many methods are used to synthesize alcohols; recall the hydration of alkenes and the hydroboration reaction discussed in Chapter 3 of the Organic Chemistry Review Notes. Another common method of generating alcohols is the reduction of carbonyl compounds. **Remember: you can recognize reducing agents by the large number of hydrogens.** Common reducing agents include $LiAlH_4$ and $NaBH_4$. Figure 5-9 illustrates the reduction of a ketone to an alcohol.

FIGURE 5-9.

Formation of alcohols by reduction.

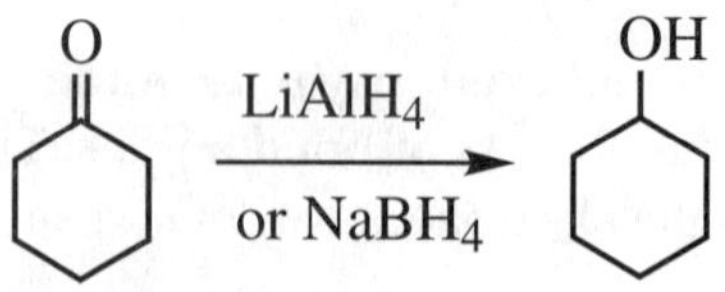

IV. Phenols

Discussion of phenols requires familiarity with benzene chemistry and acid–base theory. Phenols are special alcohols. They are **enols,** which favor the enol and not the ketone form because of aromatic stability. In addition, they are **more acidic than nonaromatic alcohols,** given the stability of the conjugate base formed on deprotonation. The resonance forms that stabilize phenol are shown in Figure 5-10.

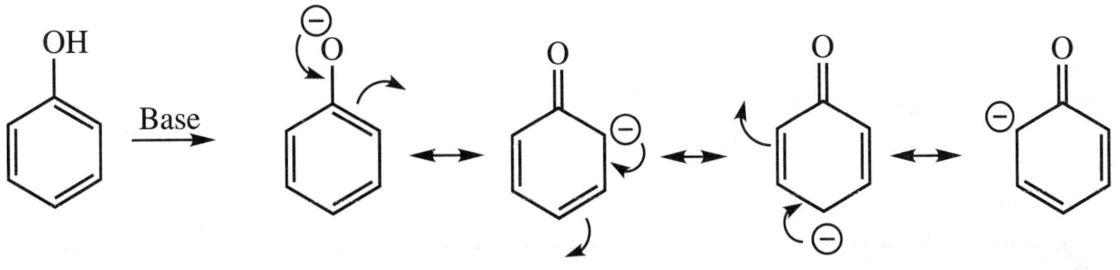

FIGURE 5-10.
Resonance forms of phenol.

Placement of electron-withdrawing groups on the ring enhance acidity. For example, phenol has a $pK_a = 9.89$, whereas the substituted phenols with electron-withdrawing nitro groups have lower pK_a values (m–NO_2 phenol: $pK_a=8.28$; o–NO_2 phenol: $pK_a=7.17$). The electron-withdrawing substituents enhance the stability of the conjugate base by the **inductive effect** (spreading the charge). The placement of these groups can also increase **resonance stability.** The anion can be stabilized through resonance with the electron-withdrawing group in the ortho and para positions (Figure 5-11). This situation will not occur when the group is in the meta position.

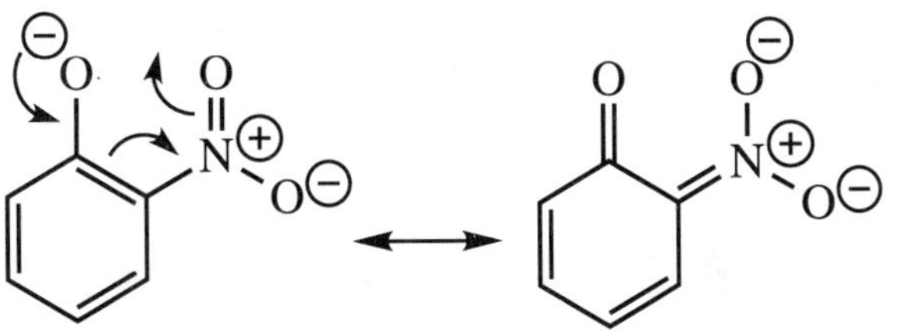

FIGURE 5-11.
Resonance stability of an electron-withdrawing group in the ortho position. Substitution of electron-withdrawing group increases acidity.

SECT. III
ORGANIC
CHEMISTRY
REVIEW
NOTES

573

6

Carbonyl Compounds

Compounds

HIGH-YIELD TOPICS	**I.** Physical Characteristics and Properties
	II. Keto–Enol Tautomerism
	III. Key Reactions

The carbonyl compounds have many similar properties and reactions based on the chemistry of the carbonyl group that they share. Throughout the following review, consider the similarities and differences among the reactions of the aldehydes, ketones, and carboxylic acids and their derivatives based on the carbonyl group and the structural differences between the molecules. (See the review of nomenclature for these compounds in the Appendix.)

I. Physical Characteristics and Properties

Carbonyl compounds have a π-bond and a σ-bond formed between the carbon and the oxygen. The chemistry of these compounds is dictated by their structure and by the dipole between the electronegative oxygen and the partially positive sp^2 carbon. Figure 6-1 illustrates the bonds and resonance forms of the carbonyl group. Note that the carbonyl carbon is electrophilic and the carbonyl oxygen is nucleophilic.

FIGURE 6-1.
Bonds and resonance forms of the carbonyl group.

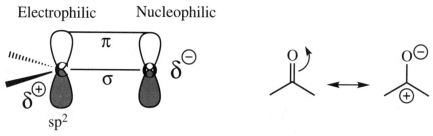

A major set of the reactions of the carbonyl compounds involves the nucleophilic attack of the carbonyl group electrophilic carbon. The consequences of nucleophilic attack depend on the type of carbonyl compound involved (with or without a good leaving group).

A. Structure

The carbonyl carbon is sp^2 hybridized, which makes the carbonyl structure **planar** with bond angles of 120°. The electrophilic nature of the carbonyl carbon is explained by looking at Figure 6-1. Note that the resonance form for the carbonyl group has a positive charge on the carbon, which renders the carbon susceptible to nucleophilic attack.

B. Melting and Boiling Points

Carbonyl compounds have higher boiling points than comparable alkanes. This difference relates to the enhanced **dipole–dipole interactions** between molecules with carbonyl groups.

Ketones lack intermolecular hydrogen bonding because they do not have hydrogens associated with oxygen. Thus, ketones have lower boiling and melting points than comparable alcohols.

Hydrogen bonding does occur for carboxylic acids. These hydrogen bonds must be overcome for boiling to occur. Thus, **carboxylic acids have higher melting and boiling points than aldehydes or ketones.** In addition, because the carboxylic acids have strong dipole–dipole interactions, they **have higher melting and boiling points than alcohols of comparable length.**

II. Keto–Enol Tautomerism

Carbonyl compounds with hydrogens on the α-carbon (carbon next to the carbonyl carbon) are rapidly interconvertible between a keto form and an enol form. Recall that an enol is a structure with an $-OH$ group attached to a doubly bonded carbon. The –ene suffix is indicative of a carbon–carbon double bond, and the –ol is used for the alcohol group. The keto form contains a carbonyl group.

The rapid interconversion between the keto form and the enol form is referred to as **tautomerism.** This interconversion occurs between compounds with structures that differ greatly in the arrangement of atoms but exist in easy and rapid equilibrium. As is true of keto–enol tautomerism, most tautomerisms involve structures that differ in the point of attachment of hydrogen. Typically, the equilibrium of this interconversion overwhelmingly favors the structure in which hydrogen is bonded to carbon (keto form). **The keto form is also more stable than the enol form.**

Figure 6-2 illustrates **keto–enol tautomerism,** a process that can be catalyzed by base or acid. Note that whether catalyzed in base or acid, the process starts with the carbonyl group in the form of a ketone. A hydrogen is extracted from the α-carbon and intermediates form. The result is a structure with a double bond and a hydroxyl group—the enol form. **Remember: the keto form is more stable than the enol form, and rapid interconversions between these two forms occur.**

FIGURE 6-2.
Keto–enol tautomerism catalyzed in acid or base.

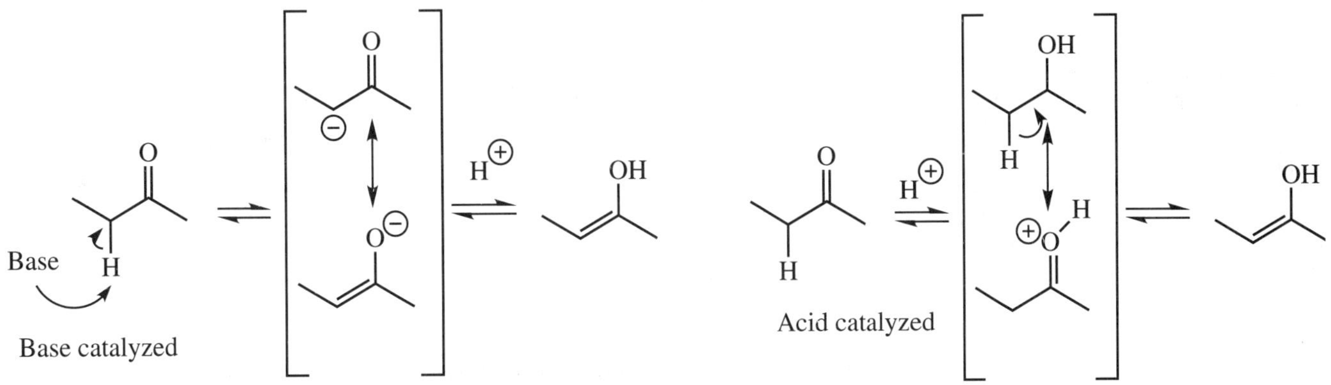

Base catalyzed

Acid catalyzed

A. Carboxylic Acids

These compounds are **acidic because of the delocalization of the electrons** of the conjugate base (carboxylate ion) over the two oxygens and the carbonyl carbon.

SECT. III
ORGANIC
CHEMISTRY
REVIEW
NOTES

575

Recall that inductive effects can enhance acidity by further polarizing the O–H bond and stabilizing the conjugate base.

If a group is close enough or is connected through an electron cloud, an electronegative moiety will enhance acidity of the carboxylic acid by helping to stabilize the conjugate base. In Figure 6-3, the electron-withdrawing nitro group removes electron density from the ring and stabilizes the anion formed after deprotonation.

FIGURE 6-3.
How an electron-withdrawing group increases acidity.

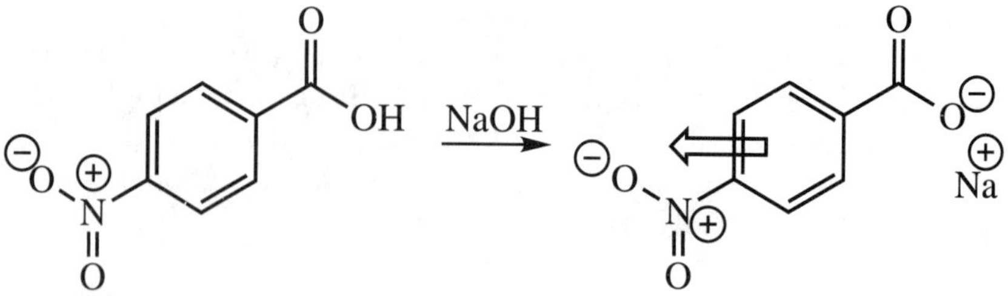

When comparing the acidity of carboxylic acids with electron-withdrawing halides attached near the carbonyl carbon, remember these general rules:

1. **The more halides attached to the acid molecule, the stronger the acid.**

2. **The closer the halide atoms are attached to the carboxylic acid functional group, the stronger the acid.**

B. Amides

These compounds also have a carbonyl group. **Amides are considered functional derivatives of carboxylic acids because instead of the −OH group of the acid, they have a −NH$_2$ group.** Like the carboxylic acids, they have **high melting and boiling points because of hydrogen bond formation.** Amides have the ability to form intermolecular hydrogen bonds as long as there is a hydrogen on nitrogen. Figure 6-4 shows the intermolecular hydrogen bonding possible with amides and the resonance forms associated with amides.

FIGURE 6-4.
Hydrogen bonding and resonance structures associated with amides.

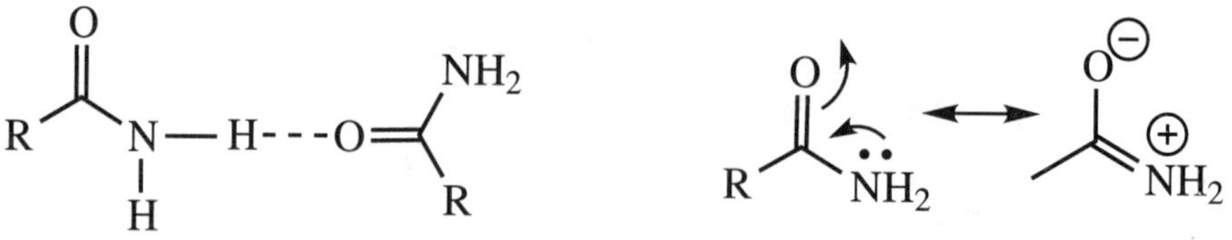

These compounds are also unique in the ability of the nitrogen to donate electrons and form a π-bond with the carbonyl carbon. This electron donation stabilizes the resonance hybrid. The C–N bond is said to have partial double-bond character. Thus, it does not rotate as easily as a normal C–N single bond. This characteristic has important implications in the structure of peptides and proteins with amide bonds between the individual amino acids.

C. Acidity of α-Protons in Carbonyl Compounds and the Enolate Ion

The protons α to the carbonyl (except for carboxylic acids and amides) are slightly acidic. The pK_a of the proton in this position varies from 17 to 30, depending on the type of carbonyl compound. The anion at this position, the **enolate ion,** is stabilized through resonance, allowing for delocalization of the negative charge.

The formation of the enolate ion (Figure 6-5) should look familiar; compare it to the keto–enol interconversion reviewed previously (see Figure 6-2). The enolate ion is critical in organic chemistry because it is a **good nucleophile.** The importance of this ion in chemical reactions is discussed subsequently.

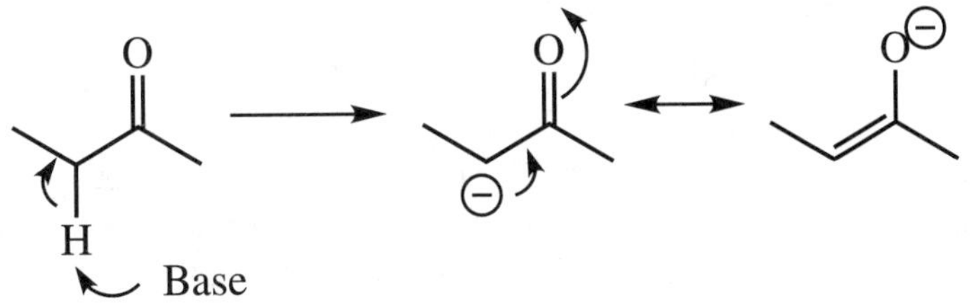

FIGURE 6-5.
Formation of the enolate ion by extraction of proton α to the carbonyl.

III. Key Reactions

A. Overview

The basic reactions of carbonyl compounds involve **nucleophilic additions and substitutions, reductions, and reactions involving enolates.**

Figure 6-6 illustrates the paths and possible results of nucleophilic attack: **nucleophilic addition (aldehydes and ketones)** and **nucleophilic substitution (carboxylic acids).** Direct addition and conversion of the carbonyl to another species are shown along **path A.** Displacement of a leaving group is shown along **path B.** Both paths go through a tetrahedral (sp^3) intermediate. The nucleophile can attack from either face of the sp^2 hybridized carbon and the π-electrons shift to the oxygen, giving it a negative charge.

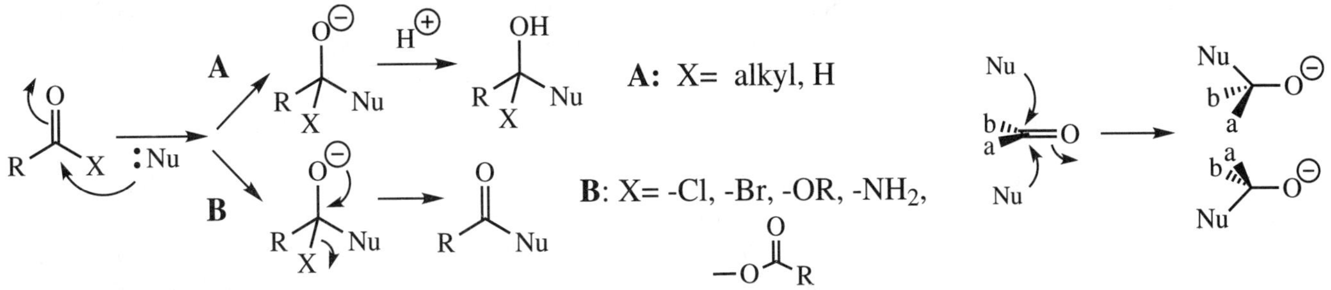

A: X= alkyl, H

B: X= -Cl, -Br, -OR, -NH₂,

FIGURE 6-6.
General types of reactions for carbonyl compounds.

By understanding that **nucleophilic attack of aldehydes and ketones tends to follow a nucleophilic addition reaction (path A)** and **nucleophilic attack of carboxylic acids tends to follow a nucleophilic substitution reaction (path B),** one can predict the products of many reactions.

Reduction (addition of H_2 across a double bond) can also occur, yielding aldehydes (under careful control) and alcohols (Figure 6-7).

Another main type of reaction is based on the **reactivity of enolates.** These ions are compounds formed from the removal of the proton α to the carbonyl. Enolates are good nucleophiles that can undergo a variety of reactions with various electrophiles.

SECT. III
ORGANIC
CHEMISTRY
REVIEW
NOTES

577

FIGURE 6-7.
Reduction of carbonyls to give
alcohols and aldehydes.

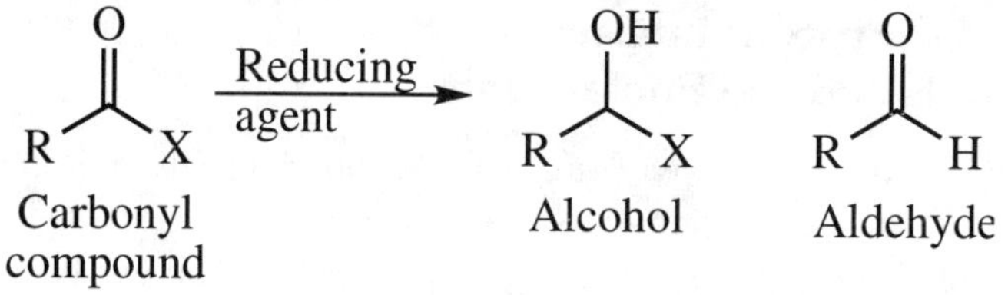

B. Nucleophilic Addition to Aldehydes and Ketones

Aldehydes and ketones possess poor leaving groups adjacent to the carbonyl, which dictates the outcome of their reactions.

1. Addition of Strong Nucleophiles

Nucleophiles can add to the carbon and form a wide variety of alcohols, a process that follows the mechanism of nucleophilic addition shown in Figure 6-6. Nucleophiles, such as Grignards (RMgBr), organocuprates (R_2CuLi), and acetylides (Figure 6-8), are needed for these reactions to occur. Addition is favored because of the poor leaving groups of the aldehydes and ketones. In each example in Figure 6-8, note: (1) that a ketone is attacked by a strong nucleophile and an alcohol is formed, and (2) that a group has been added to the carbonyl carbon.

FIGURE 6-8.
Various nucleophilic
addition reactions.

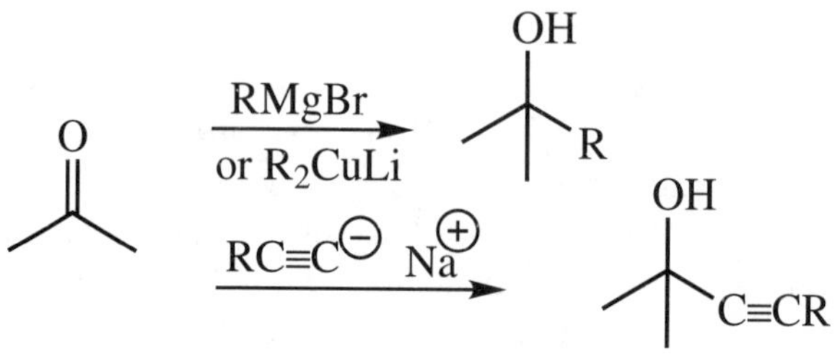

2. Hemiacetal/Hemiketal and Acetal/Ketal Formation

These reactions involve the attack of the electrophilic carbon by an alcohol. When a single alcohol molecule undergoes nucleophilic addition and adds to the carbonyl group, **a hemiacetal** (if starting compound is an aldehyde) or a **hemiketal** (if starting compound is a ketone) forms. The addition of a second alcohol molecule by nucleophilic addition gives **the acetal or ketal.** These reactions can be catalyzed by acid or base.

Study the reaction mechanism in Figure 6-9. Note that the acid protonates the carbonyl of the ketone and the alcohol attacks the electrophilic carbon, leading to the production of the hemiketal. Hemiketals and hemiacetals generally are too unstable to be isolated. The reaction can continue with transfer of a proton to the −OH group and elimination of water. The carbon is then attacked by another alcohol molecule to form the ketal. If the starting compound is an aldehyde, a hemiacetal and an acetal form according to the reaction mechanism just described.

FIGURE 6-9.
Hemiketal and ketal formation.

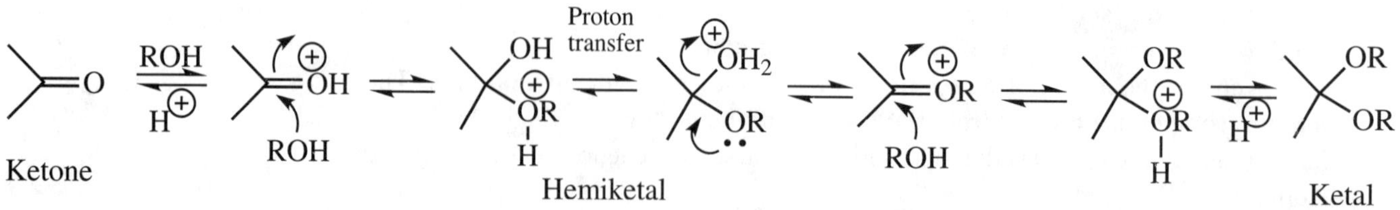

Reaction arrows indicate that the reactions are readily reversible. To favor one side over the other, the conditions must be carefully controlled. Excess alcohol shifts the reactions to the right. The addition of water and acid shifts the reactions to the left and restores the carbonyl. The acid is a catalyst and is neither consumed nor generated.

3. **Addition of Amines**

Aldehydes and ketones can be attacked by amines, resulting in imines and iminium ions (Figure 6-10). **An imine is a compound that contains a carbon–nitrogen double bond.** Note how these reactions differ from the classic nucleophilic addition reactions discussed previously. After the initial attack of the amine, a proton is transferred and water is displaced in a manner similar to acetal or ketal formation.

FIGURE 6-10.

Addition of amine to a carbonyl yields an imine.

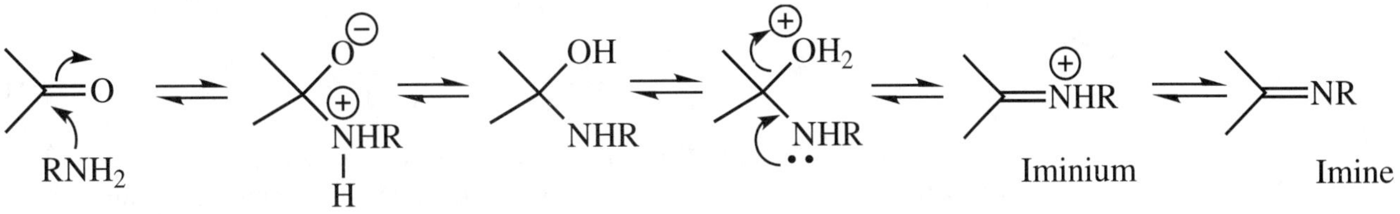

C. Nucleophilic Substitution to Carboxylic Acid Derivatives

Various types of nucleophilic substitutions are illustrated in Figure 6-11. You can see that a range of nucleophiles react readily with these compounds. **The products of nucleophilic substitution reactions include carboxylic acids, acid chlorides, amides, esters, ketones, and anhydrides.** All of the reactions go through a **tetrahedral intermediate.** The leaving group is then expelled. The reactivity of the carbonyl is directly related to the quality of X as a leaving group. Remember from $S_N1,2$ that the more stable anions are better leaving groups. The reactivity order of leaving groups, from high to low, is shown in Figure 6-12.

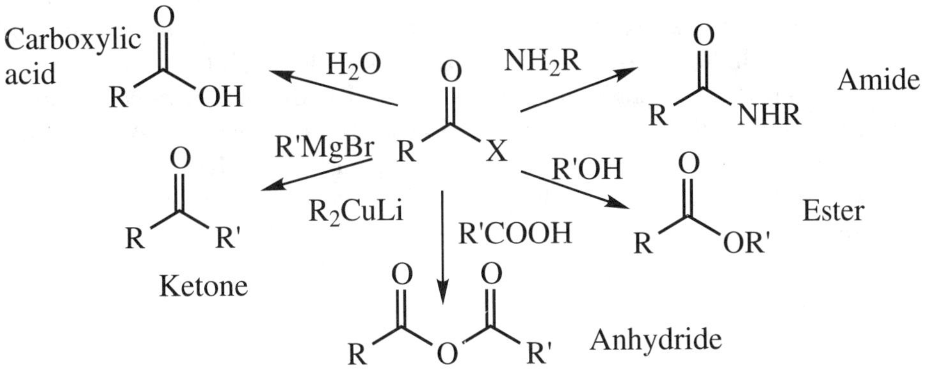

FIGURE 6-11.

Various products of nucleophilic substitution reactions. Note the production of various carboxylic acid derivatives.

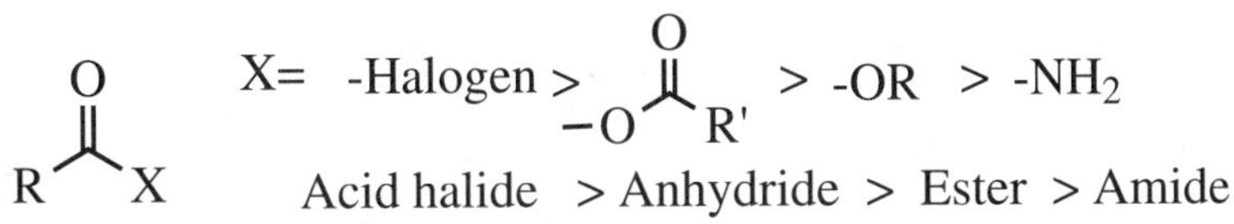

FIGURE 6-12.

Leaving group strength in nucleophilic substitution reactions.

As demonstrated in Figure 6-11, carboxylic acid derivatives can be synthesized through nucleophilic substitution. These reactions occur most readily from **acid chlorides,** which can be synthesized from the reaction of the carboxylic acid with $SOCl_2$ or PCl_3, using a mechanism similar to that for generating alkyl halides from alcohols (see Chapter 5 III A of the Organic Chemistry Review Notes).

SECT. III
ORGANIC
CHEMISTRY
REVIEW
NOTES

579

D. Reduction of Carbonyl Compounds

Carbonyl compounds are reduced by agents that deliver hydrides (H^-), such as **lithium aluminum hydride (LiAlH₄), sodium borohydride (NaBH₄), borane (BH₃), and their derivatives.** These reagents have certain selectivities, with the exception of **LiAlH₄, which is the strongest reducing agent** and reduces acids, aldehydes, and ketones down to an alcohol. LiAlH₄ reduces amides and nitriles to amines. Ketones reduce to secondary alcohols and aldehydes, and carboxylic acid derivatives reduce to primary alcohols. The more sterically hindered agents [such as LiAlH(O*t*Bu)₃] are not able to deliver the hydride as effectively as LiAlH₄, and thus are considered milder reducing agents. Consequently, they are able to reduce carboxylic acid derivatives to aldehydes without further reduction to the alcohol (Figure 6-13).

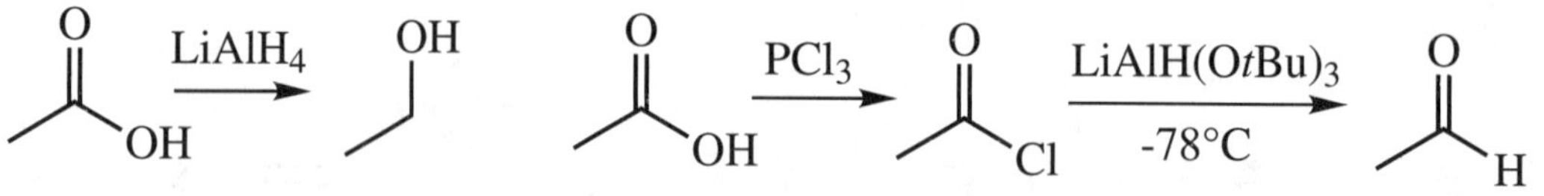

FIGURE 6-13.
Reduction of carboxylic acid to alcohol by LiAlH₄ (right), and conversion of a carboxylic acid to an acid chloride followed by reduction to an aldehyde by a mild reducing agent (left).

Catalytic hydrogenation can also be used to reduce carbonyl compounds to alcohols (from ketones, aldehydes, esters, and the like) and amines (from amides, nitriles). Heterogeneous catalysts such as Ni and Pt are often used. Note that any double bonds contained in the carbonyl compounds are reduced as well.

E. Formation of Carbonyl Compounds

Aldehydes and ketones can be synthesized by various methods discussed previously, including the **oxidation of alcohols** (see Chapter 5 III E of the Organic Chemistry Review Notes) and the **oxidation of alkenes** (ozonolysis, see Chapter 3 II D of the Organic Chemistry Review Notes).

Oxidation of alcohols and aldehydes by the strong oxidant CrO₃ yields carboxylic acids.

The **Grignard synthesis reaction is another way to synthesize carboxylic acids.** The **Grignard reagent,** one of the most useful and versatile reagents in organic chemistry, **has the general formula RMgX and the general name alkylmagnesium halide.** Basically, it is prepared by adding MgX to an alkyl group.

When the Grignard reagent is reacted with carbon dioxide, the alkyl group adds to the carbon–oxygen double bond of carbon dioxide. In the presence of mineral acid, the carboxylic acid is synthesized. Figure 6-14 shows how a Grignard reagent containing a phenyl group reacts with carbon dioxide in the presence of acid. The phenyl Grignard acts as a nucleophile and attacks carbon dioxide at the electrophilic carbon to form the carboxylic acid. This reaction is performed by pouring the Grignard reagent on crushed dry ice (carbon dioxide), or by bubbling carbon dioxide gas into an ether solution of the Grignard reagent.

FIGURE 6-14.
Synthesis of carboxylic acids by Grignard reaction (left) and nitrile synthesis (right).

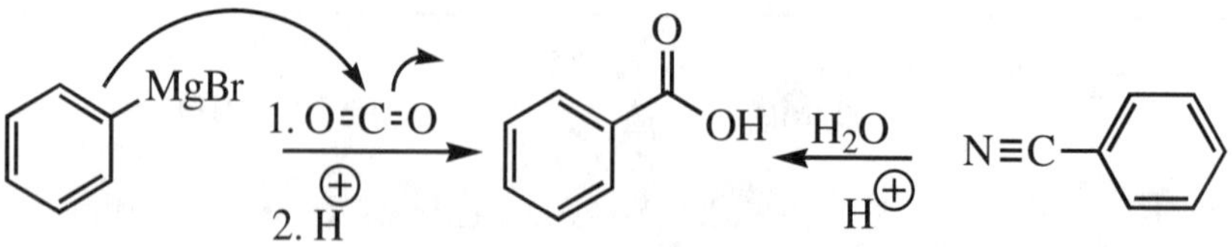

Figure 6-14 also demonstrates that **carboxylic acids can be synthesized by the hydrolysis of nitriles.** Nitriles contain an R group and a carbon atom triple bonded to a nitrogen atom (**RC≡N**), and are formed by treatment of alkyl halides with sodium cyanide in a nucleophilic substitution reaction. In the presence of water and acid, the nitrile is hydrolyzed to the carboxylic acid.

Esters are formed through acid-catalyzed attack of the electrophilic carbonyl carbon by an alcohol. Figure 6-15 shows the production of an ester by reaction of a carboxylic acid and an alcohol. In practical terms, it is easier to form esters from carboxylic acid derivatives, such as acid chlorides.

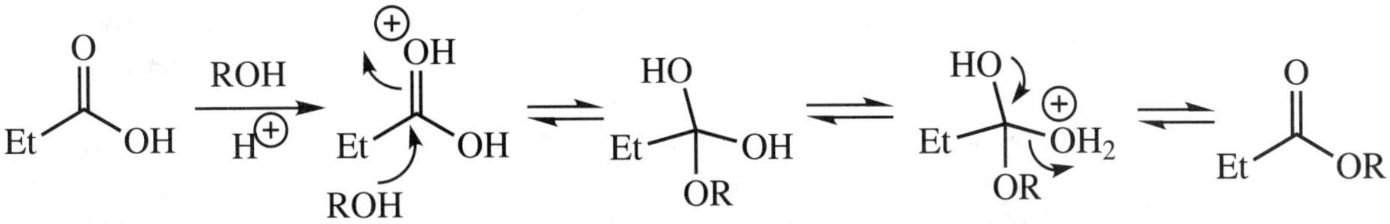

FIGURE 6-15.

Formation of esters from carboxylic acids and alcohols.

F. Reactions of Enolates

Recall that enolate ions are good nucleophiles and are important in the chemistry of carbonyl compounds. Enolate ions are often made by reacting a carbonyl compound with a base that extracts the α-proton.

1. Halogenation and Alkylation

Reactions of enolates lead to **halogenation and alkylation** of carbonyl compounds. After enolate formation, halogenation of the α-position occurs as the carbon anion attacks the halogen (Figure 6-16). Without careful control, a second halogen may add to the α-position because of the acidic α-proton that is present in the monohalogenated product.

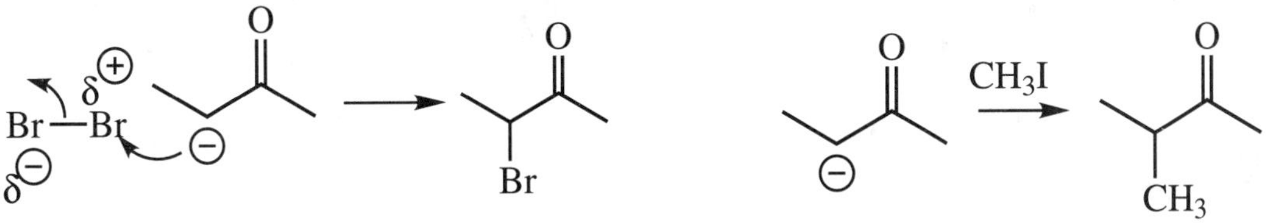

The enolate is a good nucleophile that can displace halides from alkyl halides to yield alkylated carbonyl compounds (see Figure 6-16, at right). Note that as the steric hindrance about the alkyl halide increases, the chance of E2 competing with the S_N2 alkylation increases.

FIGURE 6-16.

Halogenation and alkylation reactions involving enolates.

2. Reactions with Aldehydes and Ketones (Aldol Condensation)

Under the influence of dilute acid or base, **two molecules of aldehyde or ketone may combine. The products of this combination are β-hydroxyaldehydes or β-hydroxyketones.** This reaction is called the **aldol condensation** (Figure 6-17).

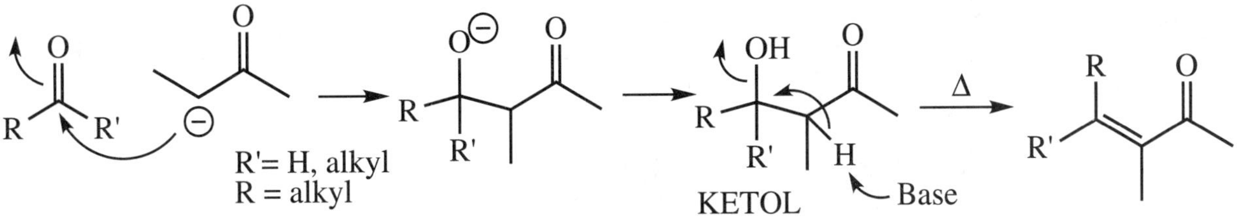

FIGURE 6-17.

Aldol condensation. Note enolate attack of carbonyl, formation of intermediate, and dehydration giving product.

This reaction occurs as follows. Remember that enolate ions are effective nucleophiles and can attack other carbonyls. As observed in other reactions, the nucleophile attacks the electrophilic carbon and forms a tetrahedral

SECT. III
ORGANIC
CHEMISTRY
REVIEW
NOTES

581

intermediate. This intermediate is a β-hydroxy carbonyl compound, known as an aldol or ketol. After heating, dehydration occurs (with acid or base catalysis) to form the more stable conjugated α,β-unsaturated carbonyl system. Deprotonation occurs because the α-proton is still acidic. Note that two carbonyl molecules have combined.

In every case, the product of this reaction results from the addition of one molecule of aldehyde or ketone to a second molecule in such a way that the α-carbon of the first becomes attached to the carbonyl carbon of the second. If both compounds contain α-protons, the result may be a mixture of products. To have more control over product formation, this reaction sometimes is carried out with one reactant that does not have α-protons.

3. **β-Keto Esters**

a. **Formation**

Enolates, being good nucleophiles, are able to react with carboxylic acid derivatives. **β-Keto esters are formed from the condensation of two esters;** one that acts as the enolate whereas the other acts as the electrophile (Figure 6-18). The initial step of this reaction yields an intermediate that has an α-proton to two carbonyl groups. A base (ethoxide) is used to deprotonate this proton. In the example in Figure 6-18, the product of the reaction can then be stabilized by resonance forms.

FIGURE 6-18.

Formation of β-keto esters by condensation of two ester molecules.

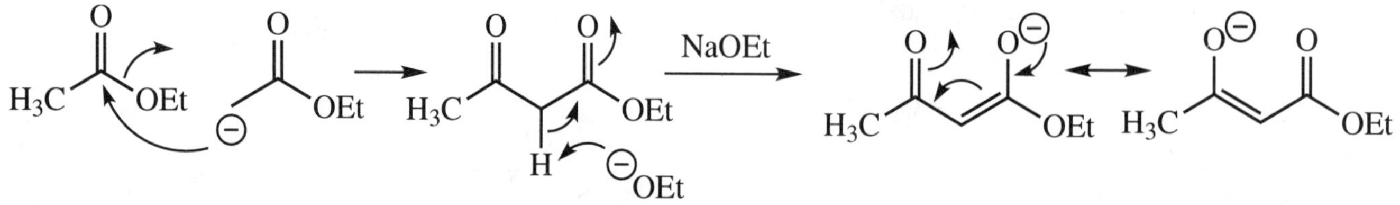

b. **Decarboxylation**

The reaction depicted in Figure 6-19 starts with hydrolysis of an ester with base, forming the β-keto acid. Remember that a β-keto acid has a keto group in position β to the carboxyl group. With protonation and heating, this species undergoes **decarboxylation,** which occurs as the six-membered, intramolecularly hydrogen-bonded intermediate forms between the two carbonyls. The enol that results quickly converts to the ketone. This reaction occurs for any dicarbonyl species in which the carbonyls are separated by an sp³ carbon and one is a protonated carboxylic acid.

FIGURE 6-19.

Decarboxylation reaction. An ester is hydrolyzed to a β-keto acid before being decarboxylated. The final product is a ketone.

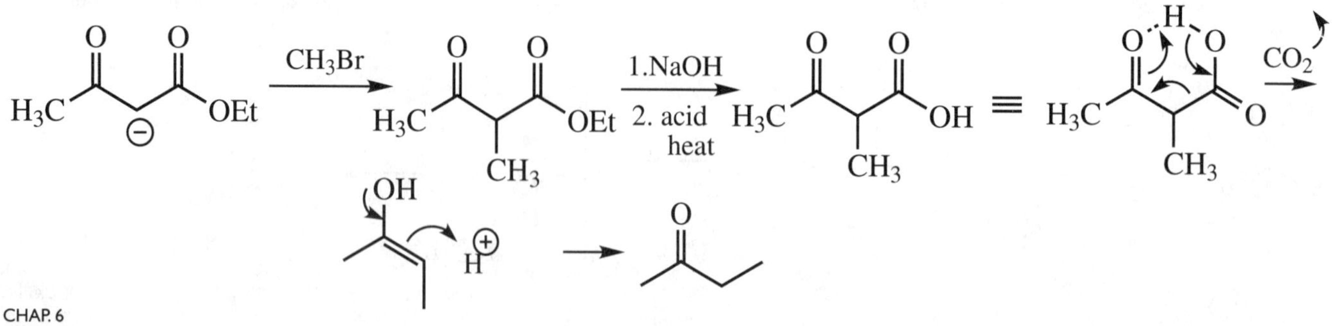

Carbohydrates

Carbohy
rates

I.	Structure and Physical Properties
II.	Key Reactions
III.	Polysaccharides

HIGH-YIELD TOPICS

From a biologic standpoint, the bonds of carbohydrates are nature's way of storing solar energy. Metabolism results in the oxidation of this stored energy and the synthesis of ATP and other high-energy molecules. Carbohydrates, commonly called sugars, are also involved in other biologically important molecules, such as nucleic acids (DNA and RNA), and in polymeric forms, such as cellulose (cell walls) and glycogen (storage form of glucose in the liver).

I. Structure and Physical Properties

Think of simple carbohydrates as polyhydroxylated aldehydes and ketones (see Chapters 5 and 6 of the Organic Chemistry Review Notes). **The simplest carbohydrates are the monosaccharides** (Figure 7-1). If the sugar contains an aldehyde group, it is an **aldose.** If it contains a keto group, it is a **ketose.** All the monosaccharides shown in Figure 7-1 are aldoses. A ketose is shown in Figure 7-2.

FIGURE 7-1.
Configuration of D- and L-glyceraldehyde and several aldohexoses.

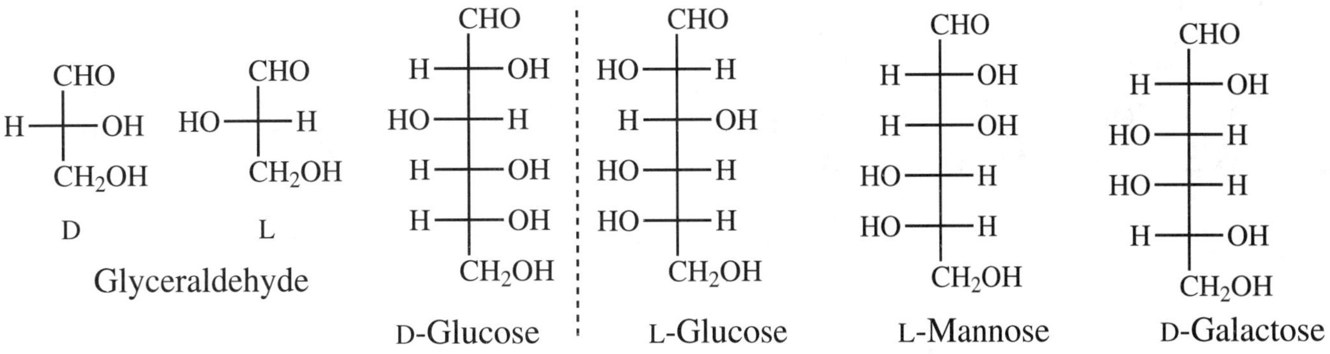

Glyceraldehyde   D-Glucose   L-Glucose   L-Mannose   D-Galactose

By convention, the monosaccharide **carbon backbone is numbered, starting from the end closest to the most highly oxidized carbon.** In Figure 7-1, carbon 1 of glucose would be the carbon with the aldehyde group at the top of the molecule. Carbon 6 would be the carbon at the bottom of the molecule (CH_2OH).

A monosaccharide is identified on the basis of the number of carbons it contains, e.g., **triose, tetrose, pentose, and hexose**. The most common monosaccharides in human diet are hexoses (glucose and fructose).

Monosaccharides are often represented as **Fischer diagrams,** and are designated D or L. These designations should **not** be confused with *d* and *l*, which designate the direction of the rotation of plane-polarized light. **The D and L designations represent the relationship of a carbohydrate to the structure of D- or L-glyceraldehyde.**

The compound glyceraldehyde (see Figure 7-1) was selected as the standard of reference for which the D and L configurations are named. Compounds related to D-glyceraldehyde are designated D, and the compounds related to L-glyceraldehyde are designated L. **All monosaccharides are named D or L on the basis of the lowest chiral center, the carbonyl group being at the top.** Thus, if −OH is on the right of the lowest chiral center, the sugar has a D-designation. The L-designation indicates that the chiral carbon farthest from the carbonyl has a hydroxy group on the left.

In Figure 7-1, note that the D-glucose has its −OH group on the right side of carbon 5 (lowest chiral center for glucose), and L-glucose has this −OH group on the left side. Check mannose and galactose to see if the correct designations are given.

By recalling the concepts of enantiomers and diastereomers (see Chapter 2 of the Organic Chemistry Review Notes), determine which of the hexoses in Figure 7-1 are enantiomers and which are diastereomers: D and L glucose are enantiomers, whereas L-glucose and D-galactose are diastereomers. L-glucose and L-mannose are also diastereomers. Note that enantiomers are D or L with the same name; diastereomers have different names.

Remember:

Epimers are diastereomers that differ in the chirality about carbon 2. L-glucose and L-mannose are epimers because they differ in the chirality of carbon 2.

Anomers are diastereomers that differ in configuration about carbon 1. Anomeric carbons are reviewed in I B.

A. Enolization to Ketoses

Aldoses can enolize to yield ketoses (see Figure 7-2). This process involves the removal of an α-proton by a base leading to the enolate and protonation to give the enediol. Tautomerization then gives the ketose. Treatment of the ketose with base reverses the reaction. The reverse reaction yields two products because of racemization of the carbon 2 position; protonation can occur on either face of the planar enolate when regenerating the aldose.

FIGURE 7-2.
Conversion of aldoses to ketoses by enolization.

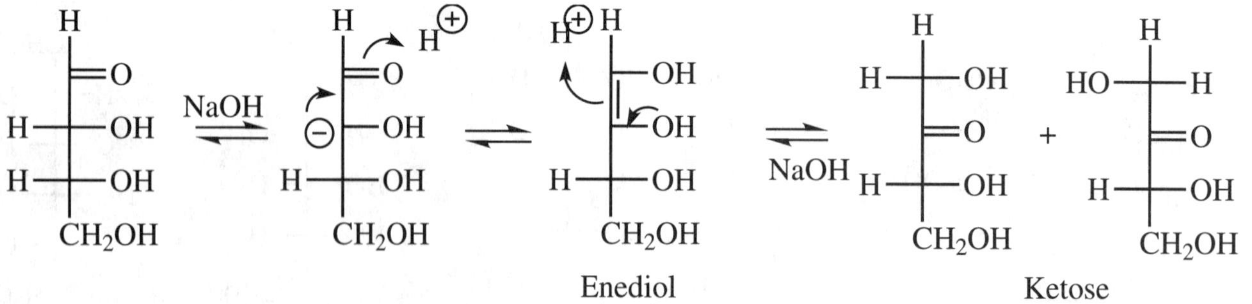

Enediol   Ketose

B. Cyclization

Sugars in solution exist in equilibrium with linear and cyclic forms, particularly true with pentoses and hexoses. Cyclization leads to the formation of hemiacetals. **Note:** This cyclization step is the same reaction as described in the discussion of hemiacetal formation in Chapter 5 of the Organic Chemistry Review Notes.

In Figure 7-3, note that the free −OH group on carbon 5 of the linear sugar forms can attack the carbonyl carbon, which has its oxygen in two different orientations. This interaction gives rise to the two different cyclic hemiacetals, an α- and a β-form. These forms are **anomers** (diastereomers that differ in configuration about carbon 1), and the carbon with the distinct stereochemistry is the **anomeric carbon.** Structurally, whether the α- or β-anomer results depends on the orientation of the aldehyde as it is attacked by the hydroxy group of the carbon.

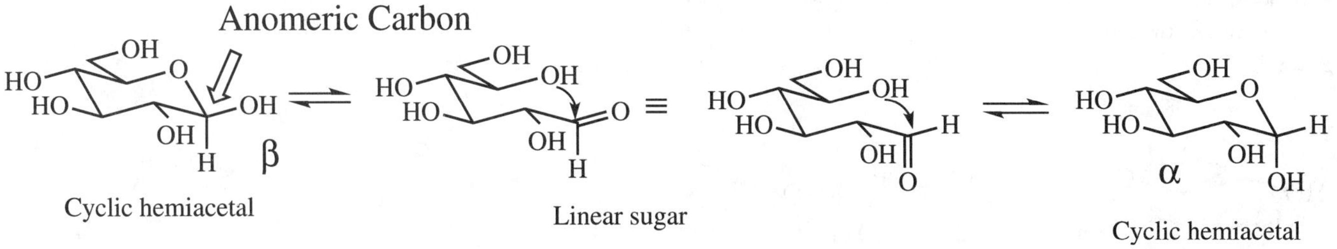

Cyclic hemiacetal

Linear sugar

Cyclic hemiacetal

D-Glucose exists in equilibrium with two cyclic forms (α and β) and the linear aldose form. At any given moment, most of the molecules are in the cyclic form; between the two cyclic forms, the β-form predominates (64% β versus 36% α). In glucose, **the β-form predominates because it is more stable.** The −OH group attached to carbon 1 of the β-anomer is in an equatorial position on the chair, which is preferable to the axial position of the −OH group of the α-anomer. If 100% α-glucose (solid) is put in solution, its optical rotation starts to change as the α and β equilibrate. This effect is called **mutarotation.**

FIGURE 7-3.
Conversion of linear forms to cyclic α- and β-hemiacetal forms. Note the involvement of the anomeric carbon in generating α- and β-forms.

II. Key Reactions

A. Glycoside Formation

Glycosides are acetals that, like normal aldehydes, are generated from the reaction of the aldehyde with an alcohol and acid (Figure 7-4). The reaction starts when an acid protonates the hydroxy group of the hemiacetal. After water leaves, a resonance-stabilized carbocation forms, the only possible carbocation that is resonance stabilized by the oxygen. The nucleophilic alcohol then attacks the carbocation from the bottom or top face, giving both α- and β-forms. Once formed, the glycoside **does not undergo mutarotation under normal conditions,** because the compound is no longer a hemiacetal.

FIGURE 7-4.
Formation of a glycoside from a cyclic hemiacetal.

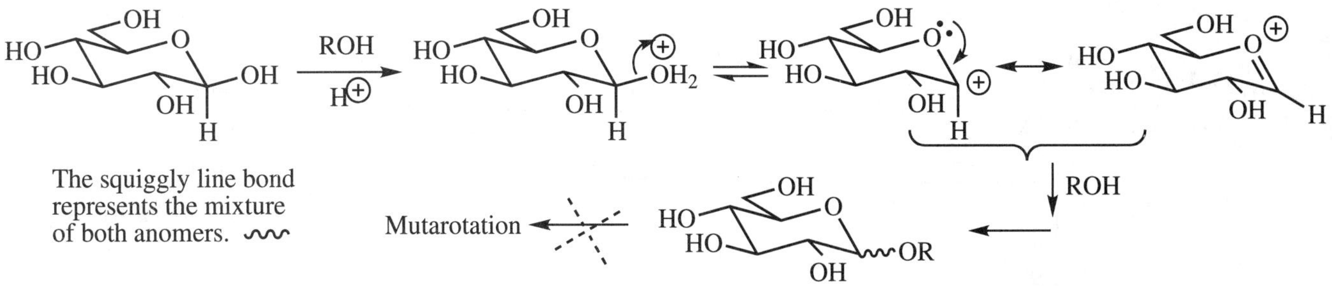

The squiggly line bond represents the mixture of both anomers. ∿

Mutarotation

Glycosides are also referred to as **nonreducing sugars.** If these compounds are tested with Tollens reagent (which identifies aldehydes by reduction of a silver salt to silver metal), they show a negative ("nonreducing") result. **In contrast, all monosaccharides are reducing sugars** and reduce Tollens reagent.

Glycosides are stable to base, but when exposed to acid and water, they revert to the sugar. The equilibrium shifts to the left, the sugar is produced, and the −OR

SECT. III
ORGANIC
CHEMISTRY
REVIEW
NOTES

585

group is released. This process is the same as the one by which polysaccharide linkages at the carbon 1 position are hydrolyzed by acid and water. The sugar then falls back into the equilibrium of α-, linear, and β-forms.

B. Ether Formation

FIGURE 7-5.

Ether formation, an example of exhaustive methylation of a glycoside.

It is easy to methylate the hydroxyl groups of a glycoside by a reaction similar to the Williamson synthesis reaction (see Chapter 5 III C of the Organic Chemistry Review Notes) called **exhaustive methylation.** The formation of ether (Figure 7-5) is an example of this process. Exhaustive methylation refers to the process in which all hydroxy groups are converted to methoxy groups.

FIGURE 7-5.
Ether formation, an example of exhaustive methylation of a glycoside.

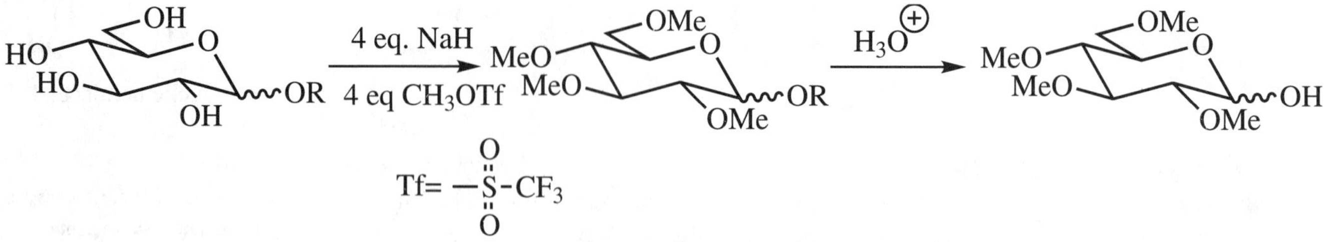

The reaction begins with interaction of the glycoside with a methoxy group bound to a leaving group (Tf, or trilate, is a good leaving group). Exhaustive methylation of the monosaccharide occurs. In the presence of acid, the alcohol group is lost and a polymethylated reducing sugar results.

FIGURE 7-6.

Formation of a polyacetylated sugar by reaction with acetic anhydride in the first step. Further reaction produces an ester by attack of an alcohol at carbon 1. Note the stereospecific formation of product.

C. Acetylation: Ester Formation

Treatment of a sugar with an excess of acetic anhydride and base (such as pyridine) results in polyacetylated sugar. The reaction, carried out at low temperatures, is stereospecific (e.g., α gives α-esters). These groups can be used for the **stereoselective formation of glycosides** (Figure 7-6).

FIGURE 7-6.
Formation of a polyacetylated sugar by reaction with acetic anhydride in the first step. Further reaction produces an ester by attack of an alcohol at carbon 1. Note the stereospecific formation of product.

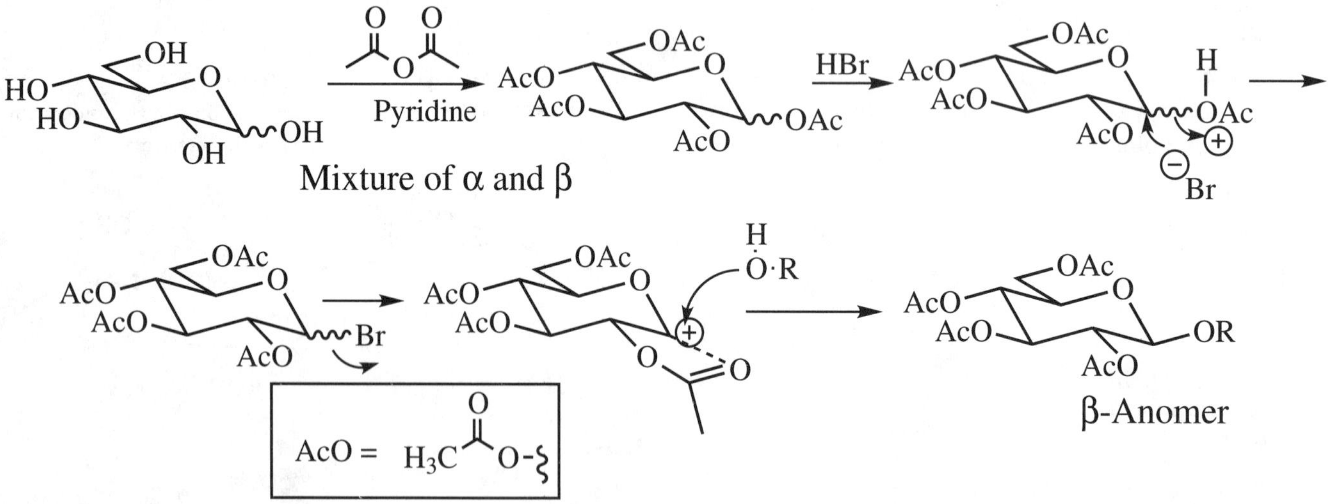

The reaction starts with the formation of a polyacetylated sugar by reacting a simple sugar with acetic anhydride and base. The acetic anhydride is the source of the acetyl groups that add on to the sugar −OH groups. Treatment of the polyacetylated sugar with HBr results in the displacement of the acetyl group on the anomeric carbon. The anomeric carbon is attacked because it is electrophilic. Bromine is a good leaving group and, under S_N1 conditions, Br leaves to give the carbocation. This carbocation is stabilized by the lone pair of electrons that the ring oxygen donates through resonance. The carbocation is further stabilized by the lone pair of electrons of the neighboring acetyl group oxygen. This interaction hinders the bottom face of the carbocation from attack, resulting in exclusive β-anomer formation because the alcohol can attack only from the top face of the carbocation.

III. Polysaccharides

Also known as glycans, polysaccharides consist of monosaccharides connected by glycosidic linkages of many varieties. These linkages can be **α or β** and they can occur between **various carbon hydroxyl groups.** For example, the hydroxyl group of carbon 1 of one sugar can bind to the hydroxyl group of carbons 3, 4, 6, and so on of another sugar.

In Figure 7-7, an α-1,4 bond connects the carbon 1 α-hydroxy group of one sugar unit to the carbon 4 hydroxy group of another. Also shown is a β-1,3 glycosidic linkage, which connects the carbon 1 β-hydroxy group of one sugar unit to the carbon 3 hydroxy group of another sugar.

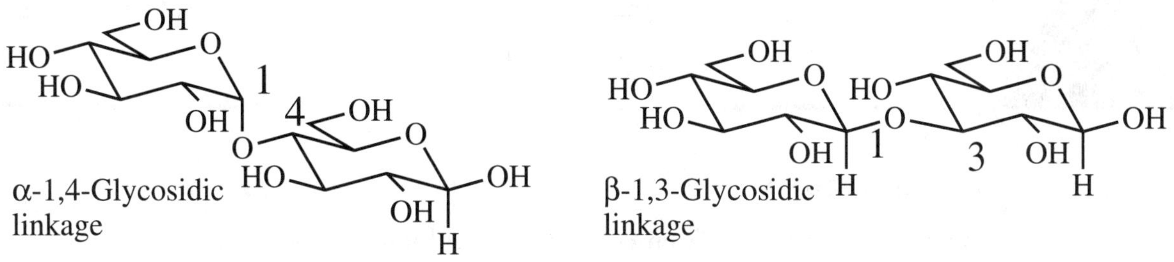

α-1,4-Glycosidic linkage

β-1,3-Glycosidic linkage

Starch consists of glucose molecules connected with α-1,4 bonds. These bonds can be hydrolyzed easily to yield monosaccharides. **Glycogen** is also a polysaccharide, but unlike starch, it is also highly branched. Some of the sugar units may contain 1,4 and 1,6 linkages, resulting in a branch point. **Cellulose** (fiber) is composed of β-linkages that cannot be broken down by human enzymes; it consists of D-glucose with β-linkages. This conformation is energetically favorable because the sugars are in chairs with the bulky groups in equatorial positions. **Glucosamines** are linkages of carbon 1 with an amine. Examples include nucleotides that link ribose and deoxyribose to bases (RNA, DNA).

FIGURE 7-7.

Glycosidic linkages. Do not memorize the structures of polysaccharides, but understand the concepts involved.

SECT. III
ORGANIC
CHEMISTRY
REVIEW
NOTES

587

Lipids

HIGH-YIELD TOPICS	**I.** Structure
	II. Fatty Acids and Triacylglycerols
	III. Steroids

I. Structure

Lipids may be isolated from cells and are soluble in nonpolar organic solvents (chloroform, diethyl ether). Lipids include compounds with different structures and functions: **fatty acids, triacylglycerols, terpenes, phospholipids, prostaglandins, waxes, and others.**

A variety of lipids are illustrated in Figure 8-1. At the far left of Figure 8-1 is the basic structure of a **fatty acid,** which contains a carboxyl group and a long hydrocarbon chain. Combining three fatty acids with the molecule glycerol yields the **triacylglyerol** (triglyceride). Note that triacylglycerols are esters of fatty acids.

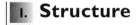

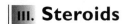

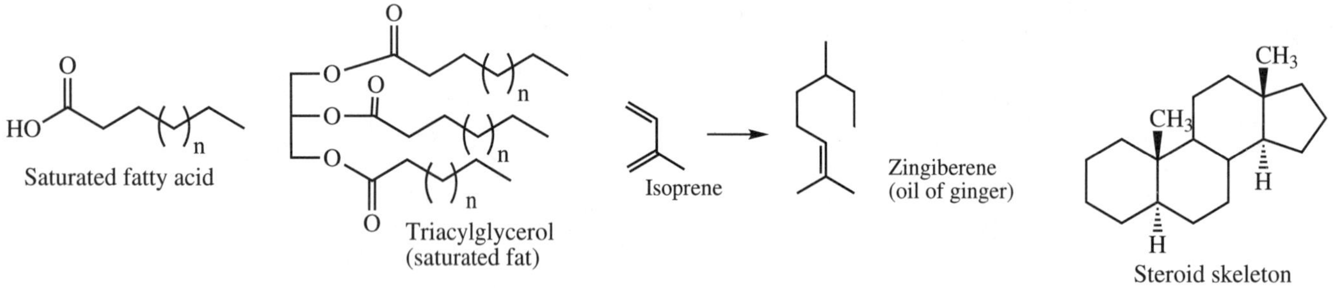

Saturated fatty acid · Triacylglycerol (saturated fat) · Isoprene · Zingiberene (oil of ginger) · Steroid skeleton

FIGURE 8-1.

Examples of lipids: fatty acid, triacylglycerol, isoprene, terpene, and steroid skeleton.

Also shown in Figure 8-1 is the structure of **isoprene,** one of nature's favorite building blocks. The five carbon-containing isoprene molecule is a diene (i.e., it has two double bonds). Isoprene units can be combined in various ways to create **terpenes,** molecules that have carbon skeletons consisting of isoprene units joined head to tail. Terpenes are found in the oils of many plants. The terpene compound in Figure 8-1 is an oil from the ginger plant.

Finally, isoprene units can be combined to create complex ring structures. Steroid compounds are made from a step-by-step combination of isoprene units; the **steroid skeleton** appears at far right in Figure 8-1.

II. Fatty Acids and Triacylglycerols

A. Structure

Fatty acids consist of a carboxylic acid group attached to a long hydrocarbon chain. If this chain does not contain multiple bonds, it is referred to as **saturated.** If the chain has multiple bonds, the structure is **unsaturated.** Triacylglycerols, esters of fatty acids and glycerol, are the form in which energy is converted for long-term storage in fat cells. Unsaturated fats (vegetable oils) are therefore triacylglycerols with unsaturated fatty acid hydrocarbon chains. The double bonds are all *cis* and generally are unconjugated. Saturated or animal fat has been implicated in the development of heart disease.

Fats are used for storage because they release more than twice the energy per gram when compared with carbohydrates. This difference is attributed to the larger number of C–H bonds in fats per molecule (and to less hydration per gram). At room temperature, saturated fats generally are solids (e.g., butter), whereas unsaturated fats typically are liquids (e.g., corn oil).

B. Saponification

Saponification involves the hydrolysis of the ester linkages of glycerides (Figure 8-2), which results in the release of the fatty acids as salts and glycerol. **The long-chain fatty acid salts are soaps.** This reaction is part of the process by which many soaps are made.

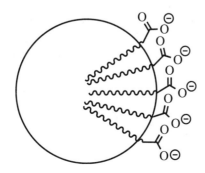

FIGURE 8-2.
Saponification of triglyceride to glycerol and fatty acid salts (soaps).

The long-chain fatty acids contain a hydrophilic (likes water) polar head group with a long hydrophobic (shies away from water) tail. At specific concentrations in aqueous solutions, these fatty acids lead to the formation of micelles.

Micelles are spherical structures made of hundreds of fatty acid soap molecules (Figure 8-3). Micelles are arranged with the polar group of the fatty acid soap molecules on the outside and the hydrophobic chains embedded on the inside, away from the water. The structure of the micelle explains how soap works. Micelles trap dirt and grease (which are hydrophobic) in the center of the micelle. The micelles are soluble in water, because the surface of the micelle contains the polar carboxylate group. Thus, micelles can wash away with water and carry dirt and grease with them.

FIGURE 8-3.
A micelle. Note the polar carboxylate groups on the outside and the nonpolar hydrocarbon chains on the inside of the structure.

SECT. III
ORGANIC
CHEMISTRY
REVIEW
NOTES

589

C. Phospholipids

Phospholipids are structures in which one of the fatty acid chains in a triacylglycerol is replaced by phosphoric acid. Therefore, phospholipids look much like triglycerides. Phosphoric acid (PO_4H_3) is a strong acid that has three free $-OH$ groups and a free oxygen atom that carries a negative charge. Phosphoric acid has the capacity to form a total of three ester bonds—an ester bond at each of its hydroxyl group sites. When an ester linkage occurs at two of its $-OH$ group sites, **phosphodiesters** form. (See Chapter 11 of the Organic Chemistry Review Notes to review how phosphoric acid can form ester linkages.)

When phosphoric acid is linked to the glyceride by forming an ester bond at one of its $-OH$ groups, the resulting molecule is **phosphatidic acid** (Figure 8-4). When phosphatidic acid is linked to an alcohol molecule, such as **choline,** by an ester linkage, the result is a **phosphodiester linkage** and a molecule known as **phosphatidyl choline.**

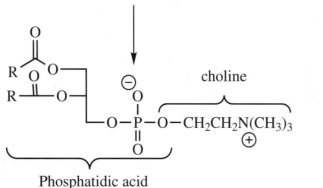

Phosphoric acid

choline

○ charged polar head group

ww hydrophobic chain

Phosphatidic acid

lipid bilayer

FIGURE 8-4.

Phosphatidic acid and choline combine to form phosphatidyl choline, an important phospholipid (left). The lipid bilayer (right) is formed by phospholipids.

The phospholipid found in cell membranes is phosphatidyl choline. The structure of this molecule (see Figure 8-4) is important because the choline/phosphate part is polar and the fatty acid chains are nonpolar. Thus, these compounds have two hydrophobic chains and a polar head group with a positive (amine) and a negative charge (phosphorus). This **"amphoteric"** nature allows for the formation of micelles and the formation of a **lipid bilayer** (see Figure 8-4), which is a critical part of cell membranes.

FIGURE 8-5.

The steroid skeleton (left), and two important steroids, cholesterol and progesterone (right).

III. Steroids

These compounds include a wide range of molecules that are essential to living organisms: **cholesterol, the sex hormones (the estrogens, testosterone, progesterone), adrenal cortex hormones, and all of their metabolites** (Figure 8-5).

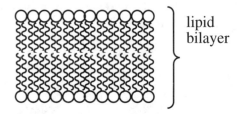

Cholesterol

Progesterone

Steroids are based on a skeleton with four basic rings (labeled A–D in Figure 8-5). For most steroids, the junctions between rings B,C and C,D are *trans* to each other. They are termed 5α or β because the type of ring junction is determined by the stereochemistry of the carbon 5 position. Do not memorize these structures; instead, understand that **the diversity of steroid compounds is based on a variety of possible ring junctions and different substituents on the basic steroid skeleton.**

Steroid hormones work by passing through cell membranes to bind to intracellular receptors of the cell. Binding initiates a cascade of chemical processes, usually within the nucleus of the cell. The reactions of steroids are as varied as the different types of structures. The functional groups attached to the steroid skeleton can undergo all of the reactions reviewed in the previous chapters.

SECT. III
ORGANIC
CHEMISTRY
REVIEW
NOTES

591

Amines

Amines

HIGH-YIELD TOPICS	**I.** Structure and Physical Characteristics
	II. Basicity
	III. Reactions

I. Structure and Physical Characteristics

The most important characteristic of amines is the lone pair of electrons. The nitrogen of amines is sp³ hybridized and the lone pair occupies one of the sp³ hybridized orbitals. The result is a **trigonal pyramidal** structure with the substituents at the base of the pyramid (Figure 9-1).

FIGURE 9-1.
The sp³ hybridized structure of amines. The lone pair of electrons occupying one of the orbitals results in a trigonal pyramidal structure. Note also the interconversion through a transition state (see text for explanation).

With four different substituents (one being the lone pair of electrons), it would seem that two separate enantiomers of amines could occur. A rapid **interconversion** takes place, however, and the energy required for this conversion is relatively low. Interconversion occurs readily at low temperatures, which means that the enantiomers cannot be resolved. The process of interconversion, **through an sp² hybridized transition state,** is depicted in Figure 9-1.

The melting and boiling points of amines are high because of hydrogen bonding. The hydrogen bonding patterns are similar to the hydrogen bonding pattern seen in water and alcohols. The effects of branching and chain length are the same as for alkanes (see Chapter 2 of the Organic Chemistry Review Notes).

II. Basicity

A. Overview

Bases are proton acceptors and electron donors. **Amines are basic because they can donate the lone pair of electrons to protons.** The basicity constant defines base strength (Figure 9-2). **A larger base constant indicates that more of the**

species exist in the protonated form, resulting in a better base; $pK_b = -\log K_b$, so the smaller the pK_b value, the stronger the base.

$$RNH_2 + HOH \rightleftharpoons \overset{\oplus}{R}NH_3 + \overset{\ominus}{O}H \qquad K_b = \frac{[\overset{\oplus}{R}NH_3][\overset{\ominus}{O}H]}{[RNH_2]}$$

FIGURE 9-2.
Relationship for K_b.

Aryl amines tend to be weaker bases. In the nonprotonated state, this molecule is stabilized by resonance with the benzene ring. When the lone pair is donated to a proton, however, it can no longer delocalize through the benzene ring and the stability of delocalization is lost (Figure 9-3).

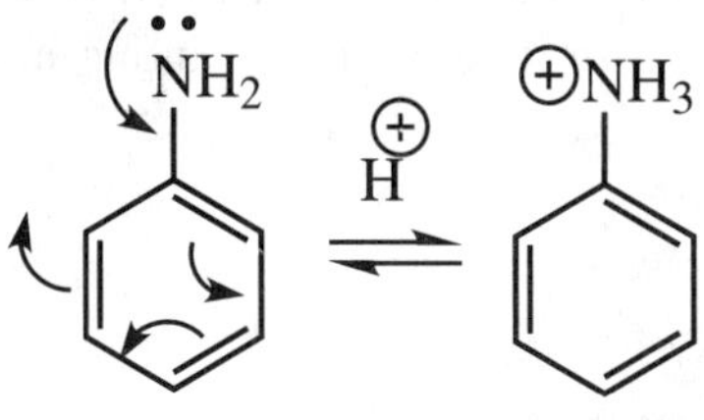

no delocalization

FIGURE 9-3.
When nonprotonated, the aryl amine is stabilized by resonance. When protonated, the lone pair is donated to the proton and delocalization is lost.

The same type of effect decreases the basicity of amide nitrogens. The nitrogens are involved in delocalization through the carbonyl. If protonation occurred, the stabilizing resonance interaction would not occur (Figure 9-4). Thus, the amide nitrogen is not basic. In actuality, when reacted with acids, the carbonyl oxygen is protonated because of the higher electron density about the oxygen.

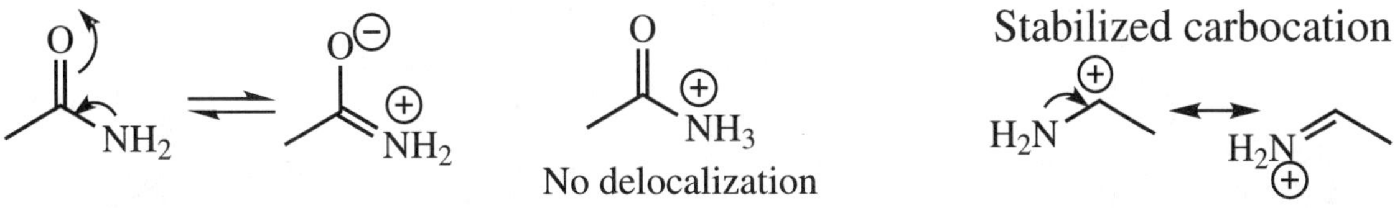

No delocalization

Stabilized carbocation

Also because of its basicity and the lone pair, **nitrogen atoms are able to stabilize adjacent carbocations,** making them easier to form. The lone pair occupies an orbital in an sp^3 hybridized nitrogen, which lines up with the empty p orbital of the adjacent carbocation and donates electrons to the C–N bond to help **spread out the charge.**

FIGURE 9-4.
Resonance forms associated with the amide bond (left). Protonation of the amine group and loss of delocalization (center). Stabilization of carbocations by nitrogen (right).

B. Governing Factors

The more highly substituted the amine with electron-releasing alkyl groups, the more basic the amine (Figure 9-5). The electron-releasing groups can stabilize the positive charge of the substituted ammonium ion. Thus, trimethylamine is a stronger base than ammonia. It is generally true that **aromatic amines are weaker bases than ammonia, given the resonance stability of aromatic compounds.**

$$(CH_3)_3N > (CH_3)_2NH > CH_3NH_2 > NH_3$$

FIGURE 9-5.
Decreasing order of base strength based on substitution of electron-releasing groups.

Hybridization also affects basicity. Consider piperidine and pyridine (Figure 9-6). Both structures possess a lone pair of electrons on the nitrogen, although the electrons in piperidine are in an sp^3 orbital, whereas those in pyridine occupy an sp^2 orbital. The increased s character of the sp^2 orbital places the electrons closer to the

SECT. III
ORGANIC
CHEMISTRY
REVIEW
NOTES

593

nucleus and therefore they are held more tightly by the nitrogen. Thus, piperidine is a stronger base because its electrons are more "available" for proton acceptance.

FIGURE 9-6.
Pyridine and piperidine. Piperidine is the stronger base because its electrons are more available for proton "acceptance."

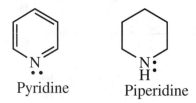

Pyridine   Piperidine

When reacted with acids, followed by repeated alkylation, amines form quaternary ammonium salts, which have the formula $R_4N^+X^-$ (X is a halogen ion). For example, if the amine RNH_2 reacts with acid (RX), R_2NH is produced. Continued alkylation with acid (RX) produces R_3N, resulting finally in the quaternary ammonium salt $R_4N^+X^-$.

III. Reactions

A. Nucleophilic Attack by Amines

Recall that in the attack of electrophiles by amines, it is the **lone pair of electrons that allows the amine to act as a nucleophile. Ammonia (with no substituents) and primary amines make the best nucleophiles because of the lack of steric hindrance.** As the level of substitution increases, the lone pair of electrons is less able to reach the electrophile to form a bond, and the amine acts more as a base than a nucleophile. As discussed previously (see Chapter 6 of the Organic Chemistry Review Notes), amines can undergo an S_N2-type attack of electrophiles and an attack of carbonyls to form imines and amides (Figure 9-7).

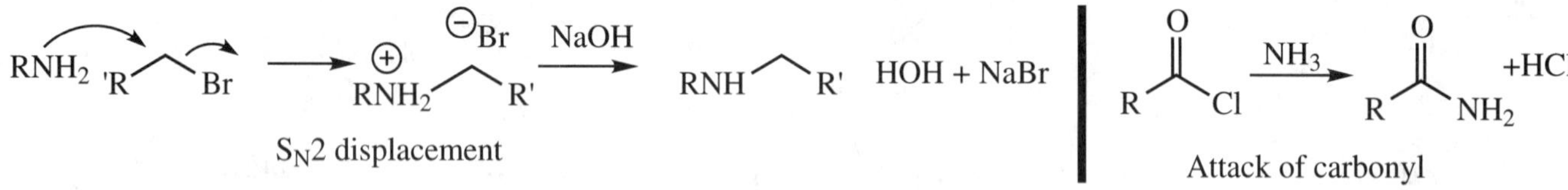

FIGURE 9-7.
Nucleophilic attack by amines. S_N2-type attack with good leaving group (left); attack of a carbonyl to form an amide (right).

B. Preparation of Amines: Reduction

As detailed in Chapter 6 of the Organic Chemistry Review Notes, the **reduction of nitriles and amides by reducing agents such as LAH results in the corresponding amines. Imines can also be reduced to amines.** This process is called **reductive amination.** Alkyl azides ($R–N_3$) can also be reduced, using LAH, to yield the amine (RNH_2).

Amino Acids and Peptides

I.	General Structure of Amino Acids
II.	Classification of Amino Acids
III.	Amino Acids as Dipolar Ions
IV.	Formation of Peptide Amide Bonds
V.	Secondary and Tertiary Structure
VI.	Enzyme Action

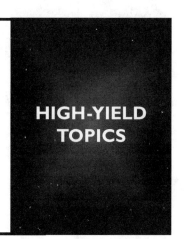

HIGH-YIELD TOPICS

I. General Structure of Amino Acids

Of the different types of biopolymers (polysaccharides, nucleic acids, and proteins), proteins have the most diverse functions. They can act as **hormones,** which bring about a specific physiologic response; enzymes that catalyze chemical reactions; and **structural elements** within our body (bones, skin, muscle); and they can be involved in transport, regulation, and a host of other processes. **Proteins are polymers of amino acid units.** Proteins can have hundreds of amino acids linked linearly by amide bonds to form complex three-dimensional structures. **Peptides,** which are smaller polymers of amino acids, often act as hormones. The specific three-dimensional structure of peptides allows for recognition of the hormone by a **receptor.** Thus, the structure and physical characteristics of the proteins and peptides are determined by the structural and physical characteristics of the basic amino acid building blocks.

Twenty naturally occurring α-amino acids are used by cells to synthesize peptides and proteins (Figure 10-1). **The primary structure of a protein is the specific linkage sequence of these amino acids.** This primary structure must be intact for the protein to function normally. A specific primary structure allows interaction of the individual amino acids in the protein such that the protein may fold in a specific manner to give rise to secondary and tertiary structure.

The amino acids differ from one another on the basis of the R-group side chain structure, which is attached to the basic amino acid skeleton. In Figure 10-1, note that each of the R-groups attaches to the amino acid skeleton to generate the 20 different naturally occurring L-amino acids.

The α-amino acids are named because of the NH_2 group attached to the α-carbon of the carboxylic acid. Like carbohydrates, they are also given the D or L

SECT. III
ORGANIC
CHEMISTRY
REVIEW
NOTES

595

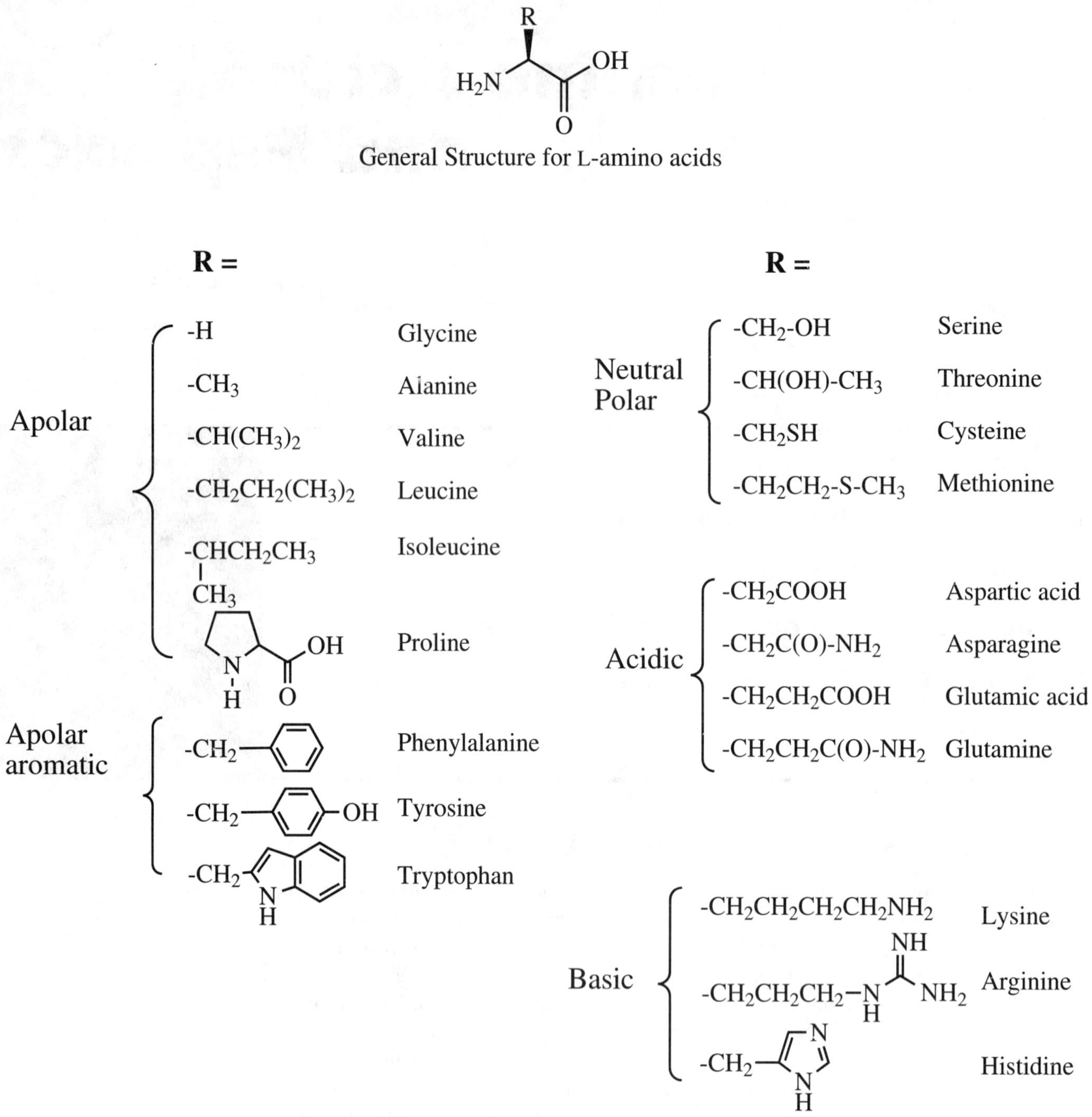

$$\text{General Structure for L-amino acids}$$

General Structure for L-amino acids

R =

Apolar
- -H — Glycine
- -CH$_3$ — Aianine
- -CH(CH$_3$)$_2$ — Valine
- -CH$_2$CH$_2$(CH$_3$)$_2$ — Leucine
- -CHCH$_2$CH$_3$ | CH$_3$ — Isoleucine
- Proline

Apolar aromatic
- -CH$_2$—⬡ — Phenylalanine
- -CH$_2$—⬡—OH — Tyrosine
- -CH$_2$— (indole) — Tryptophan

R =

Neutral Polar
- -CH$_2$-OH — Serine
- -CH(OH)-CH$_3$ — Threonine
- -CH$_2$SH — Cysteine
- -CH$_2$CH$_2$-S-CH$_3$ — Methionine

Acidic
- -CH$_2$COOH — Aspartic acid
- -CH$_2$C(O)-NH$_2$ — Asparagine
- -CH$_2$CH$_2$COOH — Glutamic acid
- -CH$_2$CH$_2$C(O)-NH$_2$ — Glutamine

Basic
- -CH$_2$CH$_2$CH$_2$CH$_2$NH$_2$ — Lysine
- -CH$_2$CH$_2$CH$_2$-N(H)-C(NH)-NH$_2$ — Arginine
- -CH$_2$— (imidazole) — Histidine

FIGURE 10-1.
The 20 α-amino acids classified by R-group. Do not memorize the structures of the amino acids or the side chains (R-groups), but be familiar with the classification groups and the side chain types.

designation (L-amino acids have the amino group on the left of a Fischer projection, D-amino acids have the amino group on the right) [Figure 10-2]. Also, as with sugars, whether an amino acid is characterized as D or L says nothing about the direction it will rotate plane-polarized light (d or l).

In most cases, D-amino acids are R (absolute configuration) and L-amino acids are S. Remember that this designation depends on the side chain priority. Amino acids are similar to sugars in that D- and L-forms of a particular amino acid are enantiomers. The exceptions to this rule include threonine and isoleucine, which contain a chiral center on the side chain, making the D- and L-forms diastereomers. Glycine has no chiral center at the α-carbon so there are no D- or L-forms. In most naturally occurring proteins, L-amino acids predominate.

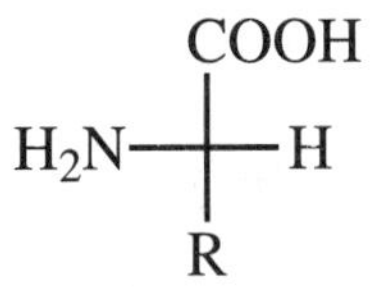

$$\text{COOH}$$
$$H_2N{-}\!\!\!\!\underset{R}{\overset{|}{\rule{0pt}{1.2em}}}\!\!\!\!{-}H$$

FIGURE 10-2.
Fischer projection of the amino acid skeleton. Note the amino group on the left, and the L-amino acid designation.

II. Classification of Amino Acids

The amino acids are classified into five different groups according to the reactivity and characteristics of the side chains (see Figure 10-1).

A. Apolar

These amino acids, with the exception of glycine, contain hydrophobic side chains and are highly inert. They have a profound effect on protein conformation because they tend to aggregate (owing to van der Waals interactions) and shy away from water. Thus, they are commonly found on the interior of proteins. Proline has a unique cyclic **imino** group and is found in regions of the amino acid chain where a turn occurs.

B. Apolar Aromatic

These side chains are also hydrophobic and relatively inert, tending to aggregate because of the van der Waals interactions. The tyrosine side chain contains a slightly acidic phenolic hydroxy group that is often involved in **hydrogen bonding.** Tryptophan contains the highly hydrophobic indole ring in which the lone pair of electrons of the nitrogen contributes to the aromatic system to give 10 π electrons [remember the formula $(4n + 2)$ π electrons].

C. Neutral Polar

These side chains are uncharged at physiologic pH, but they can also be somewhat reactive. The hydroxy group of serine is often used as **a nucleophile** in enzyme active sites. The hydroxyl group of serine can participate in hydrogen bonds. The thiol group of cysteine is also a nucleophile, but it plays a more important role in **disulfide linkages.** On treatment with a mild oxidant, disulfide linkages (cystine) can form from two cysteines with side chains in close proximity. The sulfur is a large polarizable (fluffy) atom, and thus it is able to deprotonate more readily than oxygen (thiol is a better acid than hydroxy), allowing for the easy oxidative coupling of the two atoms. Disulfide bonds (Figure 10-3) can form in proteins between cysteine molecules and often help stabilize tertiary structure (see subsequent discussion). Threonine and methionine also are polar but they are far less reactive.

FIGURE 10-3.
Disulfide linkage formation.

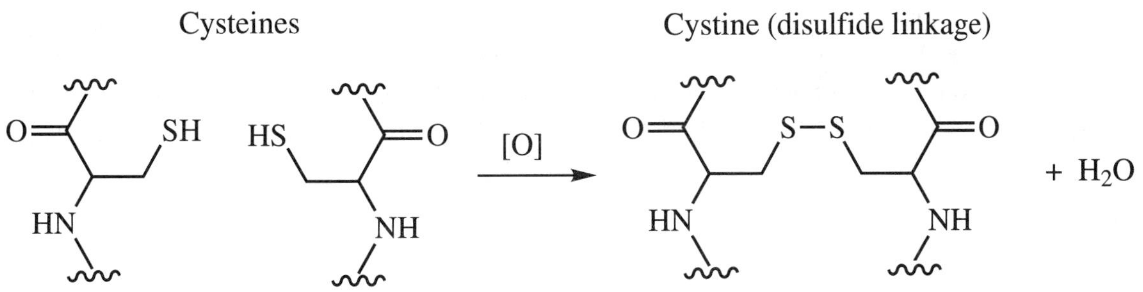

Cysteines
Cystine (disulfide linkage)

$+ H_2O$

D. Acidic Side Chains

The side chains of glutamic acid and aspartic acid are generally deprotonated at physiologic pH and thus carry a negative charge. **They often play a large role in the**

SECT. III
ORGANIC
CHEMISTRY
REVIEW
NOTES

597

active site of enzymes. Remember that these amino acids are acidic. They may act as proton donators (protonated form) or as proton acceptors (deprotonated form). Glutamine and asparagine are not truly acidic, but are placed in this group because they are derivatives of glutamic and aspartic acids; they tend to be good hydrogen bond donors and acceptors.

E. Basic Side Chains

The side chains of these amino acids are also frequently involved in the active site of enzymes. The side chain of arginine **(guanidine group)** is basic. At physiologic pH, this group is always protonated (Figure 10-4). The aromatic side chain of histidine has an **imidazole ring** (see Figure 10-4), which can act as an acid or base and is a good nucleophile. Note that both side chain functions shown in Figure 10-4 can be stabilized by resonance on protonation by an acid.

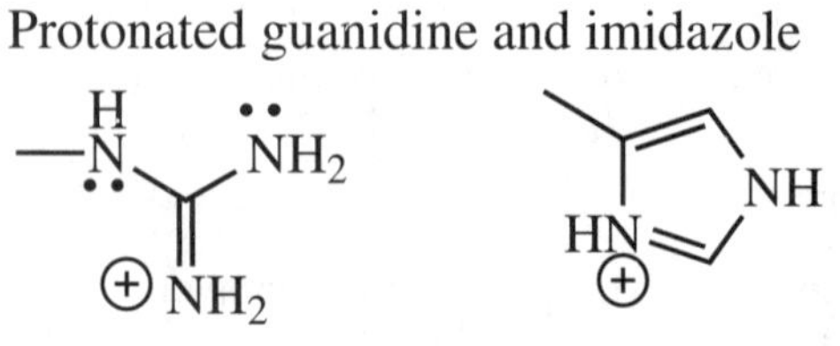

FIGURE 10-4.
Side chain group guanidine (arginine) at left; side chain group imidazole (histidine) at right. Note the possible resonance for each of these important basic side chain groups.

Protonated guanidine and imidazole

III. Amino Acids as Dipolar Ions

Amino acids in the dry solid state exist as **zwitterions or dipolar ions,** which means the amino group is protonated and the carboxyl group is deprotonated (NH_3+, COO^- on the same molecule). In solution, amino acids exist in equilibrium with protonated and deprotonated states. It is this characteristic of amino acids and their side chains that gives them their unique functional characteristics in peptides and proteins.

Whether or not the amino group, carboxyl group, and side chain group are protonated depends on the pH of the solution. **The pK_a of the carboxyl group is about 2.3. The pK_a of the amino group is generally about 9.7.** Therefore, at a pH of 2.3, about one half of the carboxyl groups of an amino acid are protonated. One would expect all of the amino groups to be fully protonated at this low pH. At pH 9.7, one half of the amino groups are deprotonated. One would expect all of the carboxyl groups to be deprotonated at this relatively high pH.

The amino acid alanine (Figure 10-5) can exist in a cationic, dipolar, or anionic state, depending on the pH of the solution. In acidic solution (pH < 2), alanine is in a cationic state because its carboxyl group is protonated and its amino group is protonated and carries a positive charge. As the pH of the solution containing alanine increases with the addition of base, the carboxyl group begins to deprotonate. By pH 2.3, one half of the carboxyl groups are deprotonated, resulting in a dipolar ion (see Figure 10-5, center). As the pH is further raised by adding more base, the amino group deprotonates next because of its higher pK_a. The deprotonation of the amino group results in alanine becoming an anion.

FIGURE 10-5.
Addition of base to a fully protonated amino acid (alanine). Note that in acidic solutions, the amino acid is fully protonated. As the pH is raised by adding base, deprotonation of the carboxyl group occurs first, producing the dipolar ion. Further deprotonation of the amino group occurs at higher pH.

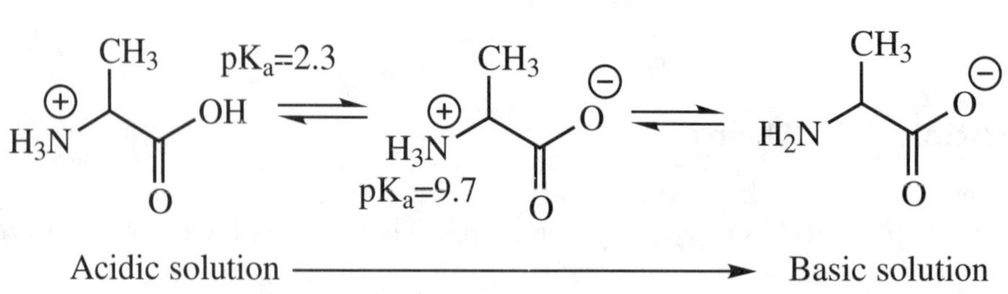

Acidic solution ⟶ Basic solution

A. Isoelectric Point

The isoelectric point is the pH at which an amino acid does not migrate in an electric field. It typically occurs where **the concentration of the dipolar ion is the greatest.** In Figure 10-5, the isoelectric point is the average of the two pK_a values, or 6.0. Remember that according to the Henderson-Hasselbalch equation (see Chapter 1 of the Organic Chemistry Review Notes), when the pH of a solution is equal to the pK_a of an acidic proton, half of the molecules are protonated and half are deprotonated.

B. Titration

By placing an amino acid solution in aqueous acid solution (pH 0), adding base, and making a plot of pH versus equivalents of base added, one obtains a graph similar to that for lysine in Figure 10-6. Lysine has a carboxyl and amino group like all amino acids, but it also has a basic side chain group containing a $-NH_2$ group. This $-NH_2$ group can be protonated and deprotonated.

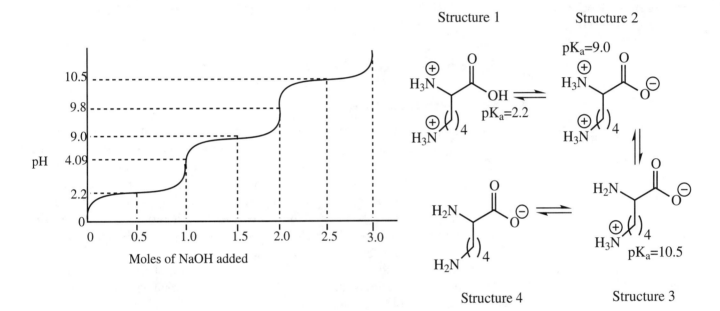

Structure 1   Structure 2

Structure 4   Structure 3

The first structure in Figure 10-6 shows lysine fully protonated. At pH 0, lysine exists as a dication because both the amino group and basic side chain NH_3 group are protonated. All the molecules look like structure 1. As base is added, the carboxyl group becomes deprotonated. After one full equivalent of base is added (1 mole of NaOH), all of the carboxyl groups are deprotonated and all lysine molecules look like structure 2. Notice that a rapid rise in pH has occurred. As more base is added, the α-amino group is deprotonated, resulting in the dipolar ion. By the time a full second equivalent of base has been added, the lysine molecules look like structure 3. As even more base is added, the side chain amine group is deprotonated, leading to the anionic form of lysine in structure 4. Lysine would be expected to be completely in a form similar to structure 4 when a total of three equivalents (3 moles of NaOH) of base are added.

The pK_a of the carboxyl group is found at the center of the first plateau of the graph, at about pH 2.3. The pK_a of the α-amino group is at the center of the second plateau of Figure 10-6, at about pH 9.7. By looking at the pH of the third plateau, one can predict the pK_a of the side chain amine group to be about 10.5. Remember that at each pK_a, about one half of the molecules are deprotonated for the group under consideration.

FIGURE 10-6.

Titration curve for the amino acid lysine. The fully protonated form deprotonates first at its carboxyl group, followed by deprotonation of its amino group and side chain basic group. Structures are shown for each step of deprotonation.

SECT. III
ORGANIC
CHEMISTRY
REVIEW
NOTES

599

IV. Formation of Peptide Amide Bonds

Different ways to make amide bonds have been discussed previously. In general, an amine is used to attack a carboxylic acid derivative that has a good leaving group, and an amide is formed. To synthesize peptides, it is often easiest to couple amino acid fragments. The carboxylic acid of one residue is activated for attack (converted to an activated carboxylic acid derivative) and the amine of the other residue is used to attack it. To ensure that the right connections take place, **protecting groups** are linked to reactive groups that are not meant to participate in the formation of amide bonds. Without this step, products other than the desired connection are possible.

Several types of protecting groups are available, including *tert*-butyl-based groups and benzyl-based groups (Figure 10-7).

FIGURE 10-7.
Protecting groups used to help form desired peptide bonds. Do not memorize these structures, but understand why they may be useful.

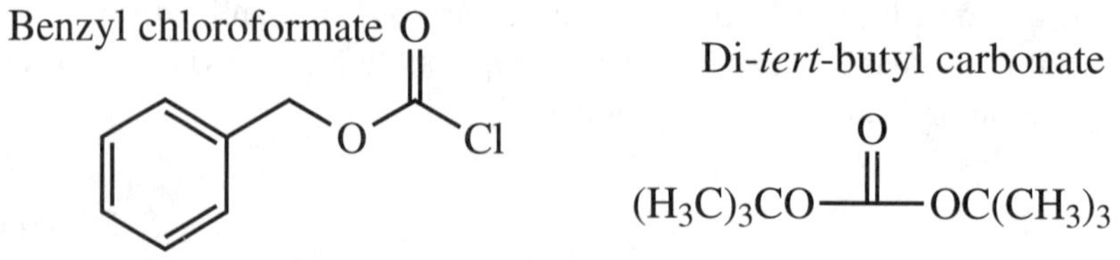

Benzyl chloroformate

Di-*tert*-butyl carbonate

V. Secondary and Tertiary Structure

A. Secondary Structure

Secondary structure is dictated by the *trans* nature of the amide bond and by hydrogen bonding along the amide-bonded main chain of the peptide or protein. Two examples are the β-pleated sheet and α-helix. Recall that through resonance, the C–N bond of an amide assumes an almost double bond-like character. Rotation about this C–N bond is more restricted than that about a normal C–N single bond. Just like alkenes, **the *trans* structure is more favored than the *cis* structure because of the higher eclipsing strain of the *cis* structure** (Figure 10-8). When the amino acid chain is spread out, the *trans* nature of the amide bonds makes the side chains alternate in terms of the side of the chain from which they protrude. The **repeat distance** is the distance between two residues appearing on the same side of the chain; in linear form, it is approximately 7.2 Å.

1. Turns

The peptide chains are not in straight lines. In many cases, the chains have up to 180° changes in direction, which are stabilized by hydrogen bonds between the proton of N–H and the oxygen of the carbonyl. The inclusion of **proline** in a peptide chain allows for *cis* amide bonds to form in the residue before it. Thus, proline is often found in regions where the turns occur. **Glycine** is also found in turn structures because it does not have a side chain to sterically hinder a turn structure from forming around it.

FIGURE 10-8.
The *trans* form of the amide bond (left) and the repeat distance (right).

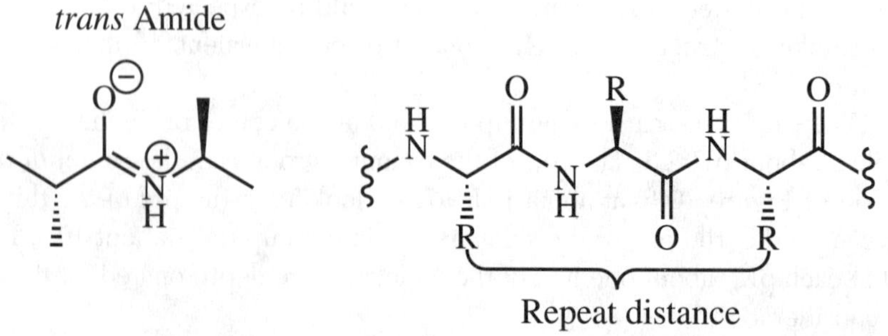

trans Amide

Repeat distance

2. β-Sheets

Antiparallel β-sheets often occur between two or more linear chains that are in close proximity. The term **antiparallel** is applied because the adjacent chains of a β-sheet run in opposite directions. **These chains are held together by hydrogen bonding** between hydrogen on nitrogen and the carbonyl oxygen. These sheets are also pleated (like a room divider) to avoid steric interactions between the side chain groups (Figure 10-9). Small to medium-sized R groups can be accommodated inside the sheet. Silk is a common example of a β-sheet structure.

3. α-Helix

The structure shown in Figure 10-9 is a **right-handed helix stabilized by hydrogen bonding of the amide hydrogens and carbonyl oxygens (dotted lines).** Note the 3.6 amino acids per turn and a rise of 5.4 Å per turn. Each amide has a hydrogen bond to another amide three residues above and below. The repeat distance is much shorter (1.5 Å) than the β-sheet because the distance along the axis of the helix is used for measurement. In this structure, the side chain groups extend out of the helix, so steric interaction between the groups is minimal.

FIGURE 10-9.
Secondary structure: the β-pleated sheet and α-helix. Dotted lines indicate hydrogen bonding.

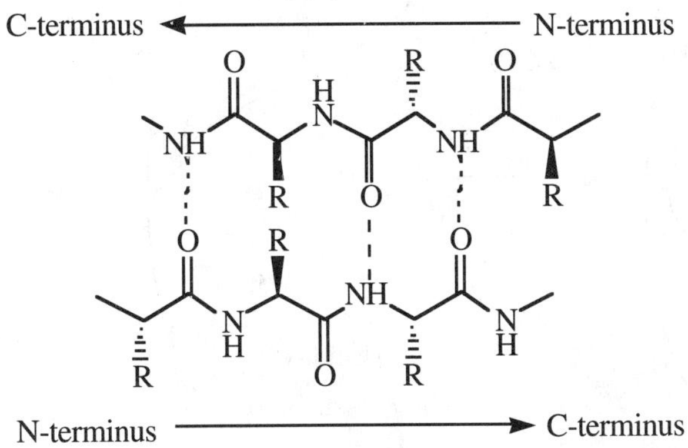

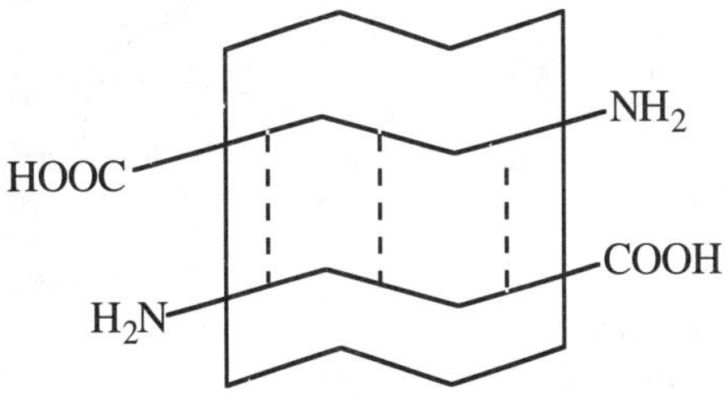

β-Antiparallel pleated sheet

α-Helix

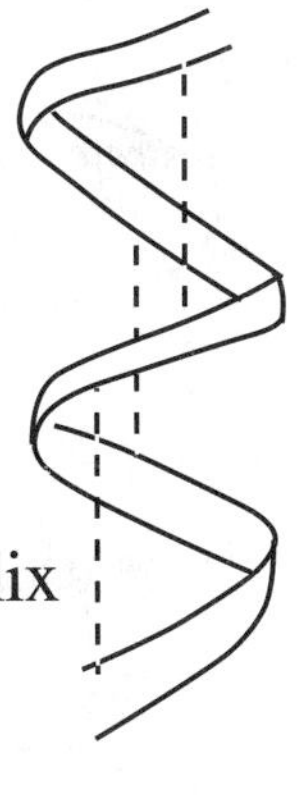

B. Tertiary Structure

Tertiary structure is the arrangement of secondary structure into a specific three-dimensional form caused by the interactions between side chains that stick out of the secondary structure. These folding processes do not occur randomly. Often, if certain residues are mutated (replaced by others or left out), the correct structure does not form and the function of the protein is destroyed.

The arrangement of these globular proteins is dictated by several factors:

1. Residues with nonpolar hydrophobic side chains are often found in the interior of the protein away from water.

2. Polar charged side chains are often found near the surface of globular proteins and are in contact with the aqueous environment. When in the interior, they may form salt bridges (protonated amine forming salt with deprotonated carboxyl) to stabilize tertiary structure.

3. Polar uncharged side chains can be found on the inside or near the surface. When in the interior, they often form hydrogen bonds with other functional groups to help stabilize tertiary structure.

SECT. III
ORGANIC
CHEMISTRY
REVIEW
NOTES

601

Tertiary structure is held together by a variety of interactions of varying strength. These include:

1. Hydrophobic interactions
2. Hydrophilic interactions
3. Hydrogen bonds
4. Disulfide linkages
5. Van der Waals forces

Individually, some of these interactions are weak. When thousands of these interactions occur together, however, a large protein can be held together.

VI. Enzyme Action

The enzyme **active site** is a catalytic cavity inside the enzyme where reactions, such as hydrolysis of amide bonds (Figure 10-10), can occur.

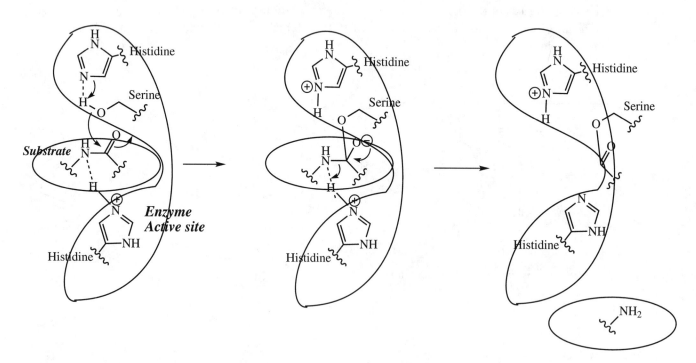

FIGURE 10-10.

Enzyme action.

First, the substrate enters the catalytic cavity and is properly aligned. In this hypothetical active site in Figure 10-10, a neutral histamine (basic imidazole group) partially deprotonates a nearby serine hydroxy side chain. This hydroxy group can attack the correctly positioned carbonyl, and the tetrahedral intermediate is formed. The C–N bond is cleaved as the nitrogen accepts a proton from another nearby protonated histidine (converting the histidine side chain to a neutral basic imidazole). In subsequent steps, a similar mechanism featuring the attack of water on the carbonyl carbon is used to release the other half of the cleaved amide bond and to restore the serine hydroxy side chain. The enzyme is ready to accept a new substrate molecule.

Remember: enzymes are catalysts. They lower the activation energy of a process by placing all of the reactive groups in the correct orientations and helping the reaction along with acidic and basic groups. In some cases, they stabilize (bind to effectively) the transition state of the reaction.

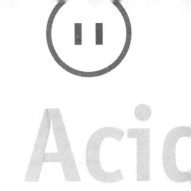

Phosphoric Acid

I. Structure and Physical Characteristics	**HIGH-YIELD**
II. Phosphate in Important Biologic Molecules	**TOPICS**

I. Structure and Physical Characteristics

Phosphoric acid is a triprotic acid that plays a key role in several biologically important molecules. It has three acidic hydrogens with pK_a of 2.2, 7.2, and 12.2, respectively. On deprotonation, the negative charge can delocalize and is stabilized. These compounds are more acidic than carboxylic acids but less acidic than sulfonic acids. They are anionic in neutral aqueous solutions, as would be expected from their pK_a values.

Mono-, di- and triesters of phosphoric acid can form when the acid is reacted with an alcohol (Figure 11-1). The mono- and di- linked phosphoric esters are highly acidic because of their remaining hydroxy groups. This acidity gives them stability in aqueous base because the negative charges on the oxygens repel the negatively charged nucleophile (^-OH).

When two or more phosphoric acid molecules link, phosphoric anhydrides form. The structure of a phosphoric anhydride is shown in Figure 11-1.

FIGURE 11-1.
Formation of phosphoric acid esters and the structure of phosphoric anhydride.

II. Phosphate in Important Biologic Molecules

For biologically important molecules, ester linkages are formed with hydroxy groups that allow the molecules to carry out their specific functions. For example, deoxyribonucleic acid (DNA) and ribonucleic acid (RNA) ribose sugars are linked together through **phosphodiester bonds** connecting the C5′ and C3′ hydroxy groups (Figure 11-2). This phosphodiester linkage forms the sugar-phosphate backbone of RNA and DNA.

SECT. III
ORGANIC
CHEMISTRY
REVIEW
NOTES

603

FIGURE 11-2.

Phosphodiester linkage. Structure of ribonucleic acid (RNA), in which two ribose sugars are linked together by a phosphate. Note that the ester is formed from the phosphoric acid and two sugar molecules.

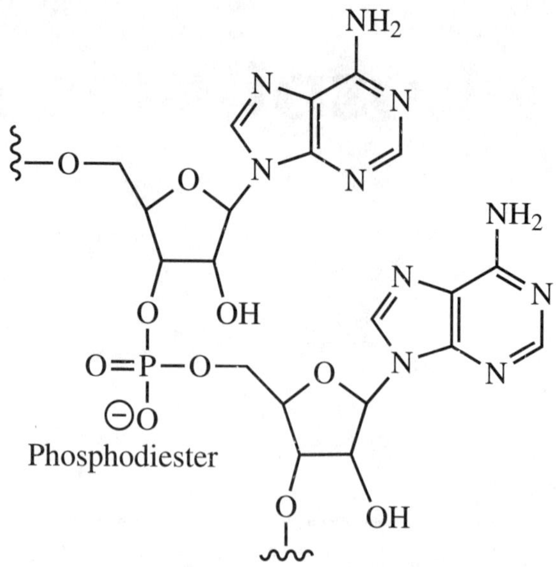

Phospholipids are also the result of phosphodiester linkages between glycerol and a small alcohol, such as choline (see Chapter 8 of the Organic Chemistry Review Notes). The charged regions of phosphatidyl choline (nitrogen and the phosphoric ester), along with the long hydrophobic tail, enable these molecules to act as boundaries in cellular systems.

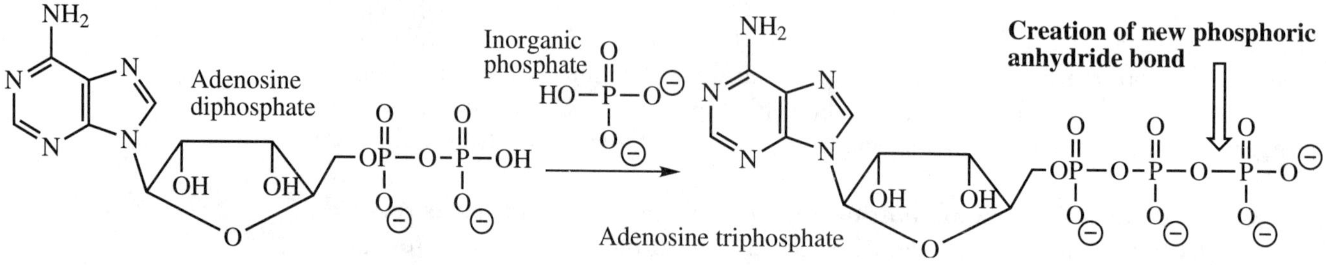

FIGURE 11-3.

Synthesis of adenosine triphosphate (ATP) from adenosine diphosphate (ADP) and inorganic phosphate. Creation of a new phosphoric anhydride bond that "stores" energy.

Phosphoric anhydrides, found in adenosine diphosphate (ADP) and adenosine triphosphate (ATP) [Figure 11-3], also play an important role in **energy storage in biologic systems.** Energy from the metabolism of glucose is **"stored"** through the chemical transformation of ADP to ATP through an endothermic reaction. This transformation creates a new **phosphoric anhydride bond.** When the energy is needed, the ATP is hydrolyzed enzymatically to yield ADP and energy that were "stored" in the bond. The hydrolysis of the triphosphate to form the diphosphate is highly exothermic. Enzymes act as catalysts, and are necessary to lower the activation energy so that hydrolysis can occur. This action results in the release of the energy stored in this bond.

Separation, Purification, and Characterization

I. Separation and Purification Techniques

II. Characterization: Infrared (IR) and Nuclear Magnetic Resonance (NMR) Spectroscopy

Clear understanding of the various separation and characterization techniques is essential, not only in terms of their performance, but also the principles behind them.

I. Separation and Purification Techniques

Purification is necessary because reactions often produce undesired side products along with the desired product. Several purification techniques are available.

A. Extraction

Extractions are used to separate compounds that have different solubilities in various solvents. Frequently, the compounds to be extracted are chemically modified to be soluble in aqueous solution or an organic solvent. For example, in a liquid-liquid extraction, two immiscible liquids, such as an aqueous solution and an organic solvent (chloroform, ethyl acetate), are often used to perform the extraction. Separatory funnels with stopcocks are useful in separating the two immiscible liquids.

Key Point: Aqueous acids extract organic bases and aqueous bases extract organic acids.

Figure 12-1 illustrates a coupling reaction of two amino acids linked to a protecting group to form a dipeptide. Note that the protecting group is linked to the carboxyl group of one amino acid and the amino group of the other amino acid. All three compounds, the two amino acids and the dipeptide, are shown. The compounds are dissolved in the organic solvent, ethyl acetate.

By adding an aqueous acid, the amino acid with the exposed amino group becomes a quaternary ammonium salt and is soluble in the aqueous phase (see Figure 12-1, at right). In the ethyl acetate phase, one can find the dipeptide and the amino acid with the exposed carboxyl group. Separation of the layers is easy because ethyl acetate is less dense than water and it is found in the top layer.

By washing the ethyl acetate with an aqueous basic solution, the amino acid with the free carboxyl group is deprotonated (see Figure 12-1, at left), charged, and becomes soluble in the aqueous layer. It is easy to separate out this aqueous layer with the separatory funnel, leaving only the desired dipeptide in the ethyl acetate, which can be isolated by evaporating the solvent.

SECT. III
ORGANIC
CHEMISTRY
REVIEW
NOTES

605

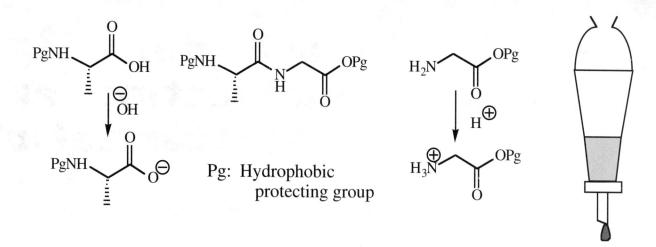

Pg: Hydrophobic
protecting group

FIGURE 12-1.

Extraction. Two amino acids, linked to a protecting group (Pg), are separated from the dipeptide formed by a coupling reaction. Note that one amino acid is converted to a quaternary ammonium salt (right), whereas the other is deprotonated (left). The amino acids are then easily separated from the dipeptide. A separatory funnel is also shown.

B. Crystallization

Recrystallization involves the purification of a solid by dissolving the solid, reducing the volume of the solution with heat, and then cooling the solution. By heating the solution, the solvent evaporates to the point where the solution is supersaturated. As the solution cools, the solubility rapidly decreases and the compound starts to precipitate.

For recrystallization to be successful, the impurities must at least be soluble in the recrystallization solvent or have a solubility that is greater than the desired compound. Otherwise, the impurities will crystallize with the desired compound.

C. Distillation

Distillation is often used to purify compounds that have different boiling points. Compounds in their liquid state are heated, and as the boiling point of the lower boiling point compound is reached, its vapors are condensed and collected.

Purifying a mixture of several compounds with different boiling points is possible by using a fractional distillation apparatus. In this apparatus, the temperature of the condensing vapor remains relatively constant until most of the lower boiling point material is evaporated from the mixture. As the temperature of the condensing vapor continues to rise, the boiling point of the higher boiling point compound is reached and the compound vaporizes. These vapors are condensed and collected in a separate flask.

When the separation of the boiling points is large, the distillation can be run under reduced pressure, which reduces the boiling points of the compounds and allows distillation to occur at lower temperatures.

Unfortunately, many liquids have significant vapor pressures at elevated temperatures. Thus, the first vapor that is condensed may contain a portion of the higher boiling point component. Repeated distillations may be necessary to increase the purity in these cases.

D. Chromatography

Chromatography involves the separation of a mixture based on certain differences in the compounds. The exploitable differences include solubility in various solvents and polarity. Chromatography generally involves a stationary and a mobile phase. The **mobile phase** carries the components of a mixture through the stationary phase, and the **stationary phase** hangs onto the components with varying affinities. The different types of chromatography are based on different types of phases, but they are all based on the same concepts.

Chromatography can be used as an analytic tool to monitor reactions or to identify products. It can also be used as a synthetic tool to purify large amounts of material.

1. Thin Layer Chromatography (TLC)

TLC is used to **monitor reaction progress and to identify specific components.** This technique is often performed with sheets of glass or plastic coated with a polar stationary phase (often silicic acid). The liquid mobile phase is a solvent. The mixture to be analyzed is spotted onto the bottom of the plate and the solvent is allowed to run up the plate by capillary action.

Generally, the stationary phase is polar, and polar compounds stick to the plate more than nonpolar compounds through dipole-dipole attractive interactions. Polar compounds tend to remain closer to the origin than nonpolar compounds. Nonpolar compounds tend not to adhere to the polar stationary phase and move farther up the plate. Thus, **the distance traveled up the plate is a reflection of the polarity of the compound.** An increase in the polarity of the solvent results in less interaction of the compounds with the stationary phase, which allows the compounds in the mobile phase to travel up the plate a greater distance.

The compounds are often visualized by looking at the plate under ultraviolet (UV) light (aromatic compounds absorb UV light) or by dipping the plate in a solution that reacts with the compounds on the plate and stains the compounds.

Figure 12-2 is a typical TLC plate used to monitor a reaction. The reaction mixture is spotted along with the starting material. The solvent is then allowed to run up the plate. The TLC shows that most of the starting material is gone and two products result. These products could then be isolated by column chromatography (see *I D 2*). In this example, the reaction components are more nonpolar than the starting materials, as shown by the fact that the products travel up the plate farther than the starting material.

FIGURE 12-2.
Thin layer chromatography.

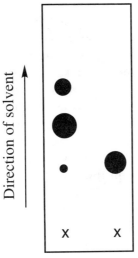

Reaction mixture   Starting material

2. Column Chromatography

In this type of chromatography, a column is packed with a stationary phase and the product mixture is loaded on top of the column. The process that follows is essentially the same as TLC, with the exception of the direction of the mobile phase (Figure 12-3). The solvent (mobile phase) runs down the column carrying the mixture while the stationary phase holds on to the compounds with varying affinities. The solvent dripping out of the column is collected in fractions, which are analyzed to determine which fraction(s) contains the desired material.

SECT. III
ORGANIC
CHEMISTRY
REVIEW
NOTES

607

FIGURE 12-3.
Column chromatography.

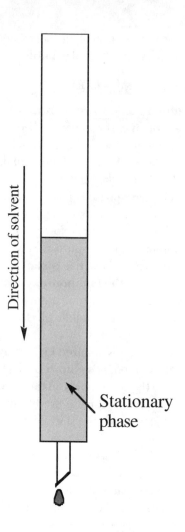

Stationary phases are of several types. **Polar stationary phases** (such as silica gel) bind more tightly to polar compounds, increasing the time polar compounds spend in the column. Not surprisingly, **solvents that are increasingly polar move the compounds more quickly through the column,** because the compounds have less interaction with the polar stationary phase and are retained in the column a shorter amount of time.

Reverse phase columns operate the opposite way: the stationary phase has higher affinity for nonpolar compounds, so the more nonpolar the mobile phase, the more quickly the compounds go through the column. **In both cases, the retention times can be altered by changing the mobile phase.**

Ion exchange chromatography can be used to separate compounds that are ionic, depending on the pH of the mobile phase. If the desired compound is an amine, the crude solution can be dissolved in an acidic solution to protonate the amine. This solution is then passed through a cation exchange column that binds cations, including the ammonium salt. The other impurities, as long as they are not cations, pass through. The column is then flushed with a salt solution that overwhelms the interactions of the stationary phase with the ammonium salt and releases the desired amine.

The same type of separation can be performed for anions, but with a different stationary phase. To remove an anion, the solution can be passed through an anion exchange column that binds the anions and lets the other compounds flow through.

Size or steric exclusion gel chromatography involves the use of stationary phase beads with little pores that allow small, light molecules to enter while letting large, heavier molecules pass between the beads. The higher the molecular weight of the molecules, the faster they pass through the column, because the higher molecular weight molecules do not have to pass through the small pores in the beads. These columns are often used to purify compounds with very different molecular weights.

3. **Gas Chromatography**

Gas chromatography involves the vaporization of a sample and its movement through a stationary phase. The mobile phase, an inert gas, carries the mixture through a column containing the stationary phase.

The compounds can be detected by a number of devices after they pass through the column. The results are given as a chromatogram (Figure 12-4), which plots time versus absorbance. This information provides the time the sample came out of the column and the relative concentration (relative peak areas). The relative concentration is proportional to absorbance.

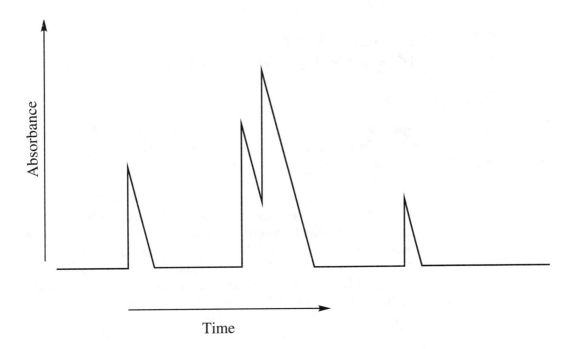

4. **High Performance Liquid Chromatography (HPLC)**

In HPLC, a mobile phase (solvent) runs through a metal-cased column that contains the stationary phase. This procedure is performed at high pressures.

A chromatogram similar to Figure 12-4 is produced by the HPLC procedure. The y-axis of the HPLC chromatogram is often absorbance of UV light, which is proportional to concentration. The area underneath the peak indicates the relative amount of material. The retention time, or the time it takes the compound to go through the column, depends on the flow rate of the mobile phase. In this way, HPLC differs from liquid chromatography, in which the retention time is based more on the composition of the solvent. In the chromatogram in Figure 12-4, the separation is not complete because of the mixing of the two middle peaks. Adjusting the conditions so that retention times are lengthened would result in a better separation.

FIGURE 12-4.

Chromatogram produced by gas chromatography or high pressure liquid chromatography of a compound.

SECT. III
ORGANIC
CHEMISTRY
REVIEW
NOTES

609

Key Points: To a point, resolution or distance between the components of a mixture through a column increases as the retention time (time the compounds spend in the column) increases. Longer interaction of the compounds with the stationary phase enhances the separation of the compounds.

Retention time can be increased by:

- decreasing the speed of the mobile phase
- changing the composition of the mobile phase
- lengthening the column

In the laboratory, chromatography can be used to determine the content of a mixture and to monitor the progress of a reaction. For analytic studies, gas chromatography, HPLC, and TLC are most often used because they are **highly sensitive** and require only **a small amount of starting material** to obtain a result. Column chromatography is often used to separate and purify larger amounts of material.

II. Characterization: Infrared (IR) and Nuclear Magnetic Resonance (NMR)

A. IR Spectroscopy

This form of spectroscopy is commonly used to determine what functional groups are present in a sample. Compared to NMR, however, IR spectroscopy does not provide as much structural information.

1. Theory

In previous chapters, bonds have been described as clouds of electrons or molecular orbitals. **For IR spectroscopy, think of the bonds as springs with natural oscillation frequencies.** All bonds have characteristic frequencies with which they stretch and bend. When the frequency of the infrared electromagnetic energy passed through a molecule is equal to the frequency of the stretches or bends of a particular bond, that energy is absorbed. It is this absorbance that can be recorded by an IR spectrometer.

Recall the formula $E = hc/\lambda = h\nu$, which implies that higher frequency means higher energy. Thus, those bonds that require more energy to stretch or bend will have higher absorbance frequencies in IR spectroscopy. The units used in IR spectroscopy are absorbances (in cm^{-1}).

"Stretchiness" depends on the strength of the bond and the masses of the atoms involved in the bond. The bonds that are most difficult to stretch are those with one heavy atom and one light atom. Thus, C–H bonds have high stretching frequencies because of a large mass difference between carbon and hydrogen. Furthermore, for C–H bonds, carbons with triple bonds ($\equiv$C–H) have higher stretching frequencies than carbons with double bonds or single bonds. This information is important, because when you look at an IR spectrum, you can predict what type of C–H bonds are in a molecule. Absorptions greater than 3000 cm^{-1} indicate multiple-bonded carbons, and absorptions below 3000 cm^{-1} indicate single-bonded carbons (Table 12-1).

Carbonyl C–O stretches are characteristic and generally occur from 1600 to 1800 cm^{-1}. Amide C=O stretches require the least amount of energy. This

TABLE 12-1. Characteristic absorbances (cm^{-1}).

Bond Type	Absorbances	Bond Type	Absorbances	
$-$C$-$H	2850–2960	$-$O$-$H	3400–3640 (very broad)	
$=$C$-$H	3020–3100	$-$N$-$H	3310–3500 (broad)	
$\equiv$C$-$H	3300			
$-$C$=$C$-$	1650–1670	C$=$O	Aldehyde	1690–1740
$-$C$\equiv$C$-$	2100–2260		Ketone	1680–1750
Aromatic ring	1600, 1500		Esters	1735–1750
			Amides	1630–1690
$-$C$\equiv$N	2210–2260	C$-$O	Ethers, esters	1080–1300

low requirement is explained by the partial single-bond character of the carbon-oxygen bond owing to resonance. Single bonds are easier to stretch than multiple bonds.

Hydrogen bonding substituents (hydroxy, amino groups) are also easy to identify because they give a broad absorbance above 3300 cm^{-1} (O–H or N–H stretch).

2. Typical IR Spectrum

The typical IR spectrum in Figure 12-5 reveals much about the ethyl ester of phenylacetic acid (Ph–CH$_2$CO–OEt). The absorbances above and below 3000 cm^{-1} indicate the presence of multiple C–H bonds. A strong carbonyl stretch at 1740 cm^{-1} indicates the presence of an ester. Medium-sized peaks at 1600 and 1500 cm^{-1} are indicative of an aromatic ring. The C–O stretches are also very strong at 1150 and 1250 cm^{-1}. Clearly, IR can be used as a tool to confirm the structure of a molecule even well after its IR spectrum has been taken and published.

FIGURE 12-5.
Typical infrared (IR) spectrum. Note the multiple bonds.

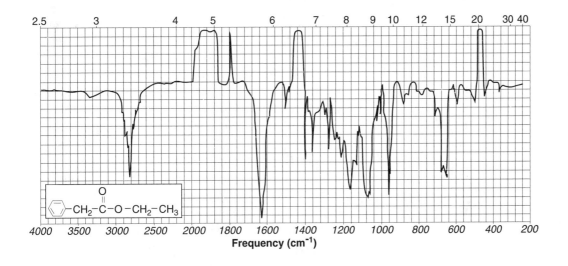

Frequency (cm^{-1})

B. NMR

1. Overview

The theory of quantum mechanics states that a nucleus with a spin number of I = 1/2 will have two degenerate or energetically equivalent states. In

SECT. III
ORGANIC
CHEMISTRY
REVIEW
NOTES

611

Figure 12-6, **position 1** shows the degenerate or energetically equivalent states. If this spinning nucleus is placed in a magnetic field, these two states will no longer be degenerate, as shown at **position 2.** The lower energy spin state will have the magnetic moment of the spinning nucleus aligned with the applied magnetic field. The higher energy spin state will have a magnetic moment aligned against the magnetic field.

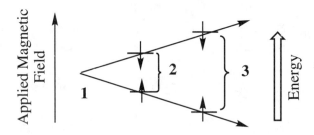

Like electrons, the nuclei of certain atoms are considered to spin. The nucleus of the hydrogen atom contains one proton that is considered to spin, and in doing so, is thought of as a tiny bar magnet.

If a sample of protons is placed in a magnetic field, some will align with and others will align against the applied magnetic field. Alignment with the field is considered more stable. Energy must be absorbed to "flip" the tiny proton magnet over the less stable alignment, against the field. If these spinning nuclei are hit with electromagnetic radiation at the correct frequency (radio frequency), the lower spin state protons can absorb the energy and "jump" to the higher spin state.

A **resonance condition** is a dynamic equilibrium that is established between the lower and higher energy spin states. This point can be detected and related to the frequency of energy that is absorbed and is necessary for resonance occur.

2.   **The NMR Spectrum**

In NMR, a substance to be studied is placed in the presence of electromagnetic radiation and a magnetic field. The electromagnetic radiation is kept at a constant frequency and the strength of the magnetic field is varied. At some value of the magnetic field strength, the energy required to "flip" the proton matches the energy of the radiation. At this point, absorption occurs and a signal is observed, which is recorded on an NMR tracing. The **NMR tracing is a plot of absorption of radiation (y-axis) versus magnetic field (x-axis).**

The frequency at which the proton comes into resonance depends on the chemical and magnetic environment surrounding it, which includes the electron density at the proton and the presence of other, nearby protons. Each proton, or each set of equivalent protons, has a slightly different environment from every other set of protons. The various electronic environments of each kind of proton accounts for the varied positions of the signals on an NMR tracing.

Four important aspects of an NMR tracing are as follows:

1.   **The number of signals** gives information on how many different "kinds" of protons are in a molecule.

2.   The **positions of the signals** tells about the electronic environment of each kind of proton.

3. The **intensities of the signals** reveals the number of each kind of proton.

4. The **splitting of a signal** into several peaks tells about the environment of a proton with respect to other, nearby protons.

3. The NMR Machine

A sample to be studied is placed in a magnetic field and irradiated with a specific frequency of electromagnetic radiation. This frequency usually is at radio frequency. The magnetic field strength is then varied. When it reaches the correct strength, the radio frequency energy is absorbed. The machine can detect this absorbance and records the frequency at which the absorbance occurs.

If electronegative groups are attached to the proton or are on an adjacent carbon, the electron density about that proton is pulled away. This **deshielding** of the proton, causing it to "feel" more of the applied magnetic field, increases the energy separation between the two spin states. In addition, the radio frequency energy needed to bring the proton resonance is higher.

A standard compound is used for comparison with the compound being studied. Tetramethyl silane (TMS) is often chosen as the internal standard. The methyl protons of this compound are highly shielded, resulting in a relatively small energy separation between the two spin states. Thus, a relatively low radio frequency energy is needed to bring the protons into resonance.

The TMS standard is arbitrarily assigned 0 hertz (Hz), and the other frequencies are reported as the number of hertz way from the TMS signal. Often, the resonances are reported as δ or parts per million (ppm).

$$\delta \text{ (ppm)} = \frac{[\text{Hz away from TMS}]}{\text{Radiofrequency of the machine}} \times 10^6$$

Thus, all NMR machines, regardless of the radio frequency used, report the same δ-values for identical compounds. The spectrum generated indicates the frequencies at which resonances occurred, and offers important information about the protons in the sample.

4. Shielding and the Chemical Shift

Electrons circulating about the proton itself generate a magnetic field. This field is aligned in such a way that it opposes the applied field. Thus, the field felt by the proton is diminished and the proton is said to be **shielded.** If the circulation of electrons (especially π-electrons) induce a field that reinforces the applied field, the proton is **deshielded.**

Compared to a "naked" proton, a shielded proton requires a higher applied magnetic field strength to provide the particular effective field strength at which absorption occurs. In essence, **shielding shifts the absorption "upfield"** (to the right on the NMR tracing). On the other hand, **deshielding shifts the absorption "downfield."** These shifts in position of NMR absorptions arising from shielding and deshielding by electrons are called **chemical shifts** (Table 12-2).

Consider an electronegative group near a proton. Electronegative groups deshield a proton, allowing the proton to "feel" more of the applied magnetic field. A larger energy separation between the spin states results (higher frequency radio energy needed for resonance to occur). The frequency at which resonance occurs is then shifted to a higher frequency relative to the TMS

SECT. III
ORGANIC
CHEMISTRY
REVIEW
NOTES

613

TABLE 12-2. Chemical shift values (δ).

Bond Type	Chemical Shift	Bond Type	Chemical Shift
$R-CH_3$	0.8–1.0	$R-O-CH_3$	3.3–3.9
$R-CH_2-R$	1.2–1.4	$R-CO-CH_3$ (ketone)	2.1–2.6
$Ph-CH_3$	2.2–2.5	RCHO (aldehyde)	9.5–9.6
$R-CH_2-Cl$	3.6–3.8	$Ph-H$	6.0–9.5
$R-CH_2-Br$	3.4–3.6	$RC\equiv CH$	2.5–3.1
$R-CH_2-I$	3.1–3.3	$R_2C=CHR$	5.2–5.7

standard (higher δ, downfield shift). **The more electronegative the adjacent group, the further downfield the signal.** Note that few protons are more highly shielded than TMS; everything else is more deshielded, and resonance occurs downfield, at a specific δ away from TMS.

The molecules that contain aromatic rings resonate far downfield. Electronegativity is not the explanation; benzene, for example, is not very electronegative. Rather, the downfield signal of these molecules is caused by π-electron clouds. The applied magnetic field induces a magnetic field in the π-electron cloud that **deshields the protons on the ring** (Figure 12-7). This effect also occurs with protons on double and triple-bonded carbons, but not to the same extent.

FIGURE 12-7.
Induction of a magnetic field in the π-electron cloud resulting from an applied magnetic field.

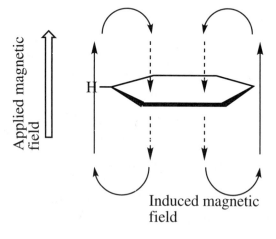

5. **Spin-Spin Splitting**

Along with the chemical environment about a proton, the magnetic environment surrounding a proton also plays a large role. **Protons can feel the different magnetic environments created by hydrogens on adjacent carbons.** If a certain proton is next to a carbon with three protons, the signal of that proton splits into a quartet. This splitting is attributable to the four ways that three protons of two different spins can be arranged: all three protons with spins aligned with the applied magnetic field; two with and one against; one with and two against; three protons with spins aligned against the applied magnetic field.

If the adjacent carbon has only two protons, the signal is split into a triplet. If the proton is flanked on both sides by carbons with protons, the splitting is more complicated and forms a multiplet. **In general, a set of n equivalent protons splits an NMR signal into n + 1 peaks;** e.g., with three adjacent, equivalent protons, the signal is split into a quartet.

Equivalent protons do not split each other. An example is the protons of a methyl group, which are chemically and magnetically equivalent. Another example is Cl–CH$_2$–CH$_2$–Cl (1,2-dichloroethane); only one signal is generated for the methylene groups.

Figure 12-8 is an NMR tracing for the molecule CH$_3$–CO–OCH$_2$CH$_2$Br, which includes two triplets and a singlet. The rise of the line above the signals is the measure of the area underneath the peak. This value is proportional to the number of protons responsible for the signal.

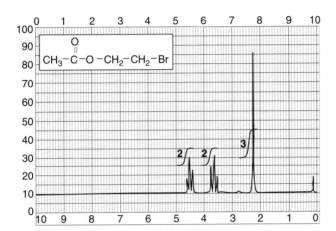

FIGURE 12-8.
A sample NMR tracing.

The integrations indicate that two protons are responsible for each of the triplets and that three protons are responsible for the singlet. The singlet is at 2 ppm, so it must be the methyl next to the carbonyl. The triplets are the methylenes with the one further downfield belonging to the CH$_2$ attached to the more electronegative oxygen.

Figure 12-9 is an NMR tracing for the molecule Ph–CH$_2$–CO–OCH$_2$CH$_3$. The combination of a triplet (integrating to three) and a quartet (two protons) suggests an ethyl group. The triplet belongs to the methyl and the downfield quartet belongs to the –O–CH$_2$– methylene. The singlet integrating to two protons is thus the benzyl –CH$_2$–, and the tallest singlet belongs to the aromatic protons.

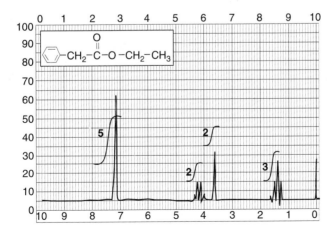

FIGURE 12-9.
A sample NMR tracing.

In summary, it is more important to understand some basic theory about this complex procedure and the principles behind what the tracings show than to be concerned with determining precise chemical structure from NMR tracings.

SECT. III
ORGANIC
CHEMISTRY
REVIEW
NOTES

615

Appendix:
Nomenclature

Nomenclature

I. General Rules for all Compounds

- **Know the names of the functional groups,** both prefixes and suffixes.

- **Find the longest carbon chain containing the highest priority functional group.** The order in decreasing priority (but not in all cases) follows:

1. Carboxylic acids and derivatives (esters, amides, nitriles, acid halides, anhydrides, and so on)

2. Aldehydes

3. Ketones

4. Alcohols

5. Amines

6. Alkynes

7. Alkenes

8. Halogens and alkyl groups

- **Number** from the end of the carbon chain, which places the highest priority functional group at the lowest numeric value.

- **List substituents alphabetically.** Use the suffix for the highest priority functional group and the prefix for the other functional groups (substituents). **Note:** sec-, iso-, and tert- are placed in alphabetical order, but di-, tri-, and tetra- are not.

II. Rules for Specific Compounds

A. Alkanes and Alkyl Halides

1. **Memorize** prefixes for carbon chains (meth-, eth-, prop-, but-, and so on)—one of the few things in organic chemistry that you need to memorize.

2. **Identify** the longest continuous carbon chain, which determines the prefix. The **suffix for all alkanes is -ane.**

SECT. III
ORGANIC
CHEMISTRY
REVIEW
NOTES

617

3. **Number** from the chain starting at the end closest to the first branch point or halogen.

- If substituents are equal distances from the opposite ends, start numbering from the substituent that is first in alphabetical order.

4. If there is more than one of a particular substituent, use di-, tri-, tetra-, and so on before the name of the substituent. (Note: This substituent does not count in the alphabetical order.)

5. **List** the substituents in alphabetical order as shown in Figure A-1. Do not use spaces, just hyphens.

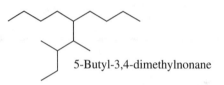

(CH₃)₂CH(CH₂)₂CH₃
2-Methylpentane

5-Butyl-3,4-dimethylnonane

2-Bromo-8-chloro-4-(1-methylpropyl)nonane

FIGURE A-1.
Examples of alkane and alkyl halide nomenclature.

6. **Complex substituents** are named starting at the atom attached to the chain. The names of these substituents are in parentheses.

7. **Common names**

These names are not official names of the International Union of Pure and Applied Chemistry (IUPAC), but are commonplace in many compounds (Figure A-2).

3-Carbon  *iso*-Propyl

4-Carbon  *sec*-Butyl *iso*-Butyl *tert*-Butyl

5-Carbon  *iso*-Pentyl *neo*-Pentyl *tert*-Pentyl

FIGURE A-2.
Common alkane names.

8. **Cyclic alkanes** (Figure A-3)

a. The base name is the cycloalkane unit.

b. The same rules apply for naming and ordering of substituents as in the linear case.

(1) Number substituents so they total to the smallest number.

(2) Order alphabetically, if possible.

FIGURE A-3.
Examples of cyclic alkane nomenclature.

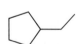
Ethylcyclopropane

1,3-Dimethylcycloheptane

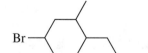
4-Bromo-2-methylpropylcyclohexane

B. Alkenes

1. **Identify** the longest carbon chain containing the double bond, which determines the prefix. The **suffix is -ene.**

2. **Number** from the end closest to the double bond.

- Multiple double bonds are numbered and the appropriate prefixes (e.g., di-, tri-, and tetra-) are applied (Figure A-4).

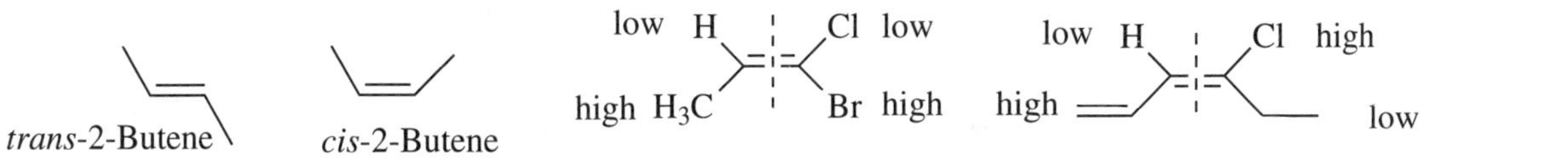

trans-2-Butene   *cis*-2-Butene

(Z)-1-Bromo-1-chloropropene   (E)-4-Chloro-1,3-hexadiene

3. **List** substituents in alphabetical order using prefixes.

4. ***Cis, trans.*** These terms identify the isomers.

- a. *cis* alkenes have the larger substituents on the same side.
- b. *Trans* alkenes have the larger substituents across the double bond.

5. **E/Z**

- a. *Cis* and *trans* are sometimes ambiguous, so IUPAC uses E (opposite) and Z (same or "Zame") designations (see Figure A-4).
- b. To designate, **prioritize the sides of each carbon of the double bond.** High priorities on the same side are Z and on the opposite side are E.

6. **Priorities** (also apply for *R/S* designation)

- a. Look at the atom attached to the double bond. Rank by atomic number.
- b. In the case of a tie, go to the next atom and rank by atomic number.
- c. Look for a point of difference such as a branch point. If there still is a tie, go to the next atom. Keep going until a higher ranking atom is found.
- d. Multiple bonds are tricky. They are counted as if they were the same number of singly bonded atoms; i.e., a $CH–CH_2$ double bond counts as 4 carbons and 3 hydrogens (Figure A-5).
- e. Remember to look for rankings according to atomic number and not total weight of the substituent group.

Lower priority   Higher priority

Higher priority   Lower priority

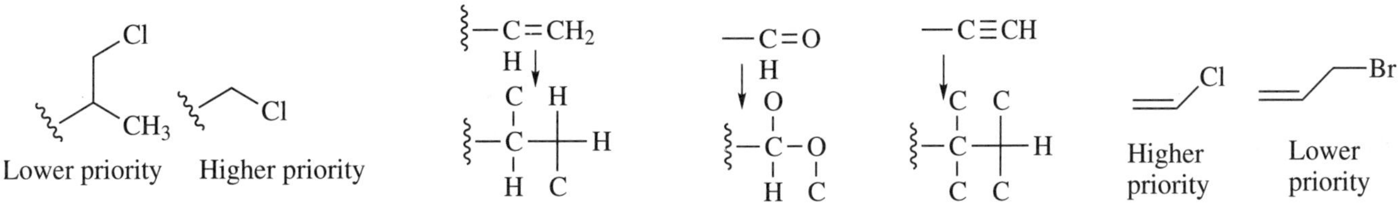

7. **Common names**

- a. Mono substituted ethylenes are vinyl (vinyl chloride or 1-chloroethene) in Figure A-5).
- b. When a methylene (CH_2) group is between the double bond and the substituent, the common name is allyl (allyl bromide or 3-bromopropene in Figure A-4). The allyl term is also used in reference to carbocations and radicals.

FIGURE A-4.
Examples of alkene nomenclature.

FIGURE A-5.
Branch point and multiple bond considerations in alkene nomenclature.

SECT. III
ORGANIC
CHEMISTRY
REVIEW
NOTES

619

C. Alkynes

1. The **rules** are the same as for alkenes, except **the suffix is -yne.**

2. **Number** from the end closest to the triple bond.

D. Benzene Compounds

1. In the absence of other functional groups, benzene is the base name.

2. **List** the substituents alphabetically and **number** the substituents so that the lowest possible numbers are used.

3. **Ortho, meta,** and **para** can be used to describe disubstituted benzene rings (Figure A-6).

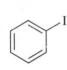

Iodobenzene

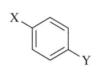

Ortho   Meta   Para

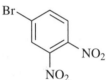

1-Bromo-3,4-dinitrobenzene

4. **Common names**

    a. When rings are substituents, the names shown in Figure A-7 are used:

    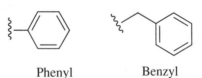

    Phenyl   Benzyl

    b. Be familiar with common names in Figure A-8. For each of the common names, substitute the given group for X in the structure. Of the names listed, the benzene carbon attached to the **X group is number 1** in the numbering scheme.

    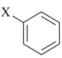

    X = CH₃, toluene; X = OH, phenol; X = NH₂, aniline; X = −CH=CH₂, styrene; X = CHO, benzaldehyde; X = COOH, benzoic acid.

E. Alcohols

1. The naming of these compounds is similar to alkanes.

    a. **Prefix** is based on the largest carbon chain containing the OH.

    b. **Suffix** is **-ol.**

2. **Numbering** begins at the end closest to the hydroxy group or amino group.

FIGURE A-6.
Nomenclature of benzene compounds.

FIGURE A-7.
Phenyl and benzyl groups.

FIGURE A-8.
Common names for benzene compounds (see text).

3. Common names

a. Primary (1°), secondary (2°) and tertiary (3°) alcohols are represented in Figure A-9.

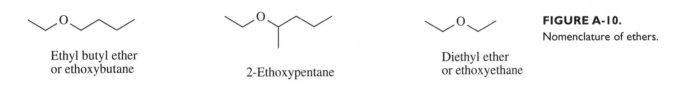

1°

2°
Isopentanol
2-propanol

3°

3-(1-Bromoethyl)-5-methyl-2-hexanol

FIGURE A-9
Examples of primary, secondary, and tertiary alcohols (left), and a branched alcohol (right).

b. Iso-, sec-, and tert- are also used to describe branching.

F. Ethers

These compounds are named by two different methods.

1. **Simple molecules:** List the alkyl groups in increasing size and add the word *ether.*

2. **More complex molecules:** Use the alkyloxyalkane method. The smaller group has the **-oxy** suffix (Figure A-10).

Ethyl butyl ether
or ethoxybutane

2-Ethoxypentane

Diethyl ether
or ethoxyethane

FIGURE A-10.
Nomenclature of ethers.

G. Ketones

1. **Identify** the longest carbon chain with the carbonyl group.

2. **Number** the chain starting at the end closest to the carbonyl.

   • Use the standard prefix for the carbon chain and **-one** as the suffix.

3. **List** the substituents in alphabetical order (Figure A-11).

FIGURE A-11.
Nomenclature of ketones.

2-Heptanone   2-Methylcyclopentanone   (Z)-Bromo-3-hexen-2-one

β   β
γ   α   α   γ

H_3C CH_3

Acetone

4. **Greek letters** are used to describe positions relative to the carbonyl (for all carbonyl compounds).

5. **Remember the common name Acet** (as in acetone), which involves CH_3CO- group.

SECT. III
ORGANIC
CHEMISTRY
REVIEW
NOTES

621

H. Aldehydes, Carboxylic Acids, and Acid Chlorides

1. **Identify** the longest carbon chain containing the aldehyde or acid.

2. **Number** the chain starting with the carbonyl carbon.

    a.   Use the standard prefix for the carbon chain.

    b.   For **aldehydes**, the suffix is **-al**.

    c.   For **carboxylic acids**, the suffix is **-ic acid**.

    d.   They can also be named (in more complicated cases) as **-carboxylic acid**.

3. **List** the substituents in alphabetical order (Figure A-12).

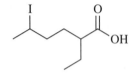

2-Ethyl-5-iodohexanoic acid

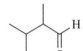

2,3-Dimethylbutanal   Acetic Acid   Butanoyl bromide   X=OH Cyclohexanecarboxylic acid
                                                         X=Cl Cyclohexanecarbonyl chloride

FIGURE A-12.
Examples of aldehyde, carboxylic acid, and acid chloride nomenclature.

4. Remember that **acet** involves a CH_3CO- (acetic acid resembles acetone, except for the hydroxy group of acetic acid).

5. **Acid chlorides** are the same as carboxylic acids, except the suffix is **-yl halide** or **-carbonyl halide**.

6. Also related are **nitriles** $(-C \equiv N)$, named the same way but the suffix is **-nitrile**.

I. Esters

1. **Identify** the alcohol section (connected to oxygen) and the carboxylic acid section (connected to the carbonyl) [Figure A-13].

FIGURE A-13.
An example of the naming of an ester compound.

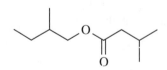

2-(Methyl)butyl 3-methylpropionate
or *sec*-Butyl 3-methylpropionate

2. **Name** the alcohol alkyl group.

3. **Finish** the name using alkyl group on the acid side and the suffix **-oate**.

4. **If substituents are attached,** number the alcohol region starting with the carbon connected to the oxygen. On the acid side, start numbering at the carbonyl carbon.

J. Amines

1. In general, amines are named by listing the alkyl substituents and ending with **-amine.**

2. For branched primary amines, the prefix **amino-** is applied, along with the position number on the chain.

3. More complex amines are named by using a combined prefix that uses the largest alkyl group as the base name (Figure A-14).

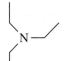 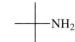

Triethylamine   *tert*-Butylamine   2-Aminobutane   2-(Ethylmethylamino) butane

FIGURE A-14.
Examples of amine nomenclature.

K. Use of Prefixes

1. **Prefixes** are used for substituents (which are lower in priority compared with the functional group on which the name is based).

2. A rough order, which may be different when applied to ring systems, follows. **Prefixes are in bold** and the list is ordered from high to low priority (high dictates the base name).

   a. Carboxylic acids: **carboxy-** and derivatives (esters, **alkoxyl-** and **carbonyl-**; amides, **amido-**; nitriles, **cyano-**; acid chlorides)

   b. Aldehydes: **formyl-**

   c. Ketones: **oxo-**

   d. Alcohols: **hydroxy-**

   e. Amines: **amino-**

   f. Alkynes

   g. Alkenes

   h. Halogens and alkyl groups

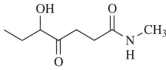

5-Hydroxy-4-oxo-*N*-methylheptamide

FIGURE A-15
An example of amide nomenclature.

3. Figure A-15 is an example to show how to name amides. The base name is the longest chain containing the amide, with the numbering starting at the carbonyl carbon. *N*- is used to describe groups attached to the nitrogen.

SECT. III
ORGANIC
CHEMISTRY
REVIEW
NOTES

623

Organic Chemistry

PRACTICE TESTS

ORGANIC CHEMISTRY PRACTICE TEST 1

Time: 45 minutes

Directions: This test contains as many organic chemistry passages as you may encounter on the real MCAT. There are also several independent multiple-choice questions at the end of this test. The time allotted approximates the time allowed on a real MCAT to solve the given number of questions. Choose one best answer for each question.

Passage I (Questions 1–8)

In order to form compound B from two other compounds, A and C, an organic chemist performed a reaction, followed by crude isolation, which led to a mixture of the three compounds in the solvent ethyl acetate (EtOAc). The extraction scheme in Figure 1 was followed to isolate the product.

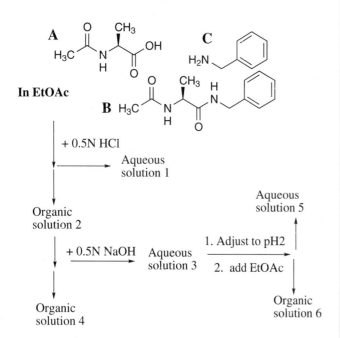

Figure 1. Extraction scheme used in isolation.

The solutions were then monitored by thin layer chromatography (TLC) to identify the contents (Figure 2). The compounds are characterized by the distance they travel up a thin layer plate using a specific mobile phase. The values are usually expressed as R_f, which is equal to the distance traveled by the compound divided by the distance traveled by the solvent.

Direction of solvent

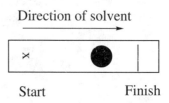

Figure 2. Thin layer chromatography plate used to identify contents of solutions.

1. Solution 1 contains which of the following compounds?

    A. A
    B. B
    C. C and A
    D. C

2. Solution 2 contains which of the following compounds?

    A. A
    B. A and B
    C. B
    D. B and C

3. Which of the following compounds is in solution 6?

4. Consider compounds A and B. Which of the following has the lowest R_f value at pH 7?

A. A
B. B
C. A and B have the same R_f.
D. It is impossible to predict the lowest value.

5. How will increasing the polarity of the TLC solvent affect the R_f values of A, B, and C?

A. All R_f values will increase.
B. All R_f values will decrease.
C. R_f value of A only will increase.
D. R_f value of C only will increase.

6. The reaction between the starting materials A and C to form B results in a(n):

A. amine.
B. ester.
C. ketone.
D. amide.

7. The ^{1}H-NMR spectra of C and A differ because of the resonances that occur at:

A. $\delta 7$–8 ppm for A with $CDCl_3$ as a solvent.
B. $\delta 7$–8 ppm for C with $CDCl_3$ as a solvent.
C. $\delta 9$–12 ppm for A with MeOD as a solvent.
D. $\delta 9$–12 ppm for C with MeOD as a solvent.

8. Methanol can dissolve compounds A, B, and C, but it is a poor solvent for extraction because it is:

A. slightly acidic.
B. slightly basic.
C. reactive with B.
D. miscible with aqueous solutions.

Passage II (Questions 9–16)

In terms of their structure and unique chemical properties, sugars are essential molecules with various biologic roles. The straight chain form of D-glucose can cyclize, forming the structures shown in Figure 3.

The cyclic isomers (α and β) are called epimers. These two forms are in a dynamic equilibrium in aqueous solution; i.e., if either α or β were isolated and then placed in an aqueous solution, the equilibrium would re-establish. The addition of methanol with acid, however, gives two different forms, and α and β are no longer interconvertible. The α-X and β-X forms can be isolated and characterized.

9. Which of the following mechanisms explains the conversion of D-glucose from the linear form to the cyclic form?

A. Intramolecular nucleophilic attack and cyclization
B. Intramolecular electrophilic attack and cyclization
C. Intramolecular addition and cyclization
D. Intermolecular addition and cyclization

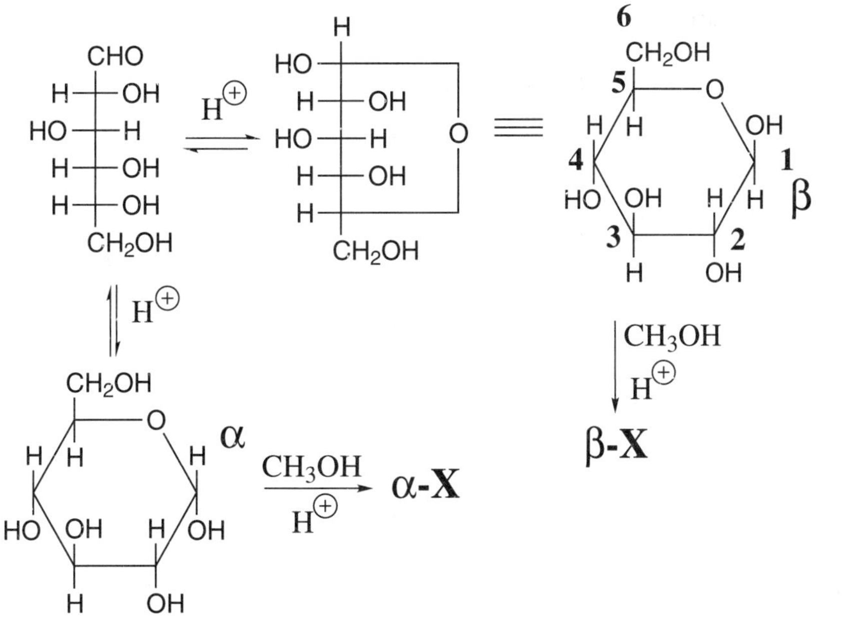

Figure 3. Cyclization of the straight chain form of D-glucose yields to cyclic isomers.

10. Diastereomers that differ in configuration only at carbon 2 of D-glucose are called:

    A. mutamers.
    B. anomers.
    C. glycosides.
    D. epimers.

11. Compound X is:

    A. a hemiketal.
    B. a hemiacetal.
    C. an acetal.
    D. none of the above.

12. How many stereocenters are found in the open chain form of D-glucose?

    A. 3
    B. 4
    C. 5
    D. 6

13. How many stereocenters are found in the cyclic pyranose form of D-glucose?

    A. 3
    B. 4
    C. 5
    D. 6

14. The interconversion of α and β anomers is also called:

    A. mutarotation.
    B. anomerism.
    C. Walden inversion.
    D. electrophilic substitution.

15. After treatment with methanol in acid, the linear sugar:

    A. can be detected.
    B. cannot be detected.
    C. will possess an extra methyl group.
    D. None of the above

16. The α-X and β-X forms are best described as:

    A. enantiomers.
    B. meso compounds.
    C. superimposable mirror images.
    D. diastereomers.

Passage III (Questions 17–24)

Stimulants of the central nervous system (CNS), such as fencamfine (Figure 4), require the proper alignment of an amine and a phenyl ring. For many compounds, the shape of a molecule as well as its chemical properties are important for the pharmacologic effects; fencamfine is no exception. Without the bridging carbon 7, the ring 1–6 would take on an entirely different shape and the compound would lose its activity.

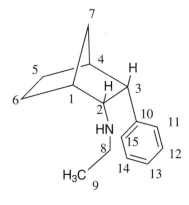

Figure 4. The CNS stimulant fencamfine.

The liver plays a large role in the metabolism of fencamfine. The liver places a hydroxy group on the aromatic ring of this compound, which renders it more water soluble and more readily excreted in the urine. Those CNS stimulants that the liver cannot hydroxylate are broken down by other metabolic pathways in the liver.

17. How may chiral carbons are found on fencamfine?

    A. 14
    B. 4
    C. 2
    D. 1

18. What is the theoretic number of stereoisomers?

    A. 8
    B. 4
    C. 16
    D. 2

19. At which pH range is fencamfine most soluble in water?

    A. < pH 3
    B. > pH 12
    C. Around pH 7
    D. < pH 3 and around pH 7

20. What is the hybridization at carbon 10?

    A. sp
    B. sp³
    C. sp²
    D. Carbon 10 is unhybridized.

21. Treatment of the compound with one equivalent of methyliodide (CH_3I) will methylate:

    A. carbon 1.
    B. carbon 13.
    C. the nitrogen.
    D. carbon 7.

22. Duplicating the hydroxylation performed by the liver in the laboratory involves several steps, beginning with an electrophilic aromatic addition. This step most likely occurs at:

    A. carbon 10.
    B. carbon 13.
    C. carbon 14.
    D. carbon 3.

23. What is the hybridization of the nitrogen?

    A. sp
    B. sp³
    C. sp²
    D. The nitrogen is unhybridized.

24. The structure of the norborane carbons 1–6 differs from the most stable conformation of cyclohexane in that:

    A. carbons 1–6 are held in a chair conformation by the carbon 7 bridge.
    B. carbons 1–6 are held in a boat conformation by the carbon 7 bridge.
    C. the nitrogen forces the chair configuration.
    D. the phenyl ring forces the boat configuration.

Passage IV (Questions 25–32)

When treated with the base lithium diisopropylamide (LDA), compound A (Figure 5) can form two different enolates. This reaction can follow one of two pathways toward B or C or B and C. Figure 6 illustrates the reaction coordinate for the formation of intermediates B or C from the starting material, compound A.

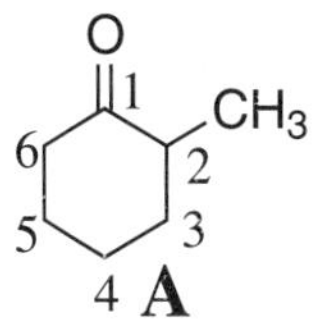

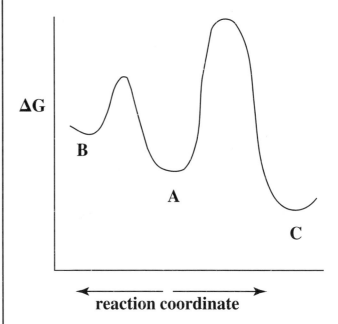

Figure 5. Compound A.

Figure 6. Formation of intermediates B and C from compound A.

After generation of the intermediate, treatment with CH_3I yields products D and E (Figure 7), based on the formation of intermediates B and C. This outcome depends on the temperatures at which the reaction takes place. The following ratios were gathered when the reaction was performed under two different conditions:

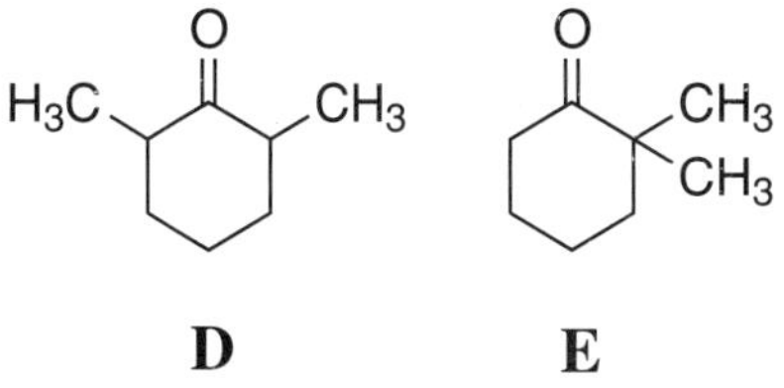

Figure 7. Treatment with CH_3I yields products D and E based on the formation of intermediates B and C.

	D	E
−78°C	95%	5%
23°C	30%	70%

25. The hydrogens α to the carbonyl are removed by base because of the:

    A.   stability of the anion at this position owing to resonance.

    B.   stability of the cation at this position owing to resonance.

    C.   stability of the radical at this position owing to resonance.

    D.   the high basicity of the hydrogens at this position.

26. Which enolate requires less activation energy to form, B or C?

    A.   B

    B.   C

    C.   B and C require the same amount of energy.

    D.   It is impossible to determine which requires less energy.

27. Which of the following compounds methylate the enolate most effectively?

    A. CH_3F

    B. CH_3Br

    C. CH_3OH

    D. CH_3I

28. When one equivalent of a methylating reagent is used, at which position(s) will deprotonation create chiral centers?

    A.   2

    B.   1

    C.   6

    D.   2 and 6

29. If one methyl group is attached to both 2 and 6, the product:

    A.   will be R absolute configuration.

    B.   will be S absolute configuration.

    C.   will be racemic.

    D.   would rotate plane-polarized light counterclockwise.

30. Which enolate is thermodynamically more stable?

    A.   B

    B.   C

    C.   B and C are equally stable

    D.   Relative stability cannot be determined

31. LDA is considered a sterically hindered base. Which proton(s) will be the easiest for LDA to extract?

    A.   2

    B.   4

    C.   6

    D.   2 and 6

32. Product E corresponds to which enolate?

    A.   B

    B.   C

    C.   B and C

    D.   Neither B nor C

Passage V (Questions 33–38)

Cocaine is no longer used widely as a local anesthetic because of allergic reactions associated with its use, its relative instability in aqueous solutions, and its high addictive potential. The first few steps in the synthesis of cocaine are shown in Figure 8.

630   **Figure 8.**   Synthesis of cocaine.

The cyclic acetal is formed in step 3. Acetals are used to mask carbonyls. They can be converted back to carbonyls and are not reactive toward a variety of reagents. This synthesis also takes advantage of the acidity of protons α to carbonyl carbons and the nucleophilic additions that can take place.

33. Not all of compound A has reacted to form B. How can you separate B from A?

    A. Acidify the mixture using dilute aqueous acid and extract with water
    B. Acidify the mixture using dilute aqueous acid and extract with ethyl acetate
    C. Make the mixture basic using dilute aqueous base and extract with water
    D. Make the mixture basic using dilute aqueous base and extract with ethyl acetate

34. Is it necessary to convert the diacid to an acid chloride (through $SOCl_2$) before converting the acids to aldehydes?

    A. No. Lithium aluminum hydride reduces acids to aldehydes.
    B. Yes. Most reducing agents reduce the acid to an alcohol.
    C. No. Lithium aluminum hydride oxidizes the acids to aldehydes.
    D. Yes. Most, if not all, oxidizing agents reduce the acid to an alcohol.

35. The strength of NaOEt as a base is sufficient to remove protons α to the carbonyl. On E, NaOEt will remove:

    A. the methyl proton on the ethoxy group.
    B. the methylene proton on the ethoxy group.
    C. the proton on the carbon between the carbonyl groups.
    D. the methylene proton on the ethoxy group and the proton on the carbon between the carbonyl groups.

36. Which of the following would occur if there was no acetal in step 3 of Figure 8?

    A. With two aldehydes, the reaction would not occur.
    B. The polarity of the second aldehyde would make the enolate less reactive.
    C. With two aldehydes, the protons between them would be more acidic than the other protons.
    D. Without protection, both aldehydes could react with two enolates.

37. In step 5 of Figure 8, the acid chloride formed from treatment of D with $SOCl_2$ is reacted with a mixture of ethyl acetate and NaOEt. What is the role of NaOEt in this reaction?

    A. It removes a proton from the ethyl group of ethyl acetate.
    B. It protonates the carbonyl of ethyl acetate.
    C. It adds another OEt group to ethyl acetate.
    D. It removes a proton on the methyl group of ethyl acetate.

38. Why is it necessary to convert the acid (D) into an acid chloride before it is attacked by the enolate?

    A. It is not necessary to make this conversion.
    B. Because chloride is a less desirable leaving group than hydroxide.
    C. Because the enolate will attack the ester before it attacks the acid.
    D. Because the hydroxide is too electronegative and it pulls too much electron density away from the carbonyl carbon.

Questions 39–40 are **NOT** based on a descriptive passage.

39. In which of the following solvents are alkenes the most soluble?

    A. Water
    B. Ethyl alcohol
    C. Carbon tetrachloride
    D. Ammonia

40. In a reaction of ethene and hydrochloric acid, the hydrogen ions act as:

    A. nucleophiles.
    B. electrophiles.
    C. carbanions.
    D. carbonium ions.

Answers and Explanations to Organic Chemistry Practice Test 1

PASSAGE I

1. **D**   Solution 1 is derived by the addition of acid. Of the compounds from which to choose, only the amine is protonated and water soluble in acidic solutions.

2. **B**   Protonation with the addition of hydrochloric acid results in the removal of the amine in aqueous solution 1, leaving compounds A and B in solution 2.

3. **B**   At this point in the purification scheme, the acid is in a protonated uncharged form and will be more soluble in the organic phase.

4. **A**   Recalling the definition of the R_f value, look for which compound travels farthest up the plate. Recall that nonpolar compounds tend to travel farther up the plate than polar compounds. At pH 7, compound A is deprotonated and charged, and will not travel up the plate as far as uncharged B.

5. **A**   Increasing the polarity of the solvent will change the migration of the solvents on the TLC plates, thus increasing all the R_f values for the compounds. An increased solvent polarity decreases binding between the compounds and the stationary phase.

6. **D**   Consider the functional groups of the compounds mentioned: a carboxylic acid and an amine. The joining of these functional groups produces an amide bond. Thus, the product is the result of amide bond formation.

7. **B**   A major structural difference between A and C is the presence of the benzene ring in C, containing aromatic protons. The aromatic protons will resonate at $\delta 7$–8 ppm. MeOD will exchange the amine and carboxylate protons and will not resonate.

8. **D**   If the organic solvent is miscible (like methanol), it cannot be separated from the aqueous solution. Thus, methanol is a poor solvent for extractions.

PASSAGE II

9. **A**   Carbohydrate chemistry is simply an application of basic alcohol chemistry. The C5 hydroxy acts as a nucleophile and attacks the C1 carbonyl to cyclize.

10. **D**   Remember some basic terms: anomers differ in configuration at carbon 1 and epimers differ in configuration at carbon 2.

11. **C**   Recall from Chapter 6 of the Organic Chemistry Review Notes that alcohols attack the electrophilic carbon of the carbonyl. In this first step, a hemiacetal is formed if the starting compound is an aldehyde. Further attack by a second alcohol produces the acetal.

12. **B**   Look for carbons attached to four different substituents. To determine how many stereoisomers are possible, remember the formula: 2^n = # stereoisomers.

13. **C**   Five carbons are attached to four different substituents. Carbons 1–5 are stereocenters. Only carbon 6 is not attached to four different substituents.

14. **A**   Mutarotation occurs as the ring is opened and closed in an equilibrium process.

15. **C**   Reaction with methanol in acid results in the formation of acetals. These acetals are glycosides generated from the reaction of the aldehyde with an alcohol and acid. Glycosides are nonreducing sugars, and possess an extra methyl group.

ANSWERS AND
EXPLANATIONS
TO ORGANIC
CHEMISTRY
PRACTICE TEST 1

632

16. **D** The two forms differ only in the stereochemistry about one carbon. Meso compounds have a plane of internal symmetry and enantiomers are nonsuperimposable mirror images.

---

17. **B** The chiral carbons are located on the molecule at carbons 1, 2, 3, and 4. Remember that chiral carbons have four different substituents.

18. **C** The theoretic number of stereoisomers is determined by taking two to the power of the number of chiral centers, which yields 2^4 or 16.

19. **A** At pH ranges less than 3, the nitrogen would be protonated and charged, rendering it polar and water soluble. Because of the benzene ring and its other hydrocarbon components, this molecule would not be soluble in water overall.

20. **C** The sp^2 hybridized carbon at position 10 is in a planar configuration. Recall that single-bonded carbons are usually sp^3 hybridized and double-bonded carbons are usually sp^2 hybridized.

21. **C** Look for the best nucleophile on the molecule. Three of the choices are carbons involved in the backbone of the molecule. The only other choice to evaluate is nitrogen, which is the best nucleophile on the compound. This is where methylation is most likely to occur.

22. **B** Look for the carbon where addition produces the least sterically hindered product. Choice D is unlikely because there are no double bonds to add across. Considering the remaining choices reveals carbon 13 is in a para position and is sterically less hindered. Carbon 13 would allow the least sterically hindered product.

23. **B** Review the chemistry of the nitrogen-containing compounds (amines) in Chapter 9 of the Organic Chemistry Review Notes. Recall that the lone pair on nitrogen occupies the fourth hybrid orbital (one of the sp^3 hybridized orbitals).

24. **B** Drawing the six-membered ring in a chair requires stretching the bridge, which does not occur.

---

25. **A** Each enolate has two different resonance forms stabilizing the anion. Removing hydrogens results in production of anions, not cations or radicals as the other choices suggest.

26. **A** Recall that the higher the hump from the starting material, the higher the activation energy. Less activation energy is required to form B than C.

27. **D** The only difference between the choices involves the leaving groups. Iodide is the best leaving group and will therefore be substituted most readily. Recall that both I and Br are good leaving groups.

28. **C** Deprotonation at position 2 will lead to two methyl groups at that position. Thus, position 2 cannot be a chiral center. Position 1 is not chiral because it contains a carbonyl. Position 6 will give rise to a chiral center with methylation and deprotonation.

29. **C** Once the enolate is formed, the methyl group is attached to either "side," yielding a racemic mixture.

30. **B** Low energy compounds generally are thermodynamically stable. Compound C is lower in energy than compound B.

31. **C** A sterically hindered base will most likely pull off a proton that is the least sterically hindered—this is found at position 6.

32. **B** The enolate that is thermodynamically more stable has the greater number of substitutions, which is reflected in the product formation.

---

33. **D** By making the mixture basic and extracting with ethyl acetate, you deprotonate the acid and make it water soluble while the product remains in the ethyl acetate layer. The other choices either do not make sense or do not allow you to separate the compounds.

34. **B** It is difficult to stop reduction of an acid at an aldehyde. Lithium aluminum hydride is a strong reducing agent and reduces acids to alcohols. To reduce an acid to an aldehyde, convert to an acid chloride, and then use a relatively mild reducing agent to reduce to the aldehyde. The amount of reducing agent should be stoichiometric and the temperature should be low.

35. **C** The proton on the carbon between the carbonyl groups is most acidic because of the stability of the enolate formed as a result of deprotonation. The methyl and methylene protons on the ethoxy group do not form enolates that are as stable.

36. **D** Unless one of the aldehydes is protected, they will both react with enolates, an unwanted response.

37. **D** NaOEt acts as a base and deprotonates the protons on the carbon α to the carbonyl carbon. In this case, the methyl group and not the ethyl group next to the oxygen is deprotonated.

38. **C** C is the best choice because the carboxylic acid is probably sufficiently acidic to protonate and quench the enolate. In addition, Cl is a better leaving group than OH.

39. **C** Hydrocarbons, such as the alkenes, are most soluble in nonpolar solvents. Water, ethyl alcohol, and ammonia have some polarity.

40. **B** The electron-deficient hydrogen ion attacks the electron-rich carbon-carbon double bond and forms a carbocation intermediate. Because the hydrogen ion seeks to gain negative charge or electrons, it is acting as an electrophile.

ANSWERS AND
EXPLANATIONS
TO ORGANIC
CHEMISTRY
PRACTICE TEST 1

634

ORGANIC CHEMISTRY PRACTICE TEST 2

Time: 45 minutes

Directions: This test contains as many organic chemistry passages as you may encounter on the real MCAT. The time allotted approximates the time allowed on a real MCAT to solve the given number of questions. Choose one best answer for each question.

Passage I (Questions 1–9)

The reaction of an aromatic aldehyde with a cyanide anion (the benzoin condensation) yields a dimer of the aromatic aldehyde. If the aromatic group is a phenyl ring, the dimer is called benzoin. A chemistry student ran this reaction with varying concentrations of reactants and measured the amount produced over time. The student could then determine the value of the rate constant of the observed rate law:

$$\text{Rate} = k[\text{benzaldehyde}]^2[\text{CN}^-]$$

$$k = \text{the rate constant}$$

The value of k was determined by measuring the rate at various concentrations of benzaldehyde and cyanide. The mechanism of the reaction is illustrated in Figure 1.

1. If the concentration of the cyanide ion is doubled, the rate of benzoin formation would:

   A. be one half the original value.
   B. remain unchanged.
   C. increase by a factor of four.
   D. double.

2. If the concentration of benzaldehyde was doubled, the rate would:

   A. double.
   B. increase by a factor of four.
   C. remain unchanged.
   D. be eight times greater than the original rate.

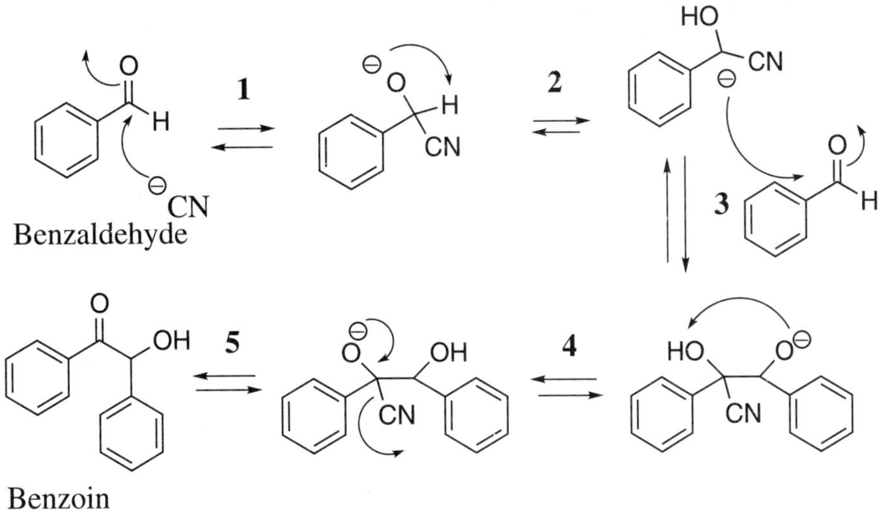

Figure 1. Mechanism of benzoin formation.

3. Which of the following experimental conditions can the student apply to change the value of the rate constant k?

  A. Changing the temperature at which the reaction was performed
  B. Changing the concentration of the reactants
  C. Changing the size of the reaction vessel without changing the volume of the solvent used
  D. No condition other than changing concentrations will change the rate constant

4. The student learns that the benzaldehyde used for the experiment was impure. Furthermore, it was determined that the impurities did not react with the cyanide ion. The calculated rate constant would then be:

  A. higher than the true value of the rate constant.
  B. lower than the true value of the rate constant.
  C. the same as the true value of the rate constant.
  D. impossible to determine with the information given.

5. Step 1 in Figure 1 changes the geometry of the carbonyl carbon from trigonal planar to:

  A. sp^2.
  B. linear.
  C. flat.
  D. tetrahedral.

6. The aromatic ring of benzaldehyde is flat and on the same plane with the aldehyde group. The best explanation for this finding is:

  A. the π-system of the aromatic ring overlaps with the π-system of the carbonyl.
  B. the π-system of the aromatic ring repulses the carbonyl.
  C. hydrogen bonding.
  D. high electronegativity of the oxygen.

7. What type of transformation is step 4 of Figure 1?

  A. Hydride shift
  B. Alkyl migration
  C. Proton transfer
  D. A reduction

8. From the proposed rate law, what is the composition of the rate-limiting step?

  A. Three molecules of benzaldehyde plus six molecules of cyanide
  B. One molecule of benzaldehyde plus two molecules of cyanide
  C. Two molecules of benzaldehyde plus two molecules of cyanide
  D. Two molecules of benzaldehyde plus one molecule of cyanide

9. The student notes that it is theoretically possible for the reaction to go backward. What is the reason that it is more difficult for CN$^-$ to attack benzoin than to attack benzaldehyde?

  A. Steric hindrance
  B. Higher electronegativity of benzoin
  C. CN$^-$ would also displace the hydroxy group
  D. None of the above. The reaction rates should be the same for the attack of benzoin and benzaldehyde.

Passage II (Questions 10–17)

In the planning stages for synthesis, chemists often conceive retrosyntheses; starting with the desired compound, disconnections are made to design a possible forward synthesis. The retrosynthesis of muscarine, the principle component of the hallucinogenic mushroom amanita muscaria, is shown in Figure 2.

The following observations were made when reactions were performed:

Observation 1: The reaction from compound A (muscarine) to compound B is methylation, which can be carried out using MeI.

Observation 2: Reduction of the amide C gives compound B.

Observation 3: The reaction of compound E with dimethylamine [$(CH_3)_2(NH)$] yields compound D via nucleophilic attack followed by opening of the ring. Compound D then closes to form the cyclic compound C.

These observations showed that the retrosynthesis of muscarine was successful when applied to the forward reaction.

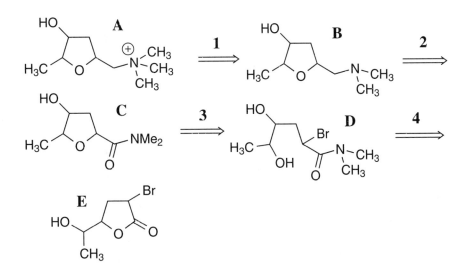

Figure 2.   Retrosynthesis of muscarine.

10. Which of the following is the major spectral characteristic that would differentiate the starting material E from the product A in infrared (IR) spectroscopy?

   A.   A strong stretch at 1750 to 1735 cm⁻¹ in the product that is not in the starting material
   B.   A strong stretch at 1750 to 1735 cm⁻¹ in the starting material that is not in the product
   C.   A stretch at 3400 cm⁻¹ that appears only in the product
   D.   A stretch at 2900 cm⁻¹ that appears only in the starting material

11. What type of intermediate is formed after nucleophilic attack of compound E by dimethylamine?

   A.   A highly substituted carbocation
   B.   A tetrahedral intermediate
   C.   An enolate
   D.   An uncharged intermediate

12. What type of functional group is present on C if sodium hydroxide is added to the lactone E?

   A.   A cyclic ether
   B.   An amine
   C.   A carboxylic acid
   D.   An alcohol

13. Which of the following reagents facilitate conversion of amide C to amine B?

   A.   LiAlH₄/ether
   B.   ⁻OH/H₂O
   C.   O₃/Zn + H₂
   D.   H₃O⁺/H₂O

14. What type of reaction will occur in the formation of D to C?

   A.   An alcohol anion will displace the nitrogen on the amide.
   B.   An alcohol anion will displace the bromide to form a four-membered ring oxirane via an SN2 reaction.
   C.   An alcohol anion will displace the bromide to form a five-membered ring oxirane via an SN2 reaction.
   D.   An alcohol anion will displace the bromide to form a five-membered ring oxirane via an E2 reaction.

15. How many stereocenters are found in muscarine?

   A.   1
   B.   3
   C.   2
   D.   4

16. The product (A) can be distinguished from the starting material (E) by examining their ¹H-NMR spectra. The chemical shift values of the protons of the methyl groups (on the nitrogen):

   A.   are lower than the chemical shift values of the protons of the methyl group of the starting material.
   B.   are higher than the chemical shift values of the protons of the methyl group of the starting material.
   C.   are the same as the chemical shift values of the protons of the methyl group of the starting material.
   D.   cannot be compared qualitatively to the chemical shift values of the protons of the methyl group of the starting material.

17. If the synthesis of muscarine involves three steps, and the yield of step 1 is 100%, that of step 2 is 60%, and that of step 3 is 50%, the overall percent yield (actual yield of product compared to the theoretic yield based on the starting material) would be:

    A.   10%
    B.   210%
    C.   40%
    D.   30%

Passage III (Questions 18–25)

E.J. Corey won the Nobel Prize in chemistry for a lifetime of creative and inventive synthetic organic accomplishments. (±)-Porantherine (1), one of the hundreds of compounds synthesized by Corey and his associates, is an example of how simple starting materials, without any chiral centers, can be combined to form a multiple stereocentered complex molecule. The initial steps in the synthesis of this compound are shown in Figure 3.

18. How many stereocenters does Porantherine (1) contain?

    A.   2
    B.   3
    C.   4
    D.   5

19. In step II, CrO_3:

    A.   oxidizes the secondary hydroxy group to a ketone.
    B.   attaches N to the same carbon as the hydroxy group.
    C.   reacts with the acetal groups.
    D.   oxidizes the hydrogen on the same carbon as the hydroxy group.

20. After examining the cyclization that occurs in step IV, what is the apparent function of the two acetal groups?

    A.   Aiding the cyclization
    B.   "Masking" the ketone functionalities and preventing the attack of a nucleophile at these positions until step IV
    C.   Improving the electrophilic nature of the positions at which they are attached
    D.   "Masking" the ketone functionalities and preventing the attack of an electrophile at these positions until step IV

21. Which of the following occurs if one equivalent of a strong base is added to the product of step IV?

    A.   The ketone is oxidized.
    B.   The ring with the nitrogen breaks.
    C.   The double bond is reduced to a single bond.
    D.   A proton α to the carbonyl is removed, resulting in an enolate.

22. The addition of an acid to Porantherine:

    A.   protonates the nitrogen.
    B.   converts the double bond to a triple bond.
    C.   removes the hydrogens on the double bond.
    D.   deprotonates the hydrogen next to the nitrogen.

23. Which of the following is the hybridization of the N in Porantherine?

    A.   sp
    B. sp^2
    C. sp^3
    D. dsp^3

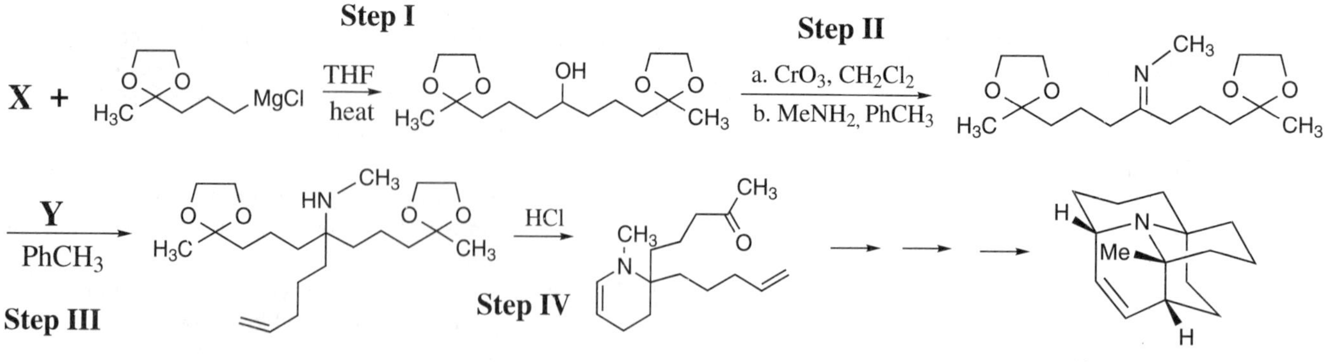

Figure 3. Synthesis of Porantherine.

24. Step III is performed using 3 moles of the product from step II and 2 moles of Y. Assuming that 1 mole of Y reacts with 1 mole of the product from step II, which of the following is the molar yield of step III if the yield is 50%?

    A. 3 moles
    B. 2 moles
    C. 1 mole
    D. Cannot be determined

25. An ^{1}H-NMR of Porantherine is performed. The protons that have resonances that are the farthest downfield, i.e., have the largest chemical shift values (δ ppm scale) are those:

    A. next to the nitrogen.
    B. on the methyl group.
    C. on the double bond.
    D. on the carbons next to the double bond.

Passage IV (Questions 26–32)

A chemistry researcher examined the free radical halogenation of methane by chlorine and bromine and noted that the free radical halogenation reaction proceeded with an initiation step and two propagation steps:

$$\text{Initiation: } X_2 \rightleftharpoons 2X\bullet$$

$$\text{Propagation 1: } X\bullet + CH_4 \rightleftharpoons HX + \bullet CH_3$$

$$\text{Propagation 2: } \bullet CH_3 + X_2 \rightleftharpoons CH_3X + X\bullet$$

The researcher then conducted experiments in which the ΔH and E_{act} (energy of activation) for the halogenation reaction by chlorine and bromine were measured. The data collected are as follows:

	ΔH(chlorine)	E_{act}(chlorine)
Initiation	58	58
Propagation 1	1	3.8
Propagation 2	−25.5	small

	ΔH(bromine)	E_{act}(bromine)
Initiation	46	46
Propagation 1	16.5	18.6
Propagation 2	−24	small

Initiation required only the activation of a few molecules. Heat or light was used to start the initiation process and a chain reaction sustained the propagation steps.

26. The homolytic cleavage of chlorine:

    A. requires more energy than the homolytic cleavage of bromine.
    B. requires less energy than the homolytic cleavage of bromine.
    C. requires the same amount of energy as the homolytic cleavage of bromine.
    D. cannot be qualitatively compared with the energy required to homolytically cleave bromine.

27. The propagation steps continue until the starting materials are consumed. Which halogenation reaction occurs faster if both are run under the same conditions (temperature, solvent, light, etc.)?

    A. Chlorination
    B. Bromination
    C. Neither. Chlorination and bromination occur at the same rate.
    D. Cannot be determined

28. Which of the following characteristics of the mass spectrums of the two halomethanes CANNOT be used to determine their identity?

    A. Different molecular ions (M^+)
    B. Different relative ratios between M^+ and $M^+ + 2$
    C. Different masses of the halogens
    D. Different mass of the methyl radical cation

29. From the data for propagation 1, which of the following halogen radicals is of higher energy?

    A. Cl•
    B. Br•
    C. Neither. They have the same energy.
    D. Cannot be determined from the information provided

30. Disregarding initiation, the overall halogenation reaction involving the homolytic cleavage of the C–H bond of methane requires:

    A. more energy when reacted with Cl•.
    B. less energy when reacted with Cl•.
    C. the same amount of energy in each case.
    D. Cannot be determined

31. The free radical reactions depend on the constant existence of a radical species. Appropriate combinations of radicals may lead to termination. Termination of the reaction will occur in which of the following radical combinations:

    I.   Cl• + Cl•
   II. Cl• + CH_3Cl
  III. •CH_3 + •CH_3

    A. I and II only
    B. I and III only
    C. II and III only
    D. I only

32. Which of the following halomethanes is more polar?

    A. Chloromethane
    B. Bromomethane
    C. Neither. Chloromethane and bromomethane have the same dipole moment.
    D. Cannot determine from the information provided

Passage V (Questions 33–40)

The β-adrenergic compounds are useful in treating a variety of medical conditions. They can provide relief of asthma through direct smooth muscle relaxation of the bronchial tree (aerosol form) and are of value in treating allergic reactions. These compounds bind to a specific receptor on the cell surface and initiate a cyclic adenosine monophosphate (cAMP) second messenger system. Successful clinical use of β-adrenergic drugs has generated interest in synthesizing these compounds in the laboratory.

One possible last step in the synthesis of the relatively selective β_2-adrenergic bronchodilator albuterol (a′-[(*tert*-butylamino)methyl]-4-hydroxy-m-xylene-a,a′-diol) (Figure 4) is the addition of *t*-butylamine to the epoxide. After running the reaction, a chemist was able to separate the starting material from the product through extraction.

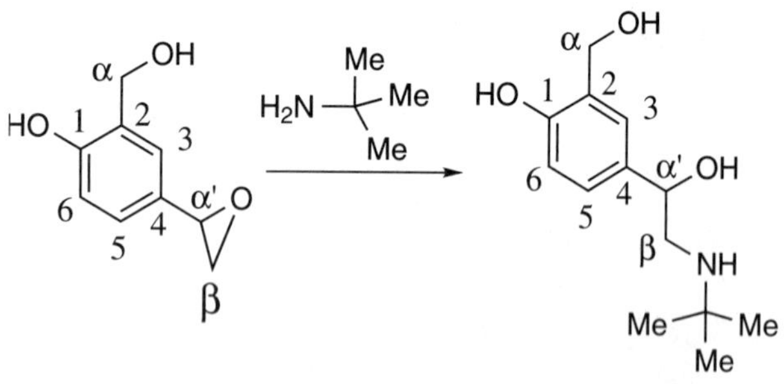

Figure 4. A step in the synthesis of albuterol.

Nucleophiles attack epoxides because of the electronegativity of the oxygen and the strain of the three-membered ring system. The nucleophile in this example has the "choice" of attacking one of two carbons of the epoxide to create two different products. The one shown, however, predominates. Note also that even a hindered nucleophile is successful at attacking the epoxide.

33. What conditions favor attack at the β-carbon of the epoxide?

    A. A small, sterically unhindered nucleophile, under mildly acidic conditions
    B. Strongly electron-donating substituents in the para position.
    C. Strongly acidic conditions
    D. A bulky base under mildly basic conditions

34. Which of the following is the mechanism for the epoxide ring opening?

    A. S_N1
    B. S_N2
    C. E1
    D. E2

35. Which site on the aromatic ring of albuterol is most susceptible to electrophilic aromatic substitution?

    A. 5
    B. 6
    C. 3
    D. None of the above. They are equally susceptible.

36. The proton of the product of the reaction that is most acidic is:

    A. on the nitrogen.
    B. on the α-carbon.
    C. the phenolic proton.
    D. of the α-carbon hydroxy group.

37. Which of the following steps ensures the successful separation of the starting material from the product through extraction?

    A. The aqueous phase should be acidic and it will contain the starting material.
    B. The aqueous phase should be acidic and it will contain the product.
    C. The aqueous phase should be basic and it will contain the product.
    D. None of the above. Extraction would not be an efficient method.

38. If the reaction is run with equal amounts of ethylamine ($EtNH_2$) and *t*-butylamine, which product predominates and why?

A. *t*-Butylamine product predominates because of a greater number of steric interactions.

B. $EtNH_2$ product predominates because of fewer steric interactions.

C. *t*-Butylamine product predominates because of enhanced nucleophilic nature of the nitrogen.

D. *t*-Butylamine and $EtNH_2$ add at about the same rate to give a 50:50 mixture of products.

39. Resonance effects indicate that the hydroxy group donates electron density to the ring. Inductively, the oxygen:

A. withdraws electron density.

B. donates electron density.

C. cancels out the resonance effect.

D. has unpredictable effects.

40. All of the following can be used as solvents for this reaction EXCEPT:

A. acetone.

B. methanol.

C. dichloromethane.

D. tetrahydrofuran.

641

Answers and Explanations to Organic Chemistry Practice Test 2

---

1. **D**   The rate of benzoin formation is determined by the rate law. Following this formula, if the cyanide concentration alone doubles, the rate of benzoin formation would double.

2. **B**   By inserting the increased concentration of reactant in the rate law formula, you arrive at a rate that increases by a factor of 4. Remember that the rate law gives [benzaldehyde]^2.

3. **A**   Rate constants generally are temperature dependent. Altering the concentration of the reactants does not change the value of the rate constant, and vessel size is irrelevant to the rate constant.

4. **B**   If the benzaldehyde was impure, the calculated concentration of the benzaldehyde would be higher than the actual concentration. Because this change does not affect the concentration of cyanide, the rate constant would be lower than the actual value.

5. **D**   In step 1, the cyanide ion attacks the carbonyl and forms an intermediate with four substituents. The hybridization of the carbon is sp^3 after CN$^-$ attack and is therefore tetrahedral. Recall the geometry associated with basic reaction intermediates.

6. **A**   The compound is stabilized through the extended conjugation of the π-system. For this to occur, the p orbitals must be lined up, which makes the aromatic ring planar and on the same plane with the carbonyl. Choice B is not the best answer because repulsion is not a factor. Choices C and D are eliminated because no significant hydrogen bonds form within the benzaldehyde molecule, and the electronegativity of the oxygen does not in itself account for the shape of this molecule.

7. **C**   Choice A is incorrect because a hydrogen ion is transferred, not the hydride, H$^-$. Choice B is incorrect because an alkyl group does not migrate in step 4. Choice D is not the best answer because no reduction occurs here.

8. **D**   Because the rate of the reaction depends on the rate-limiting step, two molecules of benzaldehyde plus one molecule of cyanide constitute the composition of the rate-limiting step. The mechanism of the reaction (Figure 1) provides the answer.

9. **A**   This reaction is an example of nucleophilic attack, and the rate therefore depends on the ease of attack. Consider the steric issues in this question. With a greater number substituents on the electrophile, the attack is more difficult.

---

10. **B**   Recall the review of IR spectral characteristics in Chapter 12 of the Organic Chemistry Review Notes. A strong stretch at 1750–1735 is indicative of a lactone or ester. This functional group is in the starting material but not in the product.

11. **B**   You are told that nucleophilic attack of compound E gives compound D, followed by ring opening. On the basis of this information and careful inspection of the retrosynthesis mechanism, you can predict that dimethylamine attacks

the carbon of the carbonyl of compound E to give an sp³ hybridized intermediate. The next step involves the breaking of the C–O bond of the lactone.

12. **C** The hydroxide adds to the most electrophilic carbon, the carbonyl, and opens the ring in a manner similar to the amide formation described previously. The hydroxide then attacks the bromine to close the ring to form compound C, a carboxylic acid instead of an amide.

13. **A** Look for a strong reducing agent. Only LiAlH₄/ether can reduce this amide to the amine; the other choices either hydrolyze or oxidize amides.

14. **C** Determine which mechanism gives the desired product (substitution or elimination). Looking at the structure of compound C, a substitution reaction likely occurs. No elimination occurs (no double bonds forming), which eliminates choice D. Choice A is incorrect because simple displacement does not occur. When evaluating choices B and C, remember that five-membered rings are more stable than four-membered rings. Thus, the alcohol anion would displace the bromide to form a five-membered ring oxirane by a substitution mechanism.

15. **B** Recall that stereocenters or chiral centers are marked by carbons attached to four different substituents. The three carbons are marked in the following diagram:

16. **B** The protons on the nitrogen are farther downfield because of the electron-withdrawing effect of the N+ (see the review NMR spectra and the principle of chemical shift in Chapter 12 of the Organic Chemistry Review Notes).

17. **D** If you have 100 moles of starting material, your yield after step 1 would be 100%, or 100 moles. After step 2, your yield would be only 60 moles. After step 3, your yield would be 50% of 60 moles, or 30 moles, which is only 30% of the original starting material. Therefore, the overall percent yield is 30%.

18. **C** The number of carbons attached to four different substituents determines the number of chiral or stereocenters. An interesting feature of this synthesis is how starting materials with no chiral centers can be turned into a molecule with four chiral centers.

19. **A** CrO₃ is an oxidizing agent. It is useful in oxidizing a secondary alcohol to a ketone. The ketone formed is then susceptible to nucleophilic attack by methylamine. Choices B and C can be eliminated because they do not describe oxidation reactions. Choice D is incorrect because CrO₃ does not oxidize hydrogen.

20. **B** Acetals are typically used as protecting groups for carbonyls. The acetals are not susceptible to attack and yield the corresponding carbonyl on treatment with acid. Choices A and C incorrectly describe the properties of acetyl groups. In choice D, the terms nucleophile and electrophile are reversed. As stated, this answer is incorrect.

21. **D** When given a strong base, try to find a proton that can be removed easily by the base. Recall that the hydrogen attached to the α position is the most acidic proton of the molecule and is the easiest to remove. Addition of base does not oxidize the ketone or break the ring. Strong base also does not lead to reduction of the double bond.

22. **A** The addition of acid to this compound tends to result in its protonation. The nitrogen is the most basic atom of the molecule. Choices B, C, and D are incorrect because the addition of acid alone does not lead to triple bond formation, and the acid will not lead to deprotonation.

23. **C** Recall that the nitrogen of amines is sp³ hybridized and the lone pair occupies one of the sp³ hybridized orbitals. In the structure of this molecule, the lone pair of N occupies the fourth sp³ orbital.

24. **C** Y is the limiting reagent. Therefore, you need only to consider the number of moles of the limiting reagent present: 50% of 2 moles is 1 mole.

25. **C** Recall from Chapter 12 of the Organic Chemistry Review Notes that the protons of the double bond are highly deshielded and are the farthest downfield.

PASSAGE IV

26. **A** Refer to the data tables and note that the energy of activation of homolytic cleavage of chlorine is higher than that of bromine.

27. **A** The energy of activation of the propagation steps is lower for chlorine; thus, chlorination occurs faster.

28. **D** Unlike the characteristics in Choices A to C, which indicate the presence of different halogens, the methyl radical cation has the same mass in either case, and thus, cannot be used to determine the identity of the unknown halomethanes. (See the review of mass spectroscopy in Chapter 12 of the Organic Chemistry Review Notes.)

29. **A** That Cl• is higher in energy is reflected by the lower E_{act} of the homolytic cleavage of the C–H bond of methane.

30. **C** The ΔH of the cleavage is different for each halogen, but this fact does not change the amount of energy required to break the bond. Note that the chlorine radical is of higher energy, and it is easier for this radical to break the bond.

31. **B** Termination occurs when two radicals come together. Both statements I and III demonstrate this process; choice B is the best answer.

32. **A** Recall the concepts of polarity and electronegativity of atoms within molecules. Chlorine is more electronegative than bromine, which makes chloromethane more polar than bromomethane.

PASSAGE V

33. **D** Steric hindrance prevents attack at α position. Remember that basic conditions favor nucleophilic attack. Choices A and C are incorrect because bulky bases are favored in mild basic conditions. Choice B is incorrect, in part, because at the β position away from the ring, the electron donating/withdrawing properties of groups attacking the ring are not as important as the nature of the nucleophile and the conditions in which nucleophilic attack occurs.

34. **B** Choices C and D are eliminated because double bonds are not formed. S_N2 is favored over S_N1 (choice A) because the nucleophile is strong and is a primary amine. Recall that the lone pair electrons allow the amine to act as a nucleophile, and ammonia (no substituents) and primary amines make the best nucleophiles because of the lack of steric hinderance. As the level of substitution increases, it becomes increasingly difficult for the lone pair electrons to reach the electrophile to form a bond. Also recall that amines tend to undergo S_N2 reactions, and an inversion of stereochemistry occurs after nucleophilic attack because of the Walden inversion.

35. **B** Phenols activate ortho and para positions toward electrophilic attack, making position 6 the most susceptible to electrophilic substitution.

36. **C** The phenoxide anion is stabilized through resonance effects. Therefore, the phenolic hydrogen is the most acidic proton.

37. **B** An acidic aqueous phase contains the product with a protonated nitrogen. Extraction back into the organic phase is possible by making the solution more alkaline, until the isoelectric point of the molecule is reached.

38. **B** Ethylamine has fewer steric interactions when it attacks the electrophile. Like S_N2 reactions, the less bulk the nucleophile possesses, the better nucleophile the compound can be.

39. **A** Because oxygen is more electronegative than C, electrons are inductively pulled out of the ring. In this case, however, resonance predominates over inductive effects. The net result of the hydroxy substituent is electron donation to the ring.

40. **B** A reagent that gives an undesired side reaction in this situation cannot be used. Such a reagent is often a reactive compound. Methanol may open the epoxide and cause undesirable side reactions (although the rate is slow).

ANSWERS AND
EXPLANATIONS
TO ORGANIC
CHEMISTRY
PRACTICE TEST 2

644

ORGANIC CHEMISTRY PRACTICE TEST 3

Time: 45 minutes

Directions: This test contains as many organic chemistry passages as you may encounter on the real MCAT. The time allotted approximates the time allowed on a real MCAT to solve the given number of questions. Choose one best answer for each question.

Passage I (Questions 1–9)

Three amino acids (**A, B,** and **C**), illustrated in Figure 1 at pH = 7, are isolated from protein X. The only amino acids found in this protein, **A, B,** and **C,** are found in the ratio of 5:3:2. Electrophoresis was performed on protein X.

Electrophoresis can be used to separate proteins or fragment of proteins by their overall charge and size. Negatively charged molecules are attracted to the cathode and positively charged molecules are attracted to the anode. Reverse-phase liquid chromatography can also be used to separate charged molecules, such as those shown in Figure 1.

The hydrolysis of an amide bond displayed in Figure 2 is similar to the reaction used to break apart protein X, although the hydrolysis of protein X was acid catalyzed. When subjected to hydrolytic proteases, a similar mechanism is involved in breaking the amide bond.

1. If protein X is subjected to electrophoresis at pH = 7, where does protein X migrate?

   A. Anode
   B. Protein X does not migrate.
   C. Cathode
   D. Protein X is unstable at pH = 7.

2. Protein X is completely hydrolyzed, and the pH is lowered to 2. The products of this hydrolysis are subjected to electrophoresis. If some migration occurs toward the cathode, it would most likely be amino acid:

   A. A
   B. B
   C. C
   D. D

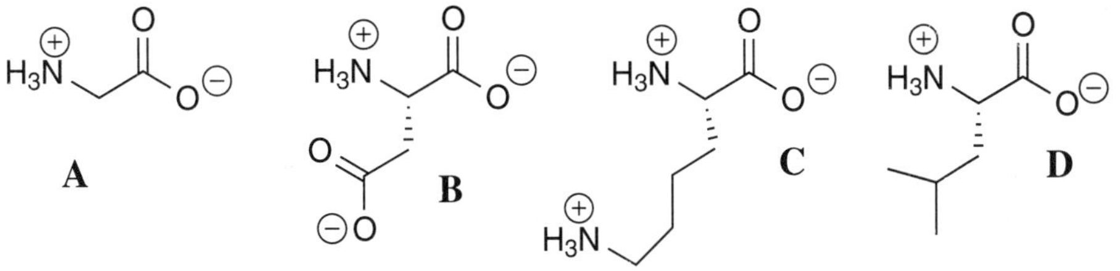

Figure 1. Amino acids **A, B,** and **C** found in protein X. A fourth molecule, D, is also shown.

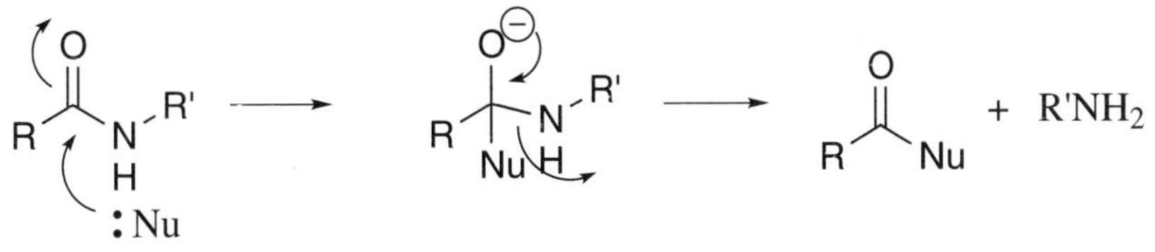

Figure 2. Hydrolysis of an amide bond.

645

3. Amino acid **B** at pH = 2 is titrated with base. Where does **B** act as a good buffer?

   A. $pH = pK_1$
   B. $pH = 7$
   C. $pH = 1 \times 10^{-7}$
   D. $pH = 2 + \log(10^7)$

4. Which of the following protein X components, at pH 7, migrates to the anode?

   A. **A**
   B. **B**
   C. **C**
   D. **A** and **B**

5. At pH = 7, amino acid **A** is known as:

   A. an enolate ion.
   B. antiperiplanar.
   C. zwitterionic.
   D. isoelectronic.

6. Which of the following molecules has the longest retention time when subjected to reverse-phase liquid chromatography?

   A. **A**
   B. **B**
   C. **C**
   D. **D**

7. A small protein **Z**, consisting of all L-amino acids (*R*-absolute stereochemistry), forms an α-helix. If all of the residues of protein **Z** are converted to their D-counterparts (*S*-absolute stereochemistry) to form protein **Y**, what would you predict about the tertiary structure of **Y**?

   A. **Y** is also an α-helix.
   B. **Y** is a β-sheet.
   C. **Y** is a linear peptide chain.
   D. **Y** is a left-handed helix.

8. Some of the most effective inhibitors mimic the transition state of the base-catalyzed hydrolysis of the amide bond. This transition state would therefore resemble:

   A. sp^2 hybridized carbon with two C–O bonds.
   B. carbonyl carbon converted to an sp^3 hybridized carbon.
   C. sp hybridized carbon.
   D. carbocation.

9. If protein X contains some residues with hydrophobic side chains, such as valine, isoleucine, and leucine, in addition to **A, B,** and **C,** describe the organization of these residues in the protein when it is placed in water.

   A. **A, B,** and **C** on the outside; valine, isoleucine, and leucine on the inside
   B. **A, B,** and **C** on the inside; valine, isoleucine, and leucine on the outside
   C. Side chains of all amino acids directed outward, toward the water
   D. Side chains of all amino acids directed inward, away from the water

Passage II (Questions 10–16)

Phenol (Figure 3), when compared with the proton of benzene, has a low pK_a (~10). The presence of the hydroxy group dramatically increases the tendency for electrophiles to add to the benzene ring. If the hydrogen of the phenol hydroxy group is substituted, the benzene ring is still activated toward electrophilic aromatic substitution. The electrophiles tend to react at specific positions on the phenol ring. When the ring is substituted by a nitro group, the pK_a of the phenolic hydrogen is diminished.

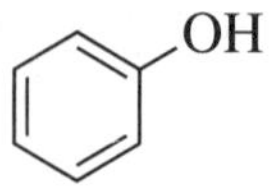

Figure 3.   Phenol.

Phenols favor the enol form because of aromatic stability. The ketone form, which is not aromatic, is less favored. Phenol can also be used for polymerization. The earliest black plastic telephones as well as the hard black handles on frying pans are made from a polymer of formaldehyde (methanal) with phenol.

10. The pK_a of phenol is low because:

    A. the hydrogen is sterically unhindered.
    B. the anion formed is stabilized by delocalization into the benzene ring.
    C. the cation formed is stabilized by delocalization into the benzene ring.
    D. None of the above are true (a pK_a of 10 is NOT low for an alcohol).

11. Electrophiles will attack phenol at:

    A. ortho and meta.
    B. para and meta.
    C. meta only.
    D. ortho and para.

12. Which of the following reagents most likely alkylates the phenolic oxygen?

   A. CH_2Cl_2
   B. $CHCl_3$
   C. ICH_3
   D. None of the above

13. At which positions on the ring, if substituted with NO_2, do you expect to find the largest decrease in pK_a?

   A. ortho and meta
   B. meta and para
   C. ortho and para
   D. Any position

14. Which of the following compounds initiates the polymerization described in the passage?

   A. Benzoyl peroxide
   B. Aluminum chloride
   C. Potassium hydroxide
   D. Aluminum chloride and potassium hydroxide

15. Which of the following conditions would you use to separate phenol from a reaction mixture by extraction, assuming that you want the phenol in the water layer?

   A. Acetone and water at pH 6
   B. Diethyl ether and water at pH 8
   C. Chloroform and water at pH 11
   D. Dichloromethane and water at pH 7

16. Which of the following conditions is best for separating phenol from a reaction mixture by extraction, assuming that you want phenol in the organic layer?

   A. Benzene and water at pH 10
   B. Acetone and water at pH 10
   C. Chloroform and water at pH 11
   D. Benzene and water at pH 4

Passage III (Questions 17–24)

Carbonyl compounds exist in a dynamic equilibrium with their keto and corresponding enol forms. Typically, the keto form dominates; however, the amount of the enol form in the equilibrium is noticeable in some cases. For example, 2,4-hexadione has a keto-enol ratio of 76:24. A pictorial explanation for this relatively large enol portion of the equilibrium is provided in Figure 4.

Carbonyl compounds with hydrogens on the α-carbon are rapidly convertible with an enol form. This rapid interconversion is known as tautomerism. The enolization can be catalyzed by either acid or base.

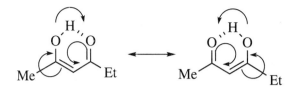

Figure 4. Structures associated with the keto-enol forms of 2,4-hexadione.

17. The ketone and enol forms are called:

   A. epimers.
   B. enantiomers.
   C. tautomers.
   D. mutamers.

18. Which of the following explains why the keto form dominates this equilibrium?

   A. Carbon is more electronegative than oxygen.
   B. The C=O bond π-bond is stronger than C=C π-bond.
   C. LeChatelier's principle favors the less stable compound.
   D. The oxygen cannot form π-bonds.

19. The proton nuclear magnetic resonance (NMR) spectrum of 2,4-pentadione displays:

   A. two singlets, one at 2 ppm and the other at about 3–4 ppm.
   B. one singlet at about 2 ppm.
   C. three singlets, two at 2 ppm, the other at about 3–4 ppm.
   D. two quartets (2 ppm) and 1 doublet (3–4 ppm).

20. The enol form of 2,4-pentadione is stabilized by:

   A. electron delocalization.
   B. the conjugated π-system.
   C. the existence of two resonance forms.
   D. all of the above.

21. Further stability on this enol form is imparted by:

   A. a cyclic transition state held together by a hydrogen bond.
   B. an sp^2 σ-bond.
   C. terminal methyl groups withdrawing electron density.
   D. both **A** and **C**.

647

22. Why does the enol form of 2,4-cyclohexadien-1-one dominate the equilibrium?

    A. The enol form has more hydrogen bonding.
    B. The enol form has less hydrogen bonding.
    C. The enol form is aromatic and therefore is more stable.
    D. The keto form is highly water sensitive.

23. The temperature of a solution of 2,4-pentadione is decreased. How does this change affect the keto-enol ratio?

    A. The ratio increases.
    B. The ratio decreases.
    C. The ratio remains the same.
    D. The effect cannot be predicted.

24. If the ethyl group in 2,4-hexadione is replaced by a phenyl group, the enol is:

    A. stabilized because of extended conjugation.
    B. destabilized because of extended conjugation.
    C. stabilized because of reduced resonance.
    D. destabilized because of reduced resonance.

Passage IV (Questions 25–32)

The Robinson ring annulation (Figure 5) is a carbonyl condensation that forms a ring. Intramolecular reactions occur relatively rapidly, and when the number of carbons and/or oxygens is sufficient to form a five- or six-membered ring, ring formation is highly favored over the condensation of two different molecules.

The methyl groups of the ring junction indicate that the ring junction is *trans*. Furthermore, it is energetically favorable for both rings to be in chair conformations (Figure 6).

Although the overall reaction in Figure 5 appears complex, the mechanism is simple. Compound 1 is converted to the diol and compound 2 forms. The diol is then oxidized by HIO_4 to the di-aldehyde, resulting in compound 3. Treat-

ment with base forms an enolate and attacks the other aldehyde to close the ring. Products **4a** and **4b** are formed.

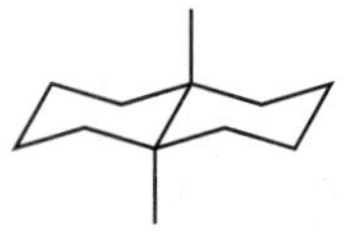

Figure 6.   Energetically favorable chair conformations.

25. Which of the following reagents **X** will yield the *cis* diol?

    A. $LiAlH_4$
    B. $KMnO_4$
    C. OsO_4
    D. $KMnO_4$ and OsO_4

26. The bulk of the phenyl ring forces the phenyl ring to:

    A. be in the equatorial position.
    B. be in the axial position.
    C. switch between axial and equatorial with no difficulty.
    D. force the ring junction to become *cis*.

27. The two hydroxy groups:

    A. occupy equatorial positions.
    B. occupy axial positions.
    C. occupy one axial and one equatorial position.
    D. are enantiomers.

28. Which of the following reagents would convert **1** to **3** without first forming the diol?

    A. HIO_4
    B. O_3, Zn/H_2O
    C. $CO_2/base$
    D. $O_3/NaIO_4$

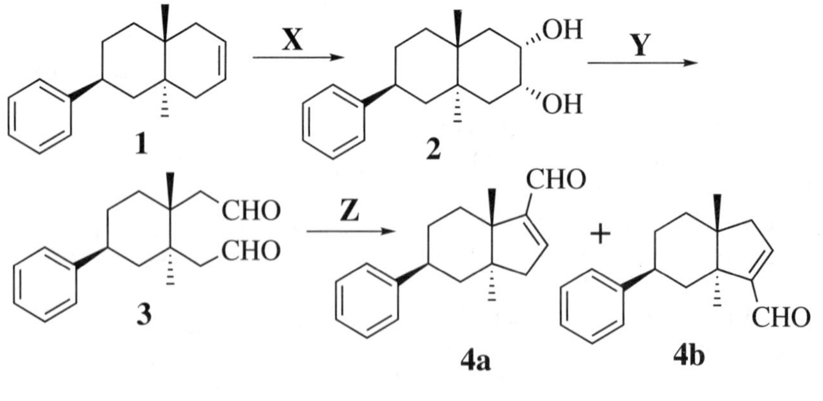

Figure 5.   Robinson ring annulation.

29. What type and how much of reagent **Z** is necessary for rings to form?

    A.   A hindered acid, 1 equivalent
    B.   A hindered base, 1 equivalent
    C.   Hindered acid, 2 equivalents
    D.   Hindered base, 2 equivalents

30. Which of the following explains why two different products, **4a** and **4b,** are formed?

    A.   Selective deprotonation does not occur.
    B.   Selective dehydroxylation does not occur.
    C.   Through resonance, the intermediates switch from the intermediate of one product to the intermediate of the other.
    D.   None of the above.

31. The driving force for the elimination of water and the formation of the double bond after condensation is:

    A.   formation of an aromatic system.
    B.   reduction of steric hindrance.
    C.   removal of the destabilizing oxygen and hydrogens.
    D.   formation of a resonance-stabilized conjugated π system.

32. Under which of the following circumstances will this compound NOT show a net rotation of plane-polarized light?

    A.   When the ring junction is *cis* and the hydroxy groups are *trans* with respect to each other
    B.   When the ring junction is *cis* and the hydroxy groups are *cis* with respect to each other
    C.   When the ring junction is *trans* or the hydroxy groups are *trans* with respect to each other
    D.   When the ring junction is *cis* or the hydroxy groups are *trans* with respect to each other

Passage V (Questions 33–40)

Drug companies create hundreds of analogs of an active compound to improve certain characteristics. By placing substituents on drug **X** (Figure 7), a drug company could alter the activity of the drug against a certain enzyme.

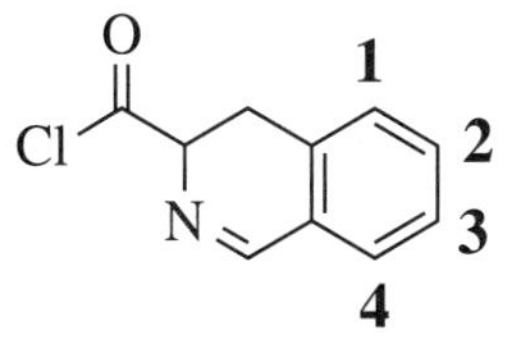

Figure 7.   Structure of drug X.

The results of several analogs of the drug are displayed in Table 1. Each position is presented with several possible substituents and their IC_{50} values (IC_{50} = concentration of the drug needed to inhibit the enzyme by 50%).

TABLE I. Analogs of drug X.

Position and Substituent	IC_{50} (μM)
1F	0.315
2F	0.138
3F	3.13
4F	0.230
1,4F$_2$	0.010
1Me	0.300
2Me	3.13
3Me	4.13
4Me	0.138
1,4Me$_2$	0.50
4Et	0.65
1Cl	0.58
2Cl	0.32
3Cl	4.13
4Cl	1.93
1,4Cl$_2$	0.048
4OMe	0.650
4OH	1.30
4NO$_2$	61.3
4NH$_2$	167.0
X	0.53

33. In all cases, substitution at positions **2** and **3**:

    A.   reduces the activity of the compound without regard to the electronic characteristics of the substituent.
    B.   increases the activity of the compound without regard to the electronic characteristics of the substituent.
    C.   maintains the same level of reverse transcriptase inhibitory activity.
    D.   cannot be qualitatively determined.

649

34. Apparently, most of the electron-withdrawing groups at position **1** or **4**:

   A. decrease the activity of the compound.
   B. increase the activity of the compound.
   C. keep activity the same as for **Z**.
   D. have no predictable effect on the activity of the compound based on the data provided.

35. Analysis of the data suggests that the size of the substituent is an important factor in the drug's action on the enzyme. This effect is displayed by the fact that:

   A. the nitro group is electron withdrawing but the activity of the derivative is low.
   B. the ethyl group at position **4** decreases activity.
   C. the ethyl group at position **4** increases activity.
   D. the nitro group is electron withdrawing but the activity of the derivative is low, and the ethyl group at position **4** decreases activity.

36. The low activity of the 4-NH_2 derivative can be explained by:

   A. its size.
   B. the electronegative nature of NH_2.
   C. the electron-donating nature of NH_2.
   D. both **A** and **C**.

37. A butyl group at position **4** would:

   A. increase activity of the compound.
   B. decrease activity of the compound.
   C. maintain the same level of activity.
   D. form a drug that would likely be effective against bacteria.

38. What effect seems to dictate the high level of activity of the halogens at **1** and **4**?

   A. Resonance effects
   B. Inductive effect
   C. Inhibitive effects
   D. Substitutive effects

39. Why is there a loss of activity when the OH group is placed on the ring and a gain in activity when the methoxy group is placed on the ring?

   A. The methoxy group is more electron donating.
   B. The hydroxy group is more electron donating.
   C. The methoxy group resembles the ethyl group in size and shape and the ethyl group substitution only slightly decreases the activity.
   D. Both **B** and **C**

40. A more accurate idea of the electronic effect of substituents on the ring could be gained by:

   A. using ethyl groups as substituents.
   B. using ethoxy groups as substituents.
   C. using iodine, bromine, or both as substituents.
   D. using two nitro groups as substituents.

ANSWERS AND
EXPLANATIONS
TO ORGANIC
CHEMISTRY
PRACTICE TEST 3

650

Answers and Explanations to Organic Chemistry Practice Test 3

1. **C** First, determine the net charge of the protein at pH = 7. Because the ratio of the amino acids is 5:3:2, the net charge of protein X will be negative at neutral pH. Amino acid **A** has no net charge at pH 7 (carboxyl group negative, amino group positive). Amino acid **B** has a net negative charge at neutral pH, because it has two deprotonated carboxyl groups. Amino acid **C** has a net positive charge at pH 7, because of the two protonated amino groups, although there are more amino acid B residues than amino acid **C** residues in the protein. Because of the net negative charge for the protein, it is attracted to the positive terminal (cathode).

2. **B** Negatively charged molecules are attracted to the cathode. Amino acid **B** has the greatest chance of migrating to the cathode because it has two carboxyl groups (these are negatively charged when not protonated). Recall that the pK_a for the carboxyl group is about 2.3, and at this point, about one half of these groups are protonated. Choices **A** and **D** have only an amino and carboxyl group, and are less likely than amino acid **B** to carry any negative charge. Choice **C** can be eliminated, because amino acid **C** carries a strong positive charge at neutrality.

3. **A** A buffer resists changes in pH. When the $pH = pK_1$, the [acid]/[base] = 1, so a small change in either acid or base will not make a significant change in the pH.

4. **C** The anode is negatively charged. Assuming neutral pH (pH = 7), the positively charged amino acid will migrate to the anode. Amino acid **C** has a positive charge at neutral pH.

5. **C** Amino acids that are dipolar ions (i.e., NH_3^+ and COO^- on the same molecule) are zwitterions. The isoelectric point is the pH at which there is no net migration of the amino acid in an electric field. Enolate ion and antiperiplanar are terms that have nothing to do with amino acids and charged side groups.

6. **D** Recall that in reverse-phase liquid chromatography, differences in polarity separate compounds. Molecule D is the least polar and will therefore have a longer retention time in the column.

7. **D** When viewed in a Fischer projection, the L-amino acids have their amino group on the left and the D-amino acids have the amino group on the right. The L and D forms of an amino acid are generally enantiomers. Thus, when a protein constructed of D-amino acids folds up, you expect it to form the mirror image of the L-amino acid-containing protein. You are told that the L-amino acid protein formed an α-helix. Replacement of the L-amino acids with their D-amino acid counterparts yields the mirror image structure, a left-handed helix.

8. **B** Generally, a nucleophile attacks the electrophilic carbonyl carbon of the amide, which is a tetrahedral transition state.

9. **A** **A, B,** and **C** are charged and hydrophilic. Valine, isoleucine, and leucine are hydrophobic and will bury the side chains in the protein to avoid contact with water.

SECT. III
ORGANIC
CHEMISTRY
PRACTICE
TEST 3

651

10. **B** Several resonance forms can be drawn for phenol when it is deprotonated. The anion formed is stabilized by delocalization into the benzene ring.

11. **D** The hydroxyl group is a strong activating ortho–para director. The lone pair of electrons on the oxygen can donate electrons into the ring to help stabilize the carbocation intermediate.

12. **C** To alkylate the phenolic oxygen ICH_3 as a reagent would result in S_N2 substitution on the methyl group. Choices **A** and **B** do not have an appropriate leaving group allowing substitution.

13. **C** Placement of electron-withdrawing groups (NO_2) on the ring enhances acidity. The addition of electron withdrawing groups enhances the stability of the conjugate base by the inductive effect. The location of placement of these groups also affects acidity. In the ortho and para positions, the anion can be stabilized through resonance with the electron withdrawing group. This stabilization will not occur when the group is in the meta position.

14. **D** Initiating the polymerization reaction is an electrophilic aromatic substitution process, which is best catalyzed by Lewis acids and bases (choices B and C).

15. **C** At high pH, phenol is safely above its pK_a and is most water soluble. Chloroform and water are immiscible. Thus, at a high pH, such as pH 11, the phenol is most water soluble and will dissolve in the water layer. Phenol will clearly separate from the chloroform layer.

16. **D** Benzene and water are virtually immiscible, and phenol is most water insoluble at pH at which it still has its hydrogen (acidic pH).

17. **C** Recall the process of keto-enol tautomerization. Tautomers are a form of isomers, yet they are interconvertible with one another. Enantiomers are non-superimposable mirror images. Epimers are carbohydrates that differ about carbon 2.

18. **B** The carbonyl form is more stable than the enol. The carbonyl π-bond is stronger than the carbon-carbon π-bond of the enol because of the greater electronegativity of oxygen.

19. **A** Recall nuclear magnetic resonance (NMR) spectra and the principles behind NMR. The two methyl groups associated with 2,4-pentadione are magnetically equivalent with no splitting. Thus, it will form two singlets.

20. **D** All of these factors contribute to the stability of the enol. Thus, choice **D** is the best answer.

21. **A** Choice **C** is eliminated because methyl groups do not withdraw electron density. Therefore, choice **D** is not the best answer. A short-lived hydrogen bond does form to stabilize the transition state. Although the energy of the interaction is small (i.e., to the energy of a bond), the hydrogen bond does make a difference and provides further stability.

22. **C** Draw the structure of 2,4-cyclohexadien-1-one. Note that it is aromatic and stabilized by resonance. Also note that the enol form of this molecule is phenol. Hydrogen bonds may be short-lived contributors to the transition states of some enols, but they alone do not explain the stability of the enol form of the molecule in question.

23. **A** With a lower temperature, less energy is available to convert the ketone to the enol. Thus, the keto:enol ratio increases.

24. **A** Both enol forms are more highly stabilized in the enol versus the ketone form (especially the form on the right side of Figure 4) because of extended conjugation opportunities. Choice **B** is incorrect because extended conjugation increases stability. Choices **C** and **D** are incorrect because resonance increases with the addition of phenol.

25. **D**   Oxidizing agents B and C both result in a *cis* diol. LiAlH$_4$ is a reducing agent.

26. **A**   Movement into the equatorial position allows the bulk of the phenyl ring to minimize 1,3-diaxial interactions. Axial position causes more steric interactions.

27. **C**   Recall the chair forms for six-membered rings. The *cis* diol on a chair ring has one group axial and one group equatorial.

28. **B**   A special reagent is needed to convert to an aldehyde without becoming an alcohol. With NaIO$_4$, carboxylic acids are formed.

29. **B**   The focus of this question is whether an acid or a base is needed. A base, which is strong enough to abstract a proton, is appropriate to carry out this reaction. Only one enolate per molecule is necessary.

30. **A**   The difference between **4a** and **4b** centers on the fact that selective deprotonation by base does not occur. Both protons are chemically equivalent, although one may be slightly more hindered than the other, and the base cannot differentiate.

31. **D**   Resonance-stabilized products are favored. The formation of products with lower energy is usually favored (unless the conditions are adjusted otherwise). Choice **A** is not as good an answer as choice **D** in that aromaticity is not as important as resonance in terms of stability. Steric issues are difficult to determine because the molecules are so bulky. Choice **C** is incorrect because oxygen and hydrogen are not destabilizing.

32. **B**   This compound is a *meso* compound if both the ring junction is *cis* and the hydroxy groups are *cis* with respect to each other. Under these conditions, the compound would show no net rotation of plane polarized light.

33. **A**   Substitution at positions 2 and 3 decreases activity regardless of what substituent is placed. A decrease in activity is reflected in higher IC$_{50}$ values.

34. **B**   The electron-withdrawing groups, such as the halogens, show low IC$_{50}$ values in positions 1 and 4. Recall that a low IC$_{50}$ value means higher activity.

35. **D**   Choices **A** and **B** are true. The nitro group is larger than the Me group, and some unfavorable charge interactions may occur because of the structure of the nitro group.

36. **C**   Size is not a factor because of the structural similarity of NH$_2$ to Me. This fact eliminates choices **A** and **D**. The electron donating character of the amine is the best explanation for the low activity of this group. Choice **B** is incorrect because the amine group chemistry is based on the basicity and electron-donating properties of the amino nitrogen, not the electronegativity of the nitrogen.

37. **B**   Butyl and ethyl behave similarly; if ethyl decreases the activity, then so will butyl. Thus, choices **A** and **C** are incorrect. Choice **D** is unsupported and should be eliminated.

38. **B**   The halogens play an inductive role. Halogens cannot donate or remove electrons through a resonance mechanism, so choice **A** is not the best answer. Choice **C** goes against the tone of the question. Choice **D** is irrelevant and is unsupported by the data provided.

39. **D**   Adding a hydroxy to the ring decreases activity. This effect suggests that the hydroxy group donates electrons to the ring. Choice **C** is reasonable and is difficult to eliminate. Choice **A** is not the best answer because addition of the methoxy group increases activity. Both choices **B** and **C** may play a role, although the data are not sufficient to strictly define the role of each factor. Therefore, choice **D** is the best answer.

40. **C**   Using the halogens iodine and bromine as substituents creates a natural progression of electronegativities, clarifying the role of the electronic effect. A progression of trends would not be as clear with the use of ethoxy, nitro, or ethyl groups.

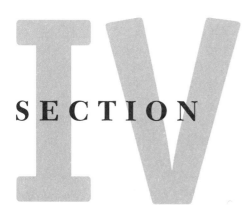

SECTION IV

Preparation for Verbal Reasoning and the Writing Sample

....

A. **The Verbal Reasoning Section: Information and Strategies**

B. **Verbal Reasoning Practice Tests**

C. **The Writing Sample: Basic Strategies and Sample Student Essays**

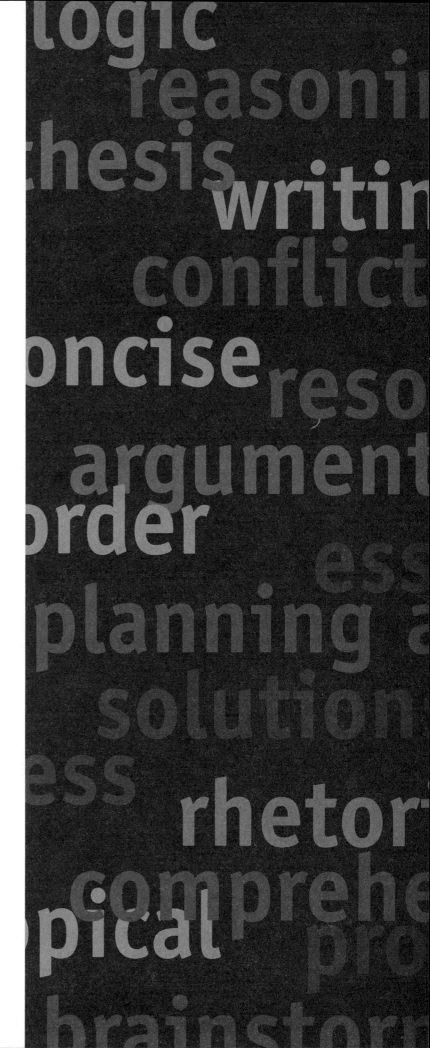

The Verbal Reasoning Section:

INFORMATION AND STRATEGIES

verbal

reasonir

The Verbal Reasoning Section: Information and Strategies

I. Format and Content of the Verbal Reasoning Section

INTRODUCTORY REMARKS

Most experts agree that the Verbal Reasoning test has become the most difficult section of the MCAT. Most of the students that you will compete against are strong readers. The competition is tough, and the Verbal Reasoning test is difficult to prepare for. On the Verbal Reasoning section of the MCAT, you have 85 minutes to read 9 passages, 500–600 words each, and answer 6–10 multiple-choice questions that follow each passage. The passages are complex and cover subjects that you may not be familiar with. Recent MCAT passages have emphasized philosophy, the arts, history, the humanities, and the social sciences.

Some students have difficulty completing the Verbal Reasoning section, because they read too slowly. Frequently, this problem occurs in students in which English is their second language. In addition, students who finish the Verbal Reasoning section may do so at the expense of rushing and carelessness. This section of the book helps you understand the structure of the Verbal Reasoning test and tune into useful strategies. Following this section are three full-length Verbal Reasoning practice tests, so that you can practice the strategies discussed. The most effective way to improve verbal reasoning skills is to practice verbal reasoning passages. Focus on accuracy and timing.

THE VERBAL
REASONING
SECTION:
INFORMATION
AND STRATEGIES

658

FORMAT

The Verbal Reasoning section of the MCAT is the first of four general sections administered. You are given 85 minutes to complete this section, which contains approximately 9 passages that are 500–600 words in length. Each passage is followed by a set of 6–10 multiple-choice questions; there is a total of 65 questions.

The difficulty level of the multiple-choice questions is averaged, and an average difficulty level is assigned to each set of questions. Although sets of questions in the Verbal Reasoning section often progress from least to most difficult, each passage will contain both easy and more difficult questions.

CONTENT

TOPICS COVERED

The passages in the Verbal Reasoning section are taken from a variety of disciplines in the social sciences, humanities, and natural sciences (**Note:** There are no passages covering the biological or physical sciences). The following disciplines may appear on the test:

- **Social sciences,** including anthropology, archeology, business, economics, government, history, political science, law, psychology, and sociology

- **Humanities,** including architecture, art, art history, dance, ethics, literary criticism, music, philosophy, religion, and theater

- **Natural sciences,** including astronomy, botany, computer science, ecology, geology, meteorology, natural history, and technology

The passages address many fields, and thus a wide variety of information is covered. However, you are not expected to have knowledge in any of these areas. The Verbal Reasoning section is designed to test your ability to read and comprehend information and then evaluate and apply this information. **All of the information you need to answer the questions is contained in the passage.**

TYPES OF PASSAGES

There are three types of passages that appear on the test:

1. **Narrative.** This type of passage is a record of events and activities that occurred during a given time period. A narrative usually tells a story.

2. **Expository/Informative.** This type of passage provides information about a subject.

3. **Argumentative.** This type of passage presents and defends a position on a controversial topic. An argument may contain inductive reasoning, deductive reasoning, or both, and points in the argument may be explicitly or implicitly stated. (See V, Types of Reasoning in an Argument, for additional information.)

II. Skills that are Tested

The Verbal Reasoning section is designed to test your reading comprehension and reasoning skills. The authors of the test have written questions to assess your abilities in four areas: **comprehension, evaluation, application,** and **incorporation of new information.**

COMPREHENSION

Comprehension skills are measured by questions that address the passage. Comprehension questions ask about information provided in the passage; the position taken by the author of the passage and evidence used to support that position; and assumptions made by the author or conclusions that are, or could be, drawn. On the Verbal Reasoning section, you are expected to be able to:

1. **Identify the central issue or thesis** of the passage

2. **Identify the reasons or evidence** offered in support of a thesis

3. **Identify background knowledge** contained in the passage or question that is relevant to a particular interpretation

4. **Determine the meaning of significant terminology or vocabulary** from the context of the passage

5. **Recognize an accurate paraphrase of complex information** presented in the passage

6. **Identify comparative relationships among ideas** or pieces of information contained in the passage

7. **Identify assumptions** (stated or unstated) contained in the passage

8. **Recognize appropriate questions of clarification that follow the passages**

EVALUATION

Evaluation skills are your abilities to make a judgement about an author's argument. An author uses inductive reasoning, deductive reasoning, or both (see V, Types of Reasoning in an Argument) when presenting evidence in support of the position being argued. Evaluation questions require you to consider the reliability, credibility, relevance, sufficiency, or accuracy of the evidence provided by the author. An evaluation question may ask you to determine the soundness or validity of the argument. On the Verbal Reasoning section, you are expected to be able to:

1. **Judge the soundness of an argument** or a step of reasoning presented in the passage

2. **Judge the credibility of a source**

3. **Judge whether or not a conclusion is based on the evidence provided** in the passage

4. **Appraise the strength of the evidence** for a generalization, conclusion, or claim

5. **Distinguish between supported and unsupported claims**

6. **Judge the relevance of information** to an argument or claim

APPLICATION

Application questions require you to think and analyze the author's message and solve a related problem, interpret a hypothetical situation, identify a probable cause of an event, or identify a general theory or model that is applicable. On the Verbal Reasoning section, you are expected to be able to:

1. **Predict a result based on the content of the passage** and specific facts about a hypothetical situation

2. **Use the information presented in the passage to solve a specified problem**

3. **Identify the probable cause of a particular event** or result based on information presented

THE VERBAL
REASONING
SECTION:
INFORMATION
AND STRATEGIES

660

4. **Determine the implications of conclusions** or results that would occur in "real-life" situations

5. **Recognize the scope of application** of hypotheses, explanations, and conclusions

6. **Identify a general theory or model based on the information provided**

INCORPORATION OF NEW INFORMATION

In this category, the question provides additional information. You need to reconsider the author's argument in light of this new information. As you answer these questions, you are expected to think beyond the information that the author presented. On the Verbal Reasoning section, you are expected to be able to:

1. **Judge the bearing of new evidence on conclusions** presented in the passage

2. **Recognize methods or results that would challenge hypotheses,** models, or theories originally presented in the passage

3. **Determine how a conclusion from the passage can be modified** to be consistent with the new information

4. **Recognize plausible, alternative hypotheses** or solutions

III. Question Types

Questions on the Verbal Reasoning section can be categorized in several ways. The best way to categorize a question is by the skill they test (i.e., comprehension, evaluation, application, or incorporation of new information) as shown in section II. You also can organize questions in the following manner: **fact questions,** which test your comprehension of the material explicitly stated in the passage; **inference questions,** which test your ability to comprehend the information presented, draw conclusions about this information, and answer questions using these conclusions; and **main idea questions,** which require you to identify the central theme of the passage. Regardless of the way you classify questions, it is important to recognize key words and phrases in the questions that indicate the type of information being sought.

FACT QUESTIONS

This type of question requires you to report information that was specifically stated in the passage. The idea contained in the correct answer is stated openly (although not usually in the same words) in one or more of the paragraphs of the passage. You must either recall what was written in the passage or go back to the passage and locate the idea. You do not need to make any assumptions—you only need to regurgitate the information you read. Fact questions test your comprehension skills.

Look for the following phrases (or phrases that are similar) that often appear in the stem of a fact question:

- According to the passage . . .
- The author states, says, asserts, claims or declares . . .
- The passage states, says, asserts, claims or declares . . .
- According to the author . . .

TRAPS TO AVOID

Trap: Reading your own ideas into the passage or into the question and answer.
Stick with the facts presented in the passage, even if you are convinced that those facts are

incorrect or outdated. You are not tested on your knowledge about a subject, only on your ability to read and comprehend the information presented.

Trap: Looking for a complicated answer. Generally, fact questions are straight-forward and relatively simple. Do not make your task more difficult by "reading into" possible choices and then confusing yourself. Look for the obvious.

Trap: Choosing answers that appear to be taken word-for-word from the passage. If you encounter choices that look as if the passage has been quoted, be very wary. Often, a word or two has been changed so that, despite "looking" correct, the answer is actually wrong. If you read carefully, you will note the inaccuracy of the choice and then be able to select the correct answer.

INFERENCE QUESTIONS

Inference questions require you to understand what the passage implies, rather than what it states specifically. You are required to make assumptions and to draw conclusions based on the facts presented in the passage. This type of question tests your ability to reason (from evidence presented to conclusions drawn) and to draw principles from the generalized statements in the passage. Thus, to answer an inference question correctly, you must first know the basic facts of the passage, and then you must organize appropriate facts into principles and draw a conclusion that corresponds with one of the answer choices. Inference questions are found in questions that test comprehension, evaluation, and application skills.

Look for the following phrases (or phrases that are similar) that often appear in the stem of an inference question:

- The passage suggests or implies . . .

- It is the author's opinion or view . . .

- One can assume . . .

- It is the purpose of . . .

- One can conclude . . .

- It can be deduced or reasonably inferred . . .

- The author most likely believes . . .

- **OR,** any question that requires you to provide a reason for a statement or belief of the author

- **OR,** any question that requires you to categorize the author's ideas according to various philosophies that are offered as the answer choices

TRAPS TO AVOID

Trap: Assuming that the answer can be found directly in the passage. It is important to realize that although all of the necessary information to answer a question correctly is contained in the passage, you must think beyond the facts and draw a conclusion based on the facts.

Trap: Inserting your own opinions. Although you must infer what the passage implies, your inference must be based on the material provided in the passage. Eliminate personal biases and focus on ideas and information in the passage.

MAIN IDEA QUESTIONS

Main idea questions require you to determine the central thesis of the passage or the key concept or assumption in the author's thought process. Main idea questions require you (1) to know the facts of the passage, (2) to organize those facts into the basic principles of

THE VERBAL
REASONING
SECTION:
INFORMATION
AND STRATEGIES

662

the passage, (3) to draw appropriate conclusions regarding the relationship or importance of the principles to each other, and (4) to determine the central thesis of the passage based on the relative importance of the principles contained therein. Primarily, these questions test comprehension skills.

Look for the following phrases (or phrases that are similar) that often appear in the stem of a main idea question:

- The passage is primarily concerned with . . .

- The central idea . . .

- If you were to sum up the passage . . .

- The main thought . . .

- . . . best describes the passage . . .

- The primary point . . .

TRAPS TO AVOID

Trap: Failing to include specific key facts in your decision-making process. Before answering a main idea question, write one or two words in the margin that summarize the thought contained in each paragraph. Then, add up the words you wrote and select the words (i.e., ideas) that are repeated most often. One of the answer choices should closely approximate the words or ideas that you believe are the central theme of the passage.

Trap: Thinking that main idea questions are easy, because essentially you are being asked to give a title to the passage. These questions are often difficult. However, if you avoid flowery or stylistic answers and stick to the main concepts contained in the passage, you should (with practice) answer correctly most of the time.

IV. Question Format

There are two types of questions: multiple-choice and extended multiple-choice questions.

MULTIPLE-CHOICE QUESTIONS

Multiple-choice questions test any of the four skills discussed in II, Skills that are Tested. There are four answer choices following each question (i.e., choices A–D). Always use the process of elimination to answer a question. For example, if you eliminate one of the four choices, your chance at correctly answering a question based on educated guessing increases from 25% to 33%. If you eliminate two choices, your chance at correctly answering a question based on educated guessing alone increases to 50%. Frequently, several answer choices may be correct (i.e., true) statements. However, **only one of the choices is the best correct statement.** Always evaluate each choice to find the single best answer. If you are impulsive and do not evaluate each answer choice, you may erroneously choose a correct statement that is not the best correct statement.

EXTENDED MULTIPLE-CHOICE QUESTIONS

Extended multiple-choice questions test any of the four skills discussed in II, Skills that are Tested. In this format, the question is always followed by three statements (I, II, and III). Choose the statement(s) that are correct, and then choose the right answer. Again, there will be four choices (A–D) following each question. For example, choice A in the answer key may state that statement I is correct; choice B may state that statements I and II are correct; choice C may state that statement III is correct; and choice D may state that statements I, II, and III are correct. Take a look at this sample question:

1. According to the passage, the author asserts that:

    I. medicine is expanding faster than the ethical issues it provokes.
   II. we may endanger those who follow us.
  III. some issues are better left unknown.

    A. I only
    B. I and II only
    C. III only
    D. I, II, and III

Evaluate each statement based on its own merit. If one of the statements is false or does not appropriately answer the question, eliminate it. After eliminating the statement, eliminate the other answer choices that include the statement. With this approach, you use the statements strategically to eliminate answer choices. Remember, with each answer choice eliminated, your odds for answering a question correctly improve dramatically.

V. Understanding Arguments

The Verbal Reasoning section often focuses on argumentative discourse. This section of the book will help you understand the basic structure of an argument, which will help you to better comprehend reading passages and the questions that follow them.

STRUCTURE OF AN ARGUMENT

The **beginning** of an argument introduces the subject, identifies the controversy, states the author's position, and indicates how the position will be defended.

The **middle** of an argument provides relevant background information, conveys the points to be considered, argues various points, and acknowledges counterarguments.

The **end** of an argument restates the position, summarizes the arguments advanced, persuades the reader to accept the position, and indicates what needs to be done.

TYPES OF REASONING IN AN ARGUMENT

DEDUCTIVE REASONING

In a deductive argument, the premises make the claim (conclusion) inevitable. The claim does not extend beyond the information provided in the premises. Deductive arguments are valid or invalid.

INDUCTIVE REASONING

In an inductive argument, the premises are provided to support the conclusion. The claim (conclusion) extends beyond the evidence provided in the passage. If the evidence is true, the claim is more probable. Inductive arguments are strong or weak.

DIFFERENTIATING BETWEEN DEDUCTIVE AND INDUCTIVE ARGUMENTS

There is a great tip to help determine if deductive or inductive reasoning is being used in a passage or question: Determine if it makes more sense to add the word *certainly* or *probably* before the conclusion. The word *probably* signals inductive reasoning, whereas the word *certainly* signals deductive reasoning.

THE VERBAL
REASONING
SECTION:
INFORMATION
AND STRATEGIES

664

VI. Key Strategies

The Verbal Reasoning test may be the most difficult section of the MCAT. You are competing with students from around the country, many of whom are strong readers. Your performance is based on how your raw score compares to other MCAT examinees. The only way to separate yourself from other students is to answer more questions correctly than they do. You can improve your score by practicing Verbal Reasoning section timing, mastering basic strategies, practicing as many Verbal Reasoning tests as possible, and maximizing your reading comprehension skills.

The following provides simple strategies to increase your reading speed and comprehension ability. Although this information is basic, it is very helpful. Remember, practice as many reading passages as you can get your hands on. In this book, three full-length verbal reasoning tests are provided. Two practice tests are in this section, and a third test is in the sample full-length MCAT at the end of this book.

TIMING

You are severely punished for not completing the Verbal Reasoning section. Your score is based on the number of questions answered correctly. **There is no penalty for guessing, so you should answer every question on the test.** However, you will probably correctly answer approximately 25% of questions on which you randomly guessed (four choices per question). Because the Verbal Reasoning section is very competitive, guessing on many questions means that most likely, you will not do well. Often, students do not complete this section because they mismanage their time. If you follow this simple approach, you have a better chance of completing the test.

Most recently, there have been 9 passages on the test. Divide the total time allotted by the number of passages (i.e., 85 minutes divided by 9 passages). This equation allows you approximately 9 minutes per passage, with approximately 4 minutes left over to either check your work or to go back and solve any question you are not sure if you answered correctly, any question left unanswered, or both.

After completing three passages, check the time. If at the end of the third passage you are more than 27 minutes into the test (i.e., 3 passages multiplied by 9 minutes per passage), you are working too slowly. At that point, adjust your pace and speed up.

HOW TO APPROACH THE READING PASSAGES

There are two basic techniques for approaching passages in the Verbal Reasoning section.

APPROACH 1

Skim the question stems, read the passage, and then carefully read the questions.

Read through the questions before reading the passage. Underline stems, key phrases, main ideas, and important words such as *except, only, always, inferred,* and *conclusion.*

Read the passage. Keep an eye out for the key words and stems from the questions, and mark (i.e., underline, circle, note in margins) the passage accordingly.

Reread each question carefully and look back at the passage. Usually, the marks you made bring you right back to the part of the passage where the topic of the question is discussed.

APPROACH 2

Read the passage, then answer the questions.

Read the passage first, underlining or circling key ideas and main points, and making brief notes summarizing material in the margins.

Then, read the questions and then refer back to your highlights and margin notes to answer the questions.

Most students prefer approach 1, in which question stems are previewed before the passage is read. Other students find this technique distracting and prefer to start reading the passage before looking at the questions. Try both approaches with a few verbal reasoning practice exams to find out which approach works best for you.

Regardless of the approach you choose, you should practice reading passages and answering questions as much as possible. Practice will hone your comprehension skills and help you read more efficiently.

ADDITIONAL TIPS

The following are five additional tips that apply to any reading strategy:

1. As you read a passage, mark (underline or circle) key areas such as shifts in tone or content, places where conclusions are drawn or suggested, and points of strong factual evidence. Note key words such as *however, yet, furthermore* and so on. Also, jot a few words next to each paragraph, stating the content of the paragraph. These strategies help you quickly retrieve information when you return to a passage to find answers to questions.

2. As you are reading, ask yourself: What is the main idea of the passage? What is the purpose of the passage? What implications can be drawn from the argument given in the passage? Thinking about these questions as you the passage will help you answer the questions that follow the passage.

3. Always read questions carefully, and be aware of answers choices that contain words such as *always, every, never, only, totally,* and *wholly.* Frequently, a passage may state that *generally* "something" is true, and then the question will be worded that the "something" is *always* true. The words *generally* and *always* are not synonymous. Thus, depending on the question and information provided in the passage, the answer that contains the word *always* is incorrect.

4. Select the single best answer based on the information from the passage or on principles derived from the information, not from previous knowledge.

5. If you are confused by a question or cannot answer it quickly, mark your best choice in the test booklet and on your Scantron sheet. Marking the question with a circle or question mark will remind you to return to it later. Move on to the next question and return to the troublesome questions after you have completed the entire Verbal Reasoning test.

STRATEGIES FOR IMPROVING READING SPEED AND EFFICIENCY

It is important to understand some basic strategies that may help you read faster and more efficiently.

The difference between an average MCAT Verbal Reasoning performance and a superior performance can be determined by the following three strategies:

1. **Preview what you read**

2. **Make a mental picture of the dialogue or flow of a passage**

3. **Read at a variable speed**

Recent reading studies show that superior readers do not necessarily read faster or with more effort than other readers. Superior readers know what to read and are able to form a mental picture of the flow of information in the passage. Also, strong readers know how to appropriate attention to the various aspects of the passage.

THE VERBAL
REASONING
SECTION:
INFORMATION
AND STRATEGIES

666

Many students perform better on the Verbal Reasoning section by skimming the topic sentences of each paragraph to preview the passage. This preview allows the student to form a mental picture of the flow of the passage. Previewing provides a great deal more in results than the few seconds of time it requires. After previewing, begin reading the passage. Feel free to read at a variable speed. Speed up if you understand or are familiar with the material. Slow down if the discussion gets complicated.

Some students perform poorly on or fail to complete the Verbal Reasoning section because they read too slowly. Why is it that many students read so slowly? There are many reasons, including that they may be reading word-for-word, they may be vocalizing words as they read, they may be regressing and looking back in the passage as they are reading, they may find the topic boring and difficult to concentrate on, or their minds may wander as they are reading.

SOLUTIONS

The following are solutions to the problems described in the preceding section.

Read for main ideas. The test writers create questions based on the concepts, ideas, and tone of a passage. They rarely test you on the meaning of specific words. Do not focus on trivia.

Focus on the topic sentence of each paragraph. In over 75% of expository passages in the Verbal Reasoning section, a topic sentence is the first or last sentence of each paragraph. By focusing on topic sentences, you are more likely to grasp the important idea(s) of the paragraph. Also, **look for words with a strong directional clue.**

Concentrate on comprehension. If you are a student who completes verbal reasoning practice tests but answers many questions incorrectly, you must focus on improving your reading comprehension. Reading comprehension can be improved by reading the passage and immediately afterward reviewing those parts of the passage that are ambiguous or unclear. Do not waste time rereading the entire passage! Immediately after reviewing the selected parts of the passage, recite to yourself the take-home message of the passage.

Do not worry about reading fast (within reasonable limits). Studies show that as you increase your reading speed (within reasonable ranges), your comprehension actually increases! This increased comprehension occurs because you often become more focused and can concentrate better. Slow reading may invite a loss of concentration and distraction.

Be sensitive to the tone and position of the author. Frequently, awareness of the tone will help you address the questions that follow the passage. Many students can use the process of elimination to arrive at the best answer to a question simply by understanding the tone or position the author takes when presenting an issue.

TYPES OF COMPREHENSION

Be aware of the type of comprehension that is troublesome for you. There are two basic types of comprehension: **receptive and reflective comprehension.** Practice building skills in the area that is difficult for you.

Receptive comprehension is the ability to understand factual information such as names, specific statements, dates, and so on. Most premedical students are good at answering receptive comprehension questions, because this type of comprehension is frequently required in science courses. The answers to receptive comprehension questions are clearly stated in the passage. You only need to find them! Using the question stem skimming strategy will make receptive comprehension easy because before you read the passage, you have already previewed the questions. When you find a fact in the passage that you know will be asked about, circle or underline it.

Reflective comprehension is more difficult for most students. Reflective comprehension is the ability to understand main ideas, inferences, and implications of a passage. If your reflective comprehension is weak, improve it by reading practice reading comprehension passages and creating a written outline of the main ideas, key points, significance, and implications of each passage. Although this technique seems painful, thinking about the passages and outlining them should improve your reflective comprehension skills. In fact, this technique is how many authors create the multiple-choice questions that follow the passages!

BASIC PRINCIPLES WORTH REPEATING

Choose the most appropriate answer for each question. Remember, the answer choices often contain more than one choice that is a correct statement. You always want to use the process of elimination to arrive at the single best correct statement.

Do not expect answers to follow the order of the text.

Do not be disturbed if the passages present subjects in fields other than your expertise. Generally, MCAT passages are selected from topics you know little about. You are not being tested on your knowledge of a given subject, only on your ability to comprehend the passages written. **Conversely, if a passage addresses a topic with which you are familiar, do not allow your knowledge about the topic to influence your choice of an answer.** Answer the questions based on the passage (i.e., the text and principles you derive from the text), not on the basis of your opinions or assumptions.

Do not waste time on questions that you do not understand or that you have difficulty answering. Mark your best guess, move on to the next question, and return to the troublesome question only after you have completed the entire exam.

Practice, practice, and practice some more. If you practice consistently from now until the MCAT, your verbal reasoning skills will improve. These improvements usually require many hours of practice.

OPPORTUNITIES FOR PRACTICE

Because the Verbal Reasoning section primarily concentrates on narrative, expository, and argumentative discourse, the best way to practice is to read as many of these types of written discourse as possible. Reading a newspaper such as the *Los Angeles Times* or the *New York Times* is great practice, particularly the editorial section. Also, try reading persuasive essays or arguments in journals or magazines such as *Time, Newsweek,* or *National Geographic.* Concentrate on sections that are approximately five paragraphs in length, because that is approximately the length of a Verbal Reasoning passage.

ADDITIONAL TIPS

The following five tips will help you practice your verbal reasoning skills:

1. Practice underlining and circling key words and phrases and making notes in the margins (as you would if you had questions to answer about the article). Do not try to speed read; instead, concentrate on efficient, focused reading.

2. Determine the tone of the article, and look for structural elements (e.g., evidence, conclusions).

3. When you are finished reading an article, pretend as if you are telling someone about the article. Briefly summarize the article, list relevant points discussed by the author, review assumptions made and evidence used by the author, and outline the conclusions that are (or could be) reached. Be able to paraphrase what you have read in one or two sentences.

4. Try to create questions about the article. Although this sounds easy, it often is not. If you can write 4–10 questions with reasonable answer choices, you most likely have strong reading comprehension skills. This exercise also helps you predict the types of questions that may be on the MCAT and develop a sense for what information and principles are important.

THE VERBAL
REASONING
SECTION:
INFORMATION
AND STRATEGIES

668

VII. Practice Tests

The following practice tests are designed to help you practice the strategies discussed in this section. Be sure that you assign yourself 85 minutes to complete each practice test. Answers and explanations follow each test.

Your goal is to complete each practice test within 85 minutes. A performance of approximately 65%–75% is average; 75%–80% is above average; and 80% or higher is excellent as well as safely placing you in the double-digit category (i.e., a score 10 or greater). Have fun, and good luck!

Verbal Reasoning

PRACTICE TESTS

SECT. IV
VERBAL
REASONING
PRACTICE
TEST 1

671

Time: 85 Minutes

Directions: There are 9 reading passages in this Verbal Reading Test. Each passage is followed by several questions. After reading a passage, select the one best answer to each of the questions that follow. If you are not certain of an answer, eliminate the alternatives that you know are incorrect, and then select an answer from the remaining alternatives.

Passage I (Questions 1–8)

Constructivism arose as an artistic movement in the newly born Soviet Union in the 1920s. Young artists wanted to forge a union between aesthetic and practical arts. They did not want their art to be enjoyed only by the aesthete, but wanted it to be a practical part of ordinary life. They also wanted to exploit the cutting edge of technology at the time. Like the modernists in Europe after them, constructivists looked at the dramatic advances in technology and the sciences during the preceding decades and saw a future of unlimited progress, expansion, optimism, and improvement of the standard of living.

Unlike modernists, however, constructivists did not envision the postindustrial world to be boring, boxy, and depressing. This is how we now think of "utilitarian," "practical," "pragmatic" art and architecture. The dominant images that come to mind are the clunky black shoe, the shapeless dress, concrete and steel cities, and colors of gray, black, and brown. The constructivists imagined a life transformed and transcendent.

The constructivists' ideals are evident in the models and sketches for the proposed Monument to the Third International. Although it was never completed, the monument was to be a soaring spiral of steel, cut through with panes of glass, reaching up 1312 feet above the ground. The monument was designed by Vladimir Tatlin, one of the early constructivists, and one who provided the movement with many of its slogans, among them, "Art into life" and "Not the old, not the new, but the necessary." Tatlin also designed a bicycle that was never manufactured. He called it *Letatlin*, and in the model it is a soaring invention of fabric and wood, resembling a bird with outstretched wings. Both of these structures are functional but also lyrical. They represent the constructivists' break from static art objects such as painted canvasses and their foray into the objects that surround citizens in their lives.

However, constructivists did not forsake painting entirely. Again, although they were moved by some of the same forces as European modernists, such as the departure from traditional pictorial representations and the exploration of principles of cubism, the results were quite different. Constructivist paintings are explosions of bright colors and shading, utilizing geometric shapes overlaid and bursting out of the frames. Vavara Stepanova, Lyubov' Popova, and Vasily Kandinsky all explored this kind of painting. However, most of the images of the constructivist period are not formal abstract studies; rather, the artists combine sharp-edged geometric design and words to make political statements or construct repeated patterns for book endpaper or textile design. Furthermore, true to their name, most of the artists made constructions out of wood, steel, and sometimes found objects such as wheels and gears.

The constructivist artists were the utopians of the new Soviet socialist state. They and the state shared the same values: optimism for the industrial state, equality of the masses, the banishment of bourgeois wastefulness and elitism, and the construction of a highly organized, efficient, bright, and gleaming future for Soviet citizens. The constructivists wanted their art to be a part of the life of the new Soviet citizen. The irony is that this art never made it into life. Stalin suppressed constructivism and its cousins, suprematism and futurism, and declared socialist realism the official art style of the state (e.g., as represented in posters of burly workers and trains). Stalin banished all independent art groups and replaced them with the Union of Artists. Not only was the works of constructivism not allowed to infiltrate ordinary life; it wasn't even shown until 1990 in Seattle and Minneapolis, and in the spring of 1991 it finally was exhibited in Moscow.

1. Which of the following are analogies between modernists and constructivists?

    I. Favored constructions with no adornments
    II. Painted still lifes and landscapes
    III. Positive view of industrialization

    A. I only
    B. I and II only
    C. III only
    D. I and III only

2. Which of the following would be a correct description of at least one constructivist artist?

    I. Sculptor
    II. Painter
    III. Designer

    A. II only
    B. I and II only
    C. II and III only
    D. I, II, and III

3. How does the slogan "Art into life" convey the principles of constructivism?

    A. Constructivists believed artistic creation made people feel more alive.
    B. Constructivists worked for increased museum attendance for further exposure of their art.
    C. Constructivists believed art should be integrated into the public sphere.
    D. Constructivists advocated more art education for young children.

4. How do constructivist paintings convey the principles of the movement?

    I. By breaking with traditional bourgeois elitist painting styles
    II. By using exuberant, bright colors
    III. By "constructing" images out of geometric forms

    A. II only
    B. I and III only
    C. II and III only
    D. I, II, and III

5. Which of the following is NOT common to both the Soviet state and constructivist artists in the 1920s?

    A. Both were optimistic about the state's ability to create a better life for its citizens.
    B. Both wanted to maintain a state museum.
    C. Both advocated the equality of all people.
    D. Both were influenced by rising industrialism.

6. In what way might someone criticize the *Letatlin* for not being truly constructivist?

    I. It was never used.
    II. It had an excessive and impractical design.
    III. It was named to aggrandize the artist.

    A. I and II only
    B. II only
    C. II and III only
    D. None of the above

7. What constructivist effect was accomplished by the use of found objects, as described in the fourth paragraph of the passage?

    I. Exemplifying the marriage of art and technology
    II. Making a political statement about the conditions of workers' lives
    III. Lowering the cost of materials

    A. I only
    B. II only
    C. III only
    D. I and II only

8. Which of the following is the ironic fact described by the author?

    A. Constructivist art was shown in the United States before it was shown in the Soviet Union.
    B. The fact that constructivist art ended up in museums.
    C. Constructivist art was never employed to improve the lives of Soviet citizens.
    D. Modernist realism replaced constructivist transcendence.

Passage II (Questions 9–14)

The modern university, with its system of degrees and examinations and its hierarchy of professorships, was originated in medieval Europe and fine-tuned in eighteenth-century Germany. However, the first person to develop a college of higher education is commonly believed to be

Plato. Therefore, we would owe our current system of higher education not to eighteenth-century Europe but to fourth-century B.C. Athens.

Before Plato started his school, Greek youth were taught by wandering scholars known as sophists. The students were young men from the upper classes, and they received grooming for the public lives they would have as part of the Athenian *polis*. Sophists sometimes taught such substantive subjects as astronomy, mathematics, and elementary medicine, but they specialized in rhetoric and eristic disputation, the kind of specious wrangling that would be useful for politicians, orators, and lawyers. Plato's mouthpiece, the Socrates of the Platonic dialogues, lashed out at sophists and their curriculum at every opportunity.

Eventually, a few of the sophistic teachers settled down and instituted static, one-teacher schools or colleges. Others then followed their lead. Gorgias, Antisthenes, and Isocrates were well-known leaders of static schools in Athens, and Aristophanes' play the *Clouds* suggests that Socrates, Plato's teacher, ran one as well. The teachers generally did not require fees from Athenian students, but did require fees or charge higher fees from students who were from other cities (the beginning of out-of-state tuition).

The founding date of Plato's school is controversial, but was probably around 375 B.C. Plato's school was called Academy, simply because that was the name of Plato's house. The school never had more than 100 students. Plato's school was unique in several ways. First, it had more than one teacher; in fact, there is doubt as to whether Plato himself ever taught a lecture course, because no records or notes exist. It provided continuous education. Students stayed for three or four years. We know from Aristotle's works, which are mostly culled from students' notes, that courses were taught as series of lectures and students listened to them sitting down, much as in the modern university auditorium. Aristotle and other teachers in the Academy probably also made use of an early Greek version of the blackboard.

The curriculum did not include any of the sophists' subjects until after Plato's death; then, rhetorical training for politicians and lawyers was added to make the school competitive with other schools in Athens such as Isocrates' school. Plato's educational philosophy is outlined in Book VII of his dialogue, the *Republic*. There, he outlines a program that will develop students' minds and bodies, school them in the arts of reasoning and scientific inquiry, make them strong and virtuous leaders or citizens of the state, and prepare them for a lifelong search for the truth.

9. Based on the evidence in the passage, which of the following features of modern universities probably do NOT come from Plato?

  I. Master's and doctoral degrees
 II. Financial ties to the state
III. Degree examinations

A. II only
B. I and III only
C. II and III only
D. I, II, and III

10. From the evidence in the passage, which of the following can be inferred about the nature of eristic disputation?

A. It was employed primarily in moral reasoning.
B. It was useful for settling philosophical disputes.
C. It had more to do with style than with content.
D. It was harder to learn than mathematics or astronomy.

11. Which of the following was Plato's main reason for banning sophistic teaching from his Academy?

A. To be more competitive with the sophists' schools
B. He was not concerned with his students' future political activities
C. The curriculum would take too long with those subjects added
D. None of the above

12. Which of the following is NOT a feature of Plato's Academy?

A. Students learned primarily through practical training.
B. Teachers lectured using visual aids.
C. Many records of lectures exist.
D. It was founded before the fall of Rome.

13. Which of the following is NOT a feature of the sophists?

A. Both Plato and the author of the passage disapprove of their educational techniques.
B. Sophists never taught in one place for an extended period of time.
C. They would be considered science teachers today.
D. They had only male students.

14. Which of the following is implied by the passage?

    A. Aristotle was a student at the Academy.
    B. Plato's Academy was not the first static school in Athens.
    C. Socrates was a sophist before he founded his static school.
    D. Socrates and Isocrates were related.

Passage III (Questions 15–22)

The tree from which the cocoa bean comes is known as *Theobroma cacao*, which means "the food of the gods." Countless millions would agree with this nomenclature for the chief product of the cacao tree, namely chocolate. Few other foods have inspired the same passionate devotion as chocolate has in its many forms. Books have been written celebrating its wonders, greeting cards offer support to fellow addicts, and whole stores are devoted to purveying it to the hungry masses.

Chocolate begins inside the seed pods of the cacao tree. Each pod contains 25–50 cocoa beans. These beans are scooped out with the pulp that fills the pod and are then cured to loosen the beans from the pulp. After the beans are separated, they are fermented to remove their bitter taste—something that plagues raw cocoa from start to finish of processing, as we shall see. Fermentation also develops the natural oils of the bean.

After fermentation, the beans are dried and shipped to a processor. There, they are selected and blended much as coffee beans are. Variety of blending accounts for the variety in flavor of different companies' chocolate products. The chosen beans are cleaned and roasted. The roasting process provides the dark color and distills the final chocolate flavor and aroma. It also loosens the outer shell of the bean, which is removed and discarded.

The nib, or inside of the shelled bean, consists of more than 50% cocoa butter. This is removed through pressing to make cocoa powder, but remains in solid chocolate products. To make the unsweetened chocolate bars used in cooking, the nibs are ground, which melts the cocoa butter and leaves chocolate liquor, a thick brown paste. This paste is refined through a process called conching, a finer grinding technique, and poured into molds to form bars. The more the paste is conched, the higher the quality of the chocolate that results, because conching makes the flavor smoother and less astringent.

Conching removes some more of the natural bitterness of the cocoa bean, but to be palatable, chocolate needs to be mixed with sugar, some butter, and vanilla flavoring. Vanilla and chocolate are often considered to be opposite flavors, like black and white or night and day, so it is ironic that vanilla is necessary for chocolate to attain its final flavor. Some chocolate is also mixed with milk before it is poured into molds, which makes—you guessed it—milk chocolate.

Chocolate is marketed in a wide variety of ways. Unsweetened chocolate usually comes in 8-ounce bars with 1-ounce squares. Dutch-process cocoa powder is treated with alkali to neutralize acids, resulting in a product with less bitterness but which cannot be used in recipes that require baking powder or baking soda. Chocolate chips are semisweet, teardrop-shaped morsels of chocolate. Contrary to many people's beliefs, semisweet chocolate is actually less sweet than dark chocolate. Products marked as chocolate-flavored, rather than real chocolate, consist of cocoa powder mixed with vegetable oil instead of cocoa butter. These products are nonetheless closer to real chocolate than white chocolate, which is made of solidified whole milk, sugar, and artificial flavoring. Better manufacturers sometimes add cocoa butter to white chocolate, but most of it has nothing to do with the cocoa bean.

15. Which of the following is the best title for this passage?

    A. *The Story of Chocolate*
    B. *The Food of the Gods is the Food of America*
    C. *The Problems of Bitterness in Chocolate Processing*
    D. *How to Tell Real Chocolate From the Pretenders*

16. Which of the following processes remove bitterness?

    I. Fermentation
    II. Blending
    III. Conching

    A. I and II only
    B. I and III only
    C. II and III only
    D. I, II, and III

17. Which of the following processes does NOT remove bitterness?

    I. Alkali treatments
    II. Adding vanilla flavoring
    III. Extraction of cocoa butter

    A. I and II only
    B. II only
    C. III only
    D. II and III only

675

18. Which of the following statements about cocoa butter is true?

    A.   There is more in milk chocolate than in dark chocolate.

    B.   It is what makes white chocolate a kind of chocolate.

    C.   It melts during conching.

    D.   It is missing from chocolate-flavored products.

19. Which of the following words best describe the author's style of presentation of the material in this passage?

    A.   Informational
    B.   Colloquial
    C.   Celebratory
    D.   Convoluted

20. What is chocolate liquor?

    A.   A chocolate-flavored alcoholic beverage
    B.   The raw material for cocoa
    C.   Preconched ground nibs
    D.   Cocoa butter with vanilla flavoring

21. Which of the following is implied by the passage?

    A.   Cocoa beans must be fermented before they are ground.

    B.   Cocoa beans must be conched before they are roasted.

    C.   Chocolate liquor must be molded before it is conched.

    D.   Cocoa powder must be mixed with vanilla to be legally called chocolate.

22. Which of the following is the best to eat?

    A.   Cocoa beans off the tree
    B.   Chocolate liquor after being conched multiple times
    C.   Nibs
    D.   Cocoa powder

Passage IV (Questions 23–28)

Sentimental films and television shows of the last 20 years have sometimes shown human beings communicating with chimpanzees. The claim is widely made that human trainers have successfully taught chimps to speak, using the gestural vocabulary of American Sign Language (ASL). However, these claims are somewhat exaggerated. When investigators tried to teach language to chimpanzees, they achieved only limited success. Chimps could repeat individual signs, or words, to signify objects or people, but

they could not master syntax, and this is the truly distinguishing mark of human language.

An animal might learn signs that represent "John," "Mary," "apple," and "give," and might be able to combine these signs into strings, but so far no animal has been able to master the difference between "John gives Mary an apple" and "Mary gives John an apple." Anyone with a rudimentary grasp of English knows that these two are quite different, and the difference is in the syntax. Syntax has to do not with the words or vocabulary of a particular language, but with its form (i.e., with the way in which the items in the vocabulary are put together).

Chimpanzees who know some words in ASL do not understand syntax at all. Neither do some aphasics, people who have had damage to the language centers in the brain. Aphasics often have trouble phrasing sentences or constructing original ones. On the other hand, very young children, although they do not have a sophisticated grasp of syntax, still show some command of it, as do speakers of pidgin languages. Pidgin languages are sets of words developed among people who do not share a language, yet still need to communicate (usually populations involved in trade). Both the case of children and the case of pidgin speakers show that even "primitive" human speakers of language show syntactic ability, so strongly that many linguists have concluded that syntactic ability is innate, (i.e., it is a built-in feature of the human brain that is present at birth).

Syntax appears in some unexpected places as well. Speakers of Western languages who are confronted with Chinese writing for the first time sometimes view it as a set of pictures, not a set of words. Until recently, speakers in the hearing world believed that ASL itself, as well as the world's other signed languages, were mere unstructured gesture systems with which the deaf communicated at about the same level as the chimpanzees described. However, both Chinese and ASL are fully fledged languages, complete with rules for the use of different parts of speech, varying inflections for noun cases and verb tenses, and combinatorial morphologies.

One type of study used to demonstrate the syntactic character of pictorial and gestural languages is the examination of deficits in native speakers who have suffered brain damage due to stroke. Chinese speakers who have received damage to the left hemisphere, the language center of the brain, have trouble reproducing Chinese characters, but they do not have trouble reproducing possible characters, configurations that look like Chinese characters but are not actual words (much as *bick* is a possible English word but not an actual one). Native speakers of ASL who have received left hemisphere damage can reproduce drawings and have good motor ability, but exhibit deficits in signing analogous to those of aphasic hearing individuals. Conversely, ASL speakers who have right hemisphere damage can speak perfectly well, but have trouble with drawing and with motor coordination in general. This shows that linguistic syntactic ability is a distinct capacity, guided by a uniquely designated part of the human brain.

23. Which of the following would be implied by the argument in the first two paragraphs?

    I. A person who makes grammatical mistakes does not really have a mastery of the language.
    II. A person who knows a few words in French does not know French.
    III. One cannot learn a language by studying a set of vocabulary flash cards.

    A. I and II only
    B. III only
    C. II and III only
    D. I, II, and III

24. What is the main difference between a deaf speaker's and a chimpanzee's use of ASL?

    A. A chimpanzee cannot distinguish the difference among various individual signs.
    B. The chimpanzee makes many more mistakes in usage.
    C. The deaf speaker uses signs to discuss abstract concepts.
    D. The deaf speaker employs signs according to formal rules.

25. What would an individual with damage to the left hemisphere of the brain still be able to do?

    I. Recognize written words
    II. Reproduce drawings
    III. Make lunch

    A. II only
    B. I and III only
    C. II and III only
    D. None of the above

26. Why is the result of studies with ASL speakers that is described in the last paragraph surprising?

    A. The studies with Chinese speakers suggested the opposite effect.
    B. Because ASL is a gestural language, impaired motor abilities and speech abilities should go hand in hand.
    C. ASL speakers could not recognize possible English words.
    D. Chinese speakers turned out to be better at drawing and other motor skills than ASL speakers.

27. Consider the sentence "The boy threw the ball to the girl." Which of the following shows a change only in the syntax of the sentence?

    I. To whom did the boy throw the ball?
    II. The girl threw the ball to the boy.
    III. The boy tossed the ball to the girl.

    A. I only
    B. I and II only
    C. II and III only
    D. I, II, and III

28. Which of the following is implied by the arguments in paragraphs two and three?

    A. Young children make the same kind of mistakes that chimpanzees do.
    B. One cannot teach a pigeon syntax.
    C. All fully functioning human speakers could theoretically tell the difference between "John gives Mary an apple" and "Mary gives John an apple."
    D. None of the above

Passage V (Questions 29–36)

When one thinks of modern architecture, one thinks of monumental, sprawling edifices: university libraries, churches, art museums, civic centers, skyscrapers, hotels, and shopping complexes. The sweeping, soaring, sometimes jarring forms of these buildings bear the marks of their creators' ideals and principles. However, one can also see, perhaps more clearly than in these overpowering structures, the architectural ideals of the twentieth century in the modest form of the chair.

Chairs are human in scale and are part of the daily life of everyone in our society. Architects often take on chair design as an exercise and a challenge—for the perfect chair is an elusive design goal. Most of the premier architects of the century have tried their hand at chair design. In these chairs, one can see, in small scale, the architectural philosophies of the greats.

The Bauhaus school of design is represented by the chairs of Mies vander Rohe and Charles Breuer. The guiding principle of this school was to let the materials dictate the form of the constructed object. In larger buildings, this resulted in the square boxes of steel and glass that now populate many of America's urban downtown areas. Steel has greater tensile strength than concrete, brick or wood, and so it could be used to frame and support a basic structure. Glass panes could then be stretched across the surface to form walls and windows at the same time. The whole had a lyric, formal purity, but tended to lack any human warmth.

The same disregard for the human form plagues Bauhaus' sitting devices. The Breuer chair is formally beautiful—bands of sturdy leather stretched in perpendicular planes across metal tubing to form seat and back—but is unyielding to the human form when sat upon. Morris Rietveld's wooden chair is worse—a reclining wedge of wood, the seat too long for the average human thigh, the back reclined but absolutely rigid. Another of Breuer's forms became quite popular, but cheap knock-offs were no more comfortable than the original—this was the metal *s*-shape with woven bamboo flat seat and back.

Frank Lloyd Wright, an American architect, was overshadowed by the Bauhaus denizens who arrived on American shores after World War II, but his principles continue to have a quiet influence on contemporary architects. Wright took a more Taoist approach to building. He tried to make his structures unobtrusive in their natural environment and suitable for their human inhabitants. This often required violating the Bauhaus regard for material by stretching them to their limits and beyond. The designs for Wright's famous house "Fallingwater," balanced on a boulder about a running stream in rural Pennsylvania, inspired several pages of structural objections by local inspectors, and the large concrete cantilevers that make up the main design of the house had to have additional steel supports added inside them and propping them up from below.

Wright designed all the furniture for his homes and public buildings and often built them into the walls so they would not be removed or exchanged. His chairs are frequently cradle-shaped, with padded cushions all around. Although they were undoubtedly more comfortable than Bauhaus chairs, Wright himself was never satisfied with his chair designs. He wrote that, in the quest for the perfect chair, he had discovered that human beings were most likely not designed to sit on their posteriors.

Perhaps architects have not yet found the perfect chair because different chairs work better and worse for different people in different circumstances. One needs a hard, straight chair when one needs to sit up at attention, for example in a lecture hall or at a formal tea in an elderly aunt's parlour. Large, padded, reclining chairs are best for longer durations and more relaxing activities—watching

television or curling up with a favorite book. The moral of the story is that, when dealing with human beings in all of their variety, one must pursue pluralism and tolerance rather than searching for a single ideal.

29. Why does the author write about chairs?

 A. The author has a penchant for monumental architectural forms.

 B. The author hopes architects will find the perfect chair.

 C. The author wants one to see the ideals of modern architecture in microcosm.

 D. Concentration on smaller forms helps one to ignore the variations that occur in them.

30. Which of the following is NOT a contrast the author draws between the Bauhaus architects and Frank Lloyd Wright?

 A. One's chairs are comfortable; the other's are not comfortable

 B. Materials versus use dictate form

 C. One had extensive influence, the other did not

 D. American versus European origins

31. Which of the following structures would accord with Bauhaus' principles?

 I. City skyscrapers
 II. Soft, padded chairs
 III. Shopping malls

 A. I only
 B. I and II only
 C. II and III only
 D. I, II, and III

32. From the context of the passage, which of the following can one infer are the Taoist principles referred to in the fifth paragraph?

 I. Usefulness to inhabitants
 II. Harmony with nature
 III. Place for spiritual retreat

 A. I only
 B. II only
 C. I and II only
 D. II and III only

33. Which of the following groups of terms probably best describe Bauhaus' buildings?

    A. Classical, functional, welcoming
    B. Expressive, expensive, elegant
    C. Austere, pure, urban
    D. Industrial, cramped, busy

34. Which of the following does the author believe?

    A. Human beings will never be completely satisfied.
    B. Bauhaus' architecture is superior to Wright's architecture.
    C. In design, intellectual factors are the most important.
    D. Chairs should be built into walls and not removed.

35. Which of the following best summarizes the two contrasting architectural philosophies?

    A. Form over simplicity; simplicity over form.
    B. Materials take priority over users; users take priority over materials.
    C. Comfort breeds efficiency; comfort elucidates efficiency.
    D. Usefulness above all; popularity above all.

36. The author of this passage describes his/her value system in the text of this passage. Based on these values, what kind of transportation does the author probably use?

    A. The author probably uses a utility vehicle.
    B. The author probably uses a variety of vehicles.
    C. The author probably uses only a bicycle.
    D. The author probably uses only public transportation.

Passage VI (Questions 37–43)

T.S. Eliot's *The Waste Land* could be the most inscrutable of the world's great poems. In it, Eliot weaves together bits and pieces from classic works in European literature and world religions and mythology (often in their original languages), and interweaves them with descriptions of modern, postindustrial urban landscapes. One needs patience and a good set of footnotes to work one's way through the poem, but the hard work is well repaid. Eliot's poem reveals itself as a modern myth to make sense of the recurring cycles of death and life in nature.

The classical fragments and allusions throughout the poem are all taken from fertility legends. Nearly every culture has a story allegorizing winter's death and dormancy and spring's renewal and new life. In these legends, winter, death, and sterility are symbolized by bare trees, rock, desert, dry wind, and the unforgiving sun. Spring and life are frequently symbolized by fish and fishermen. Fire and water play dual roles in the legends; both destroy but both can also purify. In most of the legends, including the Christian version, a land waits in drought for a Fisher King to come; the Fisher King must sacrifice his life in order to bring regeneration to the land and its people.

In Eliot's modern legend, the dry land is modern London. Its citizens flow over bridges (instead of water flowing under them), sighing and looking at their feet: "so many," the poem's narrator remarks; "I had not thought death had undone so many." Death recurs as an image when one man asks his neighbor, "That corpse you planted last year in your garden, Has it begun to sprout? Will it bloom this year?"

Sexual relationships in this city are empty, sterile, and fruitless. Eliot describes one young woman after one such tryst:

> She turns and looks a moment in the glass,
> Hardly aware of her departed lover;
> Her brain allows one half-formed thought to pass;
> "Well now that's done: and I'm glad it's over."

Perhaps the best representative of the sexual relationships in the poem is the woman in a bar at closing time, whose teeth are rotting and stained from the pills she has taken to induce an abortion. She dreads her husband's upcoming release from the army, because she had already borne him five children. Her companion tells her, "if you don't give it him, there's others will."

The physical landscapes in the poem are as putrid and sterile as the human ones. The "Unreal City" lies under brown fog, and the river Thames "sweats, oil and tar." In the final section of the poem, a traveler recites a painful litany in the dry, barren mountains:

> Here is no water but only rock. . .
> If there were only water amongst the rock. . .
> If there were water
> And no rock
> If there were rock
> And also water. . .
> But there is no water.

But soon a cock crows, which is an ancient sign of the departure of ghosts and evil spirits, thunder rumbles, and then comes "a damp gust, Bringing rain." The thunder speaks three Hindi words: "Datta. Dayadhvam. Damyata," which mean "Give alms; be compassionate; practice self-control." A Phoenician sailor has drowned on his way to London, representing the death by water that will bring the life-giving rain. The poem ends with the redemption purchased by the sailor's life, instruction from the thunder, and a benediction from Eliot himself. Eliot closes the poem with three repetitions of a word that serves as the formal ending for Hindu Upanishads (like an "amen"); the closest translation for the word is "the peace that passeth understanding." The very sound of the chant conveys feelings of resolution and quiet restfulness:

"Shantih shantih shantih."

37. Why is *The Waste Land* inscrutable?

    I. Some passages are in foreign languages.
    II. Eliot uses allusions to a wide variety of source material.
    III. The subject matter is too remote for modern readers.

    A. I and II only
    B. I and III only
    C. II and III only
    D. I, II, and III

38. What value is given to the death of the Phoenician sailor?

    A. Regeneration of the land
    B. Regeneration of the people
    C. Resolution
    D. Redemption

39. Which of the following characteristics do the two female characters discussed in the passage have in common?

    A. Physical disfigurement
    B. Boredom
    C. Disinterest in sex
    D. Both women study their own reflections.

40. What role does the corpse in the garden play in the poem?

    I. It is a parody of the Fisher King, the death that will bring new life.
    II. It is a parody of spring set in the dry, sterile time representing winter in the poem.
    III. It signifies the fruitlessness of the characters' attempts to generate life before the redemption.

    A. II only
    B. I and III only
    C. II and III only
    D. I, II, and III

41. In the poem, Eliot says that the Thames "sweats, oil and tar." How might the impact of industrial waste on the environment fit the poem's larger themes?

    A. Industrial pollution exemplifies mankind's responsibility for the death and sterility in the world.
    B. The leaders of industry are immoral villains causing suffering and unhappiness.
    C. Industrial toxins kill and maim plants and animals and poison the ground, causing death and sterility.
    D. Toxic chemicals burn and transform as fire does.

42. In paragraph two, the significance of fire is that:

    A. saints and religious figures were frequently burned at the stake.
    B. boiling water purifies it.
    C. fire destroys the former object, but leaves something else in its place (e.g., ashes or molten wax that has changed shape).
    D. fire and the sun are associated with summer.

43. What do the events at the end of the poem and Eliot's benediction show?

    A. Humankind has been redeemed by Christ.
    B. Eliot believes there is hope for the modern world.
    C. The Phoenician sailor will make it to port.
    D. Industrial civilization is doomed to death.

Passage VII (Questions 44–50)

Francois-Marie Arouet de Voltaire, better known to his readers as simply Voltaire, lived before the French Revolution, but in his life and in his work he prefigured many of its themes. He was born in 1694 in Paris and was raised in a well-off bourgeois family. Initially, he was to pursue a law career, but quickly abandoned it for his writing. Voltaire's life was marked by a number of banishments from France; his satirical writing carried sharp barbs and a serious message to leaders of the government from the very beginning.

During an exile in Great Britain, Voltaire was exposed to the philosophical and political writings of John Locke, and these writings had a great influence on the development of his political views. Locke was one of the founders of the classic liberal political school of the Enlightenment. Locke advocated democratic representation and limited interference by the government in private lives. Voltaire brought Locke's views to French readers in his *Let-*

ter Concerning the English Nation, and continued to develop them throughout his life in further writings.

Voltaire's most famous work, *Candide*, is a broadly satirical tale that lampoons many aspects of French society. The main character, Candide, receives his early education from Dr. Pangloss, who teaches that this is the best of all possible worlds, and that therefore everything that happens in it is for the best. This was a doctrine espoused by philosophers of the time, such as Leibniz. Candide has so many miserable encounters with evil, corruption, and human suffering in his journeys that he ends up relinquishing Pangloss' philosophy. These encounters also demonstrate to the reader the corruption of the Catholic church as well as of Judaism, the futility of war, the destructiveness of avarice, and the primitive nature of the justice system—the book includes a kangaroo trial and subsequent hanging for the crimes of uttering and listening to suspect information.

Before writing *Candide*, Voltaire had been in exile from Paris at Cirey, in Lorraine, and living with Madame du Chatelet. She was a scholar and scientist in her own right, and she and Voltaire together conducted experiments in physics and studied history and metaphysics. After her death in 1749, Voltaire traveled around Europe and finally settled on property he purchased at Ferney, once again in France, in 1755. From this time until the end of his life (23 years later in 1778, at the age of 84), Voltaire engaged aggressively in pursuing social justice and working for change in the French courts and government. He advocated public trial by jury, humane treatment of the accused, and fairness in the selection of judges; he was against the use of civil authority to punish religious crimes and advocated the institution of equitable punishment. During this time in France, civil courts were frequently used to try religious offenses, such as blasphemy and sorcery. Voltaire staged two high-profile campaigns against the treatment of religious criminals. One young man had been tortured and put to death for destroying a cross, and another, Jean Calas, had been put to death on the rack for being a Protestant, although he protested his innocence until the end. Voltaire succeeded in having the ruling against Calas overturned, the judges condemned, and the family remunerated with a royal pension. Voltaire also objected to the fact that the government had the church in its back pocket.

In his writings and in his life, Voltaire supported the ideals that would later inspire the revolutionaries in 1789. They, too, fought for equitable punishment, humane treatment of the accused, representative government, separation of church and state, and a recognition of the dignity and worth of all human beings.

44. Which of the following conclusions might one draw from the passage?

    A. Voltaire's ideas could have had more impact if he had been allowed to stay in France his entire life.

    B. Voltaire began by abandoning the law and ended up reforming it for future generations.

    C. Madame du Chatelet deserves at least half of the credit for Voltaire's ideas.

    D. Dr. Pangloss was a caricature of Voltaire.

45. Which of the following correctly describes Voltaire?

    I. Political philosopher
    II. Satirist
    III. Amateur scientist

    A. I only
    B. II only
    C. I and II only
    D. I, II, and III

46. Which of the following themes appear(s) both in *Candide* and in Voltaire's social work in the last 20 years of his life?

    I. Criticism of the church
    II. Leibnizian optimism
    III. Excessive punishment for crime

    A. II only
    B. I and II only
    C. I and III only
    D. I, II, and III

47. Which of the following people played significant roles in Voltaire's life during his exile?

    I. John Locke
    II. Madame du Chatelet
    III. Jean Calas

    A. II only
    B. I and II only
    C. II and III only
    D. I, II, and III

48. Which of the following descriptions of Voltaire is true?

    A. Although his views frequently landed him in hot water, he was eventually embraced by the royalty of France.

    B. He was influential in the initial organization of resistance during the French Revolution.

    C. He was the first to bring English ideas to France.

    D. His life was devoted to the pursuit of social justice.

49. Which of the following modern institutions reflect(s) Voltaire's ideals?

    I. Congressional approval of Supreme Court justices

    II. Laws designed to uphold Christian values

    III. Appointment of public defenders

    A. I only

    B. II and III only

    C. I and III only

    D. I, II, and III

50. The French Revolution was fought using terror, mass imprisonment, and torture of politically suspect citizens, and tens of thousands of deaths by guillotine for political crimes. Which of the ideals described in the passage were not adhered to?

    I. Equitable punishment

    II. Locke's liberalism

    III. Separation of church and state

    A. I only

    B. I and II only

    C. II and III only

    D. I, II, and III

Passage VIII (Questions 51–57)

In the farthest southwest corner of the South Island in New Zealand is a 33.5-mile hiking trail that was described in a 1908 travel article in a London magazine as "The Finest Walk in the World." The walk is called the Milford Track. It runs from the point of Lake Te Anau to the point of the Milford Sound, a fjord on the coast. Although the terrain is temperate rain forest and is truly wilderness, the walk is manageable for hikers who are less than mountaineers.

The area is lush with rain forest foliage such as lancewood, fuchsia, pepper trees, and giant ferns, but travelers do not need to worry about wild animals. The two islands of New Zealand separated from the continent of what is now Australia before mammals developed, so its native popula-

tion includes only birds, insects, and two species of bat. As a consequence, hikers need not worry about crocodiles or other reptiles, although they can be extremely bothered by sand flies. They may have the treat of seeing keas on the walk, which are the world's only mountain parrot.

The high point of the walk, both literally and figuratively, is Mackinnon Pass, which is marked with a stone cairn memorializing its discovery by Quinton Mackinnon in 1888. Mackinnon finished a job that was begun by Donald Sutherland, the man who settled the Milford Sound in 1878. The men, both native Scots, were each trying to find a route through the mountains that separated the ports of the coast from the inland farmlands. Mackinnon and his partner, Earl Mitchell, after several attempts to hack their way through the dense foliage, finally succeeded and crested the 3785-foot pass on October 17, 1888 (midspring in the southern hemisphere). Sutherland disputed Mackinnon's discovery, saying he knew of the route before Mackinnon, and persisted in referring to it as Balloon Pass, after nearby Balloon Mountain, until his death in 1912. Nevertheless, Sutherland is memorialized in Sutherland Falls, the fourth highest waterfall in the world at 1904 feet. It is a 20-minute walk off the main trail to see these falls, but if one chooses not to make it, there are many smaller falls to see, 35 of them from a single rest stop.

Travelers today have a much easier time topping the pass than Mackinnon did. The trail opened for tourism in 1908, and today nearly 10,000 people make the hike yearly. The New Zealand government strictly controls the number of people on the trail, allowing only 40 independent hikers, known as freedom walkers, and 42 members of guided groups to enter the trail daily. The group hikers are very well served by the Southern Pacific Hotel Corporation, which supplies guides and offers comfortably appointed huts at four stops along the trail for hikers to spend the night. The huts are staffed with cooks and chambermaids and equipped with dormitory-style bunk beds, pianos, books, and clothes dryers—often a necessity, due to the area's unpredictable weather. If clear skies hold, though, hikers are rewarded at the pinnacle of their walk with spectacular views of the majestic mountain range, lush greens, and sparkling waterfalls of this section of New Zealand.

51. Which of the following might bother hikers on the Milford Track?

    I. Carrion birds

    II. Inclement weather

    III. Cairns

    A. I and II only

    B. I and III only

    C. II only

    D. III only

52. Which of the following is NOT a feature of the walk?

    A. Waterfalls
    B. Sand flies
    C. Chambermaids
    D. Farmlands

53. Milford Track was called "The Finest Walk in the World." How many other features of the walk hold world distinction?

    A. 1
    B. 2
    C. 4
    D. 35

54. Based on the passage, how might one describe the landscape surrounding the walk?

    I. Verdant
    II. Mountainous
    III. Rugged

    A. I only
    B. I and II only
    C. II only
    D. II and III only

55. What would one need to bring along as a freedom walker on the Milford Track?

    I. Cookstove and food
    II. Snake-bite kit
    III. Bug spray

    A. II only
    B. I and III only
    C. III only
    D. I, II, and III

56. For what is Donald Sutherland remembered?

    A. Discovering the pass from Lake Te Anau to Milford Sound
    B. Founding Milford Sound
    C. Discovering Balloon Mountain
    D. Discovering Sutherland Falls

57. If October is midspring in the southern hemisphere, in what season is April?

    A. Winter
    B. Spring
    C. Summer
    D. Autumn

Passage IX (Questions 58–65)

In October of 1991, the federal government passed the Clean Air Act, which will have a widespread effect on automotive industries. Automobile emission standards set by the Clean Air Act require that hydrocarbon emissions be reduced by 35% and nitrogen oxide emissions be reduced by 60%. In order to comply with these standards, automobile manufacturers will have to develop changes in existing car design. They may even pursue such radical options as battery-powered or solar-powered vehicles. However, because many old cars continue to remain on the road, it could take 20 years before changes in automobile design can have their full impact on air quality. Changes in gasoline formulation, on the other hand, can have an effect immediately.

One change that has already been instituted in some parts of the country involves trapping the vapors released when cars are filled with gas. Automobile makers have considered building traps on cars themselves, but this has several disadvantages over providing traps on the pumps. First, as mentioned above, changes that only affect new cars have a delayed effect on existing air conditions. Second, retooling the gas system would cost about 50 dollars per car, a cost that would be passed on to consumers to the tune of about 600 million dollars per year. Institution of recovery traps at the pump would have an initial cost of about one billion dollars to gasoline companies. Vapor recovery traps at the pump would be effective more quickly, and would cost less to the industry in the long run.

Another change that will soon be instituted by a number of gasoline companies is the development of reformulated fuels. The changes made to existing fuel mixtures will vary among companies, but in general the following alterations will be made. First, reformulated gasoline will contain lower levels of benzene, in order to lower their toxicity. Second, they will have lower levels of aromatics and olefins, which are hydrocarbons that turn to smog when they interact with direct sunlight. Instead, gasoline manufacturers will add oxygenates. These oxygenates will boost octane levels, reduce hydrocarbons and carbon monoxides, and increase the fuel–air ratio, which in turn increases the amount of gasoline yield from crude oil. Third, the fuels will have reduced sulfur, which reduces hydrocarbon, carbon monoxide, and nitrogen oxide emissions and provides for more effective catalyst operation when the fuel is burned. Finally, gasoline manufacturers will try to reduce the Reid Vapor Pressure (RVP) of gasoline blends, which reduces the volatility of gasoline and therefore lowers the emissions of toxins from fuel evaporation.

One final change that would help air quality is if older cars were actually held to the emission standards set for them. The Arco company recently purchased 7000 cars that were built in 1970 or earlier in order to test their fuel efficiency and emissions. Statistics show that although older cars comprise 15% of vehicles on the road and only 10% of the total car miles traveled, they contribute 30% of total air pollution. Arco's study found that the 7000 cars averaged 11.9 miles per gallon, half the rate of cars that were built in 1990. Their emission of carbon monoxides was 11 times that of cars built in 1990, emission of nitrogen oxides 11 times higher, and emission of hydrocarbons 65 times higher. The good news resulting from this survey is that as these older cars age and are no longer on the road, and as they are replaced with fuel-efficient and cleaner burning vehicles, air quality should improve dramatically.

58. From the passage, which of the following can one conclude is/are harmful to the air?

   I. Benzene
   II. Oxygenates
   III. Fuel evaporation

   A. I and II only
   B. I and III only
   C. III only
   D. I, II, and III

59. According to the author, what is the main problem with older cars?

   A. They are staying on the road longer.
   B. Their emission of hydrocarbons is higher than their emission of carbon monoxides.
   C. They have poor gas mileage.
   D. They produce more than their share of air pollution.

60. Which of the following can be inferred from the final paragraph of the passage?

   A. Older cars travel 5% less distance per trip compared with newer cars.
   B. Hydrocarbon emissions are more dangerous than nitrogen oxide emissions.
   C. Air quality will probably improve within 20 years.
   D. None of the above

61. Which of the following is the best title for the passage?

   A. *Better Fuel for Better Air*
   B. *Increased Gas Mileage May Increase Your Life*
   C. *Changes in the Automotive Industry*
   D. *Carbons and You*

62. Based on the information provided in the passage, which of the following changes can be inferred to have the most impact?

   A. Fuels with reduced RVP
   B. Battery-powered cars
   C. Fuel vapor traps on new cars
   D. Improved enforcement of emissions standards for older cars

63. Which of the following alterations to gasoline mixture can reduce hydrocarbons?

   I. Reduced sulfur
   II. Higher octane levels
   III. Lower olefin levels

   A. I and II only
   B. I and III only
   C. II and III only
   D. I, II, and III

64. Which of the following can have a negative effect on air quality?

   I. Standing fuel exposed to sunlight
   II. Refueling automobiles
   III. Short, in-town automobile trips

   A. I only
   B. I and II only
   C. II and III only
   D. I, II, and III

65. According to the Clean Air Act, nitrogen oxide emissions must be reduced by a higher percentage than hydrocarbon emissions. Which of the following processes are gasoline companies most likely to concentrate on?

   A. Increased RVP
   B. Reduced sulfur
   C. Increased fuel–air ratio
   D. Lower benzene levels

Answers and Explanations to Verbal Reasoning Practice Test 1

1. **C**   Only statement III is correct. Refer to the first paragraph of the passage. Modernists only made unadorned constructions, thus, statement I is incorrect. Paragraph four supports that neither modernists nor constructivists painted pictures of objects, so statement II is incorrect.

2. **D**   Statements I, II, and III are correct. The fourth paragraph describes painters, designers of endpaper and textiles, and sculptors who make wood and steel constructions.

3. **C**   The constructivists believed that art should be integrated into the public sphere. The support for this choice is in the first and final paragraphs of the passage. Choices A, B, and D either are irrelevant or unsupported by the passage.

4. **D**   Statements I, II, and III convey the principles of the movement. The departure from tradition mentioned in paragraph four is mentioned as an ideal in paragraph five. The bright colors express the optimism described in paragraphs one and five. The geometric constructions resemble the wood and steel constructions mentioned in paragraph four.

5. **B**   Be careful with questions that have a negative word in the stem. The final paragraph gives a list of similar values of both the Soviet state and constructivist artists. This allows you to eliminate choices A, C, and D. Choice B is the best answer because the first paragraph implies that constructivists wanted to move their art out of the museum.

6. **B**   Statement II is correct. Although the *Letalin* was never used, it was still useful. The passage describes both the *Letalin* and the monument as functional. Statement III is incorrect because constructivists never said artists could not take credit for their work.

7. **A**   The passage supports that the constructivists were interested in technology. The use of found objects of a technological nature supplied the constructivists great material from which to create art. This is supported by statement I. There is not enough evidence in the passage such that statements II and III were constructivist goals.

8. **C**   The goal of bringing art into life was to improve the lives of Soviet citizens. Thus, the irony was that constructivist art was never employed in this manner. When the author mentions irony in the last paragraph, it is in relation to Stalin's suppression, not to the exhibitions.

9. **D**   Statements I, II, and III are not mentioned in the passage.

10. **C**   The second paragraph of the passage compares eristic disputation with a lawyer's or politician's rhetoric, designed to persuade but not necessarily to report the truth.

11. **D**   The fifth paragraph says sophistic subjects were added to increase competitiveness, and that Plato's curriculum was designed to build strong citizens. The

fourth paragraph says Plato's continuous, 3- to 4-year curriculum was unique. Thus, choices A, B, and C can be eliminated, leaving choice D.

12.	**A**	Paragraph four describes the lecture format of instruction, and says records exist of *Aristotle's* lectures. This allows you to eliminate choices B and C. Choice D is a correct statement, so it should be eliminated.
13.	**B**	Choices A, C, and D are supported by the passage. Choice C is not supported in its entirety, because in the third paragraph, the author mentions that some sophists eventually settled down.
14.	**B**	The third paragraph states that Socrates, Plato's teacher, had a school, and this would be earlier than the Academy. This supports choice B. The other choices are neither implied nor stated in the passage.

PASSAGE III

15.	**A**	Choice B can be eliminated, because the passage never mentions America. While bitterness and chocolate imitators are mentioned, they are not the main topics of the passage. Thus, eliminate choices C and D.
16.	**B**	Statements I and III are correct. The passage supports that blending just produces variety in flavors. Knowing that statement II is incorrect allows you to eliminate choices A, C, and D.
17.	**C**	Statement III is correct. Paragraphs five and six discuss bitterness issues and do not support statements I and II. By default, choice C is the best answer.
18.	**D**	The final paragraph uses the term cocoa butter and mentions that chocolate-flavored products use vegetable oil instead of cocoa butter.
19.	**A**	The author's style is not casual enough to be colloquial, and although the author discusses enthusiasm for chocolate, not much enthusiasm is actually displayed in the passage. The author tends to provide more information than celebration (choice C) or convolution (choice D).
20.	**C**	Chocolate liquor is discussed in the fourth paragraph. This question simply tests if you can quickly find information provided in the passage.
21.	**A**	This question uses terms that are described in the passage. The question asks you to choose a statement that is implied by the passage. None of these choices is as much implied as is either stated or not stated. Paragraph two states that fermentation occurs after the beans are separated. Thus, choice A is a correct statement. Choices B, C, and D are incorrect statements.
22.	**B**	You must assume that the best to eat would amount to that which is the most processed toward becoming chocolate. Choice B is the furthest along in the processing, and is thus the best answer.

PASSAGE IV

23.	**C**	Statements II and III are correct. Both of these parallel the case of the chimpanzees, who know words but not syntax.
24.	**D**	Syntactic rules are rules of formation. The author clearly states in the third paragraph that chimpanzees do not understand syntax. Thus, chimpanzees have difficulty with the way in which items in the vocabulary are put together (i.e., formal rules). This supports choice D. The author never states that chimpanzees make mistakes with individual signs (or words), so choice B is incorrect. Choice A is contradicted by the passage. Choice C is not discussed or supported by the passage.
25.	**C**	According to the passage, damage to the left hemisphere of the brain affects language abilities but *not* general motor skills. Refer to the final paragraph, which supports statements II and III, and makes choice C the best answer.
26.	**B**	According to this assumption, damage to the right hemisphere of the brain would impair *both* general motor abilities and motor abilities used in ASL.
27.	**B**	Statements I and II are correct. The passage describes what syntax is at the end of paragraph two. Syntactic changes are changes in grammatical form, not vocabulary. Eliminate statement III because it is a vocabulary change, thus choice B the best answer.
28.	**C**	Paragraph three claims that all human beings are born with syntactic ability, *unlike* chimpanzees. Because choice C presents an issue of syntax recognition, it

ANSWERS AND
EXPLANATIONS
TO VERBAL
REASONING
PRACTICE TEST 1

686

is the best choice. The other choices are incorrect statements or are not supported by the passage.

---

29. **C** The author points out that the architectural ideals of the twentieth century are illustrated by the form of the chair. A penchant is a leaning or inclination toward something. The author does not write about chairs because of an inclination toward monumental architectural forms. The author rejects the quest for the ideal chair in the last paragraph, and the essay emphasizes the variations in the smaller forms of the chairs.

30. **C** Choices A, B, and D are contrasts that are not contradicted by the passage. Choice C is not a contrast the author draws between the Bauhaus architects and Frank Lloyd Wright. Both architectural schools had extensive influence.

31. **A** Soft chair recliners follow Wrightian principles of catering to the user's comfort and do not have sleekly efficient design. Shopping malls have many designs, some are according to Bauhaus' principles and some are not.

32. **C** Statement III is not supported by the passage because Wright's spiritual beliefs are never discussed in the essay. Statements I and II are reasonable to infer because the passage does not mention environment and inhabitants.

33. **C** This question requires you to find the paragraph that describes Bauhaus' architecture. Paragraph three describes this architecture as urban, pure, and basically austere.

34. **A** This question is best answered by the process of elimination. The best choice is not directly stated, but inferred. The author's beliefs are best conveyed in the final paragraph of the passage. The author emphasizes the variety of people, their different needs and desires, and touches on issues of satisfaction. Choices B, C, and D are not supported by the passage.

35. **B** Choices A and C are not philosophies of the architects as discussed in the passage. Both the Bauhaus and Wright architects strove for usefulness, and neither strove in particular for popular acceptance. Choice D is incorrect because both architectural philosophies were based on the relationship among materials and form (Bauhaus) or users (Wright).

36. **B** The final paragraph of the passage shows that the author mainly values pluralism—everyone requires different things for different purposes. This value system coincides best with choice B.

---

37. **A** Statements I and II are correct. The first paragraph discusses the main issues, which support the first two statements. Statement III is incorrect, because the subject matter is not remote for modern readers.

38. **D** The death of the Phoenician sailor is discussed as representing the death by water that will bring life-giving rain. It is also made clear that the sailor's death brings redemption. The Fisher King is discussed as bringing regeneration to the land and people (choices A and B). Resolution (choice C) is discussed at the end of the passage as the result of the chant.

39. **C** The fourth paragraph discusses the two women and provides a description. There is a strong sexual tone and a clear disinterest in sex that is voiced in this paragraph. Choice A is incorrect because physical disfigurement is not discussed or implied. Although the female characters in the passage may be bored, the disinterest in sex outweighs this, and choice B can be eliminated. Choice D can be eliminated because there is no strong evidence that there is self-study of the female characters.

40. **D** Statements I, II, and III are correct. The corpse is a death that will not bring life, so therefore it is a spring planting that has no hope of blossoming. It resembles the sexual relationships in the characters' lives, in which the planter goes through the motions, but no new life can result.

41. **C** Industrial waste contributes to sterility and death, which best fits the poem's theme. The themes expressed in choices A, B, and D do not appear in the poem.

SECT. IV
VERBAL
REASONING
PRACTICE
TEST I

687

42. **C** In this question, look for an answer choice that expresses the dual roles of fire. This is important because the passage makes a point of mentioning both destruction and purification. As you evaluate the choices, only choice C includes both sacrifice (destruction) and rebirth as something new.

43. **B** The coming of rain signifies that spring will eventually come and life will regenerate again. This theme is best voiced by choice B. Note "resolution" and "quiet restfulness" used in the last paragraph. Choices A, C, and D are incorrect because they either suggest a negative ending or are relatively unsupported.

PASSAGE VII

44. **B** Review the first and fourth paragraphs. Paragraph two explains the impact of things he learned in exile on Voltaire's thought. Madame du Chatelet only assisted in the scientific experiments, and thus choice C is incorrect. Voltaire disagreed with Pangloss' stance, making choice D unlikely. Choice A is incorrect, because although Voltaire was banished from France several times, his ideas continued to have significant impact.

45. **D** Statements I, II, and III are correct. Voltaire's book about England is political philosophy, thus statement I is true. Statement II is correct, because *Candide* is satire. Finally, statement III is true, because Voltaire conducted scientific experiments with Madame du Chatelet.

46. **C** Statements I and III are true. In paragraph four, there are several prominent examples showing Voltaire's criticism of the church and his feelings about excessive punishment for crime. Leibnizian optimism, the belief that this is the best of all possible worlds, does not appear in Voltaire's work.

47. **B** Statements I and II are correct. Statement III is incorrect because Voltaire worked toward justice for Jean Calas after his return and final settlement in France.

48. **D** Voltaire fought against the rulers of France until his death. Thus, choice A is incorrect. Choice B is incorrect because Voltaire died before the start of the French Revolution. Choice C is not the best choice because the author of the passage never states that Voltaire's report on English philosophy was the first.

49. **C** Statements I and III are correct. Statement I upholds fairness in selection of judges, and statement III respects the right of an accused to a fair trial. Statement II does not respect the separation of church and state. Thus, C is the best choice.

50. **B** Statements I and II are correct. Beheading for politically suspect activities is excessive punishment for the crime. In paragraph two, the author says that Locke's theory includes advocating limited interference by the government in private lives. The author never states the revolutionaries had religious motives.

PASSAGE VIII

51. **C** Only statement II is correct. Carrion birds feed on dead mammals, and there are no native mammals on the trail. Cairns are symbolic piles of rock. Although the Milford Track has one, it is not likely to bother hikers. The final paragraph describes the rainy weather and the accommodations necessary to deal with weather situations.

52. **D** Although there are farmlands inland, they are not visible from the track. Recall that the track is in the mountains. This makes choice D the best choice as a feature that is not part of the walk. Waterfalls (choice A) and sand flies (choice B) are mentioned in the passage. The chambermaids (choice C) are discussed in the final paragraph as part of the accommodations that are offered to hikers.

53. **B** Skimming the passage carefully should help you answer this question. The keas, the world's only mountain parrot, and Sutherland Falls, the world's fourth highest falls are world distinctive features of the walk. Thus, choice B is the best answer.

ANSWERS AND
EXPLANATIONS
TO VERBAL
REASONING
PRACTICE TEST I

688

54. **B**   Statements I and II are correct. *Verdant* means lush and green. Thus, statement I is correct. You can eliminate choices C and D based on accepting statement I. Statement II is clearly supported in the passage, so choice B is the best answer. Statement III is not fully accurate, because even though the track is in the mountains, it is described in the first paragraph as a manageable walk.

55. **C**   Statement III is correct. The second paragraph states that there are no native reptiles, so eliminate statement II. The fourth paragraph explains that only group hikers stay in the huts, so eliminate statement I.

56. **B**   This is a straightforward question. Simply refer back to paragraph three in the passage. It clearly states that Donald Sutherland discovered Milford Sound.

57. **D**   The question points out that fall corresponds with spring in the southern hemisphere. From this, you should infer that the seasons are reversed from the northern hemisphere, and that April should correspond with autumn.

---

58. **B**   Statements I and III are correct. The toxicity of benzene and the harmful nature of fuel evaporation is supported in the third paragraph of the passage. Statement II is not correct because oxygenates replace harmful aromatics and olefins.

59. **D**   The final paragraph states that 10% of the cars produce 30% of total air pollution. There is no direct evidence in the passage that older cars either stay on the road longer than they used to, (or longer than other cars), or that hydrocarbon levels are higher than carbon monoxides (just that the deviation from 1990 levels is higher).

60. **C**   The final paragraph focuses on the air quality effects of having older cars on the road. You can infer from the passage that air quality will improve automatically as older cars are off the road. This makes C an excellent choice. Choice A is not supported numerically in the passage. Hydrocarbon and nitrous oxide are not compared relative to danger of their respective emissions.

61. **A**   The main point of this passage is not gas mileage, changes in automobile design, or carbons and hydrocarbons, but changes in fuel mixture to adhere to the Clean Air Act.

62. **B**   The author calls this a radical proposal in paragraph one. You should expect that battery-powered cars or solar-powered cars would each make a great impact on clean air. Looking at the choices, B is best. In a battery-powered car, you would not expect to burn fuel, and thus, you would have no emissions. The other choices might decrease emissions, but they would not eliminate them.

63. **B**   Statements I and III are correct and are discussed in the third paragraph. Higher octane levels do not reduce hydrocarbons; they are an effect of replacing aromatics and olefins with oxygenates. Thus, statement II is incorrect and choice B is the best answer.

64. **D**   Statements I, II, and III are correct. Fuel evaporation and vapors released from refueling release toxins into the air (see paragraphs two and three), and any car trip is going to release some emissions.

65. **B**   Paragraph three of the passage discusses many technical points and several different processes. Among all this information, you should note that reduced nitrogen oxide emission is discussed as a purpose for reducing sulfur in fuels. This is the only process discussed that mentions nitrogen oxide emissions.

SECT. IV
VERBAL
REASONING
PRACTICE
TEST I

689

Time: 85 Minutes

Directions: Each of the reading passages in this Verbal Reasoning test is followed by several questions. After reading a passage, select the one best answer to each of the questions that follow. If you are not certain of an answer, eliminate the alternatives that you know are incorrect, and then select an answer from the remaining alternatives.

Passage I (Questions 1–6)

It has been the inexorable process of mankind in modern history to divide itself into groups based on personal belief and conviction. In the smallest cases, such coteries include church groups, chess clubs, and innumerable other associations. On a larger scale, special interest groups and workers' associations represent a formidable force in any democratic country. But the acme of human achievement in this arena has been the creation of the political party. Its influence electorally and politically is unquestionable in most parts of the world. Taking France as an example . . .

Historically, France has been a nation of rapid, often tumultuous change. The revolution of 1789 was a catalyst of growing political discontent; but more than that, it was an event which would forever change the way the French viewed and treated their government. No longer the helpless proletariat, the French people became involved in the functioning of their country, and various parties formed to aggregate the differing views.

Instead of a bipolar system, which has become the norm in many democracies like England, France's multipolarity creates an interesting mix of smaller factions. The effect of this multitude of parties has been, historically, to moderate the referenda or election process. French policy making shows a tendency to make concessions to opposing or extreme factions in order to retain a majority. It is this sort of mitigation which has been the principle effect of multipolarity. Without a strong or absolute majority, legislation and policy making are governed by ephemeral coalitions of various parties.

If such fleeting confederations are prevalent in France's political culture, then what effect have they had on the ability of parties to function within the framework of the government? The answer is that the parties have reduced their individual powers by constantly compromising their positions. Their individual impact on government process has been lessened by the constant bargaining utilized to gain a working majority in the National Assembly.

In 1986, for example, the Assembly was divided among at least seven main parties and nonaffiliates. The net result is a dilution of party powers in the cauldron of a makeshift political center that has dominated French politics ever since the fateful day at the Bastille. This uneasy centrist coalition is a direct result of the enervated political parties which constitute it. Because no single party—Communist, Gaullist, or Socialist—has been able to secure an effective majority, the Assembly has become a battlefield of parties waging war on each other and on themselves. It is for this reason that neither right nor left has taken total control for any significant amount of time. A sort of civil disobedience prevents the Socialists from uniting with the left radicals and the UDF from allying with the National Front for any significant amount of time. This lack of unity and frequency of dispute have undoubtedly left the French government at the mercy of vagaries in its party system.

If history repeats itself, then France's memory is far too keen to allow a recurrence of its sordid past. History reminds French citizens daily that their government is a unique experiment of modern man that should be taken with a grain of salt. Skepticism and wariness are the gatekeepers of their souls, and their trust of the grand experiment is reflected in the wide disparity of party formations. To them, a party is a representation of their own narrow interests. To the government, such beliefs mean difficulty and discord. The inevitable result is a quixotic system of compromise and moderation—the French party system.

1. According to the author, French party politics can best be described as:

    A. a stable environment with little discord.
    B. an equally divided right/left system.
    C. similar in nature to other democratic models.
    D. a heterogeneous mix of many viewpoints.

2. If a strongly partisan issue were to confront the National Assembly, it would most likely be handled in which of the following ways?

    A. It would be altered to suit the tastes of smaller parties in order to gain their support.
    B. It would not be changed significantly.
    C. It would be debated endlessly and probably floored indefinitely.
    D. All of the above

3. If the French did not have such a dramatic political history of discontent, how might their party system differ today?

    I. It would consist of fewer parties.
    II. It would have stronger parties.
    III. It would have more parties.

    A. I only
    B. II only
    C. I and II only
    D. I and III only

4. According to the passage, parties have difficulty maintaining dominance in the Assembly because:

    A. they are afraid of offending other parties.
    B. they lack the political know-how.
    C. they both need and despise each other.
    D. they enjoy the melee of warring coalitions.

5. Bargaining is a key component in French politics because:

    I. it is problematic for the French government when trying to pass legislation.
    II. it prevents coalitions from disbanding too quickly.
    III. it gives smaller parties access to a system that might otherwise be dominated by larger ones.

    A. I only
    B. II only
    C. III only
    D. I and III only

6. It can reasonably be inferred from the passage that the diversity of France's party system is a result of:

    A. constant battle with hostile neighboring countries.
    B. the cynical nature of the French citizenry.
    C. histrionic mannerisms peculiar to the French.
    D. the organizational setup of the National Assembly.

Passage II (Questions 7–11)

Arising from nothing, human thought takes an incredible leap. From the abstract comes the concrete, and that which was never possible before is suddenly before our eyes. From the void of nothingness comes with shocking tangibility the real. This is the essence of mankind's power over its environment. People can place themselves in an alternate existence where all is possible. From the enigma of complex neurochemical reactions comes thought—but thought cannot be adequately explained with balanced equations and chemical interactions. From whence does this ability arise? How do we reconcile our physical existence with our metaphysical one?

The ability to conceptualize is a potent one indeed. It has allowed us to alter our existence in a profound fashion. Those animals considered our closest relatives have no such power, and it is for this reason that mankind is the most successful species on this planet. Devoid of limitations in the realm of thought, mankind can escape the confines of material existence and enter a state of limitless potential. Somewhere in the fleshy substance of the human cerebrum is this alternate universe, but where, and how?

Mankind's ability to function in the abstract is its greatest triumph. To merely *conceive* is an incredible feat. It requires an incredible array of faculties, which have never been even closely replicated. Indeed, the capacities of the human brain are only superficially understood. Without a working knowledge about the inception of thought, we continue to utilize it frequently and easily. We are the sole proprietor of our thought, and yet we have no owner's manual or instruction book on how to use it, or what makes it tick. We simply *do* it. The process is a mystery, but the ability is undeniably real. Thoughts that are without boundary are somehow contained in the physical parameters of our brain.

This dilemma has led some people to create poetic metaphors as explanatory tools. To many, the presence of a soul explains the nonrational elements in mankind's existence. Nested somewhere in this portion of our being is the source of our true nature. Thought is the outpouring of this nonrational character—it is the origin of the enigmatic processes that confound us. Such explanations aside, thought remains a mystery to the true skeptic. Somehow, biological processes transcend their seemingly mechanical role to create ideas, feelings, and perceptions. The physical properties of atoms and molecules take on a quality of the surreal—they formulate thought. Our imagination, arising from uncertain origin, opens the gates of infinity, leaving us to explore the fathomless depths of human consciousness.

7. The author's tone in this passage can most accurately be described as:

    A. judgmental.
    B. hostile.
    C. incredulous.
    D. detached.

8. In answering his own question about the origin of thought, the author concludes that:

    A. thought is best described as an element of a nonrational portion of our character.
    B. thought cannot be explained on a physical basis.
    C. thought is the result of tangible biologic processes.
    D. thought is an evolutionary adaptation expressed in its final form in the human species.

9. If a machine that could closely mimic the abstract qualities of the brain was constructed, its greatest feature would be:

    A. its ability to perceive the future.
    B. its capacity to create ideas from nothingness.
    C. its ability to solve complex mathematical equations.
    D. its ability to generate multiple scenarios simultaneously.

10. Based on the author's assertions, it can be logically concluded that:

    A. as humans we are blessed with a gift that is afforded to very few other creatures.
    B. thought requires processes that may never be fully understood.
    C. the brain is only a biologic factory, and so thought must be defined by irrational explanations.
    D. science alone will determine the avenues through which ideas originate.

11. Based on the author's conclusions, thought has most greatly affected our existence by:

    A. stimulating us to seek companionship.
    B. instilling a respect for our special place in the world.
    C. giving us the ability to perceive our surroundings better.
    D. allowing us to conceive in an infinite environment.

Passage III (Questions 12–16)

Karl Marx called religion "the opiate of the masses," a statement reflecting his conviction that religion gives easy answers to painful questions of life and death. But religion is more than just a pacifying system of beliefs; it offers its participants an unprecedented fraternal membership with millions of people—it is a powerful social force. By subscribing to a religious brotherhood, believers become part of a giant social machine capable of creating true social change. Any association with such organized factions can become a vehicle of strong social currents, which inevitably shape the context of their surroundings. By participating in a religion, people become wielders of a communal influence. They become Christians, or Muslims, or Jews, and by virtue of their sheer number, they exert powerful pressure on their society. The tenets of their religion define the way in which this pressure is manifested.

Religion can be viewed as a homogeneous microcosm of society. In it, groups of like-minded people gather to perpetuate their group characteristics. They share common traits, beliefs, and territory. By aggregating their numbers, they increase the likelihood that their voices will be heard, and thus ensure their existence.

Religion also acts as a normalizing force in society. It molds people into an image of itself, giving them a constant set of values to draw from and a model to emulate. In this fashion, its members are encouraged to become like one another, and extremism is discouraged. Such streamlining of the organizational membership increases the collective power of the whole, and maximizes its influence. With common beliefs and a polarized internal structure, the organization becomes a societal power of considerable proportions. At best, this can have positive effects on the ills that plague societies. At worst, it can create a dangerous belief in the right of its purpose, and society becomes the victim of its destructive zealotry.

Perhaps the greatest power of any religion is its tendency to freeze the status quo. Religious principles are largely immutable, and rapid change is discouraged. Societal progression, therefore, becomes a most difficult task. Subtle shifts in the culture are more easily accomplished, as they do not draw the attention of the organized religious masses as readily as major movements.

It is easy to see that the organizing forces of religion make it particularly immune to profound change. To alter the views and beliefs of individuals is a task that requires comparatively little effort. Affecting the beliefs of large numbers of people unified in a common framework is an entirely different matter. They are more likely to resist any efforts that may threaten the shared environment they cherish as sacred.

12. If a new religion was formed in a community, it would most likely attract people who:

A. have comparable values and beliefs.

B. have little in common but believe in a greater power.

C. are inclined to give credence to questionable beliefs.

D. come from a religious background.

13. Which of the following best explains how a religion tends to perpetuate itself?

A. By preventing rapid membership turnover

B. By inhibiting the destructive forces of other religions

C. By retaining a homogeneous membership

D. By quelling voices of opposition

14. According to the author, the most dangerous aspects of religion relate to:

A. the possibility that religious zealots might break off and form destructive cults.

B. their ability to deceive great numbers of people.

C. a certain inherent quality that discourages personal conviction.

D. the inertial forces of large, focused groups of believers.

15. This passage can best be described as:

I. a Marxist analysis.

II. a vindictive exposition.

III. a critique of religion.

A. I only

B. II only

C. III only

D. I and III only

16. Based on the passage, it can reasonably be inferred that a religion's power and influence are derived chiefly from:

A. the collective force conveyed by uniting great numbers of people.

B. strong-handed tactics.

C. the aggressive inclinations of a tightly organized membership.

D. unflinching stoicism.

Passage IV (Questions 17–21)

In an international order based on anarchy, nations are in a constant state of insecurity—this is the essence of the "security dilemma." However, none of the grand solutions to the problem of war and peace can at present guarantee the peace—not disarmament, not international adjudication, not collective security, not world government. And yet as a practical matter we cannot simply throw up our hands in resignation. We must focus our energies on the most promising of these solutions—collective security.

It is an excellent solution to the security dilemma in part due to its inherently stable nature. It is built on a system whereby all members (theoretically, the world) of the organization rely on all other members of the organization to come to their aid in a time of trouble. The stability arises from the desire of all the actors to maintain the peace through nonaggression. Because every state in the world subscribes to the same goal, the peace is ensured. If, for example, a power were to attempt to tip the scales in its favor, the other nations would correct the imbalance and ensure continued security. Besides providing a stable alternative to the security dilemma, it is also an excellent deterrent to aggression. When trying to reduce the likelihood of war, it is essential to reduce the incentive for conflict to the lowest possible levels. Collective security deters any state from attacking another by ensuring swift and devastating retribution for acts of aggression by other members. War is a product of conflict, and so eliminating potential conflict eliminates a precursor to war.

The basic premise of collective security states that any threatened nation will be aided by other members to swiftly halt aggression. In this way, even small, relatively powerless nations are assured security. Size is no longer an issue if the mechanism works ideally. If all nations are committed, and are willing to use force to preserve the peace, then security is no longer a matter of personal political policy, but of collaboration. No matter the size of the nation, security is an assured element in the structure of collective cooperation.

Collective security is a practical solution to the ongoing problem of war and peace. It is promising because it strikes a much needed equilibrium between aggression and cooperation. Cooperation is a much more attractive alternative in this system and hence promises to alleviate the tribulations of the security dilemma. A steady commitment from all involved nations makes this solution credible, viable, and stable.

17. It can reasonably be inferred from the passage that security is a dilemma for many countries because:

    A. there is no effective world policing system.
    B. they are constantly at war with other countries.
    C. most nations are intrinsically aggressive.
    D. they have a propensity to misread other nations' intentions.

18. According to the passage, collective security is a positive form of interaction because it:

    A. is based on the altruistic motives of benevolent governments.
    B. offers economic incentives for compliance.
    C. is not based on any ideological biases.
    D. is based on cooperation as the peacekeeping force.

19. In this model, if Russia were to attack Belgium, how would Belgium's integrity be preserved?

    A. It would not be preserved.
    B. Several nations would ally to counter the Russian threat.
    C. Belgium would be forced to make concessions to the Russians to assure its survival.
    D. Russia would be encouraged to hold free elections in Belgium.

20. Based on the author's statements, it is reasonable to conclude that a primary motive(s) for cooperation in a collective security model is/are:

    I. in most countries, a humanitarian desire to avoid conflict.
    II. the selfish need to keep any one country from growing too strong.
    III. a sense of justice for all participants.

    A. I only
    B. II only
    C. I and III only
    D. II and III only

21. Based on the passage, a potential stumbling block in a collective security policy might be:

    A. the collaboration of multiple nations.
    B. disparities in size between nations.
    C. the unwillingness to use force to deter aggression.
    D. the ambiguity of the policy itself.

Passage V (Questions 22–26)

Before we progress too much further, we as a society must consider the ramifications of our relentless pursuit of the unknown. Medicine is becoming more and more an exploratory science that seeks to unlock the secrets of life and death. The pace of our discovery outstrips the ethical guidelines that must temper our enthusiasm. We march relentlessly forward in our continuing search, giving cavalier treatment to the very issues that must shape our quest. It is a dangerous practice.

Gene therapy is one of the fastest growing regions of science, and also one of the most controversial. The closer we come to mapping the human genome, the greater our moral quandary. Already, purified genetic material is being inserted into human tissue to counter defects. Soon, all traits of *Homo sapiens* will be accurately described at the genetic level, and alterations in our most basic structures will become possible. We are building a modern-day Babylon, flirting with moral issues of a kind never before entertained by man.

From a strictly biologic standpoint, disease and dysfunction have a strong natural basis. On a planet with limited natural resources such as ours, overpopulation can lead to chronic shortages and intense stress on the biosphere. Death and disease, as much as they are feared, serve as natural balances to the forces of birth and growth. In a Darwinian sense, scourges like cancer and AIDS serve important functions in our continuing evolution. Periodic, pandemic outbreaks of disease weed out the least viable in the population. What is left is a smaller but stronger population. The more we attempt to delay and eliminate such important population checks, the more we endanger the safety of future generations. Nevertheless, as a civilized race, we take pride in the very fact the we have overcome the savage side of our natural existence. Eliminating pain and suffering has become a fixation, and we try everything possible to remove them from our lives. At the same time, we ignore their vital biologic significance.

We are approaching a revolutionary epoch in medicine. Our knowledge in this field has increased exponentially year after year. Yet, this rapid pace of advancement has not been accompanied by adequate moral–ethical review. We approach an era where it will be possible to alter our genetic makeup in ways never before imagined. Toying with the stuff of our existence, we play a risky game of profound consequence. This is a call for reticence, a cry for prudence. Without the proper guidelines, our relentless quest is doomed to wreak havoc on the very thing which it is supposed to protect—mankind itself.

22. The argument provided by the author is best described as:

  A. an appeal for improving a potentially dangerous medical system.
  B. a radical exposé on the scandals of modern medicine.
  C. an anecdotal report on the role of technology in modern medicine.
  D. a sentimental review of mankind's mortal plight.

23. Most disturbing to the author in this passage is the role of ethics in medical research and practice. He fears that:

  I. medicine is expanding faster than the ethical issues it provokes.
  II. we may endanger those who follow us.
  III. we are unraveling secrets that may be better left unknown.

  A. III only
  B. II and III only
  C. I and II only
  D. I, II, and III

24. A highly virulent virus creates a pandemic outbreak of a lethal disease, killing millions. Which of the following best describes the author's attitude about the ensuing rush to find a cure?

  A. A waste of money and vital resources—totally unnecessary
  B. A foolhardy gesture of humanitarianism
  C. A necessary evil of a civilized race
  D. A laudable effort

25. One can reasonably infer from the passage that the author fears medicine because it:

  A. creates genetic mutants.
  B. has no ethical standards whatsoever.
  C. unnaturally prolongs life in the diseased and dying.
  D. hides insidious motives of medical professionals.

26. Based on the passage, it can reasonably be stated that the author favors a type of medicine based on:

  A. sober, ethical considerations.
  B. unchecked disease propagation.
  C. technological advance.
  D. Hippocratic principles.

Passage VI (Questions 27–34)

The formation of groups has an invigorating effect in all spheres of human striving, perhaps mostly due to the struggle among the convictions and aims represented by the different groups. The Jews too form such a group with a definite character of its own, and anti-Semitism is nothing but the antagonistic attitude produced in non-Jews by the Jewish group. This is a normal social reaction. But for the political abuse resulting from it, it might never have been designated by a special name.

What are the characteristics of the Jewish group? What, in the first place, is a Jew? There are no quick answers to this question. The most obvious answer would be the following: A Jew is a person professing the Jewish faith. The superficial character of this answer is easily recognized by means of a simple parallel. Let us ask the question: What is a snail? An answer similar in kind to the one given above might be: A snail is an animal inhabiting a snail shell. This answer is not altogether incorrect, nor, to be sure, is it exhaustive; for the snail shell happens to be but one of the material products of the snail. Similarly, the Jewish faith is but one of the characteristic products of the Jewish community. It is, furthermore, known that a snail can shed its shell without thereby ceasing to be a snail. The Jew who abandons his or her faith (in the formal sense of the word) is in a similar position. He or she remains a Jew.

Difficulties of this kind appear whenever one seeks to explain the essential character of a group. The bond that has united the Jews for thousands of years and that unites them today is, above all, the democratic ideal of social justice, coupled with the ideal of mutual aid and tolerance among all people. Even the most ancient religious scriptures of the Jews are steeped in these social ideals, which have powerfully affected Christianity and Islam and have had a benign influence upon the social structure of a great part of mankind. The introduction of a weekly day of rest should be remembered here—a profound blessing to all mankind. People such as Moses, Spinoza, and Karl Marx, dissimilar as they may be, all lived and sacrificed themselves for the ideal of social justice; and it was the tradition of their forefathers that led them on this thorny path. The unique accomplishments of the Jews in the field of philanthropy spring from the same source.

The second characteristic trait of Jewish tradition is the high regard in which it holds every form of intellectual aspiration and spiritual effort. I am convinced that this great respect for intellectual striving is solely responsible for the contributions that the Jews have made toward the progress of knowledge, in the broadest sense of the term. In view of their relatively small number and the considerable external obstacles constantly placed in their way on all sides, the extent of those contributions deserves the admiration of all sincere people. I am convinced that this is not due to any special wealth of endowment, but to the fact that the esteem in which intellectual accomplishment is held among the Jews creates an atmosphere particularly favorable to the development of any talents that may exist. At the same time a strong critical spirit prevents blind obeisance to any mortal authority.

I have confined myself here to these two traditional traits, which seem to me the most basic. These standards and ideals find expression in small things as in large. They are transmitted from parents to children, they color conversation and judgment among friends, they fill the religious scriptures, and they give to the community life of the group its characteristic stamp. It is in these distinctive ideals that I see the essence of Jewish nature. That these ideals are but imperfectly realized in the group—in its actual everyday life—is only natural. However, if one seeks to give brief expression to the essential character of a group, the approach must always be by the way of the ideal.

27. The central concern of this passage is to:

   A. explain the struggle between the convictions and aims represented by different groups.
   B. define the essential characteristics of people professing the Jewish faith.
   C. propose a definition of the essence of Jewish nature.
   D. argue that expression of the essential character of a group must always be by the way of the ideal.

28. The author compares Jews and snails in support of the idea that:

   A. a Jew is a person who professes the Jewish faith.
   B. Judaism is just one faith among many.
   C. a Jew can abandon his or her faith and remain a Jew.
   D. Judaism has powerfully affected Christianity and Islam.

29. Which of the following is a claim made by the author but NOT supported in the passage by evidence, explanation, or example?

   A. Anti-Semitism is a normal social reaction.
   B. Moses, Spinoza, and Karl Marx were influenced by the tenets of Judaism.
   C. Jews are defined by the way of ideal.
   D. The beliefs of Jews have transformed history.

30. In order to apply the general views about defining groups stated in the passage to specific situations, it would be most helpful to know:

   A. the religion of the people being categorized.
   B. whether or not the people being studied come from the same geographic area.
   C. whether or not people live up to their ideals.
   D. how to determine the convictions and aims of the people being studied.

31. Which of the following claims is best supported by evidence from the passage?

   A. The most important trait of Jewish tradition is the high regard in which it holds every form of intellectual aspiration and spiritual effort.
   B. The democratic ideal of social justice is only effective when coupled with the ideal of mutual aid and tolerance among all people.
   C. The intellectual aspirations of the Jews are responsible for many of the contributions they have made to society.
   D. All of the above

32. Based on the information in the passage, it is reasonable to conclude that:

   I. it is of no consequence whether or not a Jew is religious.
   II. Jews would admire some of the ideals which Spinoza and Karl Marx espoused.
   III. Karl Marx's theories were based on tenets of Judaism.

   A. II only
   B. III only
   C. II and III only
   D. I, II, and III

33. According to the author, *anti-Semitism* was given a special name because:

    A. it was an antagonistic attitude produced in non-Jews by the Jewish group.

    B. it was so prevalent.

    C. it is markedly different from other forms of cultural or religious persecution.

    D. it resulted in political abuse.

34. Based on the passage, which of the following would be the best explanation for the contributions that the Jews have made in the intellectual arena?

    A. Superior educational backgrounds

    B. The external obstacles that they have been forced to overcome

    C. The respect for intellectual pursuit that is passed down from parents to children

    D. Their belief in democratic ideals

Passage VII (Questions 35–42)

The all too common failure to interact fruitfully with patients comes from the way a physician is taught to be a mere mechanic. In medical school we learn all about disease, but we learn nothing about what disease means to the person who has it.

In a study of folk medicine in Taiwan and among Chinese Americans, researcher Dr. Arthur Kleinman attributed the folk doctor's often surprising success to treatment of sickness in the context of the patient's psychology and culture. The strong stigma attached to mental illness in Chinese society means that a Chinese person often can only conceive of depression, for example, in terms of its physical symptoms, such as fatigue. Hence any treatment that does not allow the patient to believe in a physical cause of the problem is likely to be resisted and remain ineffective.

Kleinman points out a difference between *disease,* defined as the physical or psychiatric symptoms or damage visible to a doctor, and *illness,* the patient's subjective experience of the same sickness. The two are often remarkably different, especially when a person without scientific knowledge is treated by a Western physician.

I do not recommend going into trances or burning spirit money, but we must, like Plato's free physicians, ask patients what they think caused the problem, what threats and losses (or gains) it represents to them, and how they believe it should be treated. The typical review of systems that medical students are trained to use when questioning patients does not uncover time sequences or the meanings that events have to patients. Doctors often have no idea of the dynamics of the situation, unless patients volunteer those aspects, which they often don't do.

The best results proceed from a "negotiation" in which the practitioner's viewpoint and that of the patient come close enough together for true communication. If a person fervently believes in religious healing through the laying on of hands, the clinician must not become an obstacle and detract from that treatment's effectiveness. Even if the physician thinks such methods are useless, they are likely to help if the patient believes in them.

I often tell patients how I would treat myself if I had their illness. My choices may not include some of the things they're doing. Likewise, their choices may not include some of the things I would do. But I do not take away the benefit of their methods by saying they are no good. Instead, I work to see how our beliefs can mesh. To me the true measure of holistic medicine is how well the patient and doctor accept each other's belief system, even though their beliefs may differ. Neither one of us forces something upon the other. That way I can say, "If sometimes your beliefs don't work, try mine."

Obviously, I will try to talk patients out of spending enormous amounts of time and money on something I feel is ineffective, but where positive beliefs are involved I will try to support them. Doing what restores hope is beneficial. Similarly, a willingness to give a little will help the patient accept the doctor's beliefs, allowing the medical therapy a real chance to work. When patients have no faith in the physician's system, they will resist treatment consciously, by not taking their medicine, or unconsciously. In either case, healing will be thwarted.

35. According to the passage, Kleinman's study attributed the success of folk doctors to:

    A. the patient's belief in the burning of spirit money.

    B. sensitivity to the patient's cultural values and psychology.

    C. greater understanding of psychology.

    D. herbal remedies.

36. The central thesis of this passage is that:

    A. doctors need training in folk medicine.

    B. medical schools need to train doctors to be better "mechanics."

    C. doctors should spend less time learning about diseases.

    D. doctors are not sufficiently trained in psychology and subjectivity.

37. Based on information in the passage, which of the following statements is NOT true?

    A. Negotiation is a crucial aspect of medical treatment.

    B. Illness and disease are synonymous.

    C. Religious healing can be effective.

    D. A patient's assessment of what caused the problem and how it should be treated are relevant.

38. Adopting the author's views as presented in the passage would most likely mean acknowledging that the doctor–patient relationship should be:

    A. similar to that between parent and child.

    B. similar to that between husband and wife.

    C. consistent with that between teacher and student.

    D. equivalent to that between mechanic and customer.

39. Based on the information in the passage, the author would likely claim that someone who does NOT agree with his view of medicine is:

    A. dishonest.

    B. rebellious.

    C. creative.

    D. a conformist.

40. Adopting the author's views as presented in the passage would most likely mean acknowledging that:

    A. we must return to using folk medicine practices.

    B. separation between doctors and patients is desirable.

    C. doctors need to get in touch with their feelings and those of their patients.

    D. doctors need to prescribe a wider variety of treatments to their patients.

41. The two types of treatment discussed in the passage are:

    A. empathetic and mechanical.

    B. folk and traditional.

    C. effective and empathetic.

    D. innovative and harmful.

42. Which of the following concepts does the author illustrate with specific examples?

    A. Folk medicine works if the patient believes in its effectiveness

    B. The similarities between illness and disease

    C. The concept of negotiation between doctor and patient

    D. The ways in which doctors and medical school students are similar

Passage VIII (Questions 43–50)

The year 1815 marked the end of a period of American development. Up to this time, the life of the continent had been molded largely by forces from Europe; but with the conclusion of the war of 1812 against England, America turned in upon itself and with its back to the Atlantic, looked toward the West. The years following the Peace of Ghent are full of the din of the westward advance. In politics, the vehement struggles of Federalists and Republicans were replaced by what a contemporary journalist called "the era of good feeling." But underneath the calm surface of the first decade lay the bitter rivalry of sectional interests, which were soon to assume permanent and organized party forms. As in all postwar periods, the major political issue was that of finance. The ideas of Alexander Hamilton on protection and banking were reluctantly accepted by the Republican administration under the stress of war conditions. The tariff of 1816 had created a regime of protection under which New England turned from its shipping interests to manufacture and laid the foundations of her nineteenth-century prosperity. The old suspicions of Jefferson about a federal banking system were overcome, and in 1816 a charter replacing the one which had expired was issued for the foundation of a new Federal Bank.

The ties with Europe were slowly and inexorably broken. Outstanding disputes between England and America were settled by a series of commissions. The boundaries of Canada were fixed, and both countries agreed to a mutual pact of disarmament upon that storm center, the Great Lakes. In 1819, after straggling warfare in Spanish Florida, led by hero of New Orleans, Andrew Jackson, the Spanish government finally yielded the territory to the United States for five million dollars. Spain had withdrawn from the northern continent forever.

But the turmoils of European politics were to threaten America once again for the last time for many years to come. The sovereigns of the Old World were bound together to maintain the principle of monarchy and to cooperate in intervening in any country that showed signs of rebellion against existing institutions. The policy of this Holy Alliance had aroused the antagonism of Britain, which had refused to intervene in the internal affairs of Italy in 1821. The new crisis came in Spain. Bourbon France, burning to achieve respectability in the new Europe, sent an army across the Pyrenees Mountains to restore the Spanish monarchy. Russia would have liked to go farther. The Czar of Russia had worldwide interests, including large claims to the western coastline of North America, which he now reaffirmed by imperial decree. Rumors also spread to Washington that the reactionary powers of Europe, having supported the restoration of the Bourbons in Spain, might promote similar activities in the New World to restore Bourbon sovereignty there. In the southern portion of North America were the Spanish colonies, which had in their turn thrown off the yoke of their mother country.

The British government under Canning offered to cooperate with the United States in stopping the extension of this threatening principle of intervention to the New World. Britain announced that it recognized the sovereignty of the Latin republics in South America. Meanwhile President Monroe acted independently and issued his message to Congress proclaiming the principles later known as the Monroe Doctrine. This famous doctrine, as has been related, was at once a warning against interference on the part of any European powers in the New World and a statement of the intention of America to play no part in European politics. With this valedictory message, America concentrated upon its own affairs. A new generation of politicians was rising. The old veterans of the days of the Constitution had most of them vanished from the scene, though Jefferson and Madison lingered on in graceful retirement in their Virginian homes.

43. The best title for this passage might be:

A. *The Era of Good Feeling.*
B. *The Road to the Monroe Doctrine.*
C. *The Demise of Isolationism.*
D. *Looking Toward the West.*

44. According to the passage, which of the following was the genesis of the Monroe Doctrine?

A. The war of 1812
B. The retirement of the veterans of the Constitution
C. The Peace of Ghent
D. America's concentration on its own affairs

45. Based on the passage, which of the following countries broke with the tenets of the Holy Alliance?

A. Italy
B. Bourbon France
C. Russia
D. Britain

46. According to the author, the Peace of Ghent was responsible for which of the following events?

I. Westward expansion
II. Creation of the Federal Bank
III. The cession of Florida by the Spaniards

A. I only
B. II only
C. I and II only
D. I and III only

47. Based on the passage, which of the following was NOT a concern that led to the Monroe Doctrine?

A. The Czar of Russia's interest in portions of the western coastline of North America
B. Britain's refusal to aid the Italians in 1821
C. The French invasion of Spain in support of their monarch
D. The disarmament of the Great Lakes region

48. According to the author, the most important political problem after the war was:

A. the outstanding issues between England and the United States.
B. the fighting within the government between the Federalists and Republicans.
C. financial concerns exacerbated by the war.
D. the lack of guidance after Jefferson and Madison retired to Virginia.

49. Suppose that the United States had been awarded compensation for lost business in the treaty resulting in the Peace of Ghent. Which of the following would the author of this passage argue?

A. It resulted in a fairer treaty, based on the issues over which the war was fought.
B. The settlement inadequately compensated the British.
C. The original treaty was fair to the British and the Americans.
D. The passage does not give a clear answer about what the author would think about the equity of that outcome.

50. The word *valedictory*, as used in the last paragraph, most nearly means:

A. victorious.
B. parting.
C. strongly stated.
D. separatist.

Passage IX (Questions 51–58)

The celebrated physicist Albert Einstein is famed not only for his scientific discoveries; in his later years, he paid much attention to social and political problems. He spoke over the radio and wrote in the press. He was associated with a number of public organizations. Time and time again, he raised his voice in protest against the Nazi barbarians. He was an advocate of enduring peace, spoke against the threat of a new war, and spoke against the ambition of the militarists to bring American science completely under their control.

Soviet scientists and the Soviet people in general were appreciative of the humanitarian spirit that prompted these activities of the scientist, although his position was not always as consistent and clear-cut as might be desired. However, in some of Einstein's later utterances, there were aspects that seemed to us not only mistaken, but positively prejudicial to the cause of peace that Einstein so warmly espoused.

We feel it our duty to draw attention to this, in order to clarify so important a question as to how most effectively to work for peace. It is from this point of view that the idea of a world government, which Dr. Einstein sponsored, must be considered.

In the motley company of proponents of this idea, besides out-and-out imperialists who were using it as a screen for unlimited expansion, there were quite a number of intellectuals in the capitalist countries who were captivated by the plausibility of the idea, and who did not realize its actual implications. These pacifist and liberal-minded individuals believed that a world government would be a panacea against the world's evils and a guardian of enduring peace.

The advocates of a world government made wide use of the seemingly radical argument that in this atomic age, state sovereignty was a relic of the past; it was, as Spaak, the Belgian delegate, said in the United Nations General Assembly, an "old-fashioned" and even "reactionary" idea. It would be hard to imagine an allegation that is farther from the truth.

In the first place, the idea of a world government and superstate were by no means products of the atomic age. They were much older than that. They were mooted, for instance, at the time the League of Nations was formed.

Further, these ideas have never been progressive in these modern times. They were a reflection of the fact that the capitalist monopolies, which dominated the major industrial countries, found their own national boundaries too narrow. They needed a worldwide market, worldwide source of raw materials, and worldwide spheres of capital investment. Thanks to their domination in political and administrative affairs, the monopoly interests of the big powers were in a position to utilize the machinery of government in their struggle for spheres of influence and their efforts economically and politically to subjugate other coun-

tries, to play the master in these countries as freely as in their own.

We know this very well from the past experience of our own country. Under czarism, Russia, with its reactionary regime that was servilely accommodating to the interests of capital and its low-paid labor and vast natural resources, was an alluring morsel to foreign capitalists. French, British, Belgian, and German firms battened on our country like birds of prey, earning profits that would have been inconceivable in their own countries. They chained czarist Russia to the capitalist West with extortionate loans. Supported by funds obtained from foreign banks, the czarist government brutally repressed the revolutionary movement, retarded the development of Russian science and culture, and instigated pogroms against the Jews.

And now the proponents of a world superstate are asking us voluntarily to surrender this independence for the sake of a world government, which is nothing but a flamboyant signboard for the world supremacy of the capitalist monopolies.

51. The central point of this passage is that:

   A. world government is a worthy ideal but one unlikely to engender peace.
   B. Einstein is unqualified to discuss social and political problems.
   C. world government is a tool for unlimited expansion by capitalists.
   D. capitalism is inferior to communism.

52. The authors of this passage would most likely agree with all of the following statements EXCEPT:

   A. the ultimate goal of Einstein's proposal.
   B. Einstein's method of attaining his goal.
   C. the relevance of the sovereignty of state to the atomic age.
   D. Europeans benefited from czarism.

53. It can be inferred from the first paragraph that:

   A. Einstein is generally respected by the authors of the passage.
   B. Einstein supported a world government.
   C. Einstein took on too many social and political issues.
   D. the authors of this piece respect Einstein only for his scientific contributions.

54. The word *espoused*, as used in the last sentence of paragraph two, most closely means:

A. married.
B. spoke of.
C. supported.
D. believed in.

55. Based on the passage, which of the following would occur if world government were actualized?

I. Capitalism would be the dominant economic system.
II. Citizens would be repressed.
III. The leaders of the United States would be at the helm.

A. I only
B. II only
C. I and II only
D. I, II, and III

56. Based on the passage, the authors believe that:

A. communists should rule the world government.
B. capitalism is exploitive.
C. communism and world government are incompatible.
D. the League of Nations would not support a world government.

57. The claim that world government serves the interest of capitalists is:

A. supported in the passage by consideration of their motivations.
B. contradicted by the examples the authors provide.
C. supported by quotations from the Belgian delegate to the United Nations General Assembly.
D. supported by specific data on the raw material needs of the capitalist governments.

58. According to the author of the passage, the Soviet Union became:

A. A world superstate.
B. A mainstay of international security.
C. A czarist state.
D. A country free from the chains of extortionate loans from the United States.

Passage X (Questions 59–65)

Mohandas K. Gandhi, the great leader of India, discussing himself and wife Kasturbai . . .

About the time of my marriage, little pamphlets used to be issued, in which conjugal love, thrift, child marriages, and other such subjects were discussed. Whenever I came across any of these, I used to go through them cover to cover, and it was a habit with me to forget what I did not like and to carry out in practice whatever I liked. Lifelong faithfulness to the wife, inculcated in these booklets as the duty of the husband, remained permanently imprinted on my heart. Furthermore, the passion for truth was innate in me, and to be false to her was therefore out of the question. And then there was very little chance of my being faithless at that tender age.

But the lesson of faithfulness had also an untoward effect. "If I should be pledged to be faithful to my wife, she also should be pledged to be faithful to me," I said to myself. The thought made me a jealous husband. Her duty was easily converted into my right to exact faithfulness from her, and if it had to be exacted, I should be watchfully tenacious of the right. I had absolutely no reason to suspect my wife's fidelity, but jealousy does not wait for reasons. I must need be forever on the lookout regarding her movements, and therefore she could not go anywhere without my permission. This sowed the seeds of a bitter quarrel between us. The restraint was virtually a sort of imprisonment. And Kasturbai was not the girl to brook any such thing. She made it a point to go out whenever and wherever she liked. More restraint on my part resulted in more liberties being taken by her and in my getting more and more cross. Refusal to speak to one another thus became the order of the day with us, married children. I think it was quite innocent of Kasturbai to have taken those liberties with my restrictions. How could a guileless girl brook any restraint on going to the temple or on going on visits to friends? If I had the right to impose restrictions on her, had not she also a similar right? All this is clear to me today. But at that time I had to make good my authority as a husband!

Let not the reader think, however, that ours was a life of unrelieved bitterness. For my severities were all based on love. I wanted to make my wife an ideal wife. My ambition was to make her live a pure life, learn what I learnt, and identify her life and thought with mine.

I do not know whether Kasturbai had any such ambition. She was illiterate. By nature she was simple, independent, persevering and, with me at least, reticent. She was not impatient of her ignorance and I do not recollect my studies having ever spurred her to go in for a similar adventure. I fancy, therefore, that my ambition was all one-sided. My passion was entirely centered on one woman, and I wanted it to be reciprocated. But even if there were no reciprocity, it could not be all unrelieved misery because there was active love on one side at least.

I have already said that Kasturbai was illiterate. I was very anxious to teach her, but lustful love left me no time. For one thing the teaching had to be done against her will, and that too at night. I dared not meet her in the presence of the elders, much less talk to her. Kathiawad had then, and to a certain extent has even today, its own peculiar, useless and barbarous *purdah*. Circumstances were thus unfavourable. I must therefore confess that most of my efforts to instruct Kasturbai in our youth were unsuccessful. And when I awoke from the sleep of lust, I had already launched forth into public life, which did not leave me much spare time. I failed likewise to instruct her through private tutors. As a result Kasturbai can now with difficulty write simple letters and understand simple Gujarati. I am sure that, had my love for her been absolutely untainted with lust, she would be a learned lady today, for I could then have conquered her dislike for studies. I know that nothing is impossible for pure love.

59. What were the dual consequences of Gandhi's lessons of faithfulness?

A. His sexual passion was aroused and his role as a teacher limited.
B. Kasturbai's faithfulness seemed unlikely in the face of his own passion.
C. Their social behaviors were both limited and elaborated through a traditional Indian marriage.
D. Gandhi could not both allow his wife her independence and make her his own ideal wife.

60. In paragraph two, the definition of the word *exact* matches its context in the sentence with which of the following words?

A. Accurate
B. Painstaking
C. Demand
D. Appropriate

61. The passage suggests that Gandhi's motives were influenced by:

A. imagination and generosity.
B. ego and projection of his own values.
C. principally social constraints.
D. a burning attachment to duty.

62. Which of the following diverse elements does Gandhi say contributed to his unique behavior of playing the husband?

A. The little pamphlets and his passion for the truth
B. His youth, inexperience, and lustful passion
C. His jealousy and Kasturbai's reticence
D. All of the above

63. Which of the following elements does Gandhi NOT hold responsible for his wife's limited literacy?

A. Kasturbai herself
B. His own passion
C. The cultural restraints of Kathiawar
D. Pure love

64. Gandhi's tone in this passage is largely:

A. modest and relieved.
B. angry and resentful.
C. repentant and circumspect.
D. nostalgic and sentimental.

65. The author's principal concern in writing this passage is to explain:

A. his wife's limited literacy.
B. the influence of personal jealousy on his marriage.
C. the mixed motives he located in himself as a faithful husband.
D. the limitations of pure love.

Answers and Explanations to Verbal Reasoning Practice Test 2

1. **D**   The last sentence of paragraph two and the first sentence of paragraph three mention that the French political system is made up of a variety of parties, implying a heterogeneous mix of many viewpoints.

2. **A**   Paragraph three states that French policy is characterized by making concessions to opposing or extreme factions to retain a majority (also see paragraph four). Choice C is not the best choice because although the issue would likely be debated, there is no evidence that it would be debated endlessly or floored.

3. **C**   Statement I is correct. Paragraph two states that France is a nation of tumultuous change, and as a result, it has numerous political parties. Statement II is also correct, as paragraphs three, four, and five imply that political parties are weaker because they have to make concessions to retain a majority.

4. **C**   Choices A, B, and D are not discussed. Paragraph five states that the Assembly is an arena for various parties waging war on each other (implying they despise each other) and paragraph three mentions that the parties need each other to retain a majority.

5. **D**   Statement I is correct. Paragraph three states that legislation is governed by transitory coalitions of political parties, implying that legislation is difficult to pass because party interests are always changing. Statement III is also correct (see paragraph three).

6. **B**   Paragraph two begins to discuss why France's system is a multiparty one, but then spends the next several paragraphs describing the system. Not until the last paragraph does the author discuss possible reasons for the diversity of France's party system. Choice D is incorrect, because organization of the Assembly is the result of the party's diversity.

7. **C**   In the first paragraph, the author is clearly amazed by the human ability to think, and thus the author's tone is incredulous.

8. **B**   In paragraph one, the author states that thought cannot be explained on a physical basis (with equations or chemical interactions). Choice A is incorrect, because although the author mentions this as a possible explanation in the last paragraph, the author then rejects this, and reiterates that thought cannot be explained in a physical manner.

9. **B**   In paragraph three the author states that the ability to function in the abstract is the human being's greatest achievement.

10. **B**   This is the theme of the entire passage, and in the last paragraph, the author reiterates that somehow, biologic processes manage to create thought.

11. **D**   Choices A, B, and C are not discussed, whereas the last sentence of the passage supports choice D.

12. **A**   Paragraph two mentions that like-minded people gather to perpetuate their group characteristics.

13. **C**   Paragraph three says that members are encouraged to become similar to each other (i.e., homogeneous), and this increases the power and maximizes the influence of the

group (i.e., strengthens and perpetuates the religious group). Choice D is incorrect, because although extremism is discouraged, the passage does not state that quelling the voices of opposition is the best approach to discouraging extremism.

14. **D** Inertial forces, in this sense, mean resistance to change. From the third and last paragraphs, one can conclude that it is very difficult to change the beliefs of large groups united by common goals and beliefs.

15. **C** The passage is definitely a critique of religion, so statement III is correct. Neither statement I nor II is correct.

16. **A** Paragraph one states that religious groups are giant social machines (united by their common beliefs) which, by virtue of their large size, can induce social change.

PASSAGE IV

17. **A** Paragraph one says that none of the grand solutions can at present guarantee world peace, implying that there is currently no effective world policing system.

18. **D** Paragraphs three and four discuss that collective security is based on cooperation.

19. **B** According to the first sentence of paragraph three, the basic premise of collective security states that any threatened nation will be aided by other members to swiftly halt aggression.

20. **D** Statement I is incorrect, because the passage makes no reference to humanitarian goals. Statement II is correct. Nations do not like to go to war, and thus collective security achieves this selfish desire by ensuring peace. Statement III is also correct, because everyone who participates in the policy benefits equally (i.e., avoids war).

21. **C** Paragraph three mentions that if the program is to succeed, all nations must be willing to use force. A potential stumbling block might occur if a nation was unwilling to use force.

PASSAGE V

22. **A** Paragraph one states that medicine's technologic march is a dangerous practice, and in the last paragraph the author warns that the system needs guidelines or it is doomed to fail.

23. **D** Paragraph one supports that discoveries outstrip ethical guidelines (statement I); paragraph three supports that we endanger future generations (statement II); and paragraph two supports that the faster technology moves, the greater our moral quandary (statement III).

24. **C** Choice A is incorrect because the author does not argue against all technology and cures. Choice D is incorrect because the author is trying to raise consciousness about mankind's attempts to control all diseases. Paragraph three supports choice C. The author implies that it is wrong to try to cure all diseases, but states that as a civilized race, we take pride in our ability to try to do so.

25. **C** According to paragraph three, it can reasonably be inferred that the author fears medicine because it unnaturally prolongs life in the diseased and dying.

26. **A** This is the theme of the whole passage (see paragraphs one, two, and four).

PASSAGE VI

27. **C** The central concern of a passage is one that dominates the passage. The passage mentions choice A only in the introduction, as a way of foregrounding the discussions of Jews as a group. The author specifically states that faith is not mandatory to the definition of the essence of Jews; thus choice B is incorrect. Although the author believes choice D, it is not the central concern of the passage. Instead, it is a defense of his definition of the essence of Jewish nature.

28. **C** In paragraph two, the author provides a detailed explanation of the comparison.

29. **A** Choices B, C, and D are supported by evidence, explanation, or example. Choice B is discussed in paragraph three; choice C is discussed in paragraph five; and choice D is supported by the essay as a whole, but is discussed as a concept in the last paragraph.

ANSWERS AND
EXPLANATIONS TO
VERBAL
REASONING
PRACTICE TEST 2

704

30. **D** The author specifically states that religion and religious faith are not essential to his definition of Jewishness, thus choice A is incorrect. Geographic considerations are not mentioned in the essay, thus choice B is incorrect. Finally, in the last paragraph the au-

thor explicitly states that people in groups do not live up to their ideals in everyday life, thus choice C is incorrect.

31. **C** In paragraph three, the passage discusses that intellectual aspirations are responsible for their contributions to knowledge. There is no support for choices A and B. The author does not tell us which trait is the *most important*, thus choice A is incorrect. Likewise, the author does not restrict the effectiveness of the democratic idea to its coupling with mutual aid and tolerance; he merely notes that they are present together. Thus, choice B is incorrect.

32. **A** Statement II is correct. The author notes that Spinoza and Marx sacrificed themselves for social justice. Because the author claims the democratic ideal of social justice is a basic trait of the Jewish essence, one can deduce that, if nothing else, this trait would be admired by Jews. Statement I is not correct because the author does not state that loss of faith in inconsequential, but only that it is not important to the definition of Jewishness. Based on the passage, one cannot make any claims about the genesis of Marx's theories themselves; therefore, statement III is incorrect.

33. **D** In the first paragraph, the author states that this is probably the only reason that it was "designated by a special name."

34. **C** In paragraph four, the author discusses this belief.

35. **B** The example in paragraph two highlights the taboo nature of mental illness in Chinese society and the doctor's acknowledgment of this fact. Choice A is incorrect because it is not mentioned during the discussion of Kleinman's study. Choice C is incorrect because the author states that an understanding of psychology alone is not enough.

36. **D** Choice D is the best answer. There is no support for choices A, B, and C in the passage.

37. **B** In paragraph three the author quotes Kleinman's assertion that disease and illness are different. Choices A and C are stated in paragraph five, and choice D is discussed in paragraph four.

38. **B** The author presents the doctor–patient relationship as a partnership; thus, choice B is the best answer. Choice D is incorrect because the author states that one of the problems with the current doctor–patient relationship is the doctor's perception of his role as that of a "mechanic."

39. **D** The author is arguing for a new doctor–patient relationship in Western medicine; thus, those that disagree with him approve of the status quo and are conformists.

40. **C** There is no support for choices A, B, and D. In paragraph four, the author criticizes choice B. Choice A is incorrect because although the author sees admirable qualities in folk doctors' treatment, he does not advocate a return to it. Choice D is incorrect because the author is not criticizing the lack of treatments, but a lack of partnership between the doctor and patient and a lack of empathy on the part of doctors.

41. **A** The chief polarity discussed is empathetic versus mechanical treatment of patients. Choice B is incorrect because folk medicine only is used as an example of empathetic treatment. Choice C is incorrect because the author argues that empathetic treatment is the most effective. There is no support for choice D.

42. **C** Choices A, B, and D are not supported with specific examples. Choice D is incorrect because the author points out the differences between medical students and doctors. Choice A is incorrect because the example given, the Chinese patient, does not show that the treatment works because the patient believes in it. The paper money and trance examples do not demonstrate the concept that folk medicine works if the patient believes in its effectiveness.

43. **B** All the events discussed led to the writing of the Monroe Doctrine. Choice A is incorrect because in the first paragraph, the author debunks the concept that this was an era of good feeling by discussing the "bitter rivalry of sectional interests." Choice C is incorrect because the passage states that the United States became more isolationist. Choice D is incorrect because the passage leads up to westward expansion but does not discuss the actual movement. Westward expansion is not the only by-product of the end of the war of 1812 and the period of "American development" discussed.

SECT. IV
VERBAL
REASONING
PRACTICE
TEST 2

705

44. **D** Choice D is supported by the last paragraph. Choices A and C are incorrect because both occurred before the Monroe Doctrine. Choice B is not causally related to the doctrine.

45. **D** According to paragraph three, in 1821, Britain refused to intervene in the internal affairs of Italy.

46. **A** Statement I is true, as supported by paragraph one. The creation of the Federal Bank (statement II) was a by-product of financial crisis caused by the war, not the peace treaty. The cession of Florida by the Spaniards (statement III) was not directly related to the peace treaty.

47. **D** Choices A, B, and C are all identified in paragraph three as concerns that led to the Monroe Doctrine.

48. **C** As stated in paragraph one, the most important political problem after the war was financial concerns.

49. **D** The author of this passage makes no argument about the fairness or unfairness of the Peace of Ghent and the treaty that led to it. Thus, we can make no assumptions about his support of choices A, B, and C.

50. **B** *Valedictory* means farewell. This meaning can also be inferred contextually.

PASSAGE IX

51. **C** The central point of a passage is the one that best encapsulates the argument. Choice A is incorrect because the authors do not see world government as a worthy ideal and are not most concerned about its possibilities for creating peace. Choice B is incorrect because the authors' main focus is not a critique of Einstein's qualifications. Choice D is not addressed in the passage, except as specifically related to the Russian situation—the statement is a general pronouncement.

52. **B** The method of Einstein's goal of peace is world government, a concept with which the authors disagree; it is the *exception*. Choice A is incorrect because the authors state their support of peace in paragraph three. In paragraph five, they discuss the relevance of the state; choice C is incorrect. Choice D is supported by paragraph eight.

53. **A** Choice A is supported by paragraph one. Choice B is incorrect because world government is not mentioned in paragraph one. There is no support for choices C and D.

54. **C** *Espouse* means to take up and support or to become attached to. This meaning can be deduced from the context.

55. **C** Statements I and II are true and are supported by paragraph seven. Statement III is incorrect because the authors make no claim about which specific country would be leading the world government.

56. **B** Paragraphs seven through nine support the exploitive nature of capitalism.

57. **A** Choice A is supported by paragraph seven. There is no support for choices B, C, or D.

58. **B** Choice A is incorrect because the only world superstate mentioned is the United States. Choice C is incorrect because the revolution eliminated the czarist state. Choice D is incorrect because the passage never mentions loans from the United States. Choice B is the best answer by the process of elimination.

PASSAGE X

59. **D** Paragraph two explains that Gandhi was made insanely jealous by his ideals, ideals which he states in paragraph three that he wanted his wife to share. His wife, though, wanted to retain a sense of independence. Although Gandhi mentions his intense sexual passion, he does not say it resulted from his commitment to faithfulness. Therefore, choices A and B are not possible. Choice C is mentioned in Gandhi's piece, but not as a consequence of faithfulness.

60. **C** Refer to paragraph three. The word *exact* is in the infinitive form (to exact), indicating that *exact* is a verb. Of the choices offered, only choice C is a verb. Choices A, B, and D are adjectives.

ANSWERS AND
EXPLANATIONS TO
VERBAL
REASONING
PRACTICE TEST 2

706

61. **B** Both choices B and D are plausible, given the discussion in paragraph two. However, choice B is the best answer because of its greater precision and specificity. There is no evidence in the passage supporting choices A and C.

62. **D** Paragraph two mentions all of the items listed in choices A, B, and C. Therefore, choice D is correct.

63. **D** Choices A, B, and C are all mentioned in paragraph five. In the same paragraph, Gandhi says if his love had been more pure, then his wife could have learned more. Thus, choice D is correct—because the question asks what was *not* responsible for his wife's limited literacy.

64. **C** The melancholy tone eliminates choices A and B. Choice D is plausible, but the passage clearly conveys that Gandhi's regret has more than merely nostalgic overtones. The palpable sense of Gandhi's guilt makes choice C the best answer.

65. **C** The final sentence of the passage rules out choice D. Choice A is unlikely because the wife's literacy is not even mentioned until paragraph four. Choices B and C are both plausible, but choice C better represents the precise nature of Gandhi's commitment to faithfulness and its effects on his marriage.

SECT. IV
VERBAL
REASONING
PRACTICE
TEST 2

707

The Writing Sample

BASIC STRATEGIES

The Writing Sample: Basic Strategies and Sample Student Essays

I. Format and Purpose of the Writing Sample

TEST MECHANICS: WHAT TO EXPECT

The Writing Sample section of the MCAT requires you to write two 30-minute essays. The Writing Sample is given after lunch and before the Biological Sciences section. You will be given official lined paper and an essay topic sheet for each essay. Each essay requires you to perform three specific writing tasks (see II, Topics and Tasks). Sixty minutes is allocated for the entire section, thirty minutes to complete each essay. Test proctors allow only 30 minutes for you to work on the first essay, and then time will be called. After time is called for the first essay, no further work on it is allowed. (Note: Do not try to keep working. You will risk having your entire test voided.) Then, a 30-minute period is given for the second essay. A 10-minute break is given following collection of the essays.

PURPOSE

According to the AAMC, the Writing Sample is designed to assess your ability to develop a central idea; to synthesize concepts and ideas; to present ideas cohesively and logically; and to write clearly, following accepted practices of grammar, syntax, and punctuation that are consistent with timed, first-draft composition.

THE WRITING
SAMPLE: BASIC
STRATEGIES
AND SAMPLE
STUDENT ESSAYS

710

II. Topics and Tasks

TOPICS

The topics present short statements expressing an opinion, presenting a philosophy or observation, or describing a policy. In other words, **the statement provided always presents an idea.** This idea relates to your general experience as a human being and touches on subjects such as business, politics, ethics, art, and so on. Detailed knowledge of any subject matter is not required. The ability to think logically and to draw on your past reading or personal experience is a big asset.

Writing sample topics avoid specific areas. You are not expected to have advanced knowledge in any specific area, and you will not be tested on science. For example, none of the five following topics will be presented:

1. The technical subject matter of biology, chemistry, physics, or mathematics

2. The medical school application process or one's choice of medicine as a career

3. Social or cultural issues not generally familiar to college students

4. Religion or other controversial issues

5. Issues that may cause the applicant to dislike the morality, character, or personality of a person or group

TASKS

The writing sample topics follow a strict formula, requiring the writer to perform **three distinct tasks.** You must always perform all three tasks that the essay prompts. As shown in III, How the Writing Sample is Graded, failure to perform each of the three distinct tasks will cost you many points, and ultimately, a mediocre score. The three tasks are as follows:

1. **Thesis.** Explain, interpret, or make clear the statement provided. This includes providing examples.

2. **Antithesis.** Elaborate by describing a specific instance that contradicts the position expressed in the statement provided.

3. **Conflict resolution.** Evaluate and resolve the apparent conflict, specifically, by supplying your understanding of the greater implications.

For a better understanding of the three distinct tasks of the Writing Sample, look at the following sample statement and the directions that follow it. This essay statement is very similar to one that appeared on a recent MCAT:

A democratic government is never justified in keeping secrets from the voting public.

Write a unified essay in which you perform the following tasks: Explain what you think the above statement means. Describe a specific situation in which a democratic government might be justified in keeping secrets from the voting public. Discuss what you think determines whether or not keeping secrets from the voting public is a justifiable practice.

Comment: Note that the essay statement requires you to perform each of the three tasks outlined in this section. First, you were asked to explain what the statement means (thesis). Then, you were asked to describe a situation in which the antithesis could be true (contrary to the thesis). Finally, you were asked to achieve harmony between the thesis and antithesis (conflict resolution). Effectively addressing each of these three tasks will help you earn a high score on the Writing Sample.

III. How the Writing Sample is Graded

It is important to learn the system by which your essay is graded. It is strategic to understand how you are evaluated when writing essays. If you understand the criteria used to evaluate your essays, then you can target your essays to fulfill the criteria for a high score!

THE OVERALL SCORING PROCESS

English teachers and composition instructors—who may be more liberal about writing matters than are members of the general populace—read the essays. They are specifically trained and tested for this task. As you may remember from basic writing courses in college, these readers are critical and difficult to impress. Overall, the readers tend to feel that premedical students generally do not write well. Your job is to try to put together the best essays you can.

Two readers (graders) will review each essay independently. In cases of disagreement, a third, more senior reader will resolve the discrepancy. Each essay is given a number score between **1 (low score)** and **6 (high score)** by each grader. Number scores are combined from each of the two essays and from both of the graders. Thus, the maximum possible points you can receive is 24 (i.e., earning a score of 6 on each essay, from each grader). The minimum number of points you can receive is 4 (i.e., earning a score of 1 on each essay, from each grader). Thus, **you can receive a total score that ranges from 4 to 24.**

When a total numerical score is obtained, it is **converted to a scaled alphabetical score ranging from J to T.** Only the alphabetical score is reported on your official medical school score report form. The **minimum score is J;** the **maximum score is T;** and the **mean score has been N or O.** Scores tend to follow a distribution curve: J through M correspond to the lowest 25th percentile of students, and Q through T correspond to the top 25th percentile. (Note: Because your final score is based on your combined performance on the two essays, it is crucial that you give both essays your best effort. Also, the AAMC sends a photocopy of each essay you write to each medical school that you apply to, so they can independently evaluate your writing skills. This is another reason to take the Writing Sample seriously—the medical schools will!)

MCAT WRITING SAMPLE SCORING GUIDE: THE GRADING SYSTEM

Throughout the scoring process, which includes training, monitoring, supervising, and calibrating the official readers, the centrality of the scoring guide is constantly emphasized. Readers are told repeatedly to refer to the scoring guide as they wrestle with difficult scoring decisions.

Now that you understand how an overall score is obtained, you need to understand how each essay is evaluated. It is important that you learn what constitutes a good essay. Learning the following grading criteria is strategic, because it gives you the ability to aim for a high score. All you have to do is fulfill the criteria for a strong essay.

Score

6   **Level 6 essays** fully address all three tasks and present a thorough exploration of the topic. They show depth and complexity of thought, focused and coherent organization, and a superior control of vocabulary and sentence structure.

5   **Level 5 essays** address all three tasks and present a substantial treatment of the topic, although not as thoroughly or as effectively organized as a level 6 essay. They show some depth of thought, coherent organization, and control of vocabulary and sentence structures.

THE WRITING
SAMPLE: BASIC
STRATEGIES
AND SAMPLE
STUDENT ESSAYS

712

4   **Level 4 essays** address all three tasks but present only a moderate treatment of the topic. Similar to level 5 essays, they show clarity of thought, but they may lack complexity. These essays demonstrate coherent organization, although some digressions may be evident. The writing shows an overall control of vocabulary and sentence structure.

3   **Level 3 essays** may neglect or distort one or more of the writing tasks or present only a minimal treatment of the topic. They may show some clarity of thought but may be simplistic. Problems in organization may be evident. The essays demonstrate a basic control of vocabulary and sentence structure, but the language may not effectively communicate the writer's ideas.

2   **Level 2 essays** seriously neglect or distort one or more of the writing tasks. They demonstrate problems with organization and analysis of the topic. They may contain recurrent mechanical errors, resulting in language that occasionally is difficult to follow.

1   **Level 1 essays** demonstrate marked problems with organization and mechanics, resulting in language that is very difficult to follow. Alternatively, the essays may entirely fail to address the topic.

CRUCIAL IMPLICATIONS OF THE SCORING GUIDE

You must complete all three writing tasks. Conceivably, you can address the three writing tasks in any order. However, the most logical order to follow is the one provided in the tasks that follow the essay statement: Explain the statement, provide contrary examples, and account for the apparent contradiction.

Your task is to discuss the issue or question raised by the statement provided. **You are not being asked to argue for or against the statement.** You certainly may express your opinion, but do not allow your enthusiasm or disgust for the viewpoint expressed in the statement hamper the development of insightful examples and finely nuanced discussion, informed by a complexity of response.

Essays will not be scored on the positions taken (i.e., there is no right, wrong, politically correct, or politically incorrect answer).

Essays are judged on how thoroughly and thoughtfully they explain the statement provided and explore its meaning by addressing the second and third writing tasks.

Unity and organization are rewarded. Logic and development are required. The length of the essay, however, does not matter.

Misunderstanding the statement or the writing tasks will result in disaster. Read the prompt carefully, and also be sure you understand the writing tasks. Plan out your points before you begin to write.

Provide specific examples. Although the topic requires you to provide a specific example only in the second task of the essay, essays are much more convincing if they include specific examples in each of the three tasks.

Keep in mind the time limit as you write. You must perform all three writing tasks. It is better to give sketchy treatment to a task than to omit it entirely.

Be mindful of mechanical errors; they are important. Try to save a few minutes, so that you can proofread your essays before you turn them in. However, as the scoring guide suggests, avoiding mechanical (or stylistic) errors is far less important than completing the essay, developing strong content, and creating clear organization.

Your essay is a first draft, which means that you may cross out and make corrections as needed. You should be clear when crossing out and making corrections. Do not recopy your essay.

Spelling does not count. (Note: Be aware, however, that readers are not always able to overcome their bias against misspellings.) Poems, drawings, and essays that are illegible or in a foreign language will not be scored.

IV. How to Write an Essay: Basic Steps

PRELIMINARIES

The two most important pieces of advice to remember when writing your essay are **to plan your essay before you begin writing** and **to manage your time efficiently.** Students who perform well on the Writing Sample plan well and manage their time efficiently. There are **four steps**, or concerns, when writing an essay.

1. **Understand what the prompt means and what the essay tasks require.** This understanding includes insights into structure, content, style, mechanics, tone, audience, and format of both the prompt and the tasks.

2. **Prepare for the essay assignment.** For the MCAT Writing Sample, this preparation process includes familiarity with all the items listed above in the first step. Also, you can prepare by reviewing your past reading in literature, history, philosophy, and world affairs; reviewing, as necessary, stylistic, mechanical, and rhetorical demands of sound writing; considering invention strategies; and recognizing possible pitfalls in the writing process.

3. **Prewrite the essay.** For this step, take into consideration analysis of the prompt statement, strict adherence to the three writing tasks assigned, inclusion of possible clues in the prompt, development of ideas, and time constraints.

4. **Write the essay.** During this step, keep in mind all of the previous steps and concerns. In addition, keep in mind that your essay should have clarity, precision, logic as well as three distinct parts (thesis, antithesis, and conflict resolution).

PREWRITING AND WRITING STRATEGIES

You should spend 5 minutes prewriting, collecting your thoughts, and planning your essay. Do not just start writing! The following provides a guide for the prewriting process.

Carefully read the statement provided. Do you seem to understand it? Does it contain any clue words? **A clue word is a word that hints at the main idea or subject matter of the statement.** For example, in the statement *Justice is the interest of the stronger,* the word *justice* is an obvious clue word; this statement and its topic will require you to discuss how you determine what is fair or right in the interactions of human beings. Also, be certain to mark command words, such as compare, define, demonstrate, evaluate, isolate, trace, and so on. **A command word is a word that tells you what to do.** Marking command words helps you to focus your essay on what is being asked.

Read quickly through the instructions. Are there any surprises? Are there any clue words? Be mindful of the command words.

Think of a single word that can be used to summarize or explain the content of the statement. For example, does the concept word *justice* describe the issue contained in the statement?

Summarize or interpret the meaning of the statement in a single sentence of your own. Develop a paraphrase of the essay sentence (prompt) that you are given. This process helps you quickly begin to interpret a vague or general essay question in your own language. (Note: Do not write this sentence in your final essay, but do try to formulate it mentally.) If you can provide a one-sentence interpretation of the statement, then you can be relatively certain that you have at least a basic understanding of it. By formulating or having in mind a single sentence explanation, you are helping to impose unity and coherence on your thinking and, consequently, on your writing.

THE WRITING
SAMPLE: BASIC
STRATEGIES
AND SAMPLE
STUDENT ESSAYS

714

Brainstorm! Brainstorming is a critical step for prewriting. The following are three possible sources for brainstorming material:

1. Past reading in literature, history, philosophy, and so on

2. Familiarity with current events

3. Personal experience or imagination

The following are four additional strategies for brainstorming:

1. **Make a list of anything that comes to mind about the topic presented.**

2. **Make a tree or a spatial picture of related issues,** recognizing dominant and subordinate relationships. This is a great strategy if you are a visual person.

3. **Ask yourself the questions: Who? What? Where? When? Why?** This often helps to get ideas going.

4. **Use word association**—brainstorm with words that come to mind in response to the single sentence that you wrote earlier.

After brainstorming, look over the ideas you came up with. Have you found any important points, issues, or examples that are relevant to the statement provided (or the question asked)?

Come up with a topic sentence. By sifting through your available material, decide on the main point (or points) you want to address in your first paragraph—the paragraph that explains the statement. Can you provide a specific example in this paragraph?

Come up with an example in which the statement is not valid (i.e., a contradiction). Sift through your brainstorming material again and decide on those specific examples that you will describe, pointing to at least one example in which the statement is not valid. This strategy gives your essay complexity and sophistication. This section, the contradiction, is usually placed in the later part of the essay. Remember to be specific and interesting when discussing the contradiction.

Come up with a strong conclusion that demonstrates your understanding of the statement and its inadequacies. You should formulate a generalization or insight that will explain the contradiction that you introduced.

Write a basic outline for your essay and then quickly start writing. Keep an eye on the clock. Remember that you have used 5 minutes for prewriting and outlining, allowing 20–23 minutes for writing and 2–3 minutes to proofread and correct errors. Remember that neatness counts. Also, as you write, remember to be clear in your logic, always use evidence to support your claims, stress to the reader the importance of everything you write, and address all the elements that the three writing tasks ask you to address.

Most students have at least three paragraphs in their essays. Three paragraphs are the minimum that you can write to complete the three writing tasks. The first paragraph explains the statement and provides examples. The second paragraph provides the contradiction to the statement with a discussion and an example. The final paragraph resolves the conflict and concludes. Some students write essays with five or more paragraphs. Remember that length is not important, but quality and content are important.

BRAINSTORMING SAMPLES

The following provides two former MCAT essay statements and some approaches for brainstorming, which will help you come up with good material to write about. Read the two statements that follow, and try to come up with ideas to write about. Then, read the suggested brainstorming steps for each topic to see if you fully extracted all you could from each essay question. We will work through these together.

MCAT WRITING SAMPLE: TWO SAMPLE ESSAY TOPICS

Topic 1

Consider this statement:

In a free society, individuals must be allowed to do as they choose.

Write a unified essay in which you perform the following tasks: Explain what you think the above statement means. Describe a specific situation in which individuals in a free society should not be allowed to do as they choose. Discuss what you think determines when a free society is justified in restricting an individual's actions.

Topic 2

Consider this statement:

One must always be inflexible in matters of principle.

Write a unified essay in which you perform the following tasks: Explain what you think the above statement means. Describe a specific situation in which one might be flexible in a matter of principle. Discuss what you think determines whether one should be flexible or inflexible in matters of principle.

POSSIBLE BRAINSTORMING STEPS FOR TOPIC 1 (see IV, How to Write an Essay: Basic Steps)

1. **Clue words.** The clue words for topic 1 are *individual*, *free*, and *society*. Two main ideas seem possible: the conflict between the individual and society and the issue of personal liberty and the exercise of free will. Of course, these two ideas are deeply intertwined.

2. **Surprises.** There are no surprises in topic 1. The clue word *justified* raises the issue or concept of justice. As in this case, clue words can be found in the tasks that follow the prompt.

3. **Concept for discussion.** The concept to discuss for this passage could be justice, liberty, or social contract. Although social contract is not mentioned, it is the concept that usually describes the process whereby individuals are said to give up some of their personal liberty for the sake of the benefits and protections that a society provides.

4. **One-sentence interpretation.** A possible one-sentence interpretation of the statement: Personal liberty should always be valued over the demands of society.

5. **Sources from the humanities.** For specific examples in the essay, sources from the humanities could include *Antigone*, the *Declaration of Independence*, and the *Social Contract*. Sources from current events could include nudity, flag burning, and abortion. Sources from personal experience could include general education requirements, speeding, and controlled substances.

6. **Second writing task.** As demonstrated, there are plenty of items for discussion for the second writing task of the essay (antithesis)—or so it seems.

7. **Specific examples.** Could a specific example be the long tradition of individualism in American society? Could this example be made more specific by mentioning the *Declaration of Independence* and its promise of "inalienable rights," including liberty?

Actually, we did not do well in brainstorming for instances that could be useful examples for the second writing task. But a glance shows that we can generate any number of examples from contemplating the concept of a social contract, mentioning that our world would be a matter of "all against all" or "survival of the fittest" without a social contract to maintain check on our actions. At this point your thinking might start to move in the direction of recognizing that a society is a collection of individuals, all of whom would like to exercise a maximum amount of personal liberty. But what happens when these exercises of liberty conflict with one another?

8. **Third writing task.** We have, it seems, an idea for the third writing task (conflict resolution): A free society must allow people to do as they choose, but only to the extent that they do not interfere with the liberties of other individuals. Can we come up with a better conflict resolution? How about the idea that no society is completely free (or could ever be)? Is this better? Remember, you cannot worry about this issue too long. You have an essay to write.

POSSIBLE BRAINSTORMING STEPS FOR TOPIC 2 (see IV, How to Write an Essay: Basic Steps)

1. **Clue words.** The clue words for topic 2 are *always, inflexible,* and *principle.* The word *always* presents an opportunity for the second writing task, because few matters in life are definitive enough to be *always.* Americans typically value adaptability, so the word *inflexible* presents a similar opportunity for the second writing task. The word *principle* suggests the broad subject matter of ethics.

2. **Surprises.** There are neither surprises nor extra hints in the statement provided.

3. **Concept for discussion.** The concept to discuss for this passage could be morality, ethics, puritanism, relativity. Can you think of any other possible concepts?

4. **One-sentence interpretation.** A possible one-sentence interpretation (thesis) could be: There are some things beyond compromise, including those tenets by which we live our moral lives.

5. **Sources from the humanities.** For specific examples in the essay, sources from the humanities to use could include *Hamlet* and the Bible. Sources from current events could include recent wars, killing a burglar in one's house, and religious cults. Sources from personal experience could include relationships with people, the 1960s experience, and the political process.

6. **Second writing task.** Several possibilities seem apparent for explaining why principles must be flexible (this is useful for the second and third writing tasks): the call of a higher principle when two principles are found to be in conflict, the possible eccentricity of a cult group, the unresolvable conflicts of moral systems, the greater tolerance that comes with age, revolutionary times that overturn once stable moral ideas, the pragmatics of daily life, and so on.

7. **Specific examples.** Could you begin an essay with the idea that everyone would like to live in a world and practice a life in which principles are fixed and certain, developing this idea with reference to the Bible and to Hamlet? This would give a lead-in to the second writing task, which will show that this ideal is not always possible.

    There are a wealth of possible examples for the second writing task. You could quickly mention how Hamlet compromises his principles, how a person would kill to defend his life (and thereby violate what is, for most people, a moral principle against killing), and how increasing age tends to make a person more pragmatic. The challenge is merely choosing good examples.

8. **Third writing task.** We have essentially completed the brainstorming work necessary to write an effective essay. Perhaps we can contemplate and examine these concepts even further by pointing out: What needs to be inflexible is not our principles as much as our desire to have and live by a code of ethics. To state that principles must sometimes be flexible is not to say that they should become so flexible that they cease to exist. (This last point will be difficult to make clearly.)

How about mentioning the fall of Adam and Eve after they eat from the tree of the knowledge of good and evil? This would tie together the idea that moral ideas or principles are a kind of curse, a casting out of paradise. Moral principles are what make us distinctly human, but to have them (and to hold them) is largely responsible for the unhappiness we feel in our lives. To live somewhat reasonable lives, we must learn to be "flexibly inflexible" (or "inflexibly flexible") about our principles.

V. Sample Student Essays with Comments

GENERAL INFORMATION

In this section, a sample MCAT Writing Sample topic is presented and student essays are shown. These essays are actual essays that premedical students have written in response to the topic that follows. Following each student essay, an expert comment is provided that details what the student did well and what the student could have done better. Read each essay and comment.

While the MCAT Writing Sample was still being developed, a number of different essay formats and time limits were evaluated. One of the early, experimental formats is illustrated below. Although this particular format is no longer used, a look at some essays written by premedical students in response to it can reveal useful information for writing any essay.

SAMPLE TOPIC

Topic: A judicial scholar is quoted as saying: "It is unjustifiable to disobey the law, unless of course the law is unjust."

Tasks: Interpret and discuss what the scholar was saying in this quotation and provide an example of a situational, moral, or philosophical event familiar to you that exemplifies what the scholar is saying.

EXCERPTS FROM ACTUAL STUDENT ESSAYS (**Note:** These essays contain many errors made by the students. These errors intentionally have not been corrected.)

Student 1

The scholar in his quotation informs us that law should be adhered to, without question, unless the law, in the process of its enforcement, disadvantages a person unjustly. Laws, then, are not absolute. A law may apply to one man and not another. Moreover, the nature of enforcement of the law and the integrity of the lawmakers contributes to the credibility of a law, and from credibility is derived a validity. Both these factors contribute to whether a law should be obeyed or disobeyed.

The scholar in the quotation informs that law should be adhered to, without question, unless the law, in the process, of its enforcement, disadvantages a person unjustly. Laws, then, are not absolute. A law may apply to one man or not apply to another man in different situation. An example is murder. . .

Comment: The first problem is that student 1 became displeased with what he had written and started over. Try to plan out and know what you want to say, because false starts waste valuable time. Student 1 compounded his error by foolishly copying over part of the abandoned paragraph. Perhaps this student had a fussy concern for neatness and thought crossing out part of the first paragraph would look messy. Recopying merely wastes time, and, as in this instance, often results in unintended errors.

Student 2

> A judicial scholar is quoted as saying: "it is unjustifiable to disobey the law, unless of course the law is unjust." The unnamed scholar who delivered this quote provides an interesting insight into the field of medicine. The quote brings to light a delicate issue that is challenged many times in the career of a physician. The hefty burden (in many cases) of life, death and the seeming power to control both; collides head on with the law and its majority (democratic) rules.
>
> A classic example of the moral and constitutional dilemma a physician must face is abortion. Pro and Anti abortion groups in the United States have put incredible pressure on the physician. Both sides seemingly have justifiable reasons and causes. Antiabortion states that "abortion is murder," and pro-abortion states, "that women have the right to choose early in pregnancy." The emphasis of the quote enters when a law is passed and extenuating circumstances arise.
>
> In a state where abortions are illegal, A young junkie mother comes into the clinic. There is a possibility of deformities in the newborn, or (in this day and age) AIDS from an infected intravenous drug user. Can the doctor perform the abortion? If he does should he be arrested? The scholar that issued the opening quote of my essay would agree that the physician would be justified in performing the abortion. The really tough problem is, "who has enough wisdom and authority to make the correct decision all the time?" Just as the admissions committees at all the American Medical Schools are deciding who will and who will not make good doctors; many students are wondering who's decision is good enough. But just as the doctors today...TIME CALLED.

Comment: This response is somewhat ingenious with the use of "smuggling in of a doctor" example. Perhaps student 2 thought that the reader would be impressed by her apparent devotion to medicine. The use of doctor examples is certainly permissible, but most readers will probably appreciate a student writer who exhibits interests and knowledge outside the world of medicine. More importantly, the doctor example in this essay creates a problem with logic. The example does not relate to the issue in the statement as well as it could, making the essay weaker. Finally, note the entirely unnecessary announcement by this student that she ran out of time. Do not announce your failures to the reader.

Student 3

> "The Letter of the Law" or "Bullwinkle, gasping for breath and begging for 'rest,' strangled by Rocky"
>
> Euthanasia is an eye-brow-raising topic that has become increasingly controversial in the past decade, especially. It is, of course, not condoned by our legal system, although some cultures do practice it, elsewhere in the world. Euthanasia raises some serious moral, ethical and legal questions that cannot—like most such issues—be easily tackled. Certainly, today's physician is forced to be at least cognizant that public acceptance may be breaching current laws regarding it.
>
> When our 'judicious scholar' states, "it is justifiable to disobey the law, unless of course the law is unjust," he implies, first, that not all laws are 'good,' and, secondly, that even 'good' laws sometimes call on our greater sense of morality to override them if the situation demands.
>
> Euthanasia may or may not exemplify the latter treatment of the law. (Parking illegally to aid someone hit by a car (liability notwithstanding) may be a better example.) A recent anonymous letter by a physician confessing to his enthusiastic act prompted hot debate over this issue. However under current limitations, the law must be obeyed.

Comment: This essay has an effective initial title. Its alternate title is an attempt at humor, which would probably be welcomed by an essay reader, but may not be welcomed by a medical school admissions committee. The first paragraph is gassy and lacks rhythm. The physician example, once again, seems forced. The second paragraph contains an error in its first sentence. Student 3 inadvertently substitutes "judicious" for "judicial." The third paragraph begins by casting doubt on the author's own example. As football coaches say, "If you're going to make an error on the field, at least make it at full speed." This writer's waffling will do little to make him appear more judicious (judicial?).

Student 4

"It is unjustifiable to disobey the law, unless of course the law is unjust." What the scholar was saying in this quotation is that the only valid reason for breaking a law is if the law that is broken should not have been a law in the first place.

Laws are made to ensure order in a society and to protect the welfare of individuals in a society. There are certain laws that some people do not view as promoting the welfare of society and thus they choose to disobey these laws. In the 1960s in the United States. . . .

Comment: Student 4 is clearly adrift. No purpose is served by quoting the statement without first providing even a minimal introduction. The sentences that follow demonstrate that this writer has no clear direction in mind. The sentences show little relation to one another, which is something even the writer apparently felt because she makes almost every sentence stand as a new paragraph. This sample shows the absolute necessity of planning out a direction before putting pen to paper.

Student 5

"Please note that I have a severe spelling disorder known as surface dislexia. I apologize for the difficulty in reading.

Comment: There is never a reason to waste time by apologizing. And remember, spelling is not the key issue.

Student 6

The greatest societies in this world are the societies that have order, which in terms brings a better place to live and therefore a better atmosphere for humans to produce. This order is brought about by a mutual respect and understanding between individuals. This respect has to have some boundaries since as humans, we are not perfect, we see things in different ways. Most of these boundaries are called laws and later known as rights of the people.

In order for this "perfect" society to live with each other one must obey these laws because they are the only means by which all of us can live a better life.

Student 6 continues . . .

Some societies which are now in chaos have a tremendous disorder, nobody obeys any law and life becomes very unlivable. Fortunately our society is one of the most orderly societies in this world. But there are instances that these laws are not carefully structured even in the most orderly societies by the law makers in the sense that a moral factor, a none humanist factor is lacking. Such a law is the one by which a "vegetable" i.e. brain dead patient or similar instances are not allowed to rest in peace.

The old man in Florida that decided to end his wife's life, who was in the later stages of Alzheimer's disease thought that this law was unjust by seeing the agony of his wife. I believe this old man thinks the same way as the judicial scholar since he is a citizen who has never broken the law in any way but this one. He thought that for a better living with others, one must have order in society by obeying all laws. He probably also think that this one law makes no just therefore he felt it should not be obey.

Comment: The glaring problems throughout this essay are awkward syntax and prevalent mechanical errors. These problems tend to persuade a reader that student 6 is neither a clear nor careful thinker. In this essay, associating weak mechanics with weak thinking seems warranted. The fundamental problem is that the essay fails to make its subject clear, fails to address the parts of the topic, and never addresses the tasks until the final paragraph. In a 30-minute essay, there simply is no time for such a leisurely, slowly developing approach.

Student 7

The concept of law and how that idea manifests itself in a society is a most baffling study. From the time of the early Greek Empire and throughout the development of the Western World societies have come and gone. And though these societies have shared many things relevant to their being, how the concept of law has become manifest is one thing that has varied incredibly from our society to the next.

The judicial scholar who was quoted as saying: "it is unjustifiable to disobey the law, unless of course the law is unjust" was quite aware of a point that is to follow. He had a love for the law, and though his words sound rash and insolent, his love for the law, the True law, was so great that he could not keep from speaking those words. The point is that the law is for the benefit of the people, the people are not for the benefit of the law, and that there is a Higher Law, a law of Morality, that a law must be answerable. If any law is in conflict with the Law of Morality, then it is not unjustifiable to disobey that law.

This is precisely the idea that lead our forefathers to found this country, the United States of America, and it is this idea, this tribute to the Higher Law, the Moral Law. . . .

Comment: Student 7 seems bright. However, that brightness is well concealed under mounds of verbiage. Too much of this essay is grandiloquent generalization, and there are too many redundancies. This student needed to eliminate all of the throat-clearing and focus on the specific business as soon as possible.

Every woman has the right or choice whether to keep her baby or not. Abortion is one of the most controversial issues in the United States and many believe that the illegalization of children is unjustifiable. If abortion is illegal, then millions of unwanted babies will be born, leading to an increase in homeless and crime rates. Of course, this is not entirely if at all true, but yet many prochoice activists say this will happen. On the other hand, no one should have the right to take another's life, even before birth. Then there's the issue of when is the fetus actually a living human being. With all these problems to consider one has to make up for herself, is abortion morally wrong?

In the case of illegalizing abortion, for many this law would be unjust. In a situation of a fifteen year old high school girl who is pregnant, but is unable to legally get an abortion. She is an extremely good student and intends to go to college in two years. She finds it is impossible to go to a prestigious college and raise a child at the same time and decides that her only choice is to have an abortion. She must go above the law in order to do so. In her mind, she decides to place herself first, and believes she would be better off without a child.

Comment: What is this essay about? If you did not know the topic and tasks in advance, would you be able to detect any clear purpose in this essay? Every essay, if it is an essay at all, introduces its subject matter. Student 8 simply plunged in, seemingly unconcerned about the task of creating a focus or thesis. The essay only presents an example. But it is an example in service to what?

Student 9

...In summation, it is everyone's responsibility to uphold those laws that keep order.

Comment: Student 9 wrote a one-sentence conclusion. One sentence is never adequate for a conclusion. Also, this sentence fails to accurately summarize the quotation.

Student 10

Since the beginning of our country, our forefathers established the judicial system in order to maintain order and treat every man fairly. This was done in order to do away with the tariffs and other unjust laws which was brought upon them by Britain. Laws are made to make sure every individual is treated fairly and has full advantage in this country. But things have changed. Where some laws overprotect the criminal and making him a burden on society. A scholar once said "It is unjustifiable to disobey the law, unless of course the law is unjust." There are many examples of these unjust laws which exist from the common household law to the Federal law. Many have taken advantage of lawmaking by making the law work for them

To have a law go into effect is a long process that goes through many channels until it reaches the presidents desk. After he has signed the document, it has become the law of the land...

Comment: This is another essay in which the main problem is the writer's lack of focus. In this essay, the writing consists of a series of unrelated ideas, which indicates that the writer neither planned nor structured what he wanted to say.

You are awakened by a loud noise out in your backyard. Being scared of what might be there, you grab your gun and hide it under your robe and walk to the back sliding glass door. It's after 2 AM and dark. When you reach the back door you see a shadow of a man with a gun in his right hand. Before you stop walking, he spots you. He yells for you to open the door. He points his gun at you and threatens your life. He does not realize that you too have a gun and so lowers his and puts it back in his pants. Now is your chance, you bring out your gun and shoot him twice in the chest. You think he moves again, maybe for his gun, so you shoot him four more times.

When the police come, they pronounce the victim dead-on-arrival and then proceed to read you your rights. The law that you have disobeyed is sighted as manslaughter. You thought that you acted out of self defense, but the victim is found outside your house and the gun still in the victims pants. You are guilty.

In court you explain your side of the story to no use. You do some time in jail and become disenchanted with our legal system. Remember the quote "it is unjustifiable to disobey the law, unless of course the law is unjust." Your disobedience to the law saved your life. Your actions are justified by this. But the endangerment of your life is your illusion. Your disobedience is therefore unjustified because of your illusion. The lesson to be learned here. The next time you shoot a potential burglar, drag him in and put his gun in his hand.

Comment: This essay is creative and arresting. A reader would certainly enjoy reading it. However, the essay does not effectively respond to the topic. It is good to be creative, but creativeness should not interfere with the task. In this essay, the main discussion required for the topic is rather awkwardly plopped into the essay in the third paragraph. The essay is almost entirely anecdote. The cynical advice given at the end of the essay is not considered a good response to the demands of the topic.

Student 12

In the next few paragraphs I will discuss what the judicial scholar is trying to transmit. I will do this by giving my interpretation of the quote and then by giving an example or two.

In the quote 'it is unjustifiable to disobey the law, unless of course the law is unjust' expresses an important point that no situation can be looked at as black and white. In black and white photography there is a zonal scale of maximum black to maximum white. In between these extremes is the variation of less black or more white (gray areas). It is important to focus on these gray areas because it depends on where you are standing that defines what is just and unjust to you.

For example, many Mexican families cross this line which makes them illegal aliens, by law. In their eyes they don't look any different (no funny hair color change or face alteration.)

Depend on which side of the fence you are standing on defining your laws.

Comment: The first paragraph is entirely wasted. There is never a need to announce so boldly your intentions, especially when your intentions are merely to do what the essay topic asks. The second paragraph does not accurately state the thesis—a deep, fundamental problem. The third paragraph lacks coherence, signaling that the writer has lost control of the idea she may have initially had. The disintegration of this essay is more forcefully signaled by the final paragraph, which is a sentence fragment. There are numerous mechanical errors throughout this essay, and these also detract from the essay's effect.

> The judicial scholar is saying "it is not OK to break the law unless the law is unfair (unjust). This statement is best illustrated by the changes that took place concerning the United States segregation laws. The laws enforcing segregation were justifiable broken in that the laws were not fair. And breaking the laws forced the laws to be changed. Thus, not only is it justifiable to break an unjust law it also can cause the law to be rectified. So is it not our moral duty to break unjust laws or are the laws we think are unjust truly so?

Comment: The passage quoted is the entire essay as submitted by student 13. The entire essay consists of six relatively short sentences. Considering that the average person can write 250 words in 15 minutes, this essay is remarkably thin. The extreme brevity of this essay is a pity, because the essential ideas are present. The expression here is rather hobbled, and an unclear discussion can never be considered successful.

Student 14

> . . . However, there are instances when it is justifiable to break the law, and this is the point the scholar is making. An example will demonstrate this. If a divorced woman with several small children is continually being harassed by her abusive, alcoholic ex-husband, she has a right to protect herself and her children. If the ex-husband becomes dangerous and threatening, and the police cannot provide her protection, the woman may be justified in killing her husband if she fears for her life and her children's'. It could be argued however, the woman committed murder and therefore broke the law. In this case, I believe the law to be unjust, and therefore believe it is justifiable to disobey the law. The woman has a right to protect her loved ones and herself, if the police cannot always provide the protection.

Comment: This passage provides a lengthy example supporting the writer's understanding of the essay topic. However, for all of its length, the example is weak, because it fails to recognize that our laws establish a right to self-defense. The divorced woman described in the passage would not be disobeying the law, and thus her case is not a good illustration of the issue compassed by the statement.

Student 15

> The days of slavery in early America exemplifies the scholar's words. In the 1800s, when the Civil War was on the verge of outbreak, laws in the Northern and Southern states differed. In the North slavery was against the law, in the South . . .

THE WRITING
SAMPLE: BASIC
STRATEGIES
AND SAMPLE
STUDENT ESSAYS

724

Comment: Student 15 ended his essay without actually completing it. Completion of the essay is probably the main requirement; this essay is not complete in thought, nor is it complete linguistically, because the last sentence remains unfinished. Final impressions are important, so strive mightily to avoid leaving your reader suspended in midair.

VI. Sample Student Essays with Scores

GENERAL INFORMATION

The following essays were written in response to a topic on a recent MCAT. They exemplify the six levels of the MCAT Writing Sample Scoring Guide. Read each essay, and try to understand why each essay was scored at a particular level. Take note of what a great essay contains. Understand what a weak essay contains, or does not contain. Be certain to review the scoring criteria covered in III, How the Writing Sample is Graded.

The comment following each essay attempts to show why the essay was assigned its score. Each comment, roughly following the pattern of the scoring guide, discusses how content, organization, mechanics, and style are controlled (or are deficient) in the six sample essays. **The limited number of sample essays and comments included here cannot indicate the breadth of information or the wide variety of viewpoints possible in responding to the topic.** However, they indicate how important it is to remain focused on the tasks included in the topic and to present a reasoned discussion, making use of specific examples. The best essays are presented first, followed by progressively weaker essays.

SAMPLE STUDENT ESSAYS

Consider this statement:

Art is I; science is we.

Write a unified essay in which you perform the following tasks: Explain what you think the above statement means. Describe a specific situation in which the sentiment of the quotation would seem to be contradicted. Discuss what you think determines the proportion of individual and collective effort that goes into artistic creation and scientific discovery.

This statement sets up a strict dichotomy between art and science. It states that art is an individual pursuit while science is a collective process. This is generally true when artforms such as photography, painting, and drawing are considered. While these items may be viewed in a gallery or magazine they are considered to be the property of the artist. Ideal science, on the other hand, is the pursuit to increase our collective knowledge regarding processes. This knowledge is distributed in journals or through other media for the benefit of others. The original scientists are given credit for their work, but other laboratories are perfectly free to attempt to duplicate their work.

Contrarily many forms of artistic expression require teams of creative people. Two obvious examples are theatre and film. Each of these requires a hierarchy from producers down to technical crew. Ownership is still implied, but is often given to corporations. The individual source of the artistic "vision" is now shrouded behind rewriting and editing. There are also many examples of individual study in science. First, most great discoveries are attributed to a single figure. Second, with growing corporatization of biotechnology patents are becoming increasingly crucial to the survival of companies. Only ideal science is purely collective.

Essay 1 (Score: 6) continues . . .

Whether a process is classified as artistic or scientific cannot be simply decided by the number of participants involved in inventing it. Instead, the source of creative ideas must be examined. Good art is usually described as new or fresh. Often the source of the inspiration is seen only by the artist or artists. The source can arise individually or be the synthesis of many creative people (as writers of a screenplay). In contrast, good science follows strict rules, fulfills well-defined goals and logically builds on work previously done. Above all, it must not illogically contradict that which is already known. These requirements can be met on the individual or collective level. It is more difficult to act individually in science because of the continuity and interdependence necessary to distribute knowledge. It must be remembered that having a strict art/science dichotomy is dangerous. Art without communication with peers leads to repetition and little maturation of style. Also, science must occasionally "suspend its disbelief" and set out in directions that may at first seem illogical to avoid close minded science.

Comment: Level 6 essays are as often determined by declaration as they are by consensus, which is to say that we all have an idea of perfection, and we often want to insist that an essay is virtually perfect before we accede to giving it a score of 6. Therefore, those who train essay readers know that a lower boundary for the level 6 category must be established, encouraging readers to see that an essay can (and should) be assigned to the highest scoring category, although it may fall short of the ideal essay in several important ways. The idea is to reward the essay for what it does well. Exciting insights or ideas—labeled on the MCAT Scoring Guide as "thorough exploration" and "depth and complexity of thought"—are most commonly rewarded.

Essay 1 is far from perfect or ideal, but it should be considered a level 6 essay because of its wealth of ideas and its lack of significant defect. Note the quickness with which this essay accomplishes the first task (i.e., explaining the statement). Within two sentences, this first task has been completed. Also, note that the writer has cleverly turned the topic against itself, having observed that the last sentence of the topic essentially provides the key to understanding the quote. A bold statement of the meaning of the statement is never enough; however, this writer supplied some apt, specific examples to illustrate the meaning of the statement. The second task is handled similarly with deftness and aplomb. Note that this paragraph is the shortest of the three—as it should be. The main work should be accomplished in addressing the first and third tasks.

It is in addressing the third task that this essay soars. The third paragraph is full of ideas, any one of which could have been developed further. It is as if the writer has so much juice that only a sketchy treatment can be provided by way of detail. Still, there is enough specificity in the paragraph to supply the conceptual glue that is needed. The paragraph has some vagueness and even muddled thinking, but this occurs relatively early in the paragraph. As the paragraph proceeds, it grows stronger, producing that all-important final impression in the reader's mind. The last sentence, in fact, is a triumph, using a principle from literary criticism to explain the proper mental attitude for the scientist who would achieve a new discovery.

The content of this essay is strong, the organization is clear and logical, and the prose is correct and fluent. Only the most minor (and infrequent) mechanical errors intrude. The style is rather simple, most of the sentences having been cast as short, declarative statements. However, there is sufficient variety, such that the reader does not become bored while reading the essay. Given the sophistication of the many ideas, a reader can appreciate the simplicity and clarity with which the ideas are presented.

THE WRITING
SAMPLE: BASIC
STRATEGIES
AND SAMPLE
STUDENT ESSAYS

726

Essay 2 (Score: 5)

Art is His: Science is Ours

Typically, one thinks of science as a collaboration of knowledge. The news media makes constant reference to the "scientific community" and its discoveries. The geniuses like Michaelangelo and Van Gogh are constantly praised and admired. Our present day body of scientific knowledge is founded on the studies of countless thousands of pioneers, researchers, and technicians. However, our artistic masterpieces are the creations of individuals laboring for months or years on their own projects. Art is individualistic, while science is a coordinated, group effort.

Yet there exist contradictions. Gregor Mendel, with virtually no scientific training or schooling, while living in a monastery, performed some of the most important experiments ever conducted. He formulated the basic laws of genetics by himself, with no outside assistance. A remarkable feat for an individual. If one considers music as an artform, one can also point to bands or orchestra as being comprised of individual artists cooperating together to produce an artistic work. Their art is from a group, not just an individual.

Overall, artistic creations are the products of individuals, however. One individual conceives the idea, and even if the assistance of others is involved, the artistic work arises from this single dual or unit of individuals. A single group or individual is responsible for the creation. Science could not exist on the individual plane, however. Even Mendel did not glimpse the real significance of his work, like the discovery of the laws of heredity and its chemical basis. Those discoveries were by others, using his data and results and adding some of their own. Science is based on group discoveries and could not exist if only individuals performed experiments. Scientists, much as they would not want to admit it, need each other. Without collaboration, science would be reduced to endless repetition of experiments that were already performed, which would waste resources and time. Only through true team effort can significant discoveries be made.

Comment: Level 5 essays are typically thought of as "clearly competent." The essay may not stun the reader with originality; however, a level 5 essay is a substantial piece of work, an essay for which one should not have to make excuses. In essay 2, it is clear that the writer has control of the material, but it is also clear that there is not the same depth of thought present as in essay 1. Essay 2 is always clear. Also, in all ways, essay 2 demonstrates the writer's competence. Perhaps its most outstanding feature is the level of conciseness. Although the essay is relatively short, it accomplishes all three tasks, and does so with sufficient specific detail.

It is worth commenting on the use of detail in essay 2. The second and third writing tasks are handled chiefly through the example of Mendel's experiments in genetics. The MCAT that this student took had a Verbal Reasoning passage about Mendel. Perhaps the writer would have thought about Mendel regardless of this inclusion (or perhaps not). The important point is that the writer was thoughtful and economical enough to use an example readily at hand. More notably, the writer shows a sophistication of mind by demonstrating how his own example of Mendel's independent spirit, work, and creativity ultimately breaks down; the writer then uses this example for the contradiction of viewpoint. There is an intellectual honesty in acknowledging that the paradox of the quotation can be explored but probably never resolved. One cannot claim with perfect assurance who the individuals are that will make the best doctors. Nevertheless, one is tempted to think that someone like this writer (i.e., fair minded, reasonable, adaptable) has at least some of the qualities desired in a good doctor.

Having praised the writer of essay 2, we should note that the essay is a bit thin. There are not as many ideas or examples as a reader would like to see. Although all three writing tasks are completed, they are not as thoroughly addressed as a reader would like. Also, there is less precision in the execution of this essay. Careless errors intrude (e.g., "media makes" in the first sentence, a sentence fragment in the second paragraph). Also, the logic sometimes falters. For example, the second paragraph argues that bands and orchestras are examples of the collective nature of artistic expression. But are band members really artists, or are they merely performers?

Despite these flaws, essay 2 is a substantial piece of work, and it clearly deserves to be in the level 5 scoring category.

Essay 3 (Score: 4)

Art in its many forms is one of the most dramatic and idealistic ways in which an individual expresses personal opinions and emotions. In creating art, the artist is unrestrained and does not have to follow or abide by any set of laws or protocol. Science on the other hand is a constant accumulation of knowledge among many people studying many different things and whose experiments and theories must abide by the physical laws of nature. Therefore, the statement Art is I; science is We explains that art is a form of individual expression while science is a group effort with many people striving toward similar goals.

As romantic as this view may seem, it is not always correct. The creation of art can sometimes involve the work of many people, while certain scientific achievements may involve the hard work or inborn brilliance of one particular person. For example, many people may contribute to the artistic design of a skyscraper while one person may develop the scientific nature of its structure, such as an architect.

Therefore when one considers art or science, both can be seen as individual efforts in the hope of achieving something. In art this normally involved the expression of personal feelings while in science it is one man's hope of finding a solution.

However both artistic creations and scientific discoveries involve creations and scientific discoveries involve collective effort as well. In artistic creations other people may help the artist physically, or their thoughts and opinions may have affected the artist in some way as to influence his results. Therefore, artistic creation and scientific discovery both involve individual and collective effort, although the extent that each of these contributes can vary with every creation and discovery.

Comment: Level 4 essays are adequate. A level 4 essay never thrills a reader, but it responds to all three of the assigned writing tasks in a reasonably coherent way. Level 4 essays invariably have flaws, but the errors are not of a serious nature. Essays are usually given a score of 4 because of what they fail to do, rather than for mistakes they contain. The typical deficiencies are in the development, detail, and design of the essay.

Essay 4 is satisfactory; it addresses all parts of the topic and shows the writer's understanding of the concepts and ideas inherent within the statement provided. However, there is little complexity of thought or true insight demonstrated. The first paragraph is a series of rambling generalizations that are not very relevant. The final sentence of the first paragraph, which states the essential meaning of the quotation, fails to do so with any special grace or fluency. The many wasted sentences of the first paragraph demonstrate that the writer is struggling with the material, rather than being in command of it. The second paragraph has similar flaws. The writer points out that both art and science are products of individual and collective efforts, but there is little specificity. The writer provides an assertion, but with little support. An example is provided in the second paragraph, but it is not very helpful because it is not well explained or developed. At first glance, this example does not seem valid, proving the need for more expansion of the discussion. The final paragraph has the same vagueness and vapidity. These statements are too general; the writer fails to understand that mere assertion is not sufficient coverage and explanation for the critical eye of the reader.

The imprecision of thought in this essay is demonstrated by the imprecision of the prose. For example, the writer obviously does not understand the proper use of the comma. In addition, the writer does not have much of an ear. (Read the final sentence of the essay aloud, and you will see what I mean.) Although this essay is in no way pleasing, it does not contain serious problems. Strive to write a better essay, but if you must, you *can* settle for a score of 4. Receiving a score of 4 places you in the top half of the scoring guide, which is the main goal.

Essay 4 (Score: 3)

> As the artist molds and forms his clay, each etch and curve arises from the creative current that travels from the brain to fingertips. His minds eye sees his workpiece, while his hands deftly make it. The presence of foreign hands can only skew the artist's vision. His is a solitary creation. The scientist builds. He builds on former knowledge and adds dimension to existing theories. Where his minds eye is blind, often others can see. Science calls for cooperation, participation and team work.
>
> However, science is not a thunderous rally of intelligent minds churning on to new ideas—it takes only one to propose an idea and others to follow it through. For instance, Benjamin Franklin didn't take a lab team with him when he discovered electricity and Louis Pasteur worked diligently in his lab without the accompaniment of others.
>
> One can claim that science is art and art is science. This calls for a inclusive requirement of both individual effort and collective thinking. Each aspect deserves consideration. The art of science needs to be openly available to new ideas and insight. This is an important determinant of those who should be involved. This requires many. On the other hand, art needs to arise from the creator, who, on the critique of those more knowledgeable can refine and beautify.

Comment: Level 3 essays are weak. The weakness may result from a failure to address all three writing tasks, or it may reflect a serious lack of development. The weakness may be caused by incoherent organization or by prose that fails to make the writer's meaning clear. A score of 3 reflects jumbled thinking or an inability to express oneself clearly (neither of which is a coveted trait in today's world).

Essay 4 is a bit on the short side, considering the writer had 30 minutes to work. However, the length of any essay is only a symptom, not a disease itself. The real problem with this essay is the intense emptiness of the writing. Consider the first sentence of this essay. Is it necessary? Consider each sentence. How many of them can be eliminated? How many of the sentences can be combined (thereby eliminating some of the primer-style prose)? Many of the sentences in this essay simply need to be developed. Also, the writer could have profited by writing more considered statements rather than indulging in the fluff that pollutes this essay. This writer begins each paragraph with a howlingly bad sentence. If you have to write bad sentences, try to put them in a less emphatic position, such as in the middle of a paragraph.

The essay has mechanical problems with punctuation, particularly with the use of the apostrophe. Nevertheless, the writer avoided significant grammatical errors, mainly, because he used only the simplest sentence structures.

In conclusion, essay 4 is comprehensible and the writer does understand the quotation or the topic. However, it is a piece of writing that says almost nothing. The essay is merely a series of suggestions and half-completed ideas instead of a careful and clear analysis. Simplistic, minimal treatments of this nature can never garner a score higher than a 3.

Essay 5 (Score: 2)

Art, in general, is a very personal thing. It represents an individuals dipiction of somthing. Not just any dipiction, but an unique dipiction. If art is not unique, do we really consider it art? Science, on the other hand is not as personal as art. Our efforts to gain knowledge of science is a collective one. Science biulds on what was found by others.

There are times when art is consieved by groups of people. If, for example, several artists get together and design and biuld a statue. The unique efforts of the artests led to the creation of art. Artistic creation is usually the result of one or few artists. This is because if too many people are involved in the creation of art it loses its value, it is no longer unique. Science, on the other hand is usually based on several scientists before him. Art is not base on biulding on others work like science is.

Comment: Level 2 essays are poor—most likely because they fail to address one or more of the three writing tasks, or because they misinterpret the quotation. A much smaller proportion of essays receive a score of 2 because of numerous syntactic and mechanical errors.

Essay 5 is interesting, although a bit depressing. It demonstrates the writer's understanding of the quotation; it addresses all three writing tasks; and it presents no obvious distortion of any of the writing tasks. However, this is a poor essay. This essay is poor because of its almost total lack of analysis. The essay does not provide a clear explanation of the statement provided for analysis. A reader looks for some thoughtfulness in responding to the idea expressed in the statement. The reader is looking for insights or some reference to past reading, personal experience, or the fruits of meditation. The reader also expects some specific examples (names, dates, or events) to combine the information in the essay with previous knowledge, thereby stitching together a better understanding of the world. This essay provides very few specific examples. The reader is not informed by this essay.

The other salient flaw of this essay is the prose. Almost every sentence has a syntactic or mechanical error, and the reader is unnecessarily hobbled while reading the essay. It is difficult to understand why the errors were made and more difficult to understand how the writer failed to recognize them. The prose reflects poorly on the writer.

Essay 6 (Score: 1)

The above statement, "Art is I, science is we" I think implies the goal of those doing the work. The work being expressing, impersonating, delivering, receiving, manipulating, discovering, etc through art and/or through science. It "the statement" probably makes inferences to the attitude of the individual(s) who does the work and the attitude of who will be recognized for the work in the end. For instance, though paint is manufactured by different companies, scripts are written by authors, oft times besides the actors, the only "group" recognized or distinguished in the final exam is the painter—Michaelangelo, the actor—Susan Lucci, and the performer Milli Vanilli. In another instance both Watson and Crick were honored for their work and contribution to determine the structure of DNA which not only rendered them fame but everyone who is not a scientist benefits, criminals are found out, etc—the plural aspect of "we" for science. On the contrary, again in considering acting as the form of "art" chosen to observe, not only was Whoopi Goldberg "sore thumbed" for The Color Purple, but so were the writers, director, etc, Steven Spielberg even. In fact, whenever one name came up on the media so did the other. The art form of comedy was used to help the homeless on HBOs Comic Relief.

Comment: Level 1 essays have serious problems and may be incomprehensible. A level 1 essay may not address the three writing tasks that the topic demands; it may be inappropriately brief; it may lack any apparent structure or development; or, it may demonstrate the writer's lack of knowledge of the conventions of modern English usage. Essay 6 demonstrates most of these difficulties.

Essay 6 fails to, at least in any coherent manner, address the topic. If the reader did not know what the topic was, he would have a difficult time figuring out what this essay is about. The essay is short, and it does not appear to have any clear structure or plan. The essay is only one paragraph, and the sentence-to-sentence cohesiveness is minimal. The essay contains many specific details; however, the mere mention of names is not considered an effective manner of injecting details. The essay is relatively free of grammatical errors. However, a reader has a difficult time comprehending this essay, because the sentence structure is often garbled, and because the essay as a whole does not follow the organization suggested by the tasks of the topic. In fact, the essay fails to follow any organization at all.

VII. Practice Essay Prompts

What are MCAT essay questions like? Read the following topic statements, which are similar to those that have appeared on actual MCATs. Think about the following topics and how you would approach them. After you have reviewed all of them, look at the 10 practice essay topics (complete with writing tasks) that follow. We encourage you to practice writing some of these essays. Have your English professor, campus writing center, tutors, or friends (if they write well) evaluate your essays. Remember, practice makes perfect!

ESSAY STATEMENTS SIMILAR TO THOSE APPEARING ON RECENT MCAT EXAMS

1. *In business, quick solutions often do not address the real source of a problem.*

2. *In a free society, individuals must be allowed to do as they choose.*

3. *In education, the newest way is not always the best way.*

4. *Although it claims to promote individuality, most advertising promotes conformity.*

5. *A country must use its natural resources in a way agreeable to all its citizens.*

6. *No matter how oppressive a government, violent revolution is never justified.*

7. *Students should be more interested in the process of learning than in the facts learned.*

8. *Progress seldom comes from the deliberations of a group. Rather, progress most often comes from the creative thinking of individuals working alone.*

9. *A democratic government is never justified in keeping secrets from the voting public.*

10. *One must be inflexible in matters of principle.*

PRACTICE MCAT WRITING SAMPLE TOPICS WITH WRITING TASKS

1. **Consider this statement:** *Never say no when the world says yes.* Write a unified essay in which you perform the following tasks: Explain what you think the above statement means. Describe a specific situation in which it would be prudent to go against the opinion of the majority. Discuss what you think determines when it is wise to live only by one's own opinions.

2. **Consider this statement:** *True leadership is the ability to detect the public will and to follow it.* Write a unified essay in which you perform the following tasks: Explain what the above statement means. Describe a specific situation in which a leader has been praised for moving contrary to the public will. Discuss what you think determines the extent to which leaders should take actions independent of popular opinion.

3. **Consider this statement:** *What one generation has found valuable should prove valuable to those generations that follow it.* Write a unified essay in which you perform the following tasks: Explain what the above statement means. Describe a specific situation in which one generation has rejected the opinion of a prior one. Discuss what you think determines whether opinions will stand the test of time.

4. **Consider this statement:** *Laws are like cobwebs, which may catch small flies but let wasps and hornets break through.* Write a unified essay in which you perform the following tasks: Explain what you think the above statement means. Describe a specific situation in which the law has proved to be more powerful than a mere cobweb. Discuss what you think determines whether the law can be effective against the strong as well as the weak.

5. **Consider this statement:** *True education consists of learning principles rather than amassing facts.* Write a unified essay in which you perform the following tasks: Explain what the above statement means. Describe a specific situation in which the facts one knows could be considered more important than principles. Discuss what you think determines the relative importance of facts and the principles behind them.

6. **Consider this statement:** *If you have the moon, ignore the stars.* Write a unified essay in which you perform the following tasks: Explain what you think the above statement means. Describe a specific situation in which "to ignore the stars" would be wrong. Discuss what you think determines whether one should strive for "the stars."

7. **Consider this statement:** *Education consists mainly of what we have unlearned.* Write a unified essay in which you perform the following tasks: Explain what you think the above statement means. Describe a specific situation in which education could not be said to be a process of unlearning. Discuss what you think determines whether education is a process of learning or of unlearning.

8. **Consider this statement:** *Society has a right to extinguish whatever it deems to be contrary to its norms.* Write a unified essay in which you perform the following tasks: Explain what you think the above statement means. Describe a specific situation in which society should tolerate that which it determines to be atypical or deviant. Discuss what you think determines the degree to which a society has a right to insist that its members be homogenous.

9. **Consider this statement:** *Men who borrow their opinions can never repay their debts.* Write a unified essay in which you perform the following tasks: Explain what you think the above statement means. Describe a specific situation in which it made sense to adopt the opinion of another. Discuss what you think determines the degree to which one should do one's own thinking.

10. **Consider this statement:** *If their government displeases them, the governed have the right to replace it.* Write a unified essay in which you perform the following tasks: Explain what you think the above statement means. Describe a specific situation in which the governed would not be justified in replacing the government. Discuss what you think determines the degree to which citizens have a right to overturn their government.

THE WRITING
SAMPLE: BASIC
STRATEGIES
AND SAMPLE
STUDENT ESSAYS

732

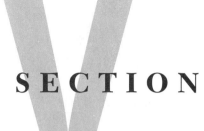

SECTION V

Sample Full-Length MCAT with Solutions and Analysis

....

A. Sample Full-Length MCAT with Answers and Explanations

B. Interpreting Test Scores

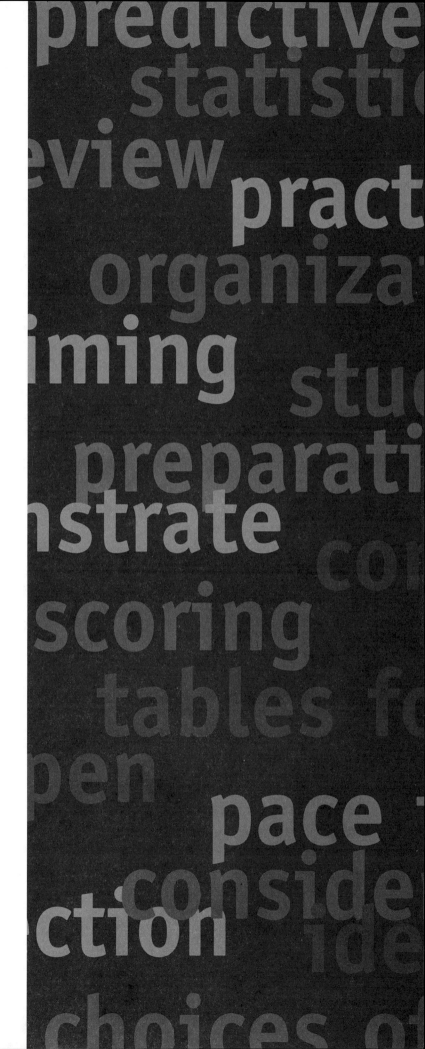

Sample
Full-Length
MCAT with
Answers and
Explanations

Verbal Reasoning

Time: 85 Minutes
Questions 1–65

VERBAL REASONING

Directions: There are nine reading passages in the Verbal Reasoning test. Each passage is followed by several questions. After reading a passage, select the one best answer to each question. If you are not certain of an answer, eliminate the alternatives that you know to be incorrect and then select an answer from the remaining alternatives.

Passage I (Questions 1–8)

After Filippo and Donatello failed to win the competition to construct the new doors for the baptistery of San Giovanni, they resolved to leave Florence and to spend several years at Rome, where they would study, the one architecture, and the other sculpture.

Filippo chose architecture as being more useful to mankind than either sculpture or painting, and he hoped that what he did as an architect would enable him to surpass both Lorenzo and Donatello. He sold a small farm that he owned at Settignano, and then in company with Donatello he left Florence for Rome. And when he walked through Rome seeing for the first time the grandeur of the buildings and the perfect construction of the churches, he kept stopping short in amazement, as if thunderstruck. He and Donatello made arrangements for taking the groundplans of the buildings and measuring the comices, and they set to work regardless of time or expense. They saw everything there was to see, both in Rome and in the countryside around, and they recorded the measurements of every good piece of work they came across.

As Filippo had no domestic ties he was able to give himself completely to his studies, not caring whether he went without food and sleep and concentrating utterly on the architecture of the past, by which I mean the good ancient orders and not the barbarous German style which was then fashionable. Filippo conceived two tremendous ambitions: first, to restore the practice of good architecture, in the belief that if he did so his name would be regarded by posterity as highly as Cimabue's and Giotto's; and secondly, if he could, to discover a way to raise the cupola of Santa Maria del Fiore at Florence which was so difficult an undertaking that after the death of Amolfo Lapi no one had ever had the courage to contemplate attempting it without allowing for vast expenditure on a wooden framework. He confided his ambition neither to Donatello nor to any other living soul although while he was in Rome he continually investigated all the problems that had been involved in vaulting the Pantheon. He noted and made drawings of all the ancient vaults and was always studying their construction. And if he and Donatello unearthed any remains, such as pieces of capitals, columns, comices, or the bases of buildings, they would start excavating and have them completely dug out in order to make a detailed examination.

There was no kind of building of which he did not make drawings: round, square, and octagonal temples, basilicas, aqueducts, baths, arches, coliseums, amphitheaters, and all the brick temples, from which he noted the methods used in binding and clamping with ties and encircling the vaults. He recorded all the methods used for binding stones together and for balancing and dovetailing them; and he investigated the reason for there being a hole hollowed out in the center and underside of all the large stones, discovering that it was for the iron used to haul them up, which we call the ulivella. He subsequently brought this into use again and employed it himself. Then he distinguished the several orders, namely, Doric, launch, and Corinthians; and his studies were so thorough and intelligent that in his mind's eye he could see Rome as it had stood before it fell into ruins.

1. The author specifically describes Filippo's:

    I. attention to detail.
    II. dedication and modesty.
    III. artistically original vision.

    A. I and II only
    B. I and III only
    C. I only
    D. I, II, and III

2. The passage can best be described as:

   A. a satire of ambition.
   B. a comparison of Donatello and Filippo.
   C. a musing on Renaissance ideals.
   D. a biography of Filippo.

3. Donatello and Filippo's dedication is best exemplified by their:

   A. lack of familial obligation.
   B. interest in understanding the accomplishments of the past.
   C. quiet rivalry with one another.
   D. endurance of poverty.

4. From the passage it can be logically concluded that:

   I. Donatello was better off financially than Filippo.
   II. Filippo was better off financially than Donatello.
   III. neither man had much interest in money.

   A. I and III only
   B. II and III only
   C. III only
   D. None of the above

5. The main problem Filippo faced in raising a cupola on Santa Maria del Fiore in Florence was:

   A. lack of technical expertise.
   B. lack of money available for the project.
   C. jealousy from other architects.
   D. fear of failure.

6. The best title for the passage is:

   A. *The Rivalry of Filippo and Donatello.*
   B. *Filippo: Renaissance Man.*
   C. *Renaissance Architecture.*
   D. *Filippo Encounters Classic Rome.*

7. The author's tone in the passage seems to be one of:

   A. scientific detachment.
   B. enthusiastic reverence.
   C. disguised envy.
   D. probing curiosity.

8. The author of the passage would probably most agree with which of these statements?

   A. It was an act of cowardice or insufficient confidence for Filippo to abandon sculpture.
   B. Filippo manifested talent, but little originality.
   C. Filippo was most interested in being fashionable.
   D. Filippo would have been a good architect had he spent more time designing buildings instead of merely doing research.

GO ON TO THE NEXT PAGE.

Passage II (Questions 9–15)

It is not alone by the rapidity of extent of conquest that we should estimate the greatness of Rome. The sovereign of the Russian deserts commands a larger portion of the globe. In the seventh summer after his passage of the Hellespont, Alexander erected the Macedonian trophies on the banks of the Hyphasis. Within less than a century the irresistible Zingis and the Mogul princes of his race spread their cruel devastations and transient empire from the sea of China to the confines of Eygpt and Germany. But the firm edifice of Roman power was raised and preserved by the wisdom of ages. The obedient provinces of Trajan and the Antonines were united by laws and adorned by arts. They might occasionally suffer from the partial abuse of delegated authority; but the general principle of government was wise, simple, and beneficent. They enjoyed the religion of their ancestors, whilst in civil honors and advantages they were exalted, by just degrees, to an equality with their conquerors.

The policy of the emperors and the senate, as far as it concerned religion, was happily seconded by the reflections of the enlightened, and by the habits of the superstitious, part of their subjects. The various modes of worship which prevailed in the Roman world were all considered by the people as equally true, by the philosopher as equally false, and by the magistrate as equally useful. And thus toleration produced not only mutual indulgence, but even religious concord.

The superstition of the people was not embittered by any mixture of theological raucous, nor was it confined by the chains of any speculative system. The devout polytheist, though fondly attached to this national rites, admitted with implicit faith the different religions of the earth. Fear, gratitude, and curiosity, a dream or an omen, a singular disorder or a distant journey, perpetually disposed him to multiply the articles of his belief and to enlarge the list of his protectors. The thin texture of the pagan mythology was interwoven with various but not discordant materials. As soon as it was allowed that sages and heroes who had lived or who had died for the benefit of their country were exalted to a state of power and immortality, it was universally confessed that they deserved, if not the adoration, at least the reverence, of all mankind. The deities of a thousand groves and a thousand streams possessed in peace their local and respective influence; nor could the Roman who deprecated the wrath of the Tiber deride the Egyptian who presented his offering to the beneficent genius of the Nile.

The visible powers of nature, the planets, and the elements were the same throughout the universe. The invisible governors of the moral world were inevitably cast in a similar mold of fiction and allegory. Every virtue, and even vice, acquired its divine representative, every art and profession its patron, whose attributes, in the most distant ages and countries, were uniformly derived from the character of their peculiar votaries. Such was the mild spirit of antiquity that the nations were less attentive to the difference than to the resemblance of their religious worship. The Greek, the Roman, and the barbarian, as they met before their respective altars, easily persuaded themselves that under various names and with various ceremonies they adored the same deities.

9. The author suggests Rome was great primarily because:

   A. it dominated its neighbors militarily.
   B. it possessed great technical ability in the arts.
   C. it governed its people fairly.
   D. it made Christianity its state religion.

10. The author believes that the practice of religion in ancient Rome was:

    I. an indulgence in superstition.
    II. psychologically necessary for some individuals.
    III. useful to the state.

    A. I, II, and III
    B. I and II only
    C. II and III only
    D. I and III only

11. Which of the following statements accurately describes the gods worshipped by the ancient Romans?

    A. They were similar to the gods worshipped by the barbarians.
    B. Some so-called gods were actually just important people.
    C. Some gods merely represented landscape features.
    D. All of the above.

12. In discussing the religious practices of the pagan world, the author's tone is primarily one of:

    A. pity.
    B. respect.
    C. condemnation.
    D. amusement.

739

GO ON TO THE NEXT PAGE.

13. The author would most likely advise a ruler to:

    A. establish a state religion.
    B. keep government and religious practices strictly separate.
    C. persecute only obnoxious religions.
    D. allow atheism.

14. The author of the passage would probably agree most strongly with which of the following statements?

    A. Rome was great because it tolerated political diversity.
    B. The greatness of Rome has been equaled or surpassed by several subsequent empires.
    C. Religion in ancient Rome did not play a major role in people's lives.
    D. It was a mistake for Rome to adopt Christianity as its state religion.

15. It can be inferred that the author would support:

    I. banning sacrifices of animals in voodoo rites.
    II. being a member of a religious organization.
    III. taxing property belonging to religious organizations.

    A. I and II only
    B. I only
    C. II only
    D. III only

Passage III (Questions 16–22)

The most striking fact about higher learning in America is the confusion that besets it. . .

The first cause of this confusion is very vulgar; it is the love of money. I do not mean, of course, that universities do not need money and that they should not try to get it. I mean only that they should have an educational policy and then try to finance it, instead of letting financial accidents determine their educational policy. Undoubtedly the love of money and that sensitivity to public demands it creates has a good deal to do with the service-station conception of a university. According to this conception a university must make itself felt in the community; it must be constantly, currently felt. A state university must help the farmers look after their cows. An endowed university must help adults get better jobs by giving them courses in the afternoon and evening. . .

Even more important than the love of money as a cause of our confusion is our confused notion of democracy. It is assumed that a student must stay in public education as long as he likes, may study what he likes, and may claim any degree. As a result, we again have the conclusion drawn that education should be immediately responsive to public opinion. But what really determines the length of free education for all? Not democratic principles, but economic conditions. Under present conditions, some kind of educational activity must be provided up to approximately the twentieth year. This means that the public junior college will become the characteristic educational institution in the United States. Free education should exist beyond the sophomore level also, but it should be open only to those who have clearly demonstrated their ability to profit by it. The only hope of securing a true university in this country is to see to it that it does not become a finishing school for students incapable of receiving intellectual training or a mere school for vocational training. A university must be a home of independent intellectual work. It cannot make its contribution to democracy on any other terms.

Another major cause of our disorder is an erroneous notion of progress—that everything is getting better from age to age. The theory of evolution got involved in our views of social and cultural progress; it gave aid and comfort to aimless experimentation and was particularly happy in its effect upon education. Evolution proves, you see, that there is steady improvement from age to age. But it shows, too, that everybody's business is to get adjusted to his environment. Obviously the way to get adjusted to one's environment is to know a lot about it. And so empiricism, having taken the place of thought as the basis of research, took its place, too, as the basis of education. It led by easy stages to vocationalism.

We begin, then, with a notion of progress and end with an anti-intellectualism which denies in effect that man is a rational animal. He can be trained to do things, but the idea that his education should consist of the cultivation of his intellect is, of course, ridiculous. . .

The people, then, do not believe in the cultivation of the intellect for its own sake. Some institutions must be strong enough and clear enough to stand firm and show our people what higher learning is. As education it is the single-minded pursuit of the intellectual virtues. As scholarship it is the single-minded devotion to the advancement of knowledge. Only if the colleges and the universities can devote themselves to these objects can we look hopefully to the future of higher learning in America.

16. The author of the passage identifies as a cause of the confusion that besets higher learning in America all of the following EXCEPT:

    A. the prevalence of the service-station conception of a university.
    B. the influence of evolutionary theory upon educational theory.
    C. the democratic system of government in the United States.
    D. the influence of empiricism on educational theory.

17. The main conclusion of the passage is that:

    A. the general public has a mistaken understanding of the proper nature of higher learning.
    B. higher learning in America is in a state of confusion.
    C. the problems facing universities today stem from a love of money.
    D. at least some universities must reaffirm the values of higher learning.

18. To which of the following would the author of this passage likely object?

    I. The determination of curriculum by a popular vote of students
    II. State-funded higher education for intellectually gifted students
    III. The teaching of evolutionary theory in universities

    A. III only
    B. I and II only
    C. I only
    D. I and III only

19. A good title for the passage is:

    A. *A Prescription for Higher Learning in America.*
    B. *The Nature of Intellectual Virtue.*
    C. *Higher Learning in America: A Bright Future.*
    D. *The Failure of Higher Learning in America.*

20. According to the passage:

    A. education and scholarship are the same thing.
    B. education and scholarship are different aspects of higher learning.
    C. education is generally more important than scholarship.
    D. empiricism is the basis of education, whereas rational thought is the basis of scholarship.

21. The author of the passage claims that a confused notion of democracy:

    A. has caused higher education to be overly responsive to public opinion.
    B. has led to the current financial crisis in higher learning.
    C. is incompatible with the cultivation of the intellect for its own sake.
    D. supports the theory of evolution as applied to education.

22. According to the passage, the theory of evolution:

    A. brought about the service-station conception of the university.
    B. encouraged experimentation in education.
    C. showed that man was a rational animal.
    D. causes the love of money.

Passage IV (Questions 23–29)

Those who opine that the age of the "Renaissance person"—the master of diverse disciplines, the boldest thinker and doer—has long since passed betray an ignorance of one of this century's greatest thinkers, Bertrand Russell. Russell's long and varied life, marked by ground-breaking contributions to philosophy, logic, and social policy, shines as brightly as the lives of the da Vincis, Newtons, and Descartes of earlier centuries.

Bertrand Russell was born in Wales in 1872. As the grandson of Lord John Russell, England's Prime Minister in the time of Queen Victoria, Russell was introduced to the upper echelon of English social and intellectual life at a very young age. Following the death of his parents when he was still young, Russell was tutored privately in Europe before returning to England at the age of eighteen to enroll in Cambridge University. There Russell excelled in mathematics and philosophy and, upon graduating, stayed on at Cambridge, first as a fellow and then as a lecturer in philosophy. It was as a lecturer that Russell and his colleague Alfred North Whitehead wrote their landmark work in mathematical logic, the *Principia Mathematica*, or *Principles of Mathematics*. The *Principia* attempted to express the major portions of mathematics in terms of pure logic. Although ultimately deemed unsuccessful, Russell and Whitehead's *Principia* remains this century's single most significant contribution to mathematical logic.

Russell's flourishing in the rarefied atmosphere of logic and mathematics was shattered by the First World War. Russell had entertained pacifist sentiments since the turn of the century, but he would probably not have opposed the war so actively had he not been exposed almost first-hand to its atrocities. Russell's opposition was vehement; he argued passionately that the possible ouster of Germany's Kaiser Wilhelm could not possibly justify the loss of millions of lives on both sides. But pacifism, even from the mouth of the internationally respected Russell, was not tolerated by an England caught up in the spirit of war. As punishment for writing supposedly libelous anti-war pamphlets and newspaper columns, Russell was dismissed from Cambridge, fined, and sentenced to six months imprisonment in 1918. Characteristically, he put the time to good use, completing both the *Introduction to Mathematical Philosophy* and *The Analysis of Mind*, the latter of which is still widely read in philosophy classes.

Russell did not return to academia until 1938. His time in between the first and second world wars was spent traveling, writing, and lecturing. Russell's proclaimed views on sexuality, marriage, and other social issues enraged the moralists of his time. He advocated, among other things, an enlightened program of sex education for all ages and a general loosening of the social restraints that prohibited sex outside of marriage. His public lecture of 1927, *Why I Am Not a Christian,* identified Russell as a prominent atheist. The public perception of Russell caused him

some trouble upon his return to academic life. In one remarkable instance, Russell was denied a position at the City College of New York by a judge who regarded him as a threat to "public health, safety, and morals." Fortunately, Cambridge University was willing to take the risk; Russell returned there in 1944 as a fellow, and remained until his death.

In 1950, Russell received the Nobel Prize in Literature. The Nobel committee described him as "a fearless champion of free speech and free thought in the West." Russell's work continued through the 1950s, and on all fronts. Indeed, in 1961 at the age of 89, Russell was jailed a second time, for the period of one week, for his participation in a demonstration for nuclear disarmament.

Russell died in 1970 at the age of 98, having witnessed the Western world's procession though an age of unprecedented technological and intellectual advance and unequaled international carnage. More than witnessing, though, Russell affected significant parts of the world we live in. Russell lived in the spirit of the Renaissance thinkers before him; he was, and will remain, a true Renaissance thinker of our own century.

23. Which of the following can be reasonably inferred from information contained in the passage?

    A. Russell vehemently protested the Second World War.
    B. Russell favored nuclear disarmament.
    C. Russell vehemently protested the Vietnam War.
    D. Russell left England as a result of being fined and imprisoned.

24. According to the passage, all of the following works were written solely by Russell EXCEPT:

    A. *Why I Am Not a Christian*
    B. *Introduction to Mathematical Philosophy*
    C. *The Analysis of Mind*
    D. *Principia Mathematica*

25. The main idea of the passage is that:

    A. Bertrand Russell suffered professionally as a result of the views he held.
    B. Bertrand Russell was a fearless champion of free speech and free thought in the West.
    C. Bertrand Russell was at least as fascinating and intelligent as da Vinci, Newton, or Descartes.
    D. Bertrand Russell was a "Renaissance person."

GO ON TO THE NEXT PAGE.

26. Information contained in the passage implies that which of the following is true?

    A. Russell was jailed for the first time after the beginning of the First World War.

    B. Russell and Whitehead wrote the *Principia Mathematica* while Russell was an undergraduate at Cambridge.

    C. The First World War broke out before Russell became a pacifist.

    D. Russell embraced atheism early in his education.

27. With the use of the word *opine,* the author of this passage means:

    A. argue.

    B. state as an opinion.

    C. deny.

    D. infer.

28. Based on information in the passage, to which of the following would Russell have likely NOT objected?

    I. The elimination of laws prohibiting adultery

    II. Eliminating the tax-exempt status enjoyed by many churches

    III. A program of sex education directed at children 4 to 6 years of age

    A. I and III only

    B. I only

    C. II and III only

    D. I, II, and III

29. Which of the following does the author of the passage identify as a cause of Russell's active opposition to the First World War?

    A. Russell's exposure at an early age to the upper echelon of English intellectual and social life

    B. Russell's conviction that all wars are morally wrong

    C. Russell's nearly first-hand exposure to the atrocities of World War I

    D. Russell's conviction that conflicts between the nations involved could be resolved more effectively through diplomacy

Passage V (Questions 30–36)

Instinct is aptly described as being an involuntary, unreasoned, inherited tendency to act or to perform a specific action under the proper internal and external stimuli. More simply, it is that natural impulse to act in a certain way.

An example of instinct in the animal world is salmon swimming hundreds of miles up mountain streams to spawn. The salmon's instinctive behavior of depositing eggs is still a mystery, though scientists, folklorists, and native people all agree that the fish answer a certain as-yet set of undiscovered (or at least not yet isolated) stimuli shared by all members of their species.

Instinct is not reflex, which is defined as a physiologically innate or even acquired "automatic" response. Reflex might involve acts as involuntary as sneezing or flinching. Reflex, however, can also be trained behavior; for instance, the hair-trigger reactions of the highly trained martial arts expert.

Where in a social structure do we locate the difference between instinct, a natural impulse, and reflex, an automatic response? A social structure offers a glaring reflection of the ethical make-up of the individuals who create that structure. The shape it takes on, along with the power it attains, reciprocally is modeled after the strength of its creators and frequently it illustrates the differences between instinct and automatic behavior, or reflex. Finally, this creative human strength suggests a singular dependence on instinctual behavior.

In *Lord of the Flies*, author William Golding attempts to evaluate the ultimate effect of social and environmental factors on individual human instinct. This highly symbolic novel, Golding once stated, "attempts to trace the defects of society back to the defects of human nature." His major premise is that the potential for certain behavior is inherent in every individual, and said behavior may readily surface if an immediate environment promotes such behavior. Thus, Golding offers environment as that specific factor delineating the activity of human instinct. Strictly reflexive behaviors suggest the singularity of unique individual action, but environment is, for Golding, that factor in the novel and in life which somehow brings us into the realm of a deeply shared instinct that is "human nature." In the novel, potential for savagely violent behavior is omnipresent in the well-bred English schoolboys, and the catalyst which brings that capability to heat and eventually detonation is the character of their immediate environment.

At the start of the narrative, a group of boys have been thrust into an entirely new and foreign situation. Their learned thought patterns cause many of them to be initially intimidated by the absence of adult supervision. Rapidly, though, the precious deficit of restrictions of various sorts provides them with the prime opportunity to liberate all inhibitions assimilated in their more familiar British societal structure. They shed all symbols of their

GO ON TO THE NEXT PAGE.

life at home—clothes, hygienic habits, mannerisms, educated speech, and eventually, all semblance of peaceful order. The defects of the society they gradually create, an anarchy overseen and promoted by a sadistic megalomaniac, can readily be traced back to the defects of their base nature, that which is no less than destructive. When the elimination of order commences, so does the extermination of any individual who impedes its very natural progression. That they throw themselves into a frenzied, ritualistic dance, and chant, and in cold blood, murder a boy while perfectly conscious of the act of attacking and killing, is irrefutable proof of what lay deep beneath the surface of their once disciplined and civilized guise—an untapped capacity for destruction of life.

30. The author's main concern in the passage is to:

   A. discuss Golding's success in developing the premise of the novel.
   B. elaborate on a simple definition of instinct.
   C. describe how easily people can behave violently.
   D. explain how every human being has the same instincts.

31. Which of the following best corresponds with the author's definition of *instinct*?

   A. Imperfect and inborn
   B. Natural and internal
   C. Involuntary and inborn
   D. Unreasonable and defective

32. According to the author, instincts:

   A. are fully controllable urges.
   B. can, if given effective stimuli, overpower learned values and behavior.
   C. wholly control the development of a society.
   D. are secondary in importance when compared to learned behavior.

33. The author considers Golding's premise:

   A. unique.
   B. illogical.
   C. extreme.
   D. credible.

34. According to the passage, it can be inferred from *Lord of the Flies* that:

   A. if stranded in the wilderness, we too would become murderers.
   B. Western society is morally defective.
   C. our environment, in part, determines how we act.
   D. man is still a beast.

35. All of the following was shed by the boys in the novel EXCEPT?

   A. Physical reminders of home
   B. Patterns of behavior
   C. Their personalities
   D. Social order

36. The shape mentioned in the fourth paragraph is the shape of:

   A. social structure.
   B. instincts.
   C. individuals who create social structure.
   D. internal or external stimuli.

744

GO ON TO THE NEXT PAGE.

Passage VI (Questions 37–43)

The worker and the master. In virtue of this monstrous system, the son of the worker, on entering life, finds no field which he may till, no machine which he may tend, no mine which he may dig, without accepting to leave a great part of what he will produce to a master. He must sell his labor for a scant and uncertain wage. His father and his grandfather have toiled to drain this field, to build this mill, to perfect this machine. They gave to the work the full measure of their strength, and what more could they give? But their heir comes into the world poorer than the lowest savage. If he obtains leave to till the fields, it is on condition of surrendering a quarter of the produce to his master and another quarter to the government and the middlemen. And this tax, levied upon him by the State, the capitalist, the lord of the manor, and the middleman, is always increasing; it rarely leaves him the power to improve his system of culture. If he turns to industry, he is allowed to work, though not always even that, only on condition that he yield a half or two-thirds of the product to him whom the land recognizes as the owner of the machine.

We cry shame on the feudal baron who forbade the peasant to turn a clod of earth unless he surrendered to this lord a fourth of his crop. We called those the barbarous times. But if the forms have changed, the relations have remained the same, and the worker is forced, under the name of free contract, to accept feudal obligations. For, turn where he will, he can find no better conditions. Everything has become private property, and he must accept, or die of hunger.

The working people cannot purchase with their wages the wealth which they have produced, and industry seeks foreign markets among the monied classes of other nations. In the East, in Africa, everywhere, in Egypt, Tonkin or the Congo, the European is thus bound to promote the growth of serfdom. And so he does. But soon he finds that everywhere there are similar competitors. All the nations evolve on the same lines, and wars, perpetual wars, break out for the right of precedence in the market. Wars for the possession of the East, wars for the empire of the sea, wars to impose duties on imports and to dictate conditions to neighboring states; wars against those "blacks" revolt! The roar of the cannon never ceases in the world, whole races are massacred, the states of Europe spend a third of their budgets in armaments; and we know how heavily these taxes fall on the workers.

Individual appropriation is neither just nor serviceable. All belongs to all. All things are for all men, since all men have need of them, since all men have worked in the measure of their strength to produce them, and since it is not possible to evaluate everyone's part in the production of the world's wealth.

All is for all! If the man and the woman bear their fair share of work, they have a right to their fair share of all that is produced by all, and that share is enough to secure them well-being. No more of such vague formulas as "The right to work," or "To each the whole result of his labor." What we proclaim is the right to well-being: well-being for all!

There must be Expropriation. The well-being for all, the end; expropriation, the means. Expropriation, such then is the problem which history has put before the men of the 20th century; the return to Communism is all that ministers to the well-being of man. But this problem cannot be solved by means of legislation. No one imagines that.

37. Based on the passage, which of the following does the author offer as the ultimate enemy of "well-being for all"?

 A. A master
 B. "Iron slaves which we call machines"
 C. The free contract
 D. The feudal lord

38. According to the author, all of the following would qualify as a result of individual appropriation of the world's wealth EXCEPT:

 A. owning an immense stock of tools and implements.
 B. collectively managed farms.
 C. indentured servitude.
 D. wars.

39. Which of the following best expresses the main idea of the passage?

 A. All men are created equal.
 B. A redistribution of society's power and wealth is the key to well-being.
 C. A society of well-being depends on group ownership of the means of production.
 D. The so-called free contract of labor depends on a monstrous system of masters and slaves.

40. In the first half of the passage, which of the following does the author identify as a condition of private property?

 A. Worker lack of power to improve his "system of culture"
 B. War making
 C. A feudal model of social and economic obligation
 D. All of the above

41. With which of the following statements would the author most strongly agree?

    A. Agricultural land should be turned over to workers who farm it.

    B. The industrial age has modeled itself on a system of social and economic inequity based on feudal exploitation.

    C. Everyone has a right to work.

    D. Workers must seize control of machines.

42. Which paraphrase below most accurately explains and expands upon the author's notion of "all things are for all men"?

    A. Everyone has the right to have work, shelter, and private property.

    B. The experience of humanity is necessarily collective and cannot, should not, be reduced to individually controlled commodity and labor exchange.

    C. Everyone in society should have equal access to the means of production.

    D. From each according to his abilities, to each according to his needs.

43. If, as the author states, "no one imagines" that the problem can be solved by legislation, how might the author imagine it could be solved?

    A. Through the further technological development of a more humane capitalism

    B. By a return of feudalism

    C. Through a social and economic revolution

    D. Via trade union negotiation with management

Passage VII (Questions 44–50)

In the aftermath of the Gulf War, the development of advanced automotive technology joins the question of what the United States should do about its cars, which consume 40% of the nation's oil. Around the world, and in California, environmental regulations are pushing clean-air technologies, with lower consumption of oil a significant side effect. Already Italy has approximately 300,000 cars powered by natural gas. Brazil, the largest automotive market in Latin America, runs almost half of its vehicles on corn, and California, home to the methanol-powered cars and buses and natural gas and propane fleets, has almost convinced car manufacturers to produce an electric car for public consumption. And now the war in the Persian Gulf oil fields makes a frontal assault on cars' oil-guzzling ways imperative.

The most immediate solution to the gasoline woes is to develop alternative fuels which are similar to, but environmentally superior and cheaper than gas. Some of the more popular options include methanol, compressed natural gas, and ethanol. Methanol will cut pollution emissions in half and can be made from natural gas, coal, or decaying organic matter. A blend of 85% methanol and 15% gasoline already is sold through ordinary pumps at some service stations. A likely favorite, the auto industry is already gearing up to produce "flex-fuel" cars to handle either gasoline or methanol. Methanol is popular because it is easily distributed and requires few vehicular modifications. It is also about to be substituted for diesel fuel in California's trucks and buses. On the down side, methanol would threaten the oil industry's market share, would require tens of billions of dollars in new refineries, and would be produced most economically in the Middle East. Compressed natural gas is cleaner than methanol, and it has the existing production and pipeline infrastructure that methanol lacks. However, it requires awkward fuel tanks that make it impractical for most family car needs. Ethanol is an alcohol fuel like methanol and is already being produced and sold in the Midwest in ethanol-gasoline blends. It is made from corn, supported by controversial government subsidies. Currently, methanol is more expensive than gasoline and no one is sure exactly how much ethanol costs because of the subsidies—but the cost of each would change if supply and demand were to change.

Perhaps the best solution is the one being pursued by some research and development companies. They are working on combining all the possible fuel alternatives, each to be used for a different purpose. "Flex-fuel!" engines in cars would run on gasoline-methanol mixes or pure methanol, the engines in buses and trucks would run on methanol blends or natural gas, and so on. This way, America could not be caught relying too heavily on any one fuel source and so another "Gulf War" in some other part of the world at some other time should be avoidable.

44. A good title for this passage is:

    A. *The Gulf War and Fuel Alternatives.*
    B. *Fuel Alternatives for Controlling Emissions.*
    C. *Fuel Alternatives and the Solution to Gasoline Woes.*
    D. *Fuel Alternatives and "Flex-Fuel" Engines.*

45. Which of the following does the author believe would be the best to develop as a solution for reducing oil dependency?

    A. Use of ethanol
    B. Use of ethanol and methanol
    C. Use of ethanol, methanol, and compressed natural gas
    D. Use of ethanol, methanol, compressed natural gas, and gasoline mixes

46. If a huge new oil field was discovered in South Dakota and the price of gasoline plunged, the author would most likely advocate:

    A. following a policy of using all possible fuel alternatives.
    B. maintaining the status quo.
    C. ceasing to import oil from the Arab nations.
    D. increasing the tax on gasoline.

47. Which of the following fuels would NOT require modification of cars?

    A. Methanol
    B. Ethanol
    C. Compressed natural gas
    D. Alcohol-gasoline mixes

48. It can be inferred from the passage that Brazil powers its cars with:

    A. ethanol only.
    B. gasoline or ethanol.
    C. methanol or ethanol.
    D. compressed natural gas or ethanol.

49. From the passage, one can conclude that the author believes that the war in the Persian Gulf:

    A. could have been avoided had the United States not been so dependent on oil.
    B. was inevitable.
    C. was good because it sparked interest in alternative fuel sources.
    D. was not a cost efficient way to settle the oil problem.

50. Which of the fuels mentioned in the passage pollutes the least when burned?

    A. Methanol
    B. Compressed natural gas
    C. Ethanol
    D. One cannot tell from the passage

Passage VIII (Questions 51–57)

One of the interesting things about human beings is that they try to understand themselves and their own behavior. While this has been particularly true of Europeans in recent times, there is no group which has not developed a scheme or schemes to explain human actions. To the insistent human query "why?" the most exciting illumination anthropology has to offer is that of the concept of culture. Its explanatory importance is comparable to categories such as evolution in biology, gravity in physics, and disease in medicine.

By "culture" anthropology, one means the total way of life of a people, the social legacy individuals acquire from their group. Or, culture can be regarded as that part of the environment that is the creation of human beings. This technical term has a wider meaning than the "culture" of history and literature. A humble cooking pot is as much a cultural product as is a Beethoven sonata. In ordinary speech, "people of culture" are those who can speak languages other than their own, who are familiar with history, literature, philosophy, of the fine arts. To the anthropologist, however, to be human is to be cultured. There is culture in general, and then there are the specific cultures such as Russian, American, British, Hottentot, Inca. The general abstract notion serves to remind us that we cannot explain acts solely in terms of the biological properties of the people concerned, their individual past experience, and the immediate situation. The past experience of other people in the form of culture enters into almost every event. Each culture constitutes a kind of blue print of all life's activities.

A good deal of human behavior can be understood, and indeed predicted, if we know a peoples' design for living. Many acts are neither accidental nor due to personal peculiarities nor caused by supernatural forces nor simple mysteries. Even we Americans who pride ourselves on our individualism, follow most of the time, a pattern not of our own making. We brush our teeth on arising. We put on pants—not a loincloth or a grass skirt. We eat three meals a day—not four, five, or two. We sleep in a bed—not in a hammock or on a sheep pelt. I do not have to know individuals and their life histories to be able to predict these and countless other regularities, including many in the thinking process of all Americans who are not incarcerated in jails or hospitals for the insane.

To the American woman a system of plural wives seems "instinctively" abhorrent. She cannot understand how any woman can fail to be jealous and uncomfortable if she must share her husband with other women. She feels it "unnatural" to accept such a situation. On the other hand, a Koryak woman of Siberia, for example, would find it hard to understand how a woman could be so selfish and so undesirous of feminine companionship in the home as to wish to restrict her husband to one mate.

All this does not mean that there is no such thing as raw human nature. The members of all human groups have about the same biological equipment. All people undergo the same poignant life experiences, such as birth, helplessness, illness, old age, and death. The biological potentialities of the species are the blocks with which cultures are built. Some patterns of every culture crystallize around focuses provided by biology: the difference between the sexes, the presence of persons of different ages, the varying physical strength and skill of individuals. The facts of nature also limit culture forms. No culture provides patterns for jumping over trees or for eating iron ore. There is thus no "either-or" between nature and that special form of nurture called culture. The two factors are interdependent. Culture arises out of human nature, and its forms are restricted both by human biology and by natural laws.

51. The author of the passage would likely agree most readily with which one of the following statements?

   A. Some cultures are inferior to others.
   B. A person biologically Swedish, but raised from infancy in a Chinese family, would manifest a Swedish style of gait and arm and hand gestures.
   C. People everywhere are all the same.
   D. Much of what we consider laws of human nature are really culturally induced beliefs.

52. The sexual morality of the Koryaks of Siberia has most likely been influenced by:

   A. their contact with Christian missionaries.
   B. their chauvinistic nature.
   C. their "instinctive" feelings of what is natural.
   D. their viewing of modern media sources.

53. The wide variations in cultural norms throughout the world demonstrate that:

   A. nothing significantly limits the forms that cultures can take.
   B. the story of the Tower of Babel in the Bible is probably true.
   C. human beings can choose to solve the problems of their existence in various ways.
   D. efforts are needed to teach backward people how to live better lives.

748

GO ON TO THE NEXT PAGE.

54. It can be inferred from the passage that Americans brush their teeth in the morning primarily because:

A. they have a biological need to brush in the morning.

B. they are expected to brush in the morning.

C. they have been influenced by clever advertisements.

D. they have copied the behavior of other countries.

55. What a person considers fit to eat depends mostly on:

A. the society in which the person grew up.

B. the society in which the person is living.

C. the society's ability to produce food.

D. the society's level of cultural advancement.

56. The most appropriate title for this passage is:

A. *How Anthropology Explains Human Behavior.*

B. *People of Culture.*

C. *People are Different.*

D. *Human Behavior.*

57. Of the following influences, which would the author likely concede to be shapers of human behavior?

I. Climate

II. Disease

III. Fate

A. III only

B. I and III only

C. II only

D. I and II only

Passage IX (Questions 58–65)

In caves lining the sandstone escarpment called the Bandiagara, which winds across 120 miles of central Mali, lie thousands of skeletons, the remains of the Tellem, a people who first appeared in what was once called French West Africa some 900 years ago. But they were not the first people to inhabit these caves. The earliest known people were what modern archaeologists have named the Toloy, who date back at least until the third century B.C. They disappeared after a few hundred years, and then more than a thousand years later, the Tellem appeared, only to be supplanted by the Dogon people of today.

The Dogon live in several hundred villages, scattered across the 5,000 miles of the high plateaus, hidden valleys, and wild cliffs. Mainly farmers, they live largely untouched by twentieth century modernization. Soil is so rare that some build their homes on top of boulders to free a few more precious feet of land for planting. The family home, or *ginna,* resembles a human body. It has a circular enclave for a head, a central clearing as a trunk, and oblong side rooms for arms. At the center of every village is the *togu na,* the men's shelter. The coolest place in town, it is an open shelter with a roof made from dried leaves eight feet thick. The roof is supported by pillars carved with representations of the eight mythical Dogon ancestors. The only other house with carved columns is the home of the *hogon,* or spiritual leader.

Most Dogon have resisted the occasional Christian missionary and remain steadfast in their belief in a complicated system of animism. Foxes tell the future, and all sorts of spirits roam the earth after dark. Even the land has spiritual meaning—prominent rocks and baobab trees have personal names like High Bosom, the Ancestor, and Small Seeds. The most sacred place for the Dogon is their burial caves. When someone dies, the Dogon grieve through dancing elaborate, masked, ritual dances. At the end of the ceremony, the dead person is tied to a wooden bier and run head-high through the village, accompanied by wailing women. The corpse is then hauled up to a cave with rope made of baobab bark. Often the Dogon use empty caves, but sometimes they appropriate Tellem burial caves, which dot the cliffside above each village.

The Dogon have touched just about every part of their countryside. Hand-laid stones mark little-used paths, stairways are attached to steep cliffs hidden by thorny brush, and deep in natural crevices there are notched logs used as ladders, their steps worn shiny from centuries of use.

58. From the passage, it can be inferred that:

A. the Tellem conquered the Toloy.

B. the Dogon conquered the Tellem.

C. the Dogon conquered the Toloy.

D. no people of the Bandiagara were conquered.

59. A good title for this passage is:

   A.   *The Mysteries of the Bandiagara.*
   B.   *The Tellem and the Dogon.*
   C.   *The Dogon People.*
   D.   *Burial Caves in Mali and Their People.*

60. The author uses the world *animism* in the third paragraph to refer to:

   A.   any non-Christian belief system.
   B.   the belief that other animals have spirits, as well as humans.
   C.   the belief that everything has a spiritual life.
   D.   any complicated belief system.

61. Using the passage as evidence, which of the following would be reasonable to conclude?

   I.   Eight is an important number to the Dogon.
   II.   Men are more important than women to the Dogon.
   III. Carved columns mark places that are important to the Dogon.

   A.   I and II only
   B.   I and III only
   C.   II and III only
   D.   I, II, and III

62. If it was discovered that the baobab tree was going extinct, it would not be surprising to discover that:

   A.   the Dogon way of life was changing.
   B.   the Dogon were going extinct.
   C.   it had little effect on the Dogon way of life.
   D.   the Dogon were becoming civilized.

63. According to the passage, what do the *ginna,* the *togu na* and the *hogon's* house have in common?

   A.   They all are shaped like bodies.
   B.   They all are types of shelter.
   C.   They all have thatched roofs.
   D.   They all have pillars.

64. The Dogon use caves for burial because:

   A.   they want to protect the corpses from wild animals.
   B.   they believe that the caves are sacred.
   C.   they want to be with their ancestors, the Tellem.
   D.   It is not clear from the passage.

65. The final paragraph of this passage gives the reader the impression that:

   A.   the Dogon are everywhere on the Bandiagara.
   B.   the Dogon have lived the same way for a long period of time.
   C.   the Dogon preserve everything.
   D.   the Dogon are afraid of being captured.

STOP. IF YOU FINISH BEFORE TIME IS CALLED, CHECK YOUR WORK. YOU MAY GO BACK TO ANY QUESTION IN THIS TEST BOOKLET.

STOP.

Physical Sciences

Time: 100 Minutes
Questions 66–142

PHYSICAL SCIENCES

Directions: Most questions in the Physical Sciences test are organized into groups, each of which is preceded by a descriptive passage. After studying the passage, select the one best answer to each question. Some questions are not based on a descriptive passage and are also independent of each other. Select the one best answer to these independent questions. A periodic table is provided for your use. You may consult it whenever you wish.

PERIODIC TABLE OF THE ELEMENTS

IA																	VIIIA
1 H 1.0	IIA											IIIA	IVA	VA	VIA	VII A	2 He 4.0
3 Li 6.9	4 Be 9.0											5 B 10.8	6 C 12.0	7 N 14.0	8 O 16.0	9 F 19.0	10 Ne 20.2
11 Na 23.0	12 Mg 24.3											13 Al 27.0	14 Si 28.1	15 P 31.0	16 S 32.1	17 Cl 35.5	18 Ar 39.9
19 K 39.1	20 Ca 40.1	21 Sc 45.0	22 Ti 47.9	23 V 50.9	24 Cr 52.0	25 Mn 54.9	26 Fe 55.8	27 Co 58.9	28 Ni 58.7	29 Cu 63.5	30 Zn 65.4	31 Ga 69.7	32 Ge 72.6	33 As 74.9	34 Se 79.0	35 Br 79.9	36 Kr 83.8
37 Rb 85.5	38 Sr 87.6	39 Y 88.9	40 Zr 91.2	41 Nb 92.9	42 Mo 95.9	43 Tc 98.0	44 Ru 101	45 Rh 102	46 Pd 106	47 Ag 108	48 Cd 112	49 In 115	50 Sn 119	51 Sb 122	52 Te 128	53 I 127	54 Xe 131
55 Cs 133	56 Ba 137	57 La 139	72 Hf 179	73 Ta 181	74 W 184	75 Re 186	76 Os 190	77 Ir 192	78 Pt 195	79 Au 197	80 Hg 201	81 Tl 204	82 Pb 207	83 Bi 208	84 Po 209	85 At 210	86 Rn 222
87 Fr 223	88 Ra 226	89 Ac 227															

58 Ce 140	59 Pr 141	60 Nd 144	61 Pm 145	62 Sm 150	63 Eu 152	64 Gd 157	65 Tb 159	66 Dy 163	67 Ho 165	68 Er 167	69 Tm 169	70 Yb 173	71 Lu 175
90 Th 232	91 Pa 231	92 U 238	93 Np 237	94 Pu 244	95 Am 243	96 Cm 247	97 Bk 247	98 Cf 251	99 Es 252	100 Fm 257	101 Md 258	102 No 259	103 Lr 260

GO ON TO THE NEXT PAGE.

Passage I (Questions 66–71)

Resistors and capacitors are two of the elementary components of an electronic circuit. A circuit containing a "black box" element is shown in Figure 1 below. In a "black box" circuit, a variety of different connections can be made between two arbitrary points. In the diagrammed circuit, a battery, B, sets up a current, I. The black box contains two points, a and b, which are connected to either resistors or capacitors. This experimental setup, diagrammed below, was used to carry out two experiments.

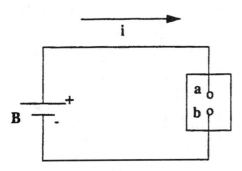

Figure 1.   A circuit containing a "black box" element.

Experiment I

Points a and b were attached to two resistors with resistances of R and $2R$, respectively.

Experiment II

Points a and b were attached to two capacitors with capacitances of C, and $2C$, respectively.

66.   In experiment I, the two resistors were connected in parallel. The current through the resistor with resistance $2R$ is what fraction of the current through the resistor with resistance R?

A.   ½
B.   1
C.   2
D.   4

67.   Based on experiment II, in which the two capacitors were connected in parallel, which one of the following statements is FALSE?

A.   The potential difference across each capacitor is the same.
B.   The magnitude of charge on each plate is the same.
C.   The effective capacitance of the two capacitors is proportional to the total charge on the combination of capacitors.
D.   The charge on each capacitor is proportional to the total voltage drop across a and b.

68.   Consider experiment II. A dielectric slab, with dielectric constant k, is placed between the plates of one of the capacitors in the circuit. In which capacitor must the dielectric slab be placed, and what must be its value so that the two capacitors have equal capacitance?

A.   C capacitor; k = ½
B.   C capacitor; k = 2
C.   2C capacitor; k = ½
D.   2C capacitor; k = 2

69.   The battery in experiment I is replaced by an alternating current source. The time dependence of the current source can be described by the following equation:

$$I = I_{max}\sin\omega t$$

In this equation, I is the instantaneous current at time t, I_{max} is the maximum current, and ω is the angular frequency of the oscillation. Which one of the following statements does NOT correctly describe the behavior of this circuit?

A.   The average power delivered over one cycle is 0.
B.   The root-mean-square (rms) current is equal to 0.707 times the maximum current.
C.   For the resistors of unit resistance and in a series configuration, the maximum current is equal to 0.707 times the rms voltage.
D.   The current averaged over one cycle is 0.

70. The resistor of resistance $2R$ in experiment I is replaced with a capacitor of capacitance C. These two elements are attached in series and allowed to reach equilibrium under the influence of the battery. After equilibrium has been reached, the battery is replaced by a resistance free wire. The resulting circuit is now referred to as an RC circuit. Which one of the following statements is NOT an accurate description of an RC circuit?

   A. The direction of current flow in the RC circuit is opposite to the current flow that occurs in the presence of the battery.

   B. The sum of the voltage drop across the resistor and capacitor is 0.

   C. At a time equal to RC after the battery has been removed, the capacitor charge is reduced to 1/e of its initial charge, where $e = 2.718$.

   D. The time required for the charge on the capacitor in an RC circuit to fall to a given fraction of its value depends on the value of the initial applied EMF.

71. Suppose that a single capacitor is present in a simple circuit. The plates of the capacitor are found to have a potential difference of 800 V. If the capacitance is found to be 1×10^{-11} farads, how much charge is stored on each plate?

   A. 8×10^{-9} C
   B. 1.25×10^{9} C
   C. 8×10^{8} C
   D. 1.25×10^{-8} C

Passage II (Questions 72–77)

The 1890s marked the beginning of the serious study of radioactivity. Radiation is the transmission of energy through space in the form of waves. Radioactive substances will spontaneously decay to emit radiation. This is not, however, the only way in which radiation can be produced. Radiation can also be produced when a cathode ray strikes various substances.

Radioactive substances can produce three different types of rays, which have been classified as alpha, beta, and gamma rays. Figure 1 demonstrates the different behavior of these types of rays when traveling in an electric field.

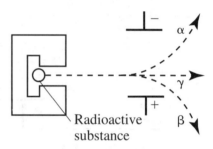

Figure 1

It is known now that an alpha ray is a helium ion (He^{2+}), and a beta ray is an electron. Elements that release alpha particles as they decay tend to change atomic number because they lose two protons as demonstrated by the following equation:

$$^{238}_{92}U \rightarrow\ ^{234}_{90}Th +\ ^{4}_{2}He$$

Elements that release beta particles also change atomic number because the source of the beta particle is the nucleus rather than an orbital. A beta particle is released when a neutron is converted to a proton. An example reaction follows:

$$^{14}_{6}C \rightarrow\ ^{14}_{7}N +\ ^{0}_{-1}\beta$$

These two types of radiation are observed for elements that vary from a stable ratio of neutrons to protons. Stable elements of low atomic mass tend to have an equal or nearly equal number of protons and neutrons. Stable elements of higher atomic mass (i.e., more than 24 protons) tend to have a greater number of neutrons than protons. The unstable elements tend to undergo radioactive decay to approach these stable ratios of neutrons to protons.

GO ON TO THE NEXT PAGE.

72. Which one of the following equations could represent the loss of a beta particle by zirconium-97?

    A. $_{97}^{40}\text{Zr} \rightarrow \ _{96}^{40}\text{Zr} + \ _{-1}^{0}\beta$

    B. $_{97}^{40}\text{Zr} \rightarrow \ _{98}^{40}\text{Zr} + \ _{-1}^{0}\beta$

    C. $_{40}^{97}\text{Zr} \rightarrow \ _{42}^{97}\text{Mo} + \ _{-1}^{0}\beta$

    D. $_{40}^{97}\text{Zr} \rightarrow \ _{41}^{97}\text{Nb} + \ _{-1}^{0}\beta$

73. What ratio of neutrons to protons should a stable isotope of gold have?

    A.   Greater than 1
    B.   Equal to 1
    C.   Less than 1
    D.   Equal to 0

74. Which of the following equations could represent the loss of an alpha particle by polonium-214?

    A. $_{84}^{214}\text{Po} \rightarrow \ _{82}^{210}\text{Pb} + \ _{2}^{4}\text{He}$

    B. $_{84}^{214}\text{Po} \rightarrow \ _{86}^{218}\text{Rn} + \ _{2}^{4}\text{He}$

    C. $_{84}^{214}\text{Po} \rightarrow \ _{86}^{210}\text{Rn} + \ _{2}^{4}\text{He}$

    D. $_{84}^{214}\text{Po} \rightarrow \ _{82}^{218}\text{Pb} + \ _{2}^{4}\text{He}$

75. What type of decay would potassium-40 be expected to undergo?

    A.   Alpha-particle emission to increase the neutron-to-proton ratio
    B.   Alpha-particle emission to decrease the neutron-to-proton ratio
    C.   Beta-particle emission to increase the neutron-to-proton ratio
    D.   Beta-particle emission to decrease the neutron-to-proton ratio

76. Which of the following is the most likely charge on a gamma ray particle?

    A. -1
    B. 0
    C. $+1$
    D. $+2$

77. Why do stable elements of high molecular weight have a greater number of neutrons than protons?

    A.   The neutrons help hold the nucleus together because of attractive forces.
    B.   The protons are attracted to the neutrons, which holds the nucleus together.
    C.   The neutrons help separate the protons, which helps decrease the amount of charge repulsion.
    D.   The extra neutrons help to hold the electrons closer to the nucleus.

Passage III (Questions 78–82)

A simple pendulum can be constructed using a small mass attached to one end of a string of negligible mass. The other end of the string is attached to a solid surface from which it can swing freely. The following experiment was performed to examine some properties of this system under collision and free fall.

Experiment

Two small spheres, A and B, of mass M and 4M, respectively, hang from the ceiling by strings of equal length, L (Figure 1). Sphere A is drawn aside so that it is raised to a height, h_o, as shown in the diagram below. After being drawn aside, sphere A is released and collides with sphere B. Once the spheres collide, they adhere to each other. This system can now be thought of as a simple pendulum system with total mass 5M. The 5M mass now travels to a maximum height, h, on the opposite side of the swing. Once it reaches maximum height, the 5M mass detaches from the string and falls to the floor under the force of gravity.

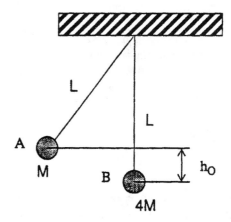

Figure 1.   The simple pendulum experiment.

78. Which of the following is the total energy of sphere A just before it is released?

    A. Mgh_o
    B. $(\frac{1}{2})Mgh_o$
    C. $4Mgh_o$
    D. $5Mgh_o$

79. As sphere A swings down towards sphere B, the potential energy of sphere A is converted into kinetic energy. If the mass of sphere A was doubled, how would the velocity of sphere A be affected just before it collides with sphere B?

    A.   It would not change.
    B.   It would double.
    C.   It would halve.
    D.   It would be four times as great.

80. The spheres stick together after the collision. What is the maximum height, h, that they can achieve?

    A. $1/2(h_o)$
    B. $1/4(h_o)$
    C. $1/5(h_o)$
    D. $1/25(h_o)$

81. Consider the path of the 5M mass described in the passage. Neglecting air resistance, which of the following statements is NOT a good representation of the ensuing trajectory as the 5M mass falls towards the ground?

    A.   The velocity along the horizontal direction is 0 throughout the trajectory.
    B.   The time it takes to fall to the ground is a function of the total height above the ground.
    C.   If the sphere has a mass of 10M instead of 5M, it would fall to the ground at the same rate.
    D.   None of the above, because statements A through C all are true.

82. Two important principles for analysis of collisions between idealized bodies are the conservation of energy and momentum. Considering these principles, all of the following statements are true EXCEPT:

    A.   conservation of energy holds whenever the work done by the nonconservative forces is 0.
    B.   when the resultant external force acting on a system is 0, the total vector momentum is conserved.
    C.   in a completely elastic collision, both the momentum and the kinetic energy are conserved.
    D.   in a completely elastic collision, the final velocities of the two colliding bodies are equal.

Passage IV (Questions 83–87)

The sulfur oxide compounds are important in both atmospheric science and industry. There are numerous sulfur oxide compounds and reactions to consider. Sulfur dioxide (SO_2) and sulfur trioxide (SO_3) react with water to give sulfurous acid (H_2SO_3) and sulfuric acid (H_2SO_4). When these compounds are present in the atmosphere, the pH of rainfall drops from approximately 5.5 to 4.0. Sulfur dioxide comes from several sources, both natural and synthetic. Natural SO_2 is emitted during volcanic eruptions. Synthetic SO_2 is given off during smelting and other industrial processes.

Smelting begins by heating metal sulfides in air as shown in reaction 1. Metal oxides are more easily reduced to the free metal.

Sulfur dioxide can be oxidized to sulfur trioxide by the path outlined in reaction 2, or by that outlined in reactions 3 through 5. Note that reactions 3 through 5 demonstrate the various steps of a mechanism. A third pathway requires dust or another solid particle to act as a catalyst for reaction 6.

Reaction 1

$$2\,ZnS(s) + 3\,O_2(g) \rightarrow 2\,ZnO(s) + 2\,SO_2(g)$$

Reaction 2

$$SO_2(g) + O_3(g) \rightarrow SO_3(g) + O_2(g)$$

Reaction 3

$$SO_2(g) + h\nu \rightarrow SO_2^+(g)$$

Reaction 4

$$SO_2^+(g) + O_2(g) \rightarrow SO_4(g)$$

Reaction 5

$$SO_4(g) + SO_2(g) \rightarrow 2\,SO_3(g)$$

Reaction 6

$$2\,SO_2(g) + O_2(g) \rightarrow 2\,SO_3(g)$$

83. Which of the following reactions has a negative entropy change?

    A.   Reaction 1
    B.   Reaction 2
    C.   Reaction 3
    D.   Reaction 5

GO ON TO THE NEXT PAGE.

84. Which of the following reactions is endothermic?

A. Reaction 2
B. Reaction 3
C. Reaction 4
D. Reaction 5

85. Which of the following species is a reactive intermediate?

A. SO_2^+
B. SO_3
C. SO_2
D. H_2SO_4

86. Why is reaction 1 an important step in the production of metals?

A. Metal sulfides are easier to reduce.
B. Metal sulfides are easier to oxidize.
C. Metal oxides are easier to reduce.
D. Metal oxides are easier to oxidize.

87. What is the difference in hydrogen ion concentration between normal rain and acid rain?

A. -9.7×10^{-5}
B. 9.7×10^{-5}
C. 1.5
D. -1.5

Questions 88 through 91 are **NOT** based on a descriptive passage.

88. An object initially at rest is dropped from a height, h. The ratio of its velocity after it has fallen half of the distance to the ground over the final velocity when it reaches the ground is:

A. 0.25
B. 0.50
C. 0.71
D. 0.87

89. A vessel is filled with a gaseous mixture of ammonia, hydrogen, and nitrogen at equilibrium. An analysis of the gases shows that $[NH_3] = 0.1M$, $[N_2] = 0.2M$, and $[H_2] = 0.3M$. The equilibrium constant for the decomposition of ammonia gas to nitrogen and hydrogen gas is best given by:

A. $(0.2)(0.3)^2/(0.1)$.
B. $(0.1)^2/(0.2)(0.3)^3$.
C. $(0.1)/(0.2)^2(0.3)^3$.
D. $(0.2)(0.3)^3/(0.1)^2$.

90. Two objects of identical mass and radius, a solid sphere and a hollow sphere, are released from rest at the top of an incline. At the base of the incline, which will have the larger linear velocity, and which will have the larger rotational kinetic energy, respectively?

A. Solid sphere, solid sphere
B. Solid sphere, hollow sphere
C. Hollow sphere, solid sphere
D. Hollow sphere, hollow sphere

91. Catalysts speed the rates of chemical reactions by lowering the activation energy associated with the reactions. Which of the following statements accurately describes an additional feature of catalysts?

A. They may alter equilibrium concentrations.
B. They favor the forward reaction.
C. The equilibrium is displaced to the more energetically favorable product.
D. The forward and backward reaction rates are accelerated equally.

Passage V (Questions 92–97)

Ammonia is a valuable raw material in the manufacturing of fertilizers and explosives. Ammonia consists of nitrogen and hydrogen atoms, and the synthesis from nitrogen and hydrogen gas is desirable and inexpensive. This synthesis was completed in 1905 by Fritz Haber and is known as the Haber process (Reaction 1).

Reaction 1

$$N_2(g) + 3 H_2(g) \rightarrow 2 NH_3(g)$$

Haber discovered the optimal temperature and pressure for the reaction. Table 1 summarizes some of the data he collected.

Table 1. Variation with temperature of the equilibrium constant for the synthesis of ammonia.

Temperature ($^\circ$C)	Equilibrium constant (K_c)
25	6.0×10^5
200	0.65
300	0.011
400	6.2×10^{-4}
500	7.4×10^{-5}

Figure 1 shows the yield of ammonia according to temperature. Figure 2 shows the mole percent of ammonia as a function of the total pressure of the system.

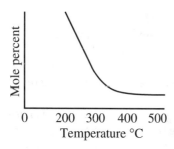

Figure 1. Mole percent of ammonia at equilibrium as a function of temperature.

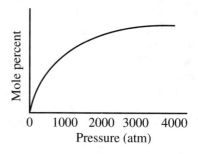

Figure 2. Mole percent of ammonia at equilibrium as a function of pressure.

Table 2 gives the boiling points for ammonia, nitrogen, and hydrogen.

Table 2. Physical properties for hydrogen, nitrogen, and ammonia.

Compound	Boiling point ($^\circ$C)
Hydrogen	−252.8
Nitrogen	−195.8
Ammonia	−33.5

92. Which of the following statements regarding the entropy of reaction 1 is true?

    A. The entropy of the reaction is positive.
    B. The entropy of the reaction is negative.
    C. The entropy of the reaction is 0.
    D. No conclusions about the entropy can be made.

93. Evaluation of the data in Figure 1 leads to the conclusion that:

    A. the yield increases with decreasing temperature because the reaction is endothermic.
    B. the yield increases with decreasing temperature because the reaction is exothermic.
    C. the yield increases with increasing temperature because the reaction is endothermic.
    D. the yield increases with increasing temperature because the reaction is exothermic.

94. Based on the data in Figure 2, what conclusion can be made?

    A. The yield increases with increasing pressure because of the favorable enthalpy change.

    B. The yield decreases with increasing pressure because of the unfavorable enthalpy change.

    C. The yield increases with increasing pressure because of the number of moles of gas produced.

    D. The yield decreases with increasing pressure because of the number of moles of gas produced.

95. If the reaction were run at $-50°C$, which of the following statements would be true?

    A. The ammonia would liquefy as it forms, pulling the equilibrium to the left.

    B. The ammonia would liquefy as it forms, pulling the equilibrium to the right.

    C. The gases would liquefy as it forms, stopping the reaction before reaching equilibrium.

    D. The ammonia would liquefy as it forms, having no effect on the equilibrium.

96. Why is the reaction run at $500°C$, rather than $25°C$, in the industrial process?

    A. A higher yield results.

    B. A faster reaction occurs.

    C. A higher yield results, and the reaction occurs faster.

    D. A slower, more controllable reaction occurs.

97. If a mixture of 1 mole H_2, 2 moles N_2, and 3 moles NH_3 were placed in an airtight container at $25°C$, what changes would occur as the system reaches equilibrium?

    A. The concentration of ammonia would increase, and the concentrations of hydrogen and nitrogen would remain the same.

    B. The concentrations of hydrogen and nitrogen would increase, and the concentration of ammonia would remain the same.

    C. The concentration of ammonia would increase, and the concentrations of hydrogen and nitrogen would decrease.

    D. The concentrations of nitrogen and hydrogen would increase, and the concentration of ammonia would decrease.

Passage VI (Questions 98–102)

Light can be defined as that part of the electromagnetic spectrum that can stimulate photoreceptors in the eye. The typical range of the normal human vision corresponds to electromagnetic radiation ranging from 400 nm (violet) to 700 nm (red). This constitutes the visible part of the electromagnetic spectrum.

There are several features of the electromagnetic spectrum that are important in understanding the properties of light. Electromagnetic radiation can be propagated through a vacuum in the form of electromagnetic waves. The energy of an electromagnetic wave is equally divided between an electric field and a mutually perpendicular magnetic field. Both of these fields are perpendicular to the direction of propagation.

All electromagnetic waves travel through a vacuum with the same speed, $c = 3.0 \times 10^8$ m/s, called the speed of light. When electromagnetic radiation travels through a transparent physical medium, it no longer travels at the speed of light. It obeys the dispersion relation, $\lambda f = v$, where λ is the wavelength, f is the frequency, and v is the speed of light. Differences in the optical density of various physical materials give rise to a value known as the index of refraction. By definition, the index of refraction, n, is the speed of light, c, through a vacuum divided by the speed of light, v, in a transparent substance.

The difference in the speed of light in different media gives rise to a phenomenon known as refraction. In refraction, bending of light occurs as it crosses obliquely from one medium to another.

98. A plane-polarized electromagnetic wave propagates in free space. This is an example of what type of wave?

    A. Standing wave

    B. Longitudinal wave

    C. Transverse wave

    D. Mechanical wave

99. Light can be piped from one point to another with little loss by allowing it to enter one end of a transparent fiber. The light undergoes total internal reflection at the boundary of the fiber and will follow its contour, emerging at its far end. Bundles of such fibers form the basis of fiber optics techniques. If one fiber with refractive index n is operated in air, what relation must the incident angle of the transported light, θ_i, satisfy in order to achieve transmission of the light along the optical fiber?

    A. $\sin\theta_i \geq 1/n$

    B. $\sin\theta_i \geq n$

    C. $\sin\theta_i \leq 1/n$

    D. $\sin\theta_i = 1/n$

100. An observer is able to measure the wavelength of a light ray as it goes from air into a medium of unknown index of refraction. The incident light ray is red, whereas the wavelength of the light in the medium is consistent with violet light. What must be the value of n?

    A.   4/7
    B.   7/4
    C.   4
    D.   7

101. In addition to waves, electromagnetic radiation can be described in terms of massless particles called photons. For an electromagnetic wave whose electric and magnetic fields oscillate at frequency, f_w, how will the frequency of its constituent photons, f_p, vary if f_w is increased?

    A.   It would increase.
    B.   It would decrease.
    C.   It would stay the same.
    D.   It is not possible to determine, because f_w and f_p are not related.

102. White light strikes a glass prism. On exiting the prism, the light beam is dispersed into a typical rainbow spectrum. The spectrum of light is then projected onto a viewing screen, such that the most refracted component of the white light is at the top of the screen. Which of the following *incorrectly* describes the behavior of the exiting and entering light rays as they related to the viewing screen?

    A.   Highest wavelength light at bottom; lowest wavelength light at top
    B.   Lowest energy light at bottom; highest energy light at top
    C.   Light waves bent away from the normal on entering the prism; light waves bent toward the normal on exiting the prism
    D.   None of the above

Passage VII (Questions 103–109)

The efficient use of solar energy relies upon efficient conversion of light energy into heat energy. One method for performing this conversion involves two types of energy exchange. First, the light energy is used to drive an endothermic reaction. This converts the light energy to chemical energy. The reverse of the endothermic reaction then occurs, releasing heat.

One such chemical system that can be used for this type of energy conversion sequence is the decomposition of sulfur trioxide. The reactions involved are shown in reactions 1 and 2.

Reaction 1

$$2\ SO_3(g) \rightarrow 2\ SO_2(g)\ +\ O_2(g)$$
$$\Delta H = 198\ kJ$$

Reaction 2

$$2\ SO_2(g)\ +\ O_2(g) \rightarrow 2\ SO_3(g)$$

One key feature for this type of solar energy conversion is that it can be a closed system. No reagents need to be added or removed. A second benefit is that reaction 2 requires the presence of a platinum catalyst. This allows the system to be used to store light energy until it is needed. Figure 1 shows how this system might be implemented.

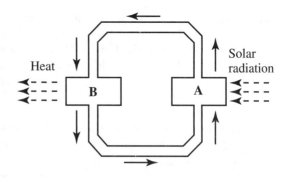

Figure 1.   Closed system for energy conversion.

103. Which of the following reactions would occur in Figure 1 at region A?

    A.   Reaction 1 only
    B.   Reaction 2 only
    C.   Reactions 1 and 2
    D.   Neither reaction 1 nor reaction 2

104. Which of the following reactions would occur in Figure 1 at region B?

   A. Reaction 1 only
   B. Reaction 2 only
   C. Reactions 1 and 2
   D. Neither reaction 1 nor reaction 2

105. The change in enthalpy, ΔH, for reaction 2 is closest to:

   A. 198 kJ.
   B. 396 kJ.
   C. −198 kJ.
   D. −396 kJ.

106. Which of the following diagrams is most likely to represent the energy of reaction 1 as the reaction proceeds?

A. 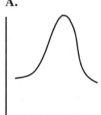 **B.**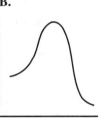

C. 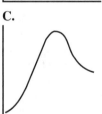 **D.**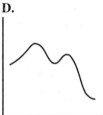

107. Which of the following diagrams is most likely to represent the energy of reaction 2 without the presence of platinum?

A. 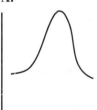 **B.**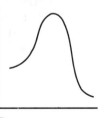

C. 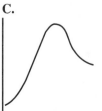 **D.**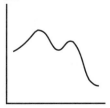

108. Which of the following diagrams is most likely to represent the energy of reaction 2 with platinum present?

A. 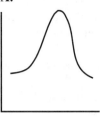 **B.**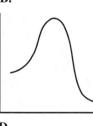

C. 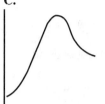 **D.**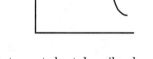

109. Which of the following statements best describes how light can drive a reaction?

   A. Light is actually used to heat up the reaction chamber, which allows the reaction to proceed.
   B. Light bounces off the molecules, pushing them together more energetically.
   C. Some molecules absorb light of certain wavelengths, becoming more energetic.
   D. Molecules all absorb light, becoming more energetic.

761

GO ON TO THE NEXT PAGE.

Passage VIII (Questions 110–114)

In 1921, Albert Einstein received the Nobel Prize for his contributions to theoretical physics, and especially for his discovery of the law of the photoelectric effect. This phenomenon, first discovered by Heinrich Hertz in 1887 and later painstakingly investigated experimentally by R. A. Millikan, refers to the observation that when light of sufficiently high energy is incident on a metal in a vacuum, the metal emits electrons.

Figure 1 depicts the apparatus used to study the photoelectric effect.

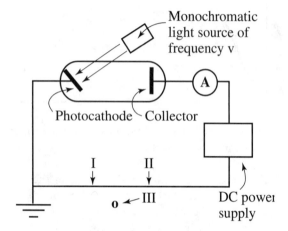

Figure 1. Apparatus used to study the photoelectric effect.

In this apparatus, the photocathode is induced to release electrons by the application of photons of frequency, v. The potential of the collector, V, measured relative to ground, can be varied continuously. The effect is described by Einstein's photoelectric equation:

$$eV = hv - W,$$

where W is the work function of the metal, and e is the charge of an electron. The work function equals the minimum energy required to eject an electron, and e has a value of 1.6×10^{-19} Coulombs. Other constants of importance are h and c: $h = 4.14 \times 10^{-15}$ eVsec, and $c = 3.00 \times 10^8$ m/s.

110. The photoelectric effect is derived under the assumption that:

A. electrons are restricted to orbits of angular momentum $nh/2\pi$ where n is an integer and h is Planck's constant.

B. electrons are associated with waves of wavelength $\lambda = h/p$, where p is the momentum.

C. light behaves like a wave.

D. light is absorbed in quanta of energy, where $E = hv$.

111. The quantity, W, in the photoelectric equation is the:

A. energy difference between the two lowest electron orbits in the atoms of the photocathode.

B. total light energy absorbed by the photocathode during the measurement.

C. minimum energy a photon must have to be absorbed by the photocathode.

D. minimum energy required to free an electron from its binding to the cathode material.

112. A metal with the work function of 3.00 eV, is used for the construction of the photocathode and collector. If violet light of wavelength 400 nm is used, will there be photoejection of electrons? [Assume 1 eV = 1.6×10^{-19} joules.]

A. Yes, because the energy of the incident photons is higher than the work function.

B. Yes, because the energy of the incident photons equals the work function.

C. No, because the energy of the incident photons is lower than the work function.

D. There is not enough information to determine an answer.

113. Electrons liberated from the metal by the photoelectric effect produce a net charge flow per unit time, or a current. Consider Figure 1 shown in the passage. Assume that the portion of the diagram lying between points I and II can be treated as an isolated wire carrying current. Which of the following statements best describes the direction of the current and the induced magnetic field at point III?

A. Current flows from point I to point II, whereas the magnetic field is directed out of the page at point III.

B. Current flows from point I to point II, whereas the magnetic field is directed into the page at point III.

C. Current flows from point II to point I, whereas the magnetic field is directed into the page at point III.

D. Current flows from point II to point I, whereas the magnetic field is directed out of the page at point III.

762

GO ON TO THE NEXT PAGE.

114. Assume that the work function of the metal and the incident frequency are matched such that there is a steady current caused by the flow of the ejected electrons. How will the intensity of the incident light beam (i.e., the number of photons per unit time that fall on the cathode) relate to the system?

A. The induced current will be proportional to the intensity of the incident light beam.

B. The induced current will be inversely proportional to the intensity of the incident light beam.

C. The kinetic energy of the photoejected electrons will be higher if the intensity of the incident light beam is increased.

D. An increase in the intensity of the incident light will decrease the work function of the metal.

Questions 115 through 118 are **NOT** based on a descriptive passage.

115. A ray of light travels from medium A into medium B. Medium B has a higher refractive index than A. Which one of the following best describes the refracted ray?

A. The ray will bend away from the normal.

B. The ray will continue along the same path as in medium A.

C. The ray will bend towards the normal.

D. The ray will not exist if the angle of incidence is greater than the critical angle.

116. A negative test charge is to be sent, moving in the vicinity of a current carrying wire. For the charge to experience a force in the same direction as the current, the motion of the charge must be directed:

A. toward the wire.

B. away from the wire.

C. opposite the current.

D. with the current.

117. Two unknown salt compounds, XY_2 and WY_2, are studied in a chemistry laboratory. Both compounds are found to have the same solubility product (K_{sp}), and both are found to dissociate completely into their respective ions when dissolved in water. Element X has a higher atomic weight than element W. Which one of the following is the best statement regarding the solubilities of these compounds?

A. More grams of XY_2 than WY_2 would dissolve at K_{sp}.

B. More grams of WY_2 than XY_2 would dissolve at K_{sp}.

C. Equal gram quantities of XY_2 and WY_2 would dissolve at K_{sp}.

D. There is not enough data to compare these two compounds.

118. Two spheres of putty, A and B, have masses M and 2M, respectively. They are hung from equal lengths of string. Sphere A is then drawn aside and raised to a height, h. It is then released and swings down, undergoing a completely inelastic collision with sphere B. The two spheres will rise to a maximum height of:

   A.   (1/9)h
   B.   (1/3)h
   C.   (1/2)h
   D.   (2/3)h

Passage IX (Questions 119–123)

Aluminum cans are the source of as much as 3 billion pounds of aluminum discarded annually. The loss of aluminum as a result of the one-time use of aluminum cans is considered by many as a waste of both precious natural resources and energy.

Aluminum is ideal for use by the beverage industry because it is nontoxic, odorless, tasteless, thermally conducting, and lightweight. Aluminum does react with strong acids and bases, which could otherwise be a problem when storing strongly acidic beverages such as carbonated sodas. However, aluminum is easily oxidized in air to Al_2O_3. A thin layer of this oxide protects the aluminum from the contents of the can.

Aluminum can be produced from bauxite by the Hall process, which is shown in Reaction 1. The ΔH for the Hall process is 1340 kJ and the ΔS is 586 J/K.

Reaction 1

$$Al_2O_3 + 3\ C(s) \rightarrow 2\ Al(l) + 3\ CO(g)$$

Figure 1 shows the type of reactor used in the Hall process.

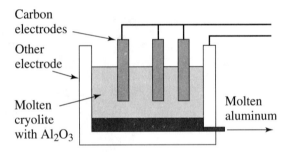

Figure 1

The recycling of aluminum requires only that the metal be heated to its melting point (660°C) with enough additional heat to melt the metal. The heat of fusion for aluminum is 10.7 kJ/mol, and the specific heat of aluminum is 0.900 J/(g°C).

119. What is the ΔG for the Hall process run at 1000°C?

   A.   1340 − (1000)(586)
   B.   1340 − (1000)(586)(1/1000)
   C.   1340 − (1273)(586)
   D.   1340 − (1273)(586)(1/1000)

GO ON TO THE NEXT PAGE.

120. What is the total energy required to recycle 1 mole of aluminum?

    A. $(27)(0.900)(600) + 10.7$
    B. $(27)(660)/(0.900) + 10.7$
    C. $(27)(0.900)(660 - 25)(1/1000) + 10.7$
    D. $(0.900)(660 - 25)$

121. Which of the following would result in the most favorable ΔG for the Hall process?

    A. Running the reaction below 0°C
    B. Running the reaction at room temperature
    C. Running the reaction at 1000°C
    D. Running the reaction at 1000°F

122. What function does carbon serve in the Hall process reactor?

    A. The carbon is the anode.
    B. The carbon is the cathode.
    C. The carbon is only a reactant.
    D. The carbon is the solvent.

123. How does the density of liquid aluminum compare with that of molten cryolite?

    A. The densities are equal.
    B. The density of aluminum is lower.
    C. The density of aluminum is higher.
    D. There is no basis to compare the densities of liquid aluminum and molten cryolite.

Passage X (Questions 124–129)

Consider a compound slab consisting of two materials having thickness W_1 and W_2, lengths L_1 and L_2, masses m_1 and m_2, cross-sectional areas A_1 and A_2, thermal conductivity k_1 and k_2, specific heats C_{p1} and C_{p2}, and coefficients of linear expansion α_1 and α_2. A compound slab is shown in Figure 1.

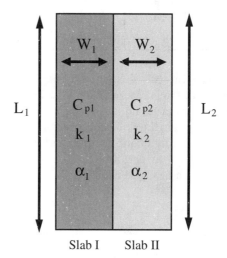

Figure 1.   Compound slab of two materials.

The quantities C_p, k, and α are important in characterizing several key thermal features of this system.

The heat capacity per unit mass of a body, called specific heat, or C_p, is the energy that must be added as heat to raise the temperature of an object one degree centigrade. The heat, Q, gained or lost by an object and the change in temperature of that object, ΔT, are related by the equation $Q = mC_p\Delta T$, where m is the mass of the object.

The transfer of energy arising from temperature differences between two adjacent objects is called heat conduction and is characterized by the constant, k. This constant is the proportionality constant in the following equation:

$$\Delta Q/\Delta t \approx (A)(\Delta T/\Delta x),$$

where ΔQ is the heat that flows per unit time Δt across a body that has a cross-sectional area A, width Δx, and a temperature difference of ΔT across its width.

Another common feature of the thermal behavior of materials is the change in size of the materials after a temperature change. In most solids, an increase in temperature is accompanied by an increase in length. This thermal expansion, ΔL, is described by the equation $\Delta L = \alpha L\Delta T$, where α is the coefficient of linear expansion, L is the original length, and ΔT is the change in the temperature.

A series of experiments were conducted. A selected set of experimentally determined values of these three constants were found and are given in Table 1:

Table 1. Experimentally determined values of α, C_p, and k.

Substance	$\alpha(°C^{-+})$	$C_p(cal/g°C)$	$k(kcal/sm°C)$
Aluminum	23×10^{-6}	0.215	4.9×10^{-2}
Copper	17×10^{-6}	0.0923	9.2×10^{-2}
Lead	29×10^{-6}	0.0305	8.3×10^{-3}
Water	51×10^{-6}	1.00(l)	4.0×10^{-4}

124. Consider the two slabs initially at thermal equilibrium with temperatures T_1 and T_2. The slabs are allowed to contact, and they reach a new thermal equilibrium. Using the slab parameters in Figure 1, which of the following quantities is important in determining the final temperature of the slabs after thermal equilibrium has been reached?

   A. k_1 and k_2
   B. α_1 and α_2
   C. W_1 and W_2
   D. m_1 and m_2

125. Consider the slabs to be long compared with their width (i.e., L >> W) and to be under a thermal gradient such that the outer surfaces of slab 1 and slab 2 are at temperatures T_1 and T_2, respectively. Which of the following describes the temperature at the interface between the two materials, T_i?

   A.   Under steady state conditions, the time rate of transfer of heat energy must be equal at the interface.
   B.   The net heat flow across the boundary must be 0.
   C.   Under steady state conditions, the net heat flow at the outer surface of slab 1 must be equal to the net heat flow at the boundary.
   D.   Under steady state conditions, the net heat flow at the outer surface of slab 2 must be equal to the net heat flow at the boundary.

126. Consider a single slab of length L at a specific temperature. Assuming no phase changes occur, which of the following compounds would show the most increase in length upon an equivalent increase in temperature?

   A.   Aluminum
   B.   Copper
   C.   Lead
   D.   Ice (water)

127. Assuming no phase changes occur, a slab made from which of the following compounds makes the best thermal insulator?

   A.   Aluminum
   B.   Copper
   C.   Lead
   D.   Ice (water)

128. A slab with a given mass undergoes a temperature increase when a given amount of heat is added. Assuming no phase changes occur, for which of the following compounds is the increase in temperature the greatest?

   A.   Aluminum
   B.   Copper
   C.   Lead
   D.   Water

129. In isotropic solids, the percent change in length for a given temperature change is the same for all lines within the solid. Every line, whether straight or curved, lengthens in the ratio α per degree temperature rise. Based on this information and the data given in the passage, what is the fractional change in volume of a sphere per degree temperature change for an isotropic solid?

   A. 2α
   B. 3α
   C. $2\pi\alpha$
   D. α

Passage XI (Questions 130–136)

The separation of isotopes of the same element is made difficult by the fact that different isotopes have the same chemical properties. A method that can be used to separate isotopes is effusion. Graham's law of effusion demonstrates the rate of effusion of a gas is inversely proportional to the square root of its molecular weight. Graham's law is shown in the following equation:

$$\frac{r_1}{r_2} = \frac{\sqrt{MW_2}}{\sqrt{MW_1}}$$

Based on this equation, a separation factor can be defined as the ratio of the square roots of the molecular weights of the compounds being studied. In addition, the larger molecular weight of the two compounds being considered is always placed in the numerator. This gives a minimum ratio value of 1. A separation factor of 1 indicates that the gases cannot be separated by effusion.

The difference in effusion of compounds with differing molecular weights allows the use of membranes to separate different isotopes. A mixture of isotopes is placed on one side of a membrane, and one of the isotopes will effuse to the other side faster than the other isotope(s). Better separation of the isotopes can be achieved by performing a multistage effusion. In fact, the separation of ^{235}U and ^{238}U to generate fuel for nuclear reactors involves a 2000-stage effusion separation.

130. Which of the following pairs of isotopes would be separated most completely by a single-stage effusion experiment?

- **A.** ^1H and ^2H
- **B.** ^1H and ^3H
- **C.** ^{16}O and ^{18}O
- **D.** ^{12}C and ^{13}C

131. Which of the following descriptions explains how the separation is achieved in the purification of uranium isotopes?

- **A.** ^{235}U effuses more slowly than ^{238}U, so ^{238}U collects on the receiving end of the apparatus, and ^{235}U remains at the starting end.
- **B.** ^{235}U effuses more quickly than ^{238}U, so ^{238}U collects on the receiving end of the apparatus, and ^{235}U remains at the starting end.
- **C.** ^{235}U effuses more quickly than ^{238}U, so ^{235}U collects on the receiving end of the apparatus, and ^{238}U remains at the starting end.
- **D.** ^{235}U effuses more slowly than ^{238}U, so ^{235}U collects on the receiving end of the apparatus, and ^{238}U remains at the starting end.

132. What effect would increasing the temperature have on the efficiency of the separation?

- **A.** There would be no effect.
- **B.** It would increase the efficiency of the separation by further slowing the effusion of the slower isotope.
- **C.** It would decrease the efficiency of the separation by slowing both isotopes.
- **D.** It would increase the efficiency of the separation by increasing the speed at which both isotopes effuse.

133. What effect would increasing the pressure on the gas mixture have on the efficiency of the separation?

- **A.** There would be no effect.
- **B.** It would increase the efficiency of the separation by further slowing the effusion of the slower isotope.
- **C.** It would decrease the efficiency of the separation by further slowing both isotopes.
- **D.** It would increase the efficiency of the separation by increasing the speed at which both isotopes effuse.

134. Which of the following statements gives the most reasonable effect on the efficiency of the separation of increasing the pressure on the empty side of the membrane?

- **A.** There would be no effect.
- **B.** It would increase the efficiency of the separation by further slowing the effusion of the slower isotope.
- **C.** It would decrease the efficiency of the separation by slowing both isotopes.
- **D.** It would increase the efficiency of the separation by increasing the speed at which both isotopes effuse.

135. What effect would increasing the temperature have on the speed of the separation?

- **A.** There would be no effect.
- **B.** It would increase the speed of the separation by further slowing the slower isotope.
- **C.** It would decrease the speed of the separation by slowing both isotopes.
- **D.** It would increase the speed of the separation by increasing the speed at which both isotopes effuse.

136. What effect would increasing the pressure on the gas mixture have on the speed of the separation?

A. There would be no effect.
B. It would increase the speed of the separation by further slowing the slower isotope.
C. It would decrease the speed of the separation by slowing both isotopes.
D. It would increase the speed of the separation by increasing the speed at which both isotopes effuse.

Questions 137 through 142 are **NOT** based on a descriptive passage.

137. Which of the following values is the current flowing through the 3-ohm resistor for the circuit shown below.

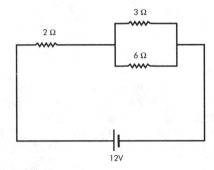

A. 2 amps
B. 3 amps
C. 4 amps
D. 6 amps

138. Which of the following groups of information must be known to determine the power output of a machine?

A. The mass and amount of work performed
B. The time required to perform work and the amount of work performed
C. The force, mass, and time required to apply force
D. The force applied and the distance over which it is applied

139. Buffer solutions are important in both inorganic and organic chemical systems. Buffer solutions resist changes in pH. Which of the following statements most accurately describes an effective buffer solution?

A. Weak acids or bases and their salts
B. Strong acids or bases
C. Strong acids or bases and their salts
D. Weak acids or bases

GO ON TO THE NEXT PAGE.

140. The simple microscope represents a special case of image formation. In the microscope, a converging lens system is used, and the object to be viewed is placed between the lens and the focal point of the lens. The image expected in this system is:

A. real, and on the same side of the lens as the object.

B. real, and on the opposite side of the lens as the object.

C. virtual, and on the same side of the lens as the object.

D. virtual, and on the opposite side of the lens as the object.

141. The process of converting $H_2O(g)$ to $H_2O(l)$ is a nonspontaneous process at a pressure of 1 atm and 373 K. Which of the following best describes why the process is nonspontaneous?

A. ΔH is greater than $T\Delta S$.

B. ΔH is positive.

C. ΔG is negative.

D. ΔH and ΔS are negative.

142. A boat travels on a lake towards the bank of the lake. Above the bank of the lake is a steep cliff. On the cliff stands an observer. As the boat approaches the cliff, it sounds its horn. Who would hear the highest perceived frequency?

A. A person standing on the boat who heard the horn.

B. The observer on the cliff who heard the horn.

C. A person standing on the boat who heard the echo of the horn.

D. All of the perceived frequencies would be the same.

STOP IF YOU FINISH BEFORE TIME IS CALLED, CHECK YOUR WORK. YOU MAY GO BACK TO ANY QUESTION IN THIS TEST BOOKLET.

Writing Sample

Time: 60 Minutes
(2 essays, separately timed, 30 minutes each)

WRITING SAMPLE

Directions: You have 30 minutes to complete Essay Topic 1. When time is called, you must stop working on this essay. Draw a line below the last sentence in Essay 1 to mark your stopping point. You then have 30 minutes to complete Essay Topic 2. You may not work on Essay Topic 1 during the second 30-minute period allotted for Essay Topic 2. Use black ink and **do not skip lines between sentences.** Illegible essays will not be scored.

ESSAY TOPIC 1

Consider this statement:

Individuals have a right to express themselves in any way they wish.
Write a unified essay in which you perform the following tasks: Explain what you think the above statement means. Describe a specific situation in which it would be appropriate for a group to stifle or restrict an individual's expression. Discuss what you think determines how much latitude an individual may have in communicating thoughts, feelings, or actions in society.

ESSAY TOPIC 2

Consider this statement:

New ideas and ways of doing things are better than the old thinking and doing.

Write a unified essay in which you perform the following tasks: Explain what you think the above statement means. Describe a specific situation in which a more traditional approach has proved superior. Discuss what you think determines whether the new or old thinking and doing should prevail.

STOP IF YOU FINISH BEFORE TIME IS CALLED, CHECK YOUR WORK. YOU MAY GO BACK TO ANY QUESTION IN THIS TEST BOOKLET.

Biological Sciences

Time: 100 Minutes
Questions 143–219

BIOLOGICAL SCIENCES

Directions: Most questions in the Biological Sciences test are organized into groups, each of which is preceded by a descriptive passage. After studying the passage, select the one best answer to each question. Some questions are not based on a descriptive passage and are also independent of each other. Select the ONE best answer to these independent questions. A periodic table is provided for your use. You may consult it whenever you wish.

PERIODIC TABLE OF THE ELEMENTS

IA																	VIIIA
1 **H** 1.0	IIA											IIIA	IVA	VA	VIA	VII A	2 **He** 4.0
3 **Li** 6.9	4 **Be** 9.0											5 **B** 10.8	6 **C** 12.0	7 **N** 14.0	8 **O** 16.0	9 **F** 19.0	10 **Ne** 20.2
11 **Na** 23.0	12 **Mg** 24.3											13 **Al** 27.0	14 **Si** 28.1	15 **P** 31.0	16 **S** 32.1	17 **Cl** 35.5	18 **Ar** 39.9
19 **K** 39.1	20 **Ca** 40.1	21 **Sc** 45.0	22 **Ti** 47.9	23 **V** 50.9	24 **Cr** 52.0	25 **Mn** 54.9	26 **Fe** 55.8	27 **Co** 58.9	28 **Ni** 58.7	29 **Cu** 63.5	30 **Zn** 65.4	31 **Ga** 69.7	32 **Ge** 72.6	33 **As** 74.9	34 **Se** 79.0	35 **Br** 79.9	36 **Kr** 83.8
37 **Rb** 85.5	38 **Sr** 87.6	39 **Y** 88.9	40 **Zr** 91.2	41 **Nb** 92.9	42 **Mo** 95.9	43 **Tc** 98.0	44 **Ru** 101	45 **Rh** 102	46 **Pd** 106	47 **Ag** 108	48 **Cd** 112	49 **In** 115	50 **Sn** 119	51 **Sb** 122	52 **Te** 128	53 **I** 127	54 **Xe** 131
55 **Cs** 133	56 **Ba** 137	57 **La** 139	72 **Hf** 179	73 **Ta** 181	74 **W** 184	75 **Re** 186	76 **Os** 190	77 **Ir** 192	78 **Pt** 195	79 **Au** 197	80 **Hg** 201	81 **Tl** 204	82 **Pb** 207	83 **Bi** 208	84 **Po** 209	85 **At** 210	86 **Rn** 222
87 **Fr** 223	88 **Ra** 226	89 **Ac** 227															

58 **Ce** 140	59 **Pr** 141	60 **Nd** 144	61 **Pm** 145	62 **Sm** 150	63 **Eu** 152	64 **Gd** 157	65 **Tb** 159	66 **Dy** 163	67 **Ho** 165	68 **Er** 167	69 **Tm** 169	70 **Yb** 173	71 **Lu** 175
90 **Th** 232	91 **Pa** 231	92 **U** 238	93 **Np** 237	94 **Pu** 244	95 **Am** 243	96 **Cm** 247	97 **Bk** 247	98 **Cf** 251	99 **Es** 252	100 **Fm** 257	101 **Md** 258	102 **No** 259	103 **Lr** 260

GO ON TO THE NEXT PAGE.

Passage I (Questions 143–149)

The female menstrual cycle is controlled by a complex series of hormones. Follicle-stimulating hormone (FSH) is known to cause growth of oocytes in the ovary and is associated with the production of estrogen. FSH is nonfunctional in the presence of peptidase. Estrogen acts to stimulate the early formation of an endometrial lining of the uterus and is functional in the presence of both peptidase and lipase. Luteinizing hormone (LH) is known to cause ovulation, which is the release of the ovum from the graafian follicle. LH is nonfunctional in the presence of peptidase but is functional in the presence of lipase. Finally, progesterone, which is produced by the corpus luteum in the ovary, stimulates the endometrium to mature and develop glandular structures. Progesterone is functional in the presence of both peptidase and lipase.

The level of the hormones associated with the functional female reproductive system in humans was studied by researchers. One hundred women who demonstrated a monthly menstrual cycle were entered into a study. Blood samples were drawn from each woman on a daily basis, and relative hormone levels were plotted on Figure 1. FSH, LH, estrogen, and progesterone levels are shown as they correlate to the day of the menstrual cycle. Day 1 is defined as the first day of menstruation. Day 28 is defined as the last day of the cycle, which is the day prior to the onset of menses.

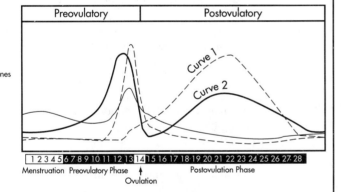

Figure 1

Fifty of the women participating in the study were given experimental drug X, and the other 50 women were given a placebo drug. Drug X was found to block the peak of LH release and had little effect on FSH levels. In addition, women who took drug X did not menstruate.

143. Based on information given in the passage, one would expect which of the following hormones to be peptide derivatives?

   A. Anterior pituitary hormones
   B. Ovarian hormones
   C. Corpus luteal hormones
   D. Thyroid hormone

144. The mechanism by which hormones produced by the corpus luteum affect levels of pituitary-produced hormones is best known as:

   A. allosteric modification.
   B. positive control.
   C. negative feedback.
   D. competitive inhibition.

145. When pregnancy occurs, the level of human chorionic gonadotropin (hCG) increases. This hormone acts most directly to sustain the release of:

   A. estrogen.
   B. progesterone.
   C. FSH.
   D. LH.

146. Based partly on the functional information provided in the passage, drug X is most likely similar in structure to which of the following hormones?

   A. Estrogen
   B. Progesterone
   C. FSH
   D. LH

147. If a patient who is enrolled in this study sustains a head injury that damages the hypothalamus, which of the following hormone levels are likely to be affected?

   I. Estrogen
   II. Progesterone
   III. FSH and LH

   A. I and II only
   B. III only
   C. I and III only
   D. I, II, and III

148. Evaluation of the curves shown in Figure 1 suggests that curve 2 most likely represents:

    A.   FSH.
    B.   LH.
    C.   estrogen.
    D.   progesterone.

149. An investigator concludes that drug X is a substance that mimics the function of estrogen. Which of the following findings LEAST supports this conclusion?

    A.   Drug X caused growth of the endometrium.
    B.   Drug X caused the development of secondary sexual characteristics in adolescent girls.
    C.   Administration of drug X decreased the levels of circulating FSH.
    D.   Administration of drug X blocked menstruation.

Passage II (Questions 150–154)

The factors that affect competing reactions are important for predicting whether a desired product can be produced. Substitution and elimination reactions frequently compete, producing complex product mixtures. Two well-known chemistry research scientists have put forth the following arguments about the competition between these reactions.

Chemist 1

The competition between substitution and elimination reactions is based entirely upon the relative basicity and nucleophilicity of the reagent used to react with the substrate. A strong base will promote elimination over substitution, and a strong nucleophile will promote substitution over elimination. Reagents that are both strong bases and strong nucleophiles will always produce a mixture of both substitution and elimination products.

Chemist 2

The competition between substitution and elimination reactions is based upon steric factors. A hindered substrate will be unable to undergo a substitution reaction and will thus eliminate. An unhindered substrate will undergo predominantly substitution because substitution occurs more rapidly than elimination under favorable conditions.

150. Whose argument would be most seriously challenged by the experimental observation that reactions between ethyl bromide and sodium hydroxide yield ethanol?

    A.   Chemist 1, because sodium hydroxide is a strong base.
    B.   Chemist 2, because ethyl bromide is a hindered substrate.
    C.   Chemist 1, because sodium hydroxide is a strong nucleophile.
    D.   Chemist 2, because ethyl bromide is an unhindered substrate.

GO ON TO THE NEXT PAGE.

151. Whose argument would be most seriously challenged by the experimental observation that solvolysis of tert-butyl bromide in water yields predominantly tert-butyl alcohol?

    A. Chemist 1, because water is a stronger base than nucleophile.

    B. Chemist 2, because tert-butyl bromide is a hindered substrate.

    C. Chemist 1, because water is a stronger nucleophile than base.

    D. Chemist 2, because tert-butyl bromide is an unhindered substrate.

152. What explanation would chemist 2 offer for the observation that 1-bromo-2,2-dimethylpropane does not perform substitution with sodium hydroxide?

    A. Hydroxide is a base and would favor elimination.

    B. The substrate is unhindered, which would favor elimination.

    C. The substrate is hindered, which would not favor substitution.

    D. The nucleophile is not strong enough to favor substitution.

153. Which of the following mechanism(s) is/are not being considered by chemist 2?

    A. E2

    B. S_N2

    C. S_N1

    D. S_N2 and E2

154. Which chemist would expect reaction between sodium hydroxide and 2-bromopropane to yield a mixture of products?

    A. Chemist 2, because 2-bromopropane is partially hindered.

    B. Chemist 1, because hydroxide is a nucleophilic base.

    C. Both chemists would expect a mixture of products for different reasons.

    D. Neither chemist would expect a mixture of products for different reasons.

Passage III (Questions 155–159)

The elderly are susceptible to fractures of the bones. This is a significant problem because a bony fracture heals slowly in elderly patients. Furthermore, the bedrest needed for older patients to heal large fractures predisposes them to other complications, including pneumonia, blood clots in the legs, deconditioning, and contracture development in the joints.

Several strategies have been developed to decrease the risk of bony fractures in the elderly. Because older patients are susceptible to osteoporosis, they are often placed on oral calcium supplements to increase total body calcium stores. The exact mechanism of osteoporosis remains unclear; however, it is known that the calcium content of the bones significantly decreases. Furthermore, it is believed that an imbalance of bone resorption to bone apposition occurs in the disease.

Another mechanism that decreases the risk of fractures in high-risk patients is hormone administration. Several hormones, including estrogen, have been used successfully to slow the bone loss associated with aging. In addition, it has been found that careful exercise in elderly patients helps to retain bone mass and density. In some patients, increased bone density and mass can result from maintaining a strict exercise program.

The cells associated with the formation and maintenance of bone have come under study as to their role in the pathogenesis of osteoporosis. Because different cells modulate the formation and resorption of bone, it may be that the disease process of osteoporosis affects the various types of cells differently.

155. Based on the description of osteoporosis given in the passage, which of the following cells are most associated with the progression of osteoporosis?

    A. Fibroblasts

    B. Osteoclasts

    C. Osteocytes

    D. Osteoblasts

156. Which of the following hormones might reverse the changes associated with osteoporosis?

    A. Testosterone

    B. Parathyroid hormone

    C. Thyroid hormone

    D. Calcitonin

157. During the early healing phase following a bony fracture, which of the following events would be expected?

    A.   Ingrowth of osteoblasts and osteoclasts
    B.   Growth of the periosteum
    C.   Activation of the growth plate
    D.   Development of haversian systems and canaliculi

158. An elderly patient suffering from osteoporosis is placed on oral calcium supplementation. Blood samples are drawn from this patient both prior to the initiation of calcium supplementation and after supplementation is begun. When comparing these two blood samples, which of the following hormone levels would be expected to decrease as a result of calcium supplementation?

    A.   Calcitonin
    B.   Adrenocorticotropic hormone
    C.   Thyroid hormone
    D.   Parathyroid hormone

159. Which of the following measurements is most likely expected in a patient suffering from an early case of rapidly progressive osteoporosis?

    A.   Elevated levels of estrogen
    B.   Elevated levels of calcitonin
    C.   Elevated levels of urinary calcium
    D.   Elevated levels of vitamin D

Passage IV (Questions 160–164)

The biologic activity of proteins is dependent on the different amino acids that comprise the primary structure of the protein. One way to classify these amino acids is based on whether the amino acid side chain is neutral, acidic, or basic. Table 1 lists the acidic and basic amino acids with the corresponding side chain pK_a.

Table 1.   Acidic and basic amino acid side chains with corresponding pK_a.

Amino acid	Side chain pK_a
Aspartate	3.96
Glutamate	4.32
Histidine	6.00
Cysteine	8.33
Tyrosine	10.11
Lysine	10.80
Arginine	12.48

The acidic and basic amino acids can be classified as hydrophilic amino acids, as can some of the neutral amino acids. The remaining neutral amino acids are classified as hydrophobic. Positive and negative interactions of amino acids with each other and their aqueous environment determine protein secondary and tertiary structure and biologic function. Proteins fold in such a way as to maximize favorable interactions, such as hydrogen bonding, ionic interactions, and Van der Waals attractions. Protein folding also minimizes unfavorable interactions, such as hydrophobic amino acid exposure to water. The tendency for hydrophobic amino acids to fold away from the aqueous environment toward the center of the protein and other hydrophobic amino acids is known as the hydrophobic effect.

160. Which of the following amino acids is the most basic?

    A.   Aspartate
    B.   Glutamate
    C.   Threonine
    D.   Arginine

161. Which of the following amino acids can be classified as acidic?

    A.   Arginine
    B.   Cysteine
    C.   Tyrosine
    D.   Aspartate

162. Which of the following is the K_a of histidine?

   A. 1×10^6
   B. 1×10^{-6}
   C. $\log(-6.00)$
   D. $\log(6.00)$

163. All acidic and basic amino acids can be classified as:

   A. charged.
   B. uncharged.
   C. hydrophobic.
   D. hydrophilic.

164. What is unfavorable about a hydrophobic amino acid being in contact with water?

   A. The water is repelled by the hydrophobic amino acid.
   B. The hydrophobic amino acid is repelled by the water.
   C. The water forms an entropically unfavorable structure to maximize hydrogen bonding with other water molecules.
   D. The water forms an entropically unfavorable structure to minimize hydrogen bonding with other water molecules.

Questions 165 through 168 are **NOT** based on a descriptive passage.

165. Eukaryotic cells possess an organelle that is required for the final stages of protein synthesis. This organelle is used to covalently modify polypeptide chains and is known as the:

   A. ribosome.
   B. rough endoplasmic reticulum.
   C. lysosome.
   D. Golgi apparatus.

166. Regulation of transcription is an important process in cells that is demonstrated by the lactose (lac) operon. In this system, a repressor protein is produced which, in the presence of lactose, no longer binds to the operator site of DNA. This is important because an unbound operator site makes the promotor available to bind:

   A. RNA polymerase.
   B. DNA polymerase.
   C. lactose.
   D. the repressor protein.

167. According to the figure below, how many asymmetric (chiral) carbons does vitamin A contain?

   A. 0
   B. 2
   C. 4
   D. 8

168. Which of the following hormones is LEAST likely to increase during a period of dehydration?

   A. Vasopressin
   B. Aldosterone
   C. Angiotensin II
   D. Oxytocin

781

GO ON TO THE NEXT PAGE.

The human pedigree describing the skeletal abnormality known as brachydactyly was first demonstrated by Farabee in 1905. Brachydactyly is a condition in which the fingers of an afflicted individual are very short. The pedigree for brachydactyly represents one of the first studies of single-gene inheritance in humans. In the pedigree shown in Figure 1, females are represented by circles and males are represented by squares. Shaded individuals are afflicted by the condition. The generation number is indicated in the far left column of the figure.

A family was studied by Dr. Farabee at the end of the nineteenth century. Five generations of this family were traced, and through good records and recall by surviving family members, the individuals demonstrating brachydactyly in the family tree were recorded. Figure 1 is a pedigree for this family. Note that in this original pedigree, Dr. Farabee did not show the marriage partners for each reproducing family member. It was assumed that each non-family marriage partner did not have brachydactyly and did not carry a gene for brachydactyly.

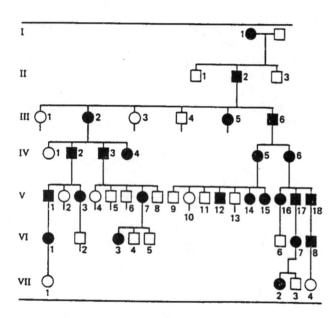

Figure 1. Original pedigree for bracydactyly.

Pedigree analysis is useful because it allows geneticists to identify the likely mode of inheritance of a particular trait and to predict the possibility of genetic transmission of a particular trait. This may be useful in counseling parents who have or carry a particular genetic condition and are concerned about transmitting this condition genetically to their offspring. One such condition, hemophilia, is passed by a sex-linked recessive transmission. Hemophilia leads to a bleeding disorder that can be fatal. Another serious condition, microcephaly, is passed by a rare autosomal recessive gene; afflicted individuals have a small head and mental retardation.

169. The mode of transmission for brachydactyly is most likely:

    A. autosomal dominant.
    B. sex-linked recessive.
    C. autosomal recessive.
    D. mediated by random mutation.

170. The pedigree shown provides classic demonstration of:

    A. the principle of segregation.
    B. nondisjunction.
    C. independent assortment.
    D. random mutations.

171. If the afflicted male in generation II of the pedigree were not shaded, the mode of transmission of brachydactyly could be:

    A. autosomal dominant.
    B. sex-linked recessive.
    C. autosomal recessive.
    D. none of these possible modes of inheritance.

172. Which of the following is expected in a pedigree demonstrating the transmission of microcephaly?

    A. Afflicted family members would likely be found in each generation.
    B. A woman carrying the microcephaly gene would always produce sons with microcephaly.
    C. Microcephaly would likely be found in offspring of heterozygous family members who intermarry.
    D. Males with microcephaly who marry a homozygous normal female would most likely produce half microcephalic sons and half normal sons.

173. Could this pedigree demonstrate the transmission of hemophilia?

    A. Yes, because the pedigree supports it.
    B. Yes, because the pedigree cannot exclude it.
    C. No, because the pedigree excludes it.
    D. There is not enough information to determine.

174. Based on the mode of inheritance, what is the expected effect if two brachydactylous individuals from this lineage were to marry and have children?

   A.   All of their children would be afflicted.
   B.   One-half of their children would be afflicted.
   C.   Three-quarters of their children would be afflicted.
   D.   One-quarter of their children would be afflicted.

Passage VI (Questions 175–179)

Natural products are often developed into new consumer products, such as pharmaceuticals, insecticides, fungicides, and agricultural chemicals. The isolation of natural products is a time-consuming and tedious task. The most common sources of natural products include plants, mushrooms, and corals. These sources all contain a large number of compounds. Isolating a single, unknown product from these sources can involve many separation and purification steps. The following diagram (Figure 1) describes a typical purification scheme.

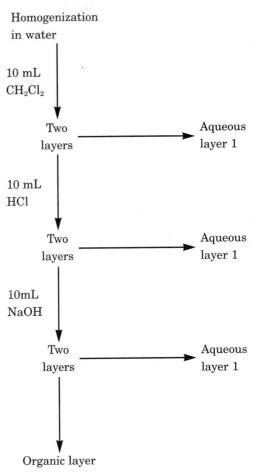

Figure 1

The homogenization step is performed to reduce the solid natural product source to small, uniform pieces to aid in the extraction steps. In the subsequent extractions, which result in two layers, the organic layer is carried on the next step, and the aqueous layers are removed and labeled for testing. The remaining steps separate the large number of chemicals into smaller classes based on their physical properties. Further steps can be performed if any of the fractions show a desired activity.

The general scheme shown in Figure 1 was performed on an extract from an as-yet-unnamed mushroom. Each fraction was then tested for various biologic activities with the following results (Table 1):

Table 1. Results of mushroom extract fractions.

Fraction	Test 1	Test 2	Test 3	Test 4
Aqueous layer 1	Positive	Negative	Negative	Negative
Aqueous layer 2	Negative	Negative	Negative	Negative
Aqueous layer 3	Negative	Positive	Negative	Negative
Organic layer	Negative	Negative	Negative	Positive

Test 1 evaluated the fraction's ability to kill gram-negative bacteria. Test 2 evaluated the fraction's ability to kill gram-positive bacteria, and test 3 evaluated the fraction's ability to kill flying insects. Finally, test 4 evaluated the fraction's ability to kill nematodes.

175. What is the purpose of the homogenization?

    A. To separate the useful parts of the natural product source from the less useful parts
    B. To make the sample uniform
    C. To make the following extraction steps easier
    D. To divide the solid into small pieces that can be strained out

176. Which of the following types of compounds will aqueous layer 3 contain?

    A. Neutral, polar compounds
    B. Basic, polar compounds
    C. Acidic, polar compounds
    D. Neutral, nonpolar compounds

177. Which of the following compounds might be found in the organic layer?

A. (benzene ring with CO_2H groups)
B. (benzene ring with NH_2 and CO_2H)
C. (steroid structure with O)
D. (cyclohexane ring with OH, HO, OH, OH groups)

178. What is the advantage of using a base in the extraction following extraction with HCl?

    A. It neutralizes the HCl.
    B. It reacts with the HCl.
    C. It neutralizes acidic components of the mixture to make them less water soluble.
    D. It neutralizes acidic components of the mixture to make them more water soluble.

179. Which of the following forms of para-aminobenzoic acid is the least water soluble?

A. (benzene with NH_2 and CO_2H)
B. (benzene with $^+NH_3$ and CO_2^-)
C. (benzene with $^+NH_3$ and CO_2H)
D. (benzene with NH_2 and CO_2^-)

GO ON TO THE NEXT PAGE.

Passage VII (Questions 180–185)

A technique to analyze the renaturation kinetics of DNA has yielded much information on DNA structure. The DNA from bacterial and eukaryotic cells are isolated. The DNA is then fragmented into small pieces of uniform size, each piece approximately 500 nucleotides in length. The temperature and ionic conditions are then manipulated to allow renaturation, and adjustments are made to ensure that one experiment can be compared with another. The fraction of the total DNA strands in solution that have been renatured is plotted as a function of the logarithm of the $C_o t$ (initial concentration of DNA in the solution multiplied by the time that the renaturation has been allowed to proceed). These results, when plotted, are know as a $C_o t$ plot. Analysis of the kinetics of the $C_o t$ plot can provide evidence about the repetitiveness of DNA sequences in DNA strands. DNA strands that contain repetitive sequences tend to renature more rapidly than sequences that are noncompetitive.

In a series of experiments, DNA from both *Escherichia coli* and calf thymus were isolated and denatured. Using the technique described above, $C_o t$ plots were generated for both the *E. coli* DNA (lighter curve) and calf thymus DNA (darker curve) and shown in Figure 1. In these curves, it was assumed that the DNA was single-stranded in the initial state and double-helical in the final state.

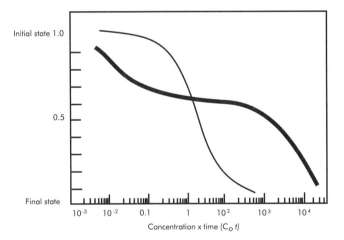

Figure 1

180. In the $C_o t$ plot for *E. coli*, the first section of the curve depicts:

   A. rapid renaturation of DNA.
   B. almost no renaturation of DNA.
   C. a slow, constant rate of DNA renaturation.
   D. DNA denaturation.

181. Which of the following statements explains how *E. coli* DNA and calf thymus DNA differ?

   A. *E. coli* DNA is found in a single, circular chromosome.
   B. *E. coli* DNA is found in the cell nucleus.
   C. *E. coli* DNA is associated with histone proteins.
   D. *E. coli* DNA is single stranded.

182. Which of the following statements best describes the kinetics of the calf thymus DNA?

   A. The population of fragments are heterogenous with respect to their kinetics.
   B. The population of fragments are homogenous with respect to their kinetics.
   C. The population of fragments are similar in heterogeneity to *E. coli* DNA fragments.
   D. The population of fragments are similar in homogeneity to *E. coli* DNA fragments.

183. Which of the following statements best explains how a $C_o t$ plot of calf liver DNA would compare with a plot for calf thymus DNA?

   A. The plots would differ because the liver DNA may be expressed differently.
   B. The plots would differ because differential translation occurs between the two cell types.
   C. The plots would be similar because the cells have the same number of chromosomes.
   D. The plots would be similar because the DNA sequence of the two cell types is the same.

184. In Figure 1, the rapid decreases that occur over time for calf thymus DNA are best explained by:

   A. rapid DNA denaturation.
   B. nonrepetitive DNA sequences.
   C. small, fragmented DNA sequences.
   D. repetitive DNA sequences.

185. Comparing *E. coli* DNA with calf thymus DNA, what conclusions can be reached based on the passage and data shown in the $C_o t$ plots?

   A. *E. coli* DNA most likely has fewer repetitive sequences than calf thymus DNA.
   B. *E. coli* DNA most likely has larger fragments of DNA that renature.
   C. *E. coli* DNA has more repetitive sequences than calf thymus DNA.
   D. *E. coli* cells most likely have fewer chromosomes than calf thymus cells.

GO ON TO THE NEXT PAGE.

Passage VIII (Questions 186–190)

Foreign chemicals, such as drugs or toxins, are metabolized by the body in many different ways. Metabolic reactions can be classified into two categories, phase I and phase II reactions. Phase I reactions (e.g., oxidation, reduction, hydrolysis) introduce or expose functional groups. Phase II reactions (e.g., sulfonation, glucuronidation, amino acid conjugation) conjugate functional groups with high-energy intermediates to increase water solubility.

Hydrophobic compounds tend to be metabolized through both phase I and phase II reactions. These molecules are not particularly water soluble and are hard for the body to excrete. These molecules can be conjugated to a hydrophilic molecule such as glucuronic acid to increase water-solubility and increase excretion. An example of a phase II reaction, glucuronide formation, is shown in Figure 1.

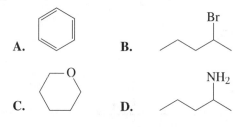

Figure 1

The resulting glucuronide conjugate is considerably more hydrophilic than the parent compound, and it can be eliminated in the urine or bile. These metabolic pathways decrease the amount of time foreign substances remain in the body, which is beneficial if the foreign molecule is a toxic substance but not beneficial if the compound is a drug.

186. The substitution reaction in the formation of the glucuronide occurs:

    A. with retention of configuration.
    B. with inversion of configuration.
    C. with racemization.
    D. with partial racemization.

187. What biologic reason can be suggested for glucuronide formation?

    A. Glucuronides tend to be less toxic.
    B. Glucuronides tend to be less water soluble and can be more easily removed from the bloodstream.
    C. Glucuronides tend to be more water soluble and can be more easily removed from the bloodstream.
    D. Glucuronides are more highly active drugs.

188. Which of the following is a phase II reaction?

    A. Oxidation of dihydropyridine to pyridine
    B. Hydrolysis of methyl acetate to acetic acid
    C. Formation of a glucuronide of N,N'-dimethylaniline
    D. Reduction of pyridine to dihydropyridine

189. What role does phosphate play in glucuronide formation?

    A. It acts as the nucleophile because of its negative charge.
    B. It acts as the substrate because of its lack of alkyl substitution.
    C. It acts as the solvent because of its proximity to the reaction.
    D. It acts as the leaving group because of its ability to delocalize the charge.

190. Which of the following molecules could possibly form glucuronides?

    A.   **B.**

    C.   **D.**

191. Which of the following statements regarding anomers is the most accurate?

    A. They are molecules that differ in configuration about a single chiral center.
    B. They are molecules that differ in different chiral centers.
    C. They are stereoisomers that rotate light in opposite directions.
    D. They are epimers in which the chiral site was formerly a carbonyl carbon.

192. An experiment is performed in which a nonpermeable, thin sheet is placed between the mesoderm and ectoderm layers of a developing amphibian, the region that ultimately gives rise to the neural tube. This procedure is performed immediately after gastrulation and prior to the formation of the neural tube. Is a neural tube expected to form?

    A. Yes, because differentiation will proceed.
    B. Yes, because induction can occur.
    C. No, because differentiation has already taken place but determination has not.
    D. No, because induction cannot occur.

193. Why do *trans* isomers of alkenes typically have lower boiling points than their corresponding *cis* isomers?

    A. The *trans* isomers have better symmetry.
    B. The *cis* isomers have better symmetry.
    C. The *trans* ismomers are less polar.
    D. The *cis* isomers are less polar.

194. Gallstones can cause the blockage of the ducts leading from the pancreas to the duodenum. In the presence of this blockage, which function of the pancreas is most impaired?

    A. Endocrine
    B. Exocrine
    C. Formation of bile
    D. Glucose storage

195. The main differences between blood types A, B, and O in humans are the glycoprotein antigens present on red blood cells. There are several similar, yet antigenically distinct, red blood cell glycoproteins in the ABO system. People with type A blood have type A antigens and antibodies against type B blood. People with type B blood have type B antigens and antibodies against type A blood. People with type AB blood are expected to have:

    A. antibodies against A antigens only.
    B. antibodies against B antigens only.
    C. antibodies against both A and B antigens.
    D. antibodies against neither A nor B antigens.

787

GO ON TO THE NEXT PAGE.

Passage IX (Questions 196–202)

The liver is an important organ that performs many diverse functions in the body. The liver is the center for detoxification, processing, and rendering harmless many toxic and otherwise harmful substances. The liver is able to perform detoxification by two major mechanisms, known as either the conjugation mechanisms or the P_{450} mechanism. In the process of conjugation, a carbohydrate-like molecule is covalently bound to the toxin, increasing its solubility and decreasing its toxicity. These conjugated compounds are then excreted in the urine. Conjugation is most often utilized by the liver to excrete lipid soluble, nonpolar molecules. The P_{450} system in the liver is an enzyme system that acts to metabolize various harmful or toxic substances, producing less harmful intermediates and ultimately a final product that is nontoxic and can be excreted in the urine or feces. The P_{450} system is inducible. Repeated exposures to chemicals that require P_{450} metabolism actually induce the synthesis of more P_{450} enzymes.

The liver is also important in filtering the blood for the purpose of removing foreign matter, antigenic compounds, and old red blood cells. An example of this important filtering role of the liver is demonstrated by the presence of special phagocytic cells. Kupffer cells are specialized macrophages found in the liver. They are adjuncts to the immune system in that they remove potentially harmful foreign microorganisms and antigens from the bloodstream.

Maintaining a storage site for glucose is an important function of the liver. In liver cells, glucose is stored as a polymerized molecule, known as glycogen. In the presence of insulin and excess glucose, glycogen formation is stimulated. Glycogen is useful to the body because it provides a short supply of glucose during periods of fasting.

196. Alcohol is considered a toxic substance by the liver. Which of the following mechanisms is most appropriate for processing alcohol in the liver?

    A. Conjugation
    B. P_{450} enzyme system
    C. Phagocytosis
    D. Direct excretion in the urine

197. Which of the following is the best mechanism by which the liver can excrete a metabolized toxin in the feces?

    A. Secrete the metabolized toxin into the bloodstream
    B. Secrete the metabolized toxin into the urine
    C. Secrete the metabolized toxin into macrophages
    D. Secrete the metabolized toxin into the bile

198. Which of the following substances tends to decrease glycogen stores and increase blood glucose?

    A. Glucagon
    B. Somatostatin
    C. Insulin
    D. Thyroid hormone

199. Which organ in the body plays an adjunctive role and aids the liver in removing and processing old red blood cells?

    A. Thymus
    B. Pancreas
    C. Adrenal medulla
    D. Spleen

200. The liver is able to effectively filter the blood shortly after it drains the digestive tract. This is useful because it allows the liver to store excess glucose and process amino acids and fats. The vessel that brings blood to the liver from the digestive tract is the:

    A. thoracic duct.
    B. hepatic vein.
    C. portal vein.
    D. hepatic artery.

201. Which of the following statements best summarizes amino acid metabolism?

    A. The liver makes urea, which is excreted in the urine.
    B. The kidney makes urea, which is excreted in the urine.
    C. The liver makes ammonia, which the kidney converts to urea and excretes in the urine.
    D. The liver makes urea, which is excreted in the bile.

202. Over a period of several months, a person takes a drug known to be metabolized by the P_{450} system of the liver. During the prolonged exposure to this drug, it most likely causes changes in which of the following liver cell process?

    A. Replication
    B. Transformation
    C. Transcription
    D. Phagocytosis

GO ON TO THE NEXT PAGE.

Passage X (Questions 203–207)

It is known that the mouse can make about 10^9 different antibodies. This number of possible antibodies is large enough to ensure that there will be an antigen-binding site to fit almost any encountered antigen. Because antibodies are proteins, and proteins are encoded by genes, the obvious question is how the mouse makes millions of different antibodies without requiring an unreasonably large number of genes. The mouse, as well as other animals, has evolved complex mechanisms to generate antibody diversity.

Antibodies, such as immunoglobulin G (IgG), are made up of two heavy chains and two light chains. Each of these chains has a constant region and a variable region. The variable regions of both the heavy and light chains comprise the antigen-binding sites.

During development of the B lymphocyte, there is DNA rearrangement, which ultimately gives rise to antibody diversity. More than one gene segment codes for each heavy and light chain. The variable regions of each heavy and light chain are encoded by many distinct gene segments, which are united into a functional gene after DNA rearrangement occurs and the variable and constant regions are brought together.

Studies have shown that the mouse inherits several hundred variable gene segments for light chains and several hundred variable gene segments for heavy chains. Through recombination of these gene segments, thousands of different combinations of heavy and light chains can be generated. In addition, the combination of different heavy and light chains during antibody assembly greatly increases antibody diversity. The mechanisms of multiple gene segments coding for each heavy and light chain, for recombination of different variable and light chains, and for differential combination of various heavy and light chains generate more than 10^7 different antibodies. The process of spontaneous mutation can increase the number of different antibodies that the mouse can make by a factor of greater than 10^2.

---

203. Which of the following statements best describes a mechanism that generates antibody diversity in the mouse?

  A. Separate gene segments that code for different parts of the variable regions can be recombined during B-cell differentiation.
  B. Light-chain genes can recombine with heavy-chain genes to create variable regions with increased diversity.
  C. Constant-region genes can recombine with light-chain genes to create diversity during B-cell differentiation.
  D. Variable-region genes can recombine with heavy-chain genes to create diversity during B-cell differentiation.

204. Which of the following statements explains why antibody diversity is necessary?

  A. An antibody may bind many different antigens.
  B. The animal must be able to generate a specific antibody for each antigen encountered.
  C. An antibody must be coded by many genes so that it can have a complex antigen-binding site.
  D. An antibody needs to possess both variable and constant regions, which allow the formation of an antigen-binding site.

205. B lymphocytes mature into antibody-producing cells. During this process of maturation, the genetic recombinations discussed in the passage occur. The mature form of the B lymphocyte that produces antibodies is the:

  A. T lymphocyte.
  B. neutrophil.
  C. macrophage.
  D. plasma cell.

206. An immature B lymphocyte is exposed to antigen X and undergoes differentiation and gene recombination. Fully mature, the cell is exposed to antigen Y. It is most likely that:

  A. the cell will undergo recombination in response to antigen Y.
  B. the cell will undergo mutation in response to antigen Y.
  C. the cell will modify the organization of its light and heavy chains in response to antigen Y.
  D. the cell will be unable to respond to antigen Y.

207. A few bacterial cells, each identical to one another, are injected into a mouse. The bacterial cells each have several different cell membrane proteins on their surface. A group of B lymphocytes begins to mature in response to the foreign bacteria. Which of the following is expected to form in response to the bacteria after maturation of the antibody-producing cells is complete?

A. One antibody that can bind and inactivate all the bacterial cell-surface proteins

B. Several different antibodies generated from each antibody-producing cell

C. One antibody that can bind and inactivate the major antigen on the bacterial cell

D. Several different antibodies, each generated from a different antibody-producing cell

---

Passage XI (Questions 208–213)

Polymerization is an industrially important reaction in which small units (monomers) are combined to form larger structures (polymers). These polymers have a host of applications in everyday life. They are components of products such as foam seat cushions, clothing, food containers, and car parts. Polymerization is characterized by three types of mechanistic steps: initiation, propagation, and termination. In initiation steps, an initial reactive species is formed from less reactive species. In propagation steps, the reactive species reacts with a less reactive species to form another (different) reactive species and less reactive products. In termination steps, two reactive species combine to form an unreactive species.

Polymers can be classified as linear polymers or cross-linked polymers. Linear polymers are formed from monomers that have only one group, thus they can only form long chains. Cross-linked polymers are formed from monomers that have more than one polymerizeable group, thus they can react to form web-like structures. In a cross-linked polymer, the polymerizeable groups can be the same or different. These two types of cross-linked polymers have vastly different physical properties, leading to different applications.

In a radical polymerization, light or heat can be used to generate the initial reactive species. One very commonly used radical initiator is azobisisobutyronitrile (AIBN), which dissociates with very little added energy. This compound forms two alkyl radicals when heated according to the following equation:

$$R\!-\!N\!=\!N\!-\!R \rightleftharpoons 2R\bullet + N_2(g),$$

where $R = (CH_3)_2C(CN)^-$.

The radical formed in the first propagation step is generally the more stable radical, when more than one are possible. Formation of a radical in the first propagation step can involve either abstraction of a hydrogen atom from alkanes or addition to alkenes. This generates new radicals, which can either propagate the reaction by reacting with other alkanes or alkenes or terminate the reaction by combining with each other.

208. Which of the following could represent the reactive species formed from ethylene after a propagation step in a reaction initiated by AIBN?

A. $H_3C\!-\!\bullet CH_2$
B. $RH_2C\!-\!\bullet CH_2$
C. $H_3C\!-\!CH_3$
D. $N_2H_2C\!-\!\bullet CH_2$

790

209. Which of the following can be used to initiate the initial reactive species in a radical polymerization?

    A.   The friction generated by rapid stirring
    B.   Vigorous shaking to mix the appropriate reactants thoroughly
    C.   An appropriate wavelength of light
    D.   Leaving all the reactants mixed together for a period of time

210. Which of the following reactive species is formed by the reaction of an initiator with propane?

    A. $H_3C-\underset{H_2}{C}-\bullet CH_2$

    B. $H_3C-\underset{H_2}{C}-CH_2N_2H_2$

    C. $H_3C-\underset{H\bullet}{C}-CH_3$

    D. $N_2H_2C-\underset{H\bullet}{C}-CH_3$

211. A termination step for a radical polymerization of ethylene initiated by AIBN might look like which of the following?

    A. $R-N=N-R \xrightarrow{h\nu} 2R^\bullet + N_2(g)$

    B. $CH_2=CH-CH_3 + R^\bullet \longrightarrow$
         $R-CH_2-CH^\bullet-CH_3$

    C. $CH_3-CH_3 + R^\bullet \longrightarrow RH + CH_3-CH_2^\bullet$

    D. $R-CH_2-CH_2^\bullet + R-CH_2-CH_2^\bullet \longrightarrow$
         $R-CH_2-CH_2-CH_2-CH_2-R$

212. Which of the following statements best explains why AIBN forms radicals so easily?

    A.   The radicals that it forms are stabilized by resonance and form easily due to their unusual stability.
    B.   The bond between the alkyl carbon atoms and the nitrogen atom is considerably weaker than a normal carbon-carbon or carbon-hydrogen bond, and it can be broken with very little energy.
    C.   The equilibrium of the reaction is disturbed by the loss of nitrogen as a gas, and more radicals are formed as the system continues to try to reach equilibrium.
    D.   The nitrogen gas that is formed is so stable that it compensates for the instability of the radicals formed.

213. Which one of the following monomers would react to form a cross-linked polymer?

    A. $CH_3-CH=CH_2$
    B. $CH_2=CH-CH(CH_3)-CH_2$
    C. $CH_2=CH-CH_3-CH=CH_2$
    D. $CH_3-CH_2-CH_2-CH_3$

Questions 214 through 219 are **NOT** based on a descriptive passage.

---

214. The greater acidity of carboxylic acids compared with alcohols arises primarily from:

    A.   the electron-donating effects of the hydroxyl group.
    B.   the electron-withdrawing effect of the carbonyl oxygen atom.
    C.   the acidity of alpha hydrogens in the carboxylic acids.
    D.   the resonance stability associated with the carboxylate ion.

215. Significant similarities have been found between the DNA contained in both bacteria and which of the following cells and structures?

    A.   Eukaryotic stem cells
    B.   Mitochondria
    C.   Golgi apparatus
    D.   Yeast cells

216. Which of the following compounds has the greatest bond angle?

    A.   Ethylene
    B.   Benzene
    C.   Acetone
    D.   Carbon dioxide

217. Which of the following best accounts for the enhanced concentration ability of the kidneys of animals that live in arid conditions?

    A.   Greater glomerular filtration
    B.   Lower levels of vasopressin
    C.   Countercurrent exchange
    D.   Long loops of Henle

218. Which of the following compounds is the strongest acid?

    A. $ClCH_2CH_2CO_2H$
    B. Cl_2CHCO_2H
    C. $CH_3CHClCO_2H$
    D. $ClCH_2CHClCO_2H$

219. During a critical period following hatching, the young of some bird species will follow the first moving object they see and form a lasting attachment to it. This kind of behavior is considered:

    A. habituation.
    B. conditioning.
    C. imprinting.
    D. instinct.

STOP. IF YOU FINISH BEFORE TIME IS CALLED, CHECK YOUR WORK. YOU MAY GO BACK TO ANY QUESTION IN THIS TEST BOOKLET.

STOP.

Answers and Explanations to Full-length MCAT

Part I: Verbal Reasoning

1. **C** Choices B and D are incorrect because Filippo's originality (statement III) is never mentioned. The author emphasizes Filippo's ambition, so choice A, which includes statement II (modesty), is also incorrect. By process of elimination, choice C is the best answer.

2. **D** Choice A is clearly incorrect because the passage is not a satire of ambition. Choices B and C are less accurate representations of the passage, making choice D the best answer.

3. **B** The emphasis of the passage is on the uniqueness of their quest to rediscover the past. The author comments little on the other features of Donatello's and Filippo's lives (choices A, C, and D).

4. **D** There is insufficient information to arrive at any of the conclusions offered.

5. **A** The passage emphasizes that during Filippo's time, the technological skills of the Romans had been lost. However, Filippo overcame this impediment by studying various ancient buildings. Choices C and D are not mentioned in the passage, and choice B impedes a solution to the main problem.

6. **D** *The Rivalry of Filippo and Donatello* (choice A), *Filippo: Renaissance Man* (choice B), and *Renaissance Architecture* (choice C) are all applicable titles for the passage. However, the main idea of the passage is the effect that rediscovering works of the past had on Filippo; *Filippo Encounters Classic Rome* is the best title for the passage.

7. **A** The passage is clearly biographical, and the author concentrates on providing facts, rather than allowing his emotions to intrude; thus choices B and C are not appropriate. Choice D may be plausible; however, the author has an informed tone, rather than a curious one.

8. **B** Choice A is not plausible because reasons other than cowardice are provided (in the first paragraph) to explain Filippo's decision to study architecture. The passage refutes choice C. Choice D is not plausible; the passage does not address the proportion of time Filippo spent on research to the time he spent actively participating in design work.

9. **C** The subject of the passage is the religious tolerance practiced in Rome, making choice C the best answer. Although choices A, B, and D are all true, they are not claims specifically made by the author of the passage.

10. **A** The second paragraph of the passage shows that the author characterizes the practice of religion in Rome as an indulgence in superstition, a psychological necessity for some individuals, and an institution that is useful for the state.

11. **D** The third and fourth paragraphs of the passage show that choice D is the best answer.

12. **B** The author's tone is neither of pity (choice A) nor of condemnation (choice C). Of the two remaining choices, choice B (a tone of respect) is more evident in the passage.

13. **D** The author's apparent sympathy for religious tolerance and manifest skepticism regarding religious beliefs (which he and the philosophers consider superstition) strongly imply that he would also be tolerant of atheism. Choices A and C are clearly incorrect

SECT. V
ANSWERS AND
EXPLANATIONS
TO FULL-LENGTH
MCAT

793

because they are not expressions of religious tolerance. Choice B is not addressed by the author. However, it seems clear in the passage that the author would not object to state-designated days for religious observance, which would eliminate choice B as a plausible answer.

14. **D** Choice D is the best answer because the author argues the wisdom of tolerance in religious affairs, not the establishment of one religion. Choice A is incorrect because religion, not political diversity, is the subject of this passage. Choice B is incorrect because the author argues in favor of the superiority of Roman greatness, not against it. Choice C is clearly incorrect because religion was a major role in the lives of ancient Romans.

15. **D** The answer choices that include statement I (choices A and B) are incorrect because the author emphasizes the virtue of tolerance. The answer choices that include statement II (choices A and C) are incorrect because the author considers all religion to be superstitious. Choice D (statement III) is the correct answer; the author views religion as a useful adjunct in governing a population, and thus would presumably not be opposed to taxing property that belongs to religious organizations.

PASSAGE III

16. **C** The author identifies a confused *notion* of democracy, not the system itself, as a cause of the problems that beset higher learning.

17. **D** The main conclusion, which is presented in the final paragraph, is that at least some universities must reaffirm the values of higher learning. Choices A, B, and C are used to support this conclusion.

18. **C** The author would object to democratic influences on educational curriculum [statement I]. The author would not object to state-funded education (in principle) [statement II] and to the teaching of evolutionary theory in universities [statement III], making any answer choices with these two statements (choices A, B, and D) incorrect.

19. **A** Because the author focuses on what must be done with higher learning in order for it to excel, *A Prescription for Higher Learning in America* is the best title for this passage. *The Nature of Intellectual Virtue* (choice B) is not a good title because the passage does not discuss intellectual virtue in any depth. *Higher Learning in America: A Bright Future* (choice C) is not a good title because the author believes that the future of higher learning in America is at risk.

20. **B** In the final paragraph of the passage, the author describes how education and scholarship are different aspects of higher learning.

21. **A** According to the author, the implications of a confused notion of democracy cause higher education to pander to the public (choice A). Financial crises (choice B), the failure to cultivate the intellect (choice C), and the acceptance of the theory of evolution (choice D) are not necessarily implications of a confused notion of democracy.

22. **B** In the fourth paragraph, the relation between the theory of evolution and educational experimentation is explicitly described.

PASSAGE IV

23. **B** Russell's participation in a protest for nuclear disarmament implies that Russell favored nuclear disarmament. Russell's pacifism does not imply an active opposition to the Second World War or the Vietnam War (choices A and C).

24. **D** The passage states that the *Principa Mathematica* was coauthored by A.N. Whitehead.

25. **D** The passage opens and closes by identifying Russell as a "Renaissance person."

26. **A** Russell was jailed as a result of his activities in opposition to the First World War, thus he was jailed after the beginning of the First World War.

27. **B** The word *opine* does not mean deny (choice C) or infer (choice D) in the context of the passage. Also, the passage does not suggest that the author's assertion is backed up by an argument (choice A).

28. **A** Although Russell was an atheist, this fact alone does not necessarily imply that he was opposed to a tax-exempt status for religious institutions.

29. **C** The passage states that Russell would most likely not have actively opposed the war had he not been exposed to its atrocities. Although Russell was a pacifist, it was more than his pacifism that caused his active opposition to the war.

30. **A** The author's main concern in the passage is the discussion of Golding's success in developing the premise of a novel. Although the author elaborates on a simple definition of instinct (choice B), it only serves as an introduction to the main topic of the passage. Choices C and D are points that are developed by Golding, not the author of the passage.

31. **C** In the first sentence of the passage, the author describes instinct as both involuntary and inborn.

32. **B** According to the passage, an individual's base nature or instincts can overpower civilized mores; this concept is exemplified in the passage, which describes the British boys becoming savages when placed in a savage environment.

33. **D** The author claims at the end of the passage that the boys' actions are "irrefutable proof" that their behavioral tendencies had always existed, which also is Golding's premise.

34. **C** Golding's premise is that different behaviors surface in different environments; therefore, our environment, in part, determines how we act.

35. **C** Golding argues that the boys' behavior was always part of their personality; their behavior simply had been buried.

36. **A** The fourth paragraph of the passage discusses the shape and strength of the social structure, which follows the same pattern as its creators.

37. **A** According to the passage, a master is the ultimate enemy of "well-being for all." Choice B, "iron slaves which we call machines," is incorrect because this quoted phrase does not appear in the passage. The free contract (choice C) as a mere instrument is not the ultimate enemy of "well-being for all." The feudal lord (choice D) is a plausible choice; however, the second paragraph describes the feudal lord only as an example of a master (and probably a less onerous one than exists in the modern world).

38. **B** The fourth paragraph makes it clear that individual appropriation would simply be a piratical taking, without any motivation for sharing behind it. A collectively managed farm (choice B) implies shared power, which is not a characteristic of individual appropriation. The remaining choices (A, C, and D) reflect the world that the author decries and the world that would still exist, even if the identity of the individual masters changed.

39. **B** All four choices reflect beliefs of the author. However, choice B is more exact and best reflects the proposed action discussed in the final three paragraphs of the passage.

40. **D** The first paragraph shows that choice A is correct. The third paragraph shows that choice B also is correct. The second paragraph demonstrates that choice C also is correct. Thus, the best answer is choice D (all of the above).

41. **B** All four choices are plausible. However, choice B is the best answer; the crux of the passage is the concept that despite small ameliorations and better living conditions, the modern world still reflects the inequities of feudalism. The second paragraph effectively expresses this concept.

42. **B** The fourth paragraph most clearly expresses the concept that what society needs is not only a more equal distribution of goods and better opportunities, but a recognition that all is to be shared. Although choices A, C, and D are plausible, they are less exact than choice B.

43. **C** It is clear, especially in the final paragraph, that the author is calling for a revolution (choice C) and breaking of all past bonds. The word *expropriation* demonstrates that the author believes that extralegal seizures would be required to change the nature of our social and economic lives. Choices A, B, and D characterize progress, which is a matter of evolutionary (or de-evolutionary) development.

44. **C** *Fuel Alternative and the Solution to the Gasoline Woes* is the best title for this passage. The first paragraph of the passage presents the problem of automotive oil consumption, and the remaining paragraphs discuss fuel alternatives.

45. **D** The final paragraph describes that the best solution to the gasoline problem is to combine all possible fuel alternatives, each to be used for a different purpose.

46. A   The final sentence indicates that the author does not favor dependence on only one fuel source; therefore, regardless of discovery of new oil fields, the author would advocate a policy in which all possible fuel alternatives are used.

47. D   Alcohol–gasoline mixes (choice D) are currently used in cars, thus modification to cars would not be required. Natural gas (choice C) requires an awkward tank, and straight alcohol fuels (choices A and B) require a "flex-fuel" engine.

48. B   Fuels made from corn are ethanols, which service half of all vehicles in Brazil. The reader can only assume that all other vehicles are gasoline-powered, otherwise the author would have mentioned the advancement in policy.

49. A   The last sentence of the passage indicates that the Gulf War could have been prevented if the United States had not relied so heavily on one fuel source.

50. D   Although the passage states that ethanol is cleaner than methanol, the cleanliness of natural gas is not mentioned.

PASSAGE VIII

51. D   Choice D states the main idea of the passage; this main idea is most persuasively expressed in the fourth paragraph, which discusses how an American woman may have an "instinctive" belief that is actually a culturally induced belief. Choice A is unlikely because the passage argues the validity of cultural responses that are different from our own (e.g., the Koryak women). Choice B is unlikely because the passage argues that behaviors and customs are culturally formed, not biologically founded. Choice C is incorrect because the author provides several examples about the differences among cultures.

52. C   Choice C is the best answer because it demonstrates that the Koryaks would defend their behavior by calling it "natural" or "instinctive," which is the same defense that other cultures use. The fourth paragraph, which discusses the Koryaks, neither mentions influences by Christian missionaries (choice A) nor influences by modern media (choice D). Also, chauvinism (choice B) is only implied in context of American women, who according to author, would narrowly call their own behavior "correct."

53. C   Choice C is the most applicable to the meaning of the passage, which is about the diversity of customs (e.g., marriage, dress, bedding, and so on) among cultures. Choice A can be eliminated because it is too general. Choice B can be eliminated because the author does not mention the Bible in the passage. Also, the author's approach is clearly scientific, and he attempts to explain matters with verifiable observations. Choice D contradicts the main point (i.e., cultures are neither advanced nor backward, merely different) of the second paragraph.

54. B   The third paragraph points out that most of our daily behaviors arise from social norms, making choice B the best answer. Choice A is incorrect because the passage demonstrates that brushing teeth is a behavior not founded in human biology or natural law. Choice C may be true, but the influence of clever advertising is not mentioned in the passage. Choice D is incorrect because it is not supported by the passage.

55. A   Choice A is the best answer because it reflects the main idea of the passage (i.e., cultural norms form our behavior). Choice B is plausible because eating patterns may change over time; however, it is not as exact of a response as choice A, which emphasizes an individual's formative years. Choice C is also a plausible answer; however, it is not the best answer because the condition it affirms is a matter of natural law, not of cultural choice ("fit to eat").

56. A   *How Anthropology Explains Human Behavior* is the best title for the passage because it is the most specific and accurate title. *People of Culture* (choice B) is contrary to the thesis of the passage. *People are Different* (choice C) and *Human Behavior* (choice D) are too vague.

57. D   Statements I and II are matters of human biology and natural law, both of which the author credits for explaining human behavior. Choice A is incorrect because it includes statement III (fate), which is a concept not credited by the author for explanatory power.

58. D Choices A and C are incorrect. According to the passage, the Tellem appeared more than a thousand years after the Toloy disappeared, and the Dogon appeared after the Tellem. Choice B is not the best answer because the passage does not mention what happened to the Tellem.

59. C *The Dogon People* is the best title because the Dogon are mentioned in every paragraph of the passage. *The Mysteries of the Bandiagara* (choice A) and *Burial Caves in Mali and Their People* (choice D) are not the best titles because the Bandiagara and the burial caves are discussed only intermittently. *The Tellem and the Dogon* (choice B) is not the best title because mention of the Tellem occurs mainly in the introduction of the passage.

60. C Choice C is the best answer because the author mentions that both foxes and the land have spiritual connections.

61. B Eight is the number of ancestral spirits as well as the depth of the roof of the *togu na* (statement I). Carved columns are found only at the *togu na* and at the home of the spiritual leader (statement III). Except for the discussion of the men's shelter, male–female relations are not mentioned (statement III).

62. C The Dogon make rope from baobab bark, but apparently they do not use the tree for actual subsistence.

63. B The *ginna*, the *togu na*, and the *hogon's* house are all types of shelter. Only the *ginna* is shaped like a body (choice A), and only the *togu na* and the *hogon's* house have pillars (choice D). The passage does not specify if the *ginna* has a thatched roof (choice C).

64. D It is not clear from the passage why the Dogon use caves for burials. The passage states that the Dogon believe that burial caves are sacred, but the passage does not specifically mention that caves in general are sacred (choice B). The passage does not mention the Dogon's wanting to protect corpses from wild animals (choice A). The passage does not mention the Dogon's relation to the Tellem (choice C).

65. B The notched logs in crevices are centuries old and are still being used by the Dogon as ladders. The passage does not mention the distribution of the Dogon people (choice A) or their disposition (choice D). There is not enough information in the passage to infer that the Dogon preserve everything (choice C).

Physical Sciences

66. A To answer this question, Ohm's law ($V = IR$) is used to compare the currents flowing through the two resistors. Using Ohm's law, one finds that half as much current flows through resistor 2R.

67. B Choices A, C, and D are all true. These choices correctly describe elements of this circuit. Choice B is false for capacitors in parallel. However, note that choice B would be true for capacitors connected in series.

68. B This question tests the understanding of capacitors and dielectrics. One should know that $k = 1$ for a vacuum, and $k > 1$ for anything else. A dielectric increases the capacitance by a factor of k. Therefore, if the two capacitors are of values C and 2C, the dielectric must go in the smaller capacitor. It can only increase the capacitance, so in the larger capacitor, it is impossible to add a dielectric and give it the same capacitance as the smaller capacitor. A dielectric of $k = 2$ in the smaller capacitor will increase its capacitance to 2C.

69. A This question asks about alternating current sources. Use the process of elimination to arrive at the best answer. Choice B is correct based on the definition of I(rms). Choice C is correct for two resistors in series, because $I_{max} = (\sqrt{2}/2)V_{rms}$. Choice D is also a correct statement. Choice A is an incorrect statement, and the answer to this question. Note that power $= P = I^2R$, and I^2 is not averaged to 0.

70. D Choices A, B, and C are all correct statements regarding RC circuits. Choice D is an incorrect statement because the decay of the stored charge on the capacitor through the resistor depends only on the time constant RC.

71. A Recall that $Q = CV$. Since $C = 1 \times 10^{-11}$ farads, and $V = 800$ volts, $Q = (1 \times 10^{-11})(800) = 8 \times 10^{-9}$ C.

SECT. V
ANSWERS AND
EXPLANATIONS
TO FULL-LENGTH
MCAT

797

72. D The important information for determining the answer to this problem is in the second equation in the passage. The loss of a beta particle increases the atomic number by one, with no change in the mass number. Remember that the atomic number is the number of protons in the nucleus, and it is written on the bottom of the atomic symbol. The mass number is the total number of protons plus neutrons.

73. A Gold should be classified as an element of higher atomic mass based on the guideline given in the passage. Its atomic number is 79, which is certainly greater than 24. Therefore, a stable isotope of gold should have a greater number of neutrons than protons, making the ratio of neutrons to protons greater than 1.

74. A The answer to this question can be modeled after the first reaction in the passage. The loss of an alpha particle results in the loss of two protons and a decrease of four in the mass number (i.e., $84 - 2 = 82$, the atomic number of lead; $214 - 4 = 210$) which corresponds to choice A. Choices B, C, and D are incorrect because they have incorrect combinations of atomic number and mass number.

75. D Potassium has an atomic number of 19, which is less than the 24 protons required to be a higher molecular weight element as described in the passage. The most favorable neutron-to-proton ratio for a light element is 1. A mass number of 40 with 19 protons means that the element has $40 - 19 = 21$ neutrons. This means the neutron-to-proton ratio is greater than 1. If this element loses a beta particle, the mass number does not change, but the atomic number increases by one. The resulting element would have $40 - 20 = 20$ neutrons. Equal numbers of protons and neutrons make a more stable light isotope. Thus, potassium-40 would be expected to undergo loss of a beta particle to decrease the neutron-to-proton ratio.

76. B A gamma particle shows no deflection in an electric field as shown in Figure 1 of the passage. The alpha particle (with a $^+2$ charge, as stated in the passage) is deflected toward the negative side of the electric field. The beta particle, with a charge of $^-1$, like any electron, is deflected toward the positive side of the electric field. It should make sense that only uncharged particles would travel without deflection. Furthermore, one should know that a gamma particle is an uncharged photon.

77. C Use the process of elimination to determine the best answer. Choice C makes the most sense. Protons carry a charge of $^+1$, whereas neutrons carry no charge. Like charges repel each other, so separating protons by putting neutrons around them decreases the amount of repulsion in the nucleus. Choice A is incorrect because neutrons are not associated with attractive forces in the nucleus. Choice B is incorrect, as protons are not attracted to neutrons. Finally, choice D can be eliminated because neutrons do not hold electrons in association with the nucleus.

78. A The total energy is the sum of potential energy and kinetic energy. Because the kinetic energy of sphere A is 0 (i.e., it is not moving), the total energy equals the potential energy. The potential energy is simply equal to mgh (mass × gravity × height).

79. A Ignoring air friction, potential energy is converted to kinetic energy as sphere A swings down toward sphere B. Using the expression PE = KE, it follows that $mgh = \frac{1}{2}(mv^2)$. Note that the mass term drops out of this relationship when solving for the velocity.

80. D The conservation of energy relationship is used to determine the velocity of sphere A just before it hits sphere B. This velocity and the conservation of momentum equation is then used to determine the final velocity of mass 5M. Finally, the conservation of energy equation is used to determine final object height. The work is as follows: $\frac{1}{2}(mv_A^2) = mgh_o \rightarrow$ solve for velocity of sphere A (v_A). Next, use $5Mv_{5M} = mv_A$. This gives the velocity of mass 5M just after the collision. Last, $\frac{1}{2}(5M)(v_{5M})^2 = (5M)gh$. Solve for h, the maximum height.

81. D Choices A, B, and C are all true statements. Choice A states that there is no component of velocity in the horizontal direction if the ball is released exactly when it reaches the maximum point in its upward swing. Choice B states that the time it takes to hit the ground is a function of the acceleration and the height above the ground. Choice C states that particles of identical mass fall to the ground at the same rate (i.e., at g).

82. D   Choices A, B, and C are true statements. Choice D is a false statement. In an inelastic collision, the colliding bodies stick together, so that their final velocities are the same. This is not the case for elastic collisions.

83. A   A reaction that loses moles of gas becomes more ordered. A reaction that gains moles of gas becomes less ordered. A negative entropy is an unfavorable entropy change, and it represents a system becoming more ordered. Reaction 1 has 3 moles of gas on the left [3 $O_2(g)$] and only 2 moles on the right [2 $SO_2(g)$].

84. B   Endothermic reactions require energy input. The two indications in the passage about energy input are the first sentence of the second paragraph and the $h\nu$ in reaction 3. The paragraph states that smelting begins by heating, as shown in reaction 1. However, reaction 1 is not offered as an answer choice. Light ($h\nu$) is also a form of energy input, so reaction 3 must be endothermic. There is no evidence presented in the passage that reactions 2, 4, or 5 are endothermic. Therefore, choice B is the best answer.

85. A   A reactive intermediate is a species that is not isolated because of its high reactivity. Reactive intermediates are used as quickly as they are produced. The only compound listed that looks reactive is the charged species. Another way to find a reactive intermediate is to add together the steps of reaction 3 to find the overall equation. The reactive intermediates will not appear in the overall equation.

86. C   This question tests information recall. In the second sentence of the second paragraph the statement is made that metal oxides are more easily reduced to the free metal.

87. A   The hydrogen ion concentration of normal rain is $10^{-5.5}$ and of acid rain is $10^{-4.0}$. The difference between normal rain and acid rain is then $10^{-5.5} - 10^{-4.0}$. The result is a negative number because $10^{-4.0}$ is larger than $10^{-5.5}$. The question is, therefore, whether the answer is -1.5 or -9.7×10^{-5}. The hydrogen ion concentration of both normal rain and acid rain is not as large as 1.5, so the smaller number (-9.7×10^{-5}) makes the most sense (even without a calculator).

88. C   Kinematic relations should be used to determine the answer to this question. Recall that $v_f^2 - v_o^2 = 2ay$. Suppose that the object, which was at rest, is dropped from a height of 10 m. Then, $v_f^2 - 0 = 2(-10 \text{m/s}^2)(-10\text{m})$, $v_f^2 = 200 \text{ m}^2/\text{s}^2$, and $v_f \approx 14$ m/s. Now, if the object falls only 5 m, $v_f^2 - 0 = 2(-10 \text{ m/s}^2)(-5 \text{ m})$, $v_f^2 = 100 \text{ m}^2/\text{s}^2$, and $v_f = 10$ m/s. The ratio of 10:14 = 0.71.

89. D   The answer to this question can be determined via the following steps. First, the reaction described in the question should be balanced. For the decomposition of ammonia, the balanced reaction is: 2 $NH_3(g) \rightarrow N_2(g) + 3H_2(g)$. Thus, $K = [H_2]^3[N_2]/[NH_3]^2$. Substituting the given concentrations, $K = (.3)^3(.2)/(.1)^2$.

90. B   The mass (m) and radius (r) of the solid and hollow spheres in this question are the same. The only difference between these two shapes is the mass distribution. The solid sphere will have the larger linear velocity because it has the most mass in its center. A hollow sphere will have a larger rotational kinetic energy because it has a greater moment of inertia (I) than a solid sphere. Recall that the moment of inertia is directly proportional to mr^2 for most shapes, including spheres. This problem can be solved by comparing how far the mass is situated from the center of each sphere. Because nearly all of the mass of a hollow sphere is located a distance (r) away from its center, this gives it a greater I.

91. D   Catalysts increase the rates of reactions by lowering the activation. Catalysts accelerate both forward and backward reaction rates equally. They do not shift the equilibrium or change equilibrium concentrations.

92. B   The reaction starts with a total of 4 moles of gaseous reactants [1 mole $N_2(g)$ + 3 moles $H_2(g)$] and ends with only 2 moles gaseous product [2 moles $NH_3(g)$]. This is entropically unfavorable because the system becomes more ordered. Entropically unfavorable processes have negative entropy changes.

93. B   The yield increases with decreasing rather than increasing temperature, so only choices A and B need to be considered. Exothermic reactions (those that give off heat) continue if the heat that is produced is removed by cooling the reaction. An endothermic

SECT. V
ANSWERS AND
EXPLANATIONS
TO FULL-LENGTH
MCAT

799

reaction that requires heat produces a higher equilibrium yield when it is heated. Do not confuse equilibrium with kinetics. Both endothermic and exothermic reactions react faster when heated, but the position of the equilibrium does not depend on the rate of the reaction.

94. C High pressure favors the side of the reaction with fewer moles of gas. This is mainly due to the large volume occupied by a mole of gas (22.4 L at STP).

95. B Because the product is liquid ammonia, removing it by condensation decreases the concentration of ammonia. Removing ammonia by condensation also tends to pull the position of the equilibrium toward the right as the system tries to replace the missing component.

96. B The reaction may have a more favorable equilibrium at low temperatures, but is impractical for industrial use because of the speed of the reaction. Heating any reaction speeds it up, although the equilibrium position may not be as favorable. Industrially, this is an acceptable trade-off because many of the reagents can be recycled.

97. C The equilibrium constant (K_c) given in the passage for 25°C and a 1-L container is 6.0 $\times$ 10^5. $K_c = [NH_3]^2/[N_2][H_2]^3$ at equilibrium, or by using the values for moles of gas in the expression, $Q = \frac{9}{2}$. This makes Q much smaller than K_c. When Q is much smaller than K_c, the reaction proceeds to the right. In this case, that means that the concentration of ammonia will increase, and the concentrations of hydrogen and nitrogen will decrease.

PASSAGE VI

98. C Light is an example of transverse wave motion, with the electric (E) and magnetic (B) fields perpendicular to each other and to the direction of travel. Sound is a longitudinal wave.

99. A This question appears complex, yet the solution is simple. Recall that $\sin\theta_c = n_r/n_i$. Thus, for the light ray to be internally reflected, $\sin\theta_i \geq n_r/n_i$. If $n_r = 1$ (air), then $\sin\theta_i \geq 1/n$ is simply the condition for total internal reflection.

100. B In a media of refractive index (n), the wavelength becomes $1/n$ times the original wavelength. Thus, for a wavelength of 700 nm to become 400 nm, the n value must have been $7/4$. This is because $[1/n](700$ nm] should equal 400 nm. $[(1)/(7/4)](700) = 400$ nm.

101. A The oscillation of E (electric field) and B (magnetic field) are at the same frequency as used for determination of the photon energy. Therefore, if f_w is increased, the frequency of the photons associated with the electromagnetic wave will increase.

102. C Choice C is incorrect if based on the principle of Snell's law. For choices A and B, note that the higher the energy or frequency of the light wave, the greater the extent to which it is refracted. Therefore, the highest frequencies and energies and the lowest wavelengths are expected to be at the top of the screen.

PASSAGE VII

103. A The passage states that light energy is used to drive an endothermic reaction. Because reaction 2 is just reaction 1 written backward, its ΔH is just the negative of that for reaction 1. The ΔH for reaction 1 is given (198 kJ), so the ΔH for reaction 2 is −198 kJ. An endothermic reaction is one that absorbs energy from the surroundings (a positive enthalpy change), so the solar energy will drive reaction 1.

104. B In compartment B, heat is given off. This indicates that the exothermic reaction occurs here. An exothermic reaction gives off heat to the system as indicated by a negative ΔH. Therefore, reaction 2 occurs in compartment B.

105. C This is a simple question. Assume that the reaction occurs as it is written. Because reaction 2 is just the reverse of reaction 1, change the sign of ΔH for reaction 1 to obtain the ΔH of reaction 2. Thus, the ΔH of reaction 2 is ⁻198 kJ.

106. C Note that reaction 1 requires energy (endothermic), because it has a positive ΔH. Therefore, the products must be higher in energy than the reactants. Only diagram C shows an endothermic reaction. Choices B and D are incorrect because they show exothermic reactions. Choice A is incorrect because the products have a similar energy content as the reactants.

107. B Without a catalyst, the energy changes in reaction 2 should simply be the reverse of the energy changes in reaction 1. The reactants are higher in energy than the products.

108. D A catalyst provides a pathway with a lower activation energy, but the reactants and the products have the same energy as in the uncatalyzed reaction. Look for a diagram with the same starting and ending heights as in diagram B but with a lower "hill."

109. C Some molecules can absorb certain wavelengths of light, which transfers the light energy to the molecule. This moves the molecule to a higher energy or excited state. This higher energy state is more reactive than the ground state of that atom because it is less stable.

PASSAGE VIII

110. D Choices A, B, and C do not deal with the photoelectric effect. Choice D is correct because absorption of light by matter in energy quanta is the assumption of the photoelectric effect.

111. D This question requires information recall. The answer simply follows from the definition given in the passage text; that is, W is the work function of the metal. Choice C is incorrect because W strictly refers to photoejection of an electron.

112. A To answer this question, the following relationship should be used: $E = h (c/\lambda)$. The values of h and c are given in the passage. The value of the wavelength should be substituted into the relationship. Solving for E, one will see that the energy of the incident photons is greater than the work function given. This means that choice A is correct, because an E value greater than the work function gives photoejection.

113. B By convention, all charge carriers are positive and current flows in the direction that these charges move. Electrons move from photocathode to the collector. Therefore, current travels from collector to photocathode. The direction of the B field comes from the right hand rule. Recall that the right hand rule states that if the fingers of the right hand are wrapped around the wire, and the thumb is pointed in the direction that the electrical current travels, the fingers curl in the direction of the induced B field. Using the right hand rule, one finds that the induced B field is directed into the page at point III.

114. A Increasing the intensity of the beam increases the frequency of the photons emitted but not their energy. Choice B is incorrect because increased light intensity gives increased current. Choices C and D are incorrect because the kinetic energy and work function do not directly relate to the intensity of the beam.

INDEPENDENT QUESTIONS

115. C This question involves classic optical refraction. A light ray always bends toward the normal when traveling from an area of lower-to-higher n value, and away from the normal when traveling from an area of higher-to-lower n value.

116. A This challenging problem can be solved in two steps. First, the direction of the magnetic field due to the wire must be determined. The right hand rule can be applied in this step. Then, the right hand rule can be applied again to find the direction of motion of the charge. Suppose the initial wire is drawn on a piece of paper vertically, with the direction of current upward. Using the right hand rule (i.e., thumb pointed in direction of current, palm around wire), the B field is found to be directed into and out of the plane of the paper. To determine the direction of the negative charge, the back of the hand is placed toward the direction of the force (back of hand for negative charge, palm for positive charge), with straightened fingers in the direction of the B field. The right thumb points in the direction that the charge travels. It may be helpful to use the choices as possible options for the direction of travel (i.e., the direction of the right thumb). The charge in this question is negative, so the direction must be reversed if the direction of current is used to apply the right hand rule. If this question was difficult, review the electromagnetism chapter in the Physics Review Notes.

117. A Note that both salts dissociate as follows: $XY_2 \rightarrow X + 2Y$, with $K_{sp} = [X][Y]^2$, and $WY_2 \rightarrow W + 2Y$, with a $K_{sp} = [W][Y]^2$. Note that the two salts dissociate similarly and share a similar ion (Y). Because it is stated that the atomic weight of X is greater than W, it makes sense that for an equal number of moles of salt dissociated, a greater number of grams of XY_2 would dissolve than WY_2.

118. A This difficult physics question can be solved in three steps. First, the conservation of energy is used to determine the velocity of M just before impact. Because $Mgh = \frac{1}{2}mv_i^2$, $v_i = (2gh)^{1/2} = (20h)^{1/2}$. In the second step, the conservation of momentum is used to determine the velocity of the masses just after the impact, v_f. $Mv_i = (M + 2M)v_f$. Solving for v_f gives $(20h)^{1/2}/3$. Finally, the conservation of energy is used again to determine the height to which the masses rise $(M + 2M)gh_f = \frac{1}{2}(M + 2M)v_f^2$. Solving for h_f gives $h_f = \frac{1}{9}h$.

SECT. V
ANSWERS AND
EXPLANATIONS
TO FULL-LENGTH
MCAT

801

119. D The first step in answering this question is remembering that $\Delta G = \Delta H - T\Delta S$. The second important consideration is that to subtract two numbers, the numbers must have the same units. The units on the given enthalpy are kJ and for the given entropy are J/K (this unit requires that the temperature be in Kelvins). Therefore $\Delta G = 1340$ kJ $-$ $(1000°C + 273)(586$ J/K$)(1$kJ/1000J$)$.

120. C The total energy required to recycle 1 mole of aluminum will be the amount of heat needed to get the metal to its melting point, plus the amount of heat needed to actually melt it. To get the metal to its melting point, look at the units on the specific heat [0.900 J/(g°C)]. To get energy out of this, the specific heat needs to be multiplied by a mass and a temperature change. The mass is simply the mass of 1 mole, or 27 g, and the temperature is 660°C, initial temperature. The initial temperature was not given in the passage, so standard conditions should be assumed. To actually melt 1 mole of aluminum, the heat of fusion (10.7 kJ/mole) must be added to the previous value. Overall, the answer is 27.0 g/mole $\times$ 0.900 J/(g°C) $\times$ (660 $-$ 25) (1 kJ/1000J) + 10.7 kJ/mole.

121. C The free energy is calculated by the equation $\Delta G = \Delta H - T\Delta S$. A favorable free energy change is a negative free energy change. To make the free energy more negative, $T\Delta S$ should be a large positive number. The largest temperature given is 1000°C (which converts to 1832°F). If you have forgotten the conversion between celsius and Fahrenheit, just compare two values you know. Since water boils at 100°C and 212°F, 100°C must be hotter than 100°F. Therefore, a reaction run at 1000°C has a higher $T\Delta S$ than a reaction run at 1000°F.

122. A The carbon is oxidized from the zero oxidation state to the +2 oxidation state. Oxidation always occurs at the anode. Two mnemonics may help you to remember which electrode is which. AN(ode) OX(idation) and a RED(uction) CAT(hode) is one. Or, simply remember that anode and oxidation both begin with vowels, and reduction and cathode both begin with consonants.

123. C This is a simple question, and Figure 1 in the passage can be used to help determine the answer. Note that the diagram shows the aluminum sinking and the cryolite floating on top. This suggests that the aluminum is more dense.

124. D To find the final temperature of the slabs after thermal equilibrium, the masses, heat capacities, and the temperature difference between the slabs must be known. Choices A B, and C are incorrect because the quantities of k, α, and W are not important in determining the final slab temperatures.

125. A In a steady-state condition, there is equal transfer of heat energy from one slab to the other. Choice A is a correct statement and is a general statement. It is supported by the concept of heat transfer, which is described in the passage. Choice B is incorrect because steady state does not necessarily mean that there is no heat flow. Choices C and D are incorrect because the net heat flow at specific regions of the slabs is not totally predictable with the information given in the passage. Notice that choices B, C, and D are emphatic statements and not difficult to eliminate.

126. D Note the formula given in the passage that describes the thermal expansion for length: $\Delta L = \alpha L \Delta T$. The question states that T is equivalent for all the choices. For slabs with equivalent lengths L, the choice with the largest value of α will have the greatest ΔL. Looking at Table 1 in the passage, ice (given in water row) has the greatest value of α.

127. D A lower k value implies higher thermal insulation. In the table, ice (water row) has the lowest k value, and it is therefore the best thermal insulator.

128. C Recall that the lower the C_p, the easier it is to warm that material per unit area. Lead is noted in Table 1 to have the lowest C_p, thus it warms the most when given a specific amount of heat energy.

129. B Note that the question makes it clear that straight lines and curved lines should be treated similarly when considering the percent change in length for a solid. The question asks about the fractional change in volume of a sphere. Volume is a three-dimensional measurement. Because it is stated that curved lines lengthen in the ratio α per degree temperature rise, the three-dimensional component suggests multiplying by three. An exponential relationship is not correct because terms with exponents were not among the answer choices. Thus, the best answer is 3α.

130. **B**   The separation factor depends on the ratio between the square roots of the molecular weight. The closer together the molecular weights are, the smaller the separation factor will be. The greatest difference in molecular weight is between ^1H and ^3H.

131. **C**   The lighter molecule will effuse faster. If this is not obvious, choose some sample molecular weights to plug into the formula given in the passage to see that if MW_1 is smaller, the ratio is greater than 1, and if it is larger, the ratio is less than 1.

132. **A**   The only variable that appears in the equation is molecular weight, therefore, temperature has no effect on the efficiency of the separation. Speed does depend on the temperature, but it cancels out in the ratio.

133. **A**   As in question 132, the only variable that appears in the equation is molecular weight. Therefore, only the molecular weight has a direct effect on the separation. Increasing pressure has no effect on the efficiency of the separation.

134. **A**   Again, because molecular weight is the only variable in the equation, only molecular weight has a direct effect. Increasing the pressure on the empty side of the membrane has no effect on the efficiency of the separation.

135. **D**   An increase in temperature (addition of heat) makes all gas molecules effuse faster. Therefore, the speed of the separation would be increased if the temperature was increased.

136. **A**   The kinetic molecular theory of gases indicates that the kinetic energy of a gas sample is dependent only on the temperature of the gas. Therefore, pressure changes will not change the speed of the separation.

137. **A**   The amount of current going through the 3-ohm resistor cannot be determined until the net current (I) travelling through the basic (series) circuit is determined. First, determine net I. Recall that Ohm's law says $V = IR$, so $I = V/R$. The figure shows that there are 12 volts, but the total (net) resistance (R) is needed. So, parallel resistor $R \rightarrow 1/R = 1/3 + 1/6 = 3/6$, so R = 2 ohms for the parallel resistor connection. This, in addition to the single 2-ohm resistor to the left of the parallel connection gives a net R = 2 + 2 = 4 ohms. Thus, the net $I = V/R = 12$ volts/4 ohms = 3 amps. Thus, a total of 3 amps enter the parallel junction, and are divided in a ratio inverse to the resistor's resistance. This means that 2 of the 3 amps would travel through the 3-ohm resistor, and only 1 amp would travel through the 6-ohm resistor. This should make sense because the 6-ohm resistor has twice the resistance of the 3-ohm resistor—it is twice as difficult to get current through it.

138. **B**   Determining the answer to this question requires knowing that power = work/time.

139. **A**   Buffer solutions are comprised of weak acids or bases and their salts. These solutions resist changes in pH. For an overview of this topic, review the chapter on buffers in the General Chemistry Review Notes.

140. **C**   A magnifying glass is often referred to as a simple microscope. In this system, a converging lens is placed nearer to an object than is its focal length from the object so that a virtual, upright image is formed on the same side of the lens. This makes sense conceptually using the example of using a magnifying glass: The image is on the same side of the lens as the object, which is the definition of a virtual image for a lens.

141. **A**   Nonspontaneous processes have positive ΔG values. Since $\Delta G = \Delta H - T\Delta S$, ΔG is positive when ΔH is greater than $T\Delta S$.

142. **C**   This challenging question requires that sound travel and the Doppler principle are understood. When the horn in sounded, a person standing on the boat hears a frequency associated with this sound. A person standing on a cliff who heard the horn from the approaching boat perceives a frequency higher than the person on the boat. This is caused by the Doppler effect. An echo of the horn heard by a person on the boat (choice C) would be perceived at an even higher frequency because the echo of the sound bounces off the cliff wall and returns toward the boat. The boat, in turn, approaches the cliff from which the echo rebounded.

Biological Sciences

PASSAGE I

143. A Anterior pituitary hormones are expected to be peptide derivatives. The passage discusses two enzymes: peptidase and lipase. Peptidase cleaves peptide bonds, and lipase degrades lipids. This question tests if you know which hormone type is a peptide (i.e., a protein that is made up of amino acids). All pituitary hormones are peptides. Hormones produced by the ovary or testes are steroids. Thyroid hormone is iodinated.

144. C The graafian follicle eventually forms the corpus luteum. The corpus luteum produces progesterone, which in turn, feeds back to the hypothalamus and pituitary to regulate (inhibit) the production and release of follicle-stimulating hormone (FSH) and luteinizing hormone (LH). This process is termed negative feedback.

145. B Human chorionic gonadotropin (hCG) sustains pregnancy by maintaining the production of progesterone by the ovary. This is a knowledge-based question. The passage does not mention hCG but does state that progesterone stimulates the endometrium to mature and develop glandular structures.

146. B Drug X is most similar in structure to progesterone. In analyzing Figure 1, one can see that drug X blocks the release of LH, which prevents ovulation. The hormone that has this same action naturally is progesterone. Progesterone acts by a negative-feedback mechanism to block LH release. Estrogen, FSH, or LH are less likely choices.

147. D A head injury damaging the hypothalamus would most likely directly affect the release of FSH and LH. Recall that the hypothalamus produces releasing factors that stimulate anterior pituitary production and the release of FSH and LH. In addition, the products that FSH and LH ultimately stimulate—estrogen and progesterone—would likely be affected. If much less FSH and LH are produced, the ovary will likely produce less estrogen and progesterone. Thus, all choices are correct (i.e., statements I, II, and III).

148. C Curve 2 most likely represents estrogen. This can be determined first by looking at curve one. This curve rises after ovulation. Therefore, curve 1 must represent progesterone, which is produced by the corpus luteum after ovulation. Curve 2 has two peaks, one before ovulation and one after ovulation. The other two curves have a single peak only prior to or at the time of ovulation. The dotted peak that just precedes ovulation is LH. This surge causes ovulation to occur. The lowest curve is FSH. This means that curve 2 is estrogen. The first peak of curve 2 corresponds to the release of estrogen that causes endometrial maturation. The second peak, which occurs with the progesterone peak, prepares the endometrium for implantation of a fertilized zygote.

149. D The finding that drug X blocked menstruation does not support the conclusion that drug X mimics estrogen. The question asks which finding *least* supports the conclusion. If drug X caused endometrial growth or secondary sexual characteristics, then it would mimic estrogen. Thus, choice A (caused growth of the endometrium) and choice B (caused secondary sexual characteristics) can be eliminated. If drug X acted like estrogen, then it would cause negative feedback control of FSH. Thus, choice C (decreased levels of circulating FSH) can be eliminated. Choice D is the best choice because blocking menstruation is a function of progesterone.

PASSAGE II

150. A Sodium hydroxide is both a strong base and a strong nucleophile. Chemist 1 indicated that such reagents would always produce a mixture of the substitution and the elimination products. Choice A is challenged the most because, as a base, sodium hydroxide would be expected to lead to formation of the elimination product. Only the substitution product is formed (ethanol). The other choices are not as clearly contradicted by the passage.

151. B Tert-butyl bromide is a tertiary substrate in which the carbon bearing the leaving group is very hindered. According to the statement of chemist 2, such substrates should undergo elimination rather than substitution. The tert-butyl alcohol observed in the experiment is a substitution product.

152. C Chemist 2 argued that the competition between substitution and elimination reactions is governed by steric factors. Although 1-bromo-2,2-dimethylpropane is a primary halide, it has a tertiary carbon adjacent to the carbon bearing the leaving group. This tertiary group hinders the nucleophile's approach to the back of the carbon bearing the leaving group, and substitution occurs very slowly.

153. **C** The arguments put forth by chemist 2 seem to ignore that some substrate can form carbocations. Carbocations can either substitute or eliminate based on the relative basicity and nucleophilicity of the reagent. Thus, a hindered substrate can undergo substitution, but by the S_N1 rather than the S_N2 mechanism.

154. **C** Chemist 1 would expect a mixture of products because sodium hydroxide is both a strong base and a strong nucleophile. Chemist 2 would expect a mixture of products because the substrate is somewhat but not highly hindered.

155. **B** The cells that are most associated with the progression of osteoporosis are osteoclasts. The progression of osteoporosis and the calcium association are discussed in the second paragraph of the passage. Osteoporosis leads to calcium being removed from bone. The cells that resorb bone are osteoclasts. Osteoblasts form bone, and osteocytes maintain bone.

156. **D** Calcitonin is a hormone that might reverse the changes associated with osteoporosis. Calcitonin decreases serum calcium by incorporating calcium into bone. Choice B (parathyroid hormone) is incorrect because parathyroid hormone tends to resorb bone. Choice A (testosterone) and choice C (thyroid hormone) are not supported by the passage.

157. **A** Ingrowth of osteoblasts and osteoclasts (choice A) would be expected during the early healing phase of a bony fracture. Following a bony fracture, bone remodeling occurs. Bone remodeling requires both osteoblast and osteoclast participation (i.e., continual new "building" and continual "destructive" repair of bone structure, respectively). Choice B (growth of the periosteum) is incorrect because although the periosteum may heal following a fracture, it is not the primary activity of early bony healing. Choice C (activation of the growth plate) is incorrect because the growth plate gives rise to long-bone growth, not fracture healing. Choice D (development of haversian systems and canaliculi) is incorrect because haversian systems form in mature bone, not early healing bone.

158. **D** Following calcium supplementation, the level of parathyroid hormone would be expected to decrease. Hormones that increase serum calcium levels, such as parathyroid hormone, decrease because an outside supply of calcium has been added. Calcitonin levels might rise in an effort to decrease serum calcium levels. Adrenocorticotropic hormone (ACTH) and thyroid hormone levels would probably not change.

159. **C** Rapidly progressive osteoporosis would lead to elevated serum calcium, which would cause calcium to be excreted into the urine. Elevated estrogen levels would be expected if estrogen was used as a treatment for osteoporosis. Calcitonin decreases serum calcium by incorporating the serum calcium into bone. Vitamin D is associated with improved calcium absorption.

160. **D** The amino acid with the highest pK_a value is the most basic. This can be determined by looking at the values in the table. Look for the side chain pK_a with the largest value; that is, arginine.

161. **D** Acidic amino acids will always have pK_a values below 7. This is because acidic amino acids have both carboxyl groups and acidic side groups. This can also be determined by looking at the values in the table. Note that only aspartate has a pK_a value below 7.

162. **B** The K_a is determined by taking the antilog of the negative pK_a (i.e., 10^{-pK_a}). This problem must be solved by the process of elimination without a calculator. Work backward by seeing which choice could produce a value of 6 when the antilog of the negative pK_a is taken. This would be 10^{-6}, or 1×10^{-6}.

163. **D** This is an information recall question. All of the acidic and basic amino acids are classified as hydrophilic in the passage.

164. **C** Contact between a hydrophobic amino acid and water is unfavorable because the water forms an entropically unfavorable structure to maximize hydrogen bonding with other

SECT. V
ANSWERS AND
EXPLANATIONS
TO FULL-LENGTH
MCAT

805

water molecules. Choice A (water is repelled by the amino acid) and choice B (the amino acid is repelled by the water) contradict basic principles of intermolecular attractions. The only repulsive force is that between like charges. Because neither water nor a hydrophobic amino acid is charged, they should not repel each other until their electron clouds are close enough to repel each other. Thus, the repulsive force between water and a hydrophobic amino acid is no greater than between two hydrophobic amino acids. The actual separation observed between water and a hydrophobic substance such as oil is caused by water organizing itself to maximize hydrogen bonds.

INDEPENDENT QUESTIONS

165. D This question tests basic cell biology knowledge. Recall that the Golgi apparatus is especially important in protein modification and processing. Choice A (ribosome) and choice B (rough endoplasmic reticulum) refer to organelles that are important in translation (protein synthesis), whereas choice C (lysosome) refers to an organelle that contains powerful digestive enzymes.

166. A Recall that RNA polymerase is responsible for transcription. RNA polymerase binds to the promoter site in the lactose (lac) operon system. Lactose acts as the inducer substance. In the absence of the inducer substance, the repressor protein binds to the operator, which blocks the binding of RNA polymerase to the promoter. In the presence of lactose, the inducer (lactose) binds to the repressor protein itself and inactivates it. DNA polymerase is involved in DNA replication and has nothing to do with the lactose operon.

167. A An asymmetric carbon or chiral carbon has four different substituents attached to it. In this molecule, there is no carbon atom with four different substituents. Thus, there are no chiral carbons.

168. D Oxytocin, produced by the posterior pituitary gland, stimulates smooth muscle contraction during labor and lactation. Of the four choices listed, oxytocin is least likely to increase during dehydration. Choices A, B, and C would be likely to increase so that body water is conserved.

PASSAGE V

169. A Notice that the trait appears in every generation; there are no skipped generations. This is classic autosomal dominant transmission. Choice B (sex-linked recessive) is false because female children of men with the condition are affected by the condition rather than just being carriers. Choice C (autosomal recessive) is false because offspring have the condition with only one parent expressing the condition. Random mutation (choice D) is rare and certainly cannot explain occurrence in each generation.

170. A The principle of segregation describes the segregation of homologous chromosomes in meiosis. Notice the segregation of the brachydactyly gene in this pedigree. Independent assortment refers to independent assortment of nonhomologous chromosomes. Nondisjunction refers to homologous chromosomes not disjoining (from each other) at the first meiotic division; this gives abnormalities of chromosomal number. Random mutations do not reappear at each generation.

171. D An autosomal dominant inheritance pattern (choice A) requires an afflicted individual in each generation. Choice B (sex-linked recessive) is incorrect because males cannot be carriers in sex-linked conditions. Autosomal recessive inheritance (choice C) is false because an unshaded male in generation II would be a carrier; his partner cannot be a carrier based on the information given in the passage. Thus, there is no way autosomal recessive transmission can work. Choice D is the only possible choice.

172. C The passage states that microcephaly is a rare, autosomal recessive trait. Choice A (affected members in each generation) is incorrect because it describes autosomal dominant traits. Choice B (woman always produces affected sons) is incorrect because only half of her sons would inherit a microcephaly gene, and they would be carriers. Choice D (males mating with homozygous normal females produce half microcephalic and half normal sons) is incorrect because all offspring of the described cross would produce carrier children (who are phenotypically normal). Choice C (microcephaly would likely be found in offspring of heterozygous family members who mate) is correct because a heterozygous cross produces some homozygous recessive offspring.

173. C Hemophilia is a sex-linked recessive trait, as mentioned in the passage. The discussion of question 169 excluded sex-linked transmission as a possible mode of inheritance.

174. C If *B* stands for the dominant brachydactyly gene, and *b* is the normal gene, the cross would likely be: Bb × Bb. Offspring genotypes and ratios would be: 1 BB, 2 Bb, 1 bb. Thus, three fourths of the offspring would be afflicted (i.e., have BB and Bb genotypes). Only the child with the bb genotype would be normal (i.e., not carry the unfortunate phenotype).

PASSAGE VI

175. B The purpose of homogenization is to make a mixture uniform (i.e., homogeneous). Homogenization is discussed in the second paragraph of the passage. Choice A is incorrect because there is no separation of useful from less useful parts in homogenization. Choice C is incorrect because homogenization does not actually make any of the following steps of the extraction easier, only more efficient. Choice D (dividing the solid into small pieces to be strained out) is not supported or implied by the passage.

176. C Acidic species have two forms: the neutral, protonated form, and the negatively charged, deprotonated form. The negatively charged form is more water soluble and is the major component when an adequate amount of base has been added.

177. C Components found in the organic layer should be relatively hydrophobic. Polar groups can be present if a significant portion of the molecule is hydrocarbon-like. Of the choices given, only choice C is significantly hydrophobic and is clearly the most soluble in the organic layer. Choices A, B, and D are not as likely because they are small molecules with polar side groups.

178. D The advantage of using a base in the extraction following extraction with hydrochloric acid is that a base will react with acidic components in the mixture to make water-soluble salts. The water-soluble salts will partition into the aqueous layer, which greatly aids in the extraction of the acidic components of the mixture.

179. A Charged species are very water soluble because of ion–dipole interactions. Thus, the form of para-aminobenzoic acid that contains neither a positive nor a negative charge would be the least water soluble species, as is shown in choice A. Choices B, C, and D are incorrect because they have charged side groups and tend to demonstrate an element of solubility in water. A substance with both a positive and a negative charge, as shown in choice B, is known as a zwitterion.

PASSAGE VII

180. C The first section of the curve in the C_0t plot for *Escherichia coli* depicts a slow, constant rate of DNA renaturation. Look at the lighter curve for *E. coli*. The flat, first section of this curve implies a slow renaturation of DNA. It slopes downward gently, so some renaturation is occurring. Choices A and B are incorrect because renaturation is occurring slowly. Choice D is incorrect because DNA denaturation is not demonstrated in the plot.

181. A This is a conceptual question. A student should know that bacterial DNA is a double-stranded, circular chromosome structure. Bacteria contain neither a nucleus, nor histone proteins (DNA-associated proteins).

182. B Notice that calf thymus DNA renatures rapidly. The passage states in the last sentence of the first paragraph that rapid renaturation is associated with repetitive sequences. Repetition implies homogeneity. One should look for homogenous fragments in the answer choices. Thus, choice A (heterogenous with respect to kinetics) can be eliminated. The DNA of *E. coli* is more heterogenous because its renaturation is slow. Thus, choices C and D are incorrect.

183. D Recall that all cells of the same animal contain the same DNA (genetic information). Cells from different individuals within the same species have very similar DNA. Similar plots are found for similar samples of DNA, which contain the same primary sequence. Choices A, B, and C are incorrect because DNA expression, translation, and chromosome number are not as relevant.

184. D As discussed in question 182, rapid changes indicate sequence repetition. This is stated in the passage at the end of the first paragraph.

185. A Because the DNA of *E. coli* is initially slow to renature, it likely has few repetitive sequences. Calf thymus DNA renatures rapidly, which suggests repetitive sequences. Chromosome number (choice D) and fragment size (choice B) are irrelevant.

SECT. V
ANSWERS AND
EXPLANATIONS
TO FULL-LENGTH
MCAT

807

186. B Figure 1 in the passage shows that the configuration at the anomeric center changed from alpha to beta. This is known as inversion of configuration. Because configuration changed, choice A is incorrect. Recall that racemization relates to enan-tiomer inter-conversion. Thus, choices C and D are incorrect because the passage gives no indication that racemization occurs, and there is no evidence for it in the diagram.

187. C The final paragraph of the passage states that the glucuronides formed in this reaction are more hydrophilic (meaning more water soluble). The passage also states that the glucuronides can be filtered from the bloodstream by the kidneys.

188. C A phase II reaction involves high-energy intermediates. Oxidation, hydrolysis, and reduction do not involve high-energy intermediates. Glucuronide formation involves uridine diphosphate (UDP)–glucuronic acid as the high-energy intermediate.

189. D The substitution occurs at the anomeric center, with part of the drug molecule acting as the nucleophile and the phosphate acting as a leaving group. Because the phosphate group has an oxygen π-bonded to the phosphorus, the leaving group is stabilized by multiple resonance forms. Choices A, B, and C should be eliminated because they label the role of the phosphate in this reaction incorrectly.

190. D To form a glucuronide, the molecule must have a nucleophilic portion. Out of the possibilities shown, the amino group (NH_2) is the most significantly nucleophilic.

191. A Choice A provides the definition of anomers. Enantiomers are nonsuperimposable mirror-image structures (stereoisomers) that rotate light in opposite directions. Epimers are diastereoisomeric aldoses (sugars) that differ in configuration about carbon 2.

192. D Basic embryologic and development concepts should be reviewed in answering this question. Recall that induction requires some physical or chemical contact between two adjacent or nearby developing tissues. Placing a nonpermeable sheet between the two tissues prevents the needed interaction from happening, thus induction, differentiation, and subsequent tissue development cannot occur.

193. C The *trans* isomers are less polar than the *cis* isomers. Consider an example of an alkene with two electronegative substituents. If these substituents were in the *trans* configuration (substituents on opposite sides of the molecule), there would be some cancelling of polarity vectors. In the *cis* configuration (substituents on same side of the molecule), there is an additive action of the polarity vectors.

194. B In this case, as in most cases, exocrine function refers to the transport of important digestive enzymes and products via ducts to a final site. Thus, if the pancreatic or common bile ducts are blocked for some reason (e.g., gallstone, tumor, inflammation), the exocrine (duct) system of the pancreas would be greatly impaired (i.e., completely shut down). The back-up of pancreatic enzymes can lead to severe problems, including enzymatic breakdown of the pancreas.

195. D This question reviews most of the important biology of the ABO blood-type system. People with type AB blood would be expected to have antibodies against neither A nor B antigens (choice D). People with blood type AB have both A and B antigens on the surface of their red blood cells (RBCs), and, hopefully, no antibodies to themselves. Antibodies to one's own RBCs leads to quick destruction of the RBCs.

196. B The P_{450} enzyme system would be the most appropriate mechanism for processing alcohol in the liver. Alcohol is a very polar molecule that is not very lipophilic. Therefore, one can assume alcohol is not metabolized via conjugation (choice A). Phagocytosis (choice C) by Kupffer cells is said to involve metabolism of foreign matter, antigens, and old red blood cells. Direct excretion of alcohol in the urine (choice D) is not supported by the passage. With a general knowledge of biology one should know that the liver metabolizes ethanol (alcohol).

197. D Secreting metabolized toxins into bile allows for the direct passage of that substance out of the gastrointestinal tract via feces transport. Bile components pass from the liver, through the bile storage and duct systems, into the intestine, and eventually out of the body through the anus. Passage of metabolized toxins via a transporter (e.g., bile) is a common occurrence.

198. A This question relates to the topic discussed in the last paragraph of the passage, but the answer comes from one's own knowledge of endocrinology (i.e., the answer is not given in the passage). Glucagon is the hormone produced by the pancreas (endocrine function) that is responsible for the removal of glucose moieties from glycogen stores in the liver. Increased glucose entry into the blood allows for increased free glucose availability to "hungry" body tissues.

199. D The spleen is the master filter and processor of old or damaged red blood cells. This is a knowledge-based question; the answer is not given in the passage. The thymus plays a role in the maturation of lymphocytes (T cells). The pancreas produces digestive enzymes, such as insulin, glucagon, somatostatin, and bicarbonate. The adrenal medulla is responsible for epinephrine and norepinephrine hormonal production.

200. C The answer to the question comes from one's basic knowledge of biology. Recall that the portal vein drains the small intestine, which is where most nutrient absorption occurs. Thus, the portal vein contains blood that is very highly concentrated with important gastrointestinal nutrients and macromolecules. The thoracic duct (choice A) drains lymphatics, and the hepatic vein (choice B) drains the liver (it connects the liver to the inferior vena cava). The hepatic artery (choice D) transports fresh, highly oxygenated blood from the aorta to the liver.

201. A Recall that the liver metabolizes amino acids and forms urea as a waste product. Urea is then excreted from the body in the urine. Choices B, C, and D describe organ functions and processes that are incorrect.

202. C The last two sentences of the first paragraph in the passage state that the P_{450} enzymes are inducible and that repeated exposure to substances requiring P_{450} metabolism can lead to additional enzyme synthesis. Thus, one could predict increased transcription of P_{450} genes in liver cells. Choices A, B, and D do not use terms that best describe how P_{450}-producing cells generate more enzyme product (i.e., the transcription of P_{450}-coding genes with subsequent translation and protein processing).

---

203. A The correct answer comes from the passage (or one's own knowledge of immunology). The last sentence of the second paragraph states that it is the variable region that provides the antigen-binding sites (i.e., specificity) for the antibody. The third paragraph overviews gene rearrangement as the source of antibody diversity. The fourth paragraph again discusses generation of antibody diversity.

204. B The statement that the animal must be able to generate a specific antibody for each antigen that is encountered (choice B) best explains why antibody diversity is important and necessary. The importance of antibody diversity is pointed out in the first paragraph of the passage.

205. D Recall that a mature B cell that secretes antibodies is called a plasma cell. T lymphocytes play many roles in the immune system but do not produce antibodies. Recall that there are three types of T cells (i.e., helper, suppressor, and killer). Neutrophils primarily act as phagocytic cells for bacteria. Macrophages are phagocytic cells for bacteria, organic matter, and cellular debris. Macrophages are also involved in presenting antigen to other cells in the immune system.

206. D Choice D (the cell will most likely be unable to respond to antigen Y) is the best answer because it is stated that the immature cell was exposed to X and matured only with previous exposure to antigen Y. That is, the cell is naive to antigen Y. It is not stated that the cell had previously been exposed to or could cross-respond to antigen Y.

207. D The injected bacterial cells are identical to each other, but each has many different potential surface antigens. Therefore, the many B cells can begin responding to the bacterial antigens. Recall that each B cell selectively responds to one specific antigenic determinant. Thus, many different specific antibodies will be produced, each of which is produced and secreted by a specific B cell.

SECT. V
ANSWERS AND
EXPLANATIONS
TO FULL-LENGTH
MCAT

809

208. B   AIBN forms two alkyl radicals (R•) when heated, as shown in the equation in the passage. One of these radicals attacks an ethylene to initiate the reaction according to the following mechanism:

$$R\bullet \qquad H_2C = CH_2 \longrightarrow RCH_2 - CH_2\bullet$$

209. C   The two methods mentioned in the passage for initiating the reactive species are light and heat. The friction generated by stirring (choice A) or shaking (choice B) would not be sufficient to initiate the reaction. However, the use of an appropriate wavelength of light would be sufficient to generate radicals. Choice D is incorrect because energy input is required for the initiation process.

210. C   Two important clues are given in the passage to determine what reactive species is formed by the reaction of an initiator with propane. First, the passage states that the radical formed in the first propagation step is generally the more stable radical when more than one are possible. Second, the last paragraph of the passage gives a clue by stating "abstraction of a hydrogen atom from alkanes." Because propane is an alkane (i.e., there are no double bonds), the product should be the radical formed by the removal of a hydrogen atom. Therefore, choices B and D can be eliminated. Because a secondary radical is more stable than a primary radical, choice C is better than choice A.

211. D   The passage states that a termination step is one in which two reactive species combine to form an unreactive species. Therefore, an example of a termination step must show two radicals reacting together on the left side of the equation to form no radicals on the right side of the equation (choice D).

212. C   Equilibria are governed by Le Chatelier's principle, which states that a system at equilibrium will act to restore equilibrium when a stress is applied to the system. Because N_2 is a gas, it will not remain in the system. This effectively results in less product available than is needed for equilibrium. Thus, the reaction proceeds to the right. Another way to show the equilibrium is via the following expression:

$$K_{eq} = [R\bullet]^2[N_2]/[R-N=N-R]$$

Because K_{eq} is a constant, if a product is removed from the system, the right side of the equilibrium expression will be too small, and the system will produce more product in an attempt to reach equilibrium. Choice A is incorrect because the radicals that form from AIBN can make resonance structures. Choices B and D are incorrect statements and are not supported by the passage.

213. C   The passage states that cross-linked polymers are formed from monomers that have more than one polymerizable group. The addition of a radical to an alkene results in a higher molecular weight species. Thus, a double bond is a polymerizable group. Choice C is the only structure with more than one double bond.

INDEPENDENT QUESTIONS

214. D   Any factor that stabilizes the conjugate base of a carboxylic acid more than it stabilizes the acid itself will increase the strength of the acid. The main reason carboxylic acids are stronger acids than the alcohols is because the carboxylic acids have resonance stability associated with the carboxylate ion. Because the carboxylate ion of an acid has more resonance stability than the acid itself, the carboxylic acids are quite strong.

215. B   The DNA of certain bacteria is similar to that found in mitochondria. Recall that there is speculation that a primitive eukaryotic cell incorporated a prokaryotic (bacteria) cell into it, allowing for new metabolic abilities and new symbiotic relations.

216. D   The bond angle of carbon dioxide is 180 degrees, which describes a linear molecule. The other molecules listed—ethylene (C_2H_4), benzene, and acetone—have bond angles of 120 degrees.

217. D   The loop of Henle contains active transport ion pumps, which provide the ability to concentrate the urine. The longer and more active the loops, the better able the animal is to form a smaller volume but more concentrated urine. Animals that live in dry regions and that can conserve water have a powerful survival advantage over those animals that cannot conserve water. Producing a highly concentrated, low-volume urine confers survival advantage. Water conservation is critical for animals living in arid regions such as the desert.

218. B This question tests one's understanding of inductive effects of halogens on acidity. Recall that the stronger the electronegativity (i.e., the more electron withdrawning) of the halogen attached, the easier it is for the acid to lose a proton (i.e., it is a stronger acid). The closer the halogen is to the acid functional group, the stronger the acid. The more halogen atoms near the acid functional group, the stronger the acid. Choice B has the most halogen atoms closest to the functional group of the acid. Note that there are two chloride atoms one carbon away from the acid group, which is more electron withdrawing than a single chloride atom adjacent to the acid group.

219. C Imprinting appears to be a genetically programmed, automatic learning process. It is logical that the newborn is equipped with this automatic learning ability to bond to with what is most likely its parent. The newborn duckling best illustrates the phenomenon of imprinting.

SECT. V
ANSWERS AND
EXPLANATIONS
TO FULL-LENGTH
MCAT

811

Interpreting
Test Scores

INTERPRETING TEST SCORES

Interpreting
Test Scores

The Full-Length Practice MCAT: A Computerized Analysis of Performance

The distribution of raw and scaled scores from the Columbia Review Full-Length Practice MCAT is estimated from the performance of thousands of premedical students who have taken this examination. Premedical students who have taken this test include students from around the country, with different backgrounds, grade point average (GPA) ranges, and aptitudes. Instead of providing variable data for different student populations taking this test, we provide an estimated MCAT score and percentile rank, based on averaging different populations of premedical students. Using the data from their performance, you can get a good idea of how ready you are to attempt the real MCAT.

Remember, most of you will need scores approaching "double-digit" in each of the three numerically scored sections to be competitive for medical school admissions. To rate your performance in the Writing Sample section, we have included some sample essays with scoring and detailed evaluation to help you critique your essays. Constructive teaching points are included with these scored, sample essays.

SCORING THE VERBAL REASONING, PHYSICAL SCIENCES, AND BIOLOGICAL SCIENCES SECTIONS OF THE PRACTICE MCAT

We have carefully evaluated each section of the practice MCAT and provide several sources of valuable information to rate your performance. Start by calculating your raw score for the Verbal Reasoning, Physical Sciences, and Biological Sciences sections. Total the number of correct responses you made in each section. Then, look at Figure 1 to determine your estimated scaled MCAT score and average estimated percentile rank.

After you have determined your scaled MCAT score, you can compare your performance with that of other students. Figures 2, 3, and 4 show a computer-generated distribution for the Verbal Reasoning, Physical Sciences, and Biological Sciences sections. These graphs show what percentage of the test-takers achieved a particular scaled score.

You may wonder how close this test is to former MCATs. Because many students find a great deal of variability in the difficulty level of the MCAT test administration to test administration, we provide a comparison of the Columbia Review full-length practice MCAT with previously released MCAT exams. Table 1 shows that the number of questions answered correctly by test-takers was about the same on the Columbia Review full-length practice MCAT as on the two most recently released MCAT exams.

Estimated Scaled Score Range	Average Estimated Percentile Rank (%)	Verbal Reasoning	Physical Sciences	Biological Sciences
		Raw Score	Raw Score	Raw Score
14-15	99+	64-65	73-77	74-77
13	98-99	62-63	67-72	69-73
12	97	60-61	61-66	65-68
11	88-96	56-59	56-60	60-64
10	74-87	52-55	51-55	54-59
9	58-73	48-51	44-50	48-53
8	42-57	44-47	37-43	43-47
7	31-41	38-43	31-36	38-42
6	18-30	33-37	27-30	33-37
1-5	0-17	0-32	1-26	0-32
		Mean 8.0	Mean 8.0	Mean 8.0

SCORING THE WRITING SAMPLE SECTION OF THE FULL-LENGTH PRACTICE MCAT

STUDENT ESSAYS WITH SCORES, COMMENTS, AND DISCUSSION

To help you grade and evaluate the quality of the Writing Sample essays you wrote on the full-length practice MCAT, a detailed evaluation of the two essay prompts is provided.

In this section, there are three essays for each of the two essay topic prompts; each essay has been written by a different student. The essays were written by students who were actually preparing for the MCAT, and these essays are good examples of the MCAT essay scoring spectrum: one superb essay (a score of 6), one good essay (a score of 4), and one poor essay (a score of 2) for each of the two essay topics. These essays were written under simulated MCAT testing and timing conditions (i.e., 30 minutes per essay). Although the students' original responses (which were handwritten) appear in a typed form, all other aspects of their essays, including errors in spelling, grammar, and punctuation, are intact. Detailed comment and discussion by a MCAT Writing Sample expert, a senior Columbia Review English instructor who is a Ph.D. in Literature and Composition and a university faculty member, follow each student essay.

FIGURE 1.

MCAT raw scores, estimated scaled score ranges, and average estimated percentile rank on the full-length practice MCAT.

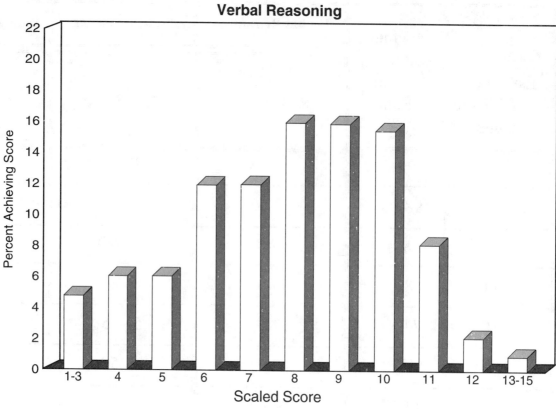

FIGURE 2.
Distribution of scaled scores for the Verbal Reasoning section of the full-length practice MCAT.

FIGURE 3.
Distribution of scaled scores for the Physical Sciences section of the full-length practice MCAT.

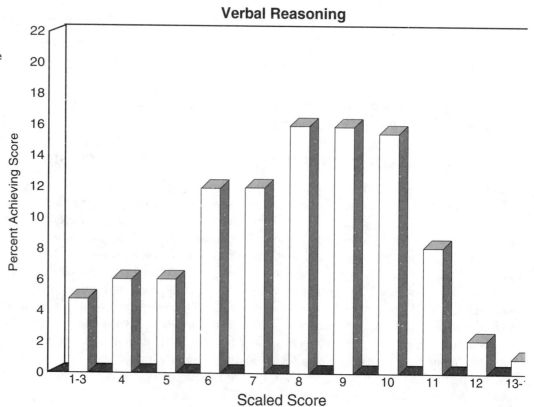

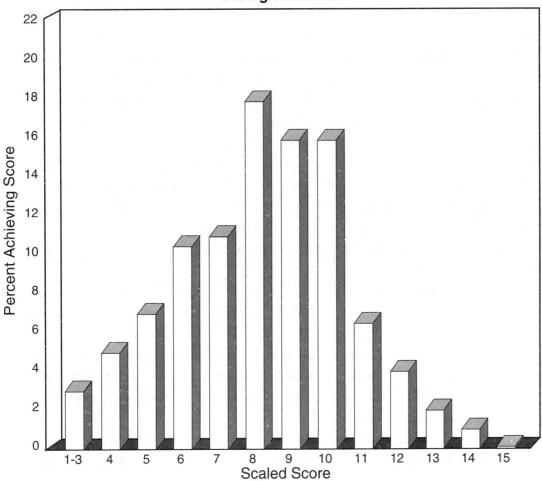

Biological Sciences

Please refer to Section IV, Part C, The Writing Sample: Basic Strategies and Sample Student Essays, for a detailed discussion of scoring criteria. Remember that you are given numerical scores for each essay (1–6), which are converted to a letter score (J–T). This letter score is the official MCAT score for the Writing Sample. Generally, outstanding essays with a score of 5 or 6 correlate with a letter score of R or T. Essays with a score of 4 or 5 usually yield letter scores of Q or R. Essays with a score of 3 or 4 frequently yield letter scores of O or P. Weak essays (score of 2 or 3) yield letter scores in the L–N range.

Remember that each category of the scoring guide stresses the necessity of completing the three writing tasks provided in the topic. Essays that fail to address all three tasks, or which neglect or distort one or more, cannot receive an upper-half score (i.e., a score of 4, 5, or 6). Writing Sample scoring also emphasizes that development or content in an essay is rewarded over clarity or precision of expression. In other words, insight or complexity of thought is more important than fine attention to grammar, punctuation, or precision of style. Spelling and neatness are not directly considered in the scoring process. However, try your best to spell and punctuate correctly and be neat.

FIGURE 4.

Distribution of scaled scores for the Biological Sciences section of the full-length practice MCAT.

Essay Topic 1

Individuals have a right to express themselves in any way they wish.

The statement means individuals have a right to free speech, action or press and cannot have these rights infringed upon by any authoritarian figure. This statement is seen most apparently in our constitution. Certain amendments say people have the right to free speech, bear arms, press, etc. In a Democratic nation, this idea of free is held as sacred and is enforced by the government. Examples of individuals expressing themselves as they wish occurs often throughout history. During the Vietnam war, citizens of the US who did not want to serve in the war because they felt the war was wrong burnt draft cards to protest the war. Protesters and picket lines form when people want to object to a certain practice, either in the workplace or due to the activities of a certain group of people. Especially when people want to oppose the government, they express their views by banding together and making petitions (environmental groups), picketing government meeting, or even burning the US flag. Even when not protesting, the idea that people can express themselves as they wish is shown. Most students at public schools can choose what clothes to wear. As a consumer, I can choose which products to buy. And there are few, if any restrictions, regarding how I should decorate my home or my belongings.

There are times, though, when it is held as justifiable to restrict an individual's expressions. Most people would agree that it would be okay to prevent Hitler from spreading his anti-Jew propaganda because of the pain caused to the Jews as a result of Hitler's views. In addition, protesters who resort to violence as an Anti-Abortion protestor who kills a doctor or bombs an abortion clinic does not have a right to express his disapproval of abortion by destroying humans and property. Finally, peoples whose expression are slanderous, vulgar or profane should not have free expression. A student who wears a hat proclaiming dominance of one race is being offensive. So too is a person who wears clothing with profanity on it, or with vulgar topics (nudity, bigotry, etc.).

People should have the ability to express themselves however they feel as long as that expression does not damage another person emotionally or physically, or damage his property. Thoughts or actions, though, may not intentionally hurt someone, or the subject may not be intending to hurt. An example is someone unknowingly wearing "gang colors" or a bandana. In these cases, expression has to still be free. Whenever people interact, there will be the possibility of inadvertently offending someone, this is natural due to the diversity in the way people think. Therefore, a persons actions, expressions, etc. may only be limited if the intent of those expressions are to cause harm or offend another person, not if the caused harm is unintended. An example of this difference is a journalist who writes an article about a Congressman intentionally slandering him and his family versus a journalist who, while studying for a report, discovers the wrongdoings of a congressman and reports them, not to hurt the congressman, but to get the truth out. Similarly, one who intentionally wears certain clothes to offend should be refrained from doing so, while one who does not should be informed of his offensive behavior and be given a choice to offend or not to offend. When determining what is offensive and what is harm, it should be left to the majority of the society.

Comment and Discussion

The MCAT Writing Sample scoring guide emphasizes that "thorough exploration of the topic" and "depth and complexity of thought" typify an essay that is awarded a score of 6. In the essay written by Student 1, substantial development is obvious. For example, consider the second paragraph, which has the assigned task of describing one specific example that would counter the sentiment of the statement provided (i.e., a contradiction). Student 1 provides three specific examples, each illustrating instances in which one might be plausibly moved to restrict free expression. Similar depth of presentation is apparent in the first paragraph. After providing some discussion of what guarantees free expression—the United States Constitution—Student 1 develops several specific examples to show how individuals have choices in their lives and, perhaps most importantly, in their daily relations with government.

The most difficult part of writing an MCAT essay is the third writing task: drawing together the argument into a conclusion. The writer is required to resolve the apparent contradiction raised through the discussions in the first two writing tasks. Student 1 does a creditable job of stating a principle to resolve the contradiction. Student 1 states that an individual has the right to free expression as long as the individual does not harm another person. Such a formulation is fairly obvious. Student 1, however, shows insightfulness by developing a complication. By posing and discussing the issue of an individual's intention, student 1 makes it clear that solely the matter of harm done as a result of an individual's expression may not be adequate to condemn that individual's free expression. Currently, the issues of offending people and free speech have collided, and our society struggles to achieve a compromise. If possible, when you write your essay, provide more than one principle to account for the contradiction raised during the discussion. Student 1 has provided only one principle to account for the contradiction, but it was clearly central to the issue discussed. If student 1 had provided more than one principle to account for the contradiction, then this essay would be considered extraordinary.

No essay is perfect and an essay does not have to be perfect to receive a score of 6. For example, this essay has several minor errors in style and punctuation as well as lapses in grammar. It would have been more artful if student 1 had avoided using the hackneyed and obvious way of beginning an essay: "The statement means…" Also, some of the examples provided are less useful or less clear than others, and some of the writer's pronouncements are contradictory to the very constitutional principles that are cited as a basis for free expression. The essay grader must keep in mind that this essay was written in only 30 minutes. This writer's accomplishment in that amount of time is well deserving of a score of 6.

Student 2 (Score: 4)

This statement infers that individuals, living in a society, have a right to communicate thoughts, feelings, or actions in any form they wish. This holds especially true here in the United States were these expressions are constituted by the First Amendment. Individuals should be free people who are allowed to do whatever they want. It is a basic human right that people have been striving for. And why should individuals have the right to do what they want? People aren't individuals in the sense of being unique if they aren't able to express themselves. Expression of actions help make people different from everybody else. Along with these differences come desires and expectations that they want to carry out to carry on with their life. As a result, individuals have a right to express themselves in any way they wish.

But what happens when these expressions bring about violence or harm to other? In this case, individuals don't have a right to do what they desire. When an individual wants to express their anger through violence, this brings about more violence in society (like brings more that are alike). This, in turn, results in a chaotic civilization, where people have a right to inflict harm on another.

With all this in mind, what determines whether individuals have a right to express themselves in any way they wish? Individuals have a basic right to express themselves that expose their uniqueness. However, they are restricted to keeping this expression within the realms of keeping a stable, civilized society. For example, if an individual wanted to express her anger over a court decision, rather than resorting to shooting another person or burning down buildings, she can express her anger through peaceful marches or writing a concerned letter to her congressmen. She can also write editorials in newspapers or magazines or appear on a talk show to express her anger. In this way, she is still able to express herself, and let her individuality be exposed and still stay within the limits of keeping social order.

Comment and Discussion

Every student who takes the MCAT should aim to receive at least a score of 4 on the two essays. A score of 4 is a top-half score, which means that the essay is adequate or satisfactory. These essays may not be brilliant, but they are evidence that the student is at least a competent writer. Student 2 demonstrates competence, but nothing more. Note the repetition in the first paragraph. More importantly, note that the first paragraph does not contain a specific example. In fact, there is not a specific example in the essay until the third paragraph. The general vagueness of the discussion does not discredit the essay, but it is not especially enlightening or persuasive. Although the scoring guide only requires that students provide one specific example when addressing the second writing task, merely providing the minimum of detail is not advised.

Note that the writer's organization is flawed. At the beginning of the second paragraph, student 2 delivers a principle—harm done to another—to explain the context in which free expression could justifiably be curtailed. No specific example is provided. In paragraph three, this same principle has been repeated, but in this case an example is provided. It would have been more effective to address the writing tasks in their natural order: first providing the specific illustration of an occasion when free expression would not be appropriate, following up with an example of the principle to account for the coexistence of sentiments in favor of free expression, and the acknowledgment that some restrictions might be necessary.

Despite the deficiencies of the essay, it is important to note that all three writing tasks have been performed, the prose is understandable, only a minimum of mechanical errors intrude, and student 2 seems to understand the issue involved and has produced an adequate discussion. Graders who score the essays are usually instructed to reward the essay according to what was well performed, rather than penalize the essay according to what has not been well performed. With this perspective, it is easy to understand why this essay earned a score of 4; it is an adequate essay, but lacks the complexity of thought or insight to be considered for a higher score.

Student 3 (Score: 2)

As individuals amidst a diverse culture, we all have our own unique ability to express ourselves. This expression through a spectrum of mediums such as art, dance, song, theatre, or in word all seek to paint a picture of that individual's thoughts and feelings. Each of us has the right to communicate the truth of ourselves in an environment that fosters the improvement of our fellow man.

On the contrary however, we have witnessed instances in history or in our own personal lives where this expression of one self has offended the other. It is true as it has been said, that you can say some pretty harsh things to the ones you love, but it has always been with the understanding that we love them. To cross the line then is for one to express geniuine human emotion, by whatever medium, so as to repress the person in opposition.

An example therefore we see is in the case of radical neo-nazi propaganda. Whether through published word or in the blood beatened eyes of hate, their right to express crosses the line. They seek the elimination of another culture, namely the Jewish through extermination, as well against the blacks who they believe are transformed monkeys. It is at the heart of this individual group expression—fear as well as the fear of the unknown, even perhaps ignorance, that sets destructive forces against their fellow, non-belligerent mankind. This my friends, is not acceptable. We therefore must attempt as a peace-loving society, to deter from this kind of expression.

The tongue, just as an utter can steer a large ship, so controls the individual expression. For a destructive fire to be set, and a society to be led off course from trying to make its citizens the best they can be, only envelopes more harm. To slander or prohibit another's God given right as a human to live or create a rift between individual's right and his right under the law is the measure of latitude about individual expression.

Comment and Discussion

According to the scoring guide, a level 2 essay seriously neglects or distorts one or more of the writing tasks. Another useful guideline from our scoring guide is that a level 2 essay demonstrates problems with organization and analysis of the topic. In this essay, it is apparent that student 3 has arguably done less than an adequate job with all three writing tasks. The third writing task is the most crucial, and in this essay, it is the most poorly handled. The essay does not contain any clearly stated principles. Student 3 comes close to clearly stating a principle in the final sentence, but this sentence (especially in a paragraph beset with mangled syntax) is too little and too late.

The grader's last impression of an essay may influence the score assigned, and the grader's first impression of an essay may influence his receptiveness to the essay. In the first paragraph, student 3 hobbles through the essay and too narrowly addresses the topic. The initial focus on artistic expression is not "wrong," but it is useless. With this approach, student 3 is in a position from which he cannot develop the essay. This essay seems to begin twice, and with only 30 minutes to complete the exercise, a writer cannot afford this approach. Every sentence must be in service of the three writing tasks.

Although the scoring guide (for all score categories) does not emphasize clarity of expression, the lack of fluency in this essay is a problem. Virtually every sentence in this essay demonstrates a problem with clarity. For example, consider the first few sentences of the third paragraph. Although a reader can understand what student 3 is attempting to convey, the reader must labor to do so. The syntax makes comprehension difficult, and this difficulty leads the reader to believe that the ideas are either unclear in the writer's mind, or that there is a sheer lack of verbal facility. The ideas, organization, and language are confusing in this essay. Student 3 fails to provide a lucid analysis, and thus the score of 2 seems appropriate.

Essay Topic 2

New ideas and ways of doing things are better than the old thinking and doing.

Student 4 (Score: 6)

New ideas are usually thought of as better than older, traditional ways because new ideas have more experience and examples with which to support them than older ideas do. This is seen in all sorts of science. In the Medieval times, all the earth was supposedly composed of the 4 humors—fire, water, air and soil. The alchemists said this was the basics of all life. But as the field of chemistry expanded, elements were discovered, and today the 4 humors are regarded as nonsense. In physics, most people believed Newtonian physics regarding the movement of masses because all the data supported Newton's results. But, as there became more information on the planets and their interactions, Einstein formulated his theory of relativity which explained the motions of objects in a way different from Newton and in a way that better supports the existing data. Finally, technology has advanced our wisdom and enabled us to make life easier and safer. Before the 1970's, seat belts were not even mandatory in all cars. But, research began to show people in accidents who wore seat belts had a better chance of surviving. As a result, seat belts are now mandatory. In addition, engineers have added air bags, and changed the structure and makeup of cars to make them safer. All this resulted from people figuring out new ways of doing things.

There are instances, though, of where the old way of doing and thinking is better. Today, people are in a hurry and everything is rushed. People do not spend time with their loved one, or sit down for the traditional 3 meals per day. Traditionally, dinner time was a time for relaxation and discussing the days events. Now, people just turn on the TV and eat in silence. This has created a society that is somewhat estranged. People do not trust others, they are quiet and keep to themselves. Even married people do not talk like they used to, and this leads to problems such as divorce. In addition, traditionally, when you pulled into a gas station or went shopping, you were treated like something special. A mechanic would check your oil, wash your windows, and check your tires while getting gas. In a store, the sales person would attend to your wishes and get to know you, understand what you want to buy and why. This made purchasing a more pleasurable experience for some. Finally, the new ideas in science have not all been beneficial. The creation of the atom bomb certainly changed many people's outlook on life and seems to have increased anxiety. Likewise, the human genome project has many ethical debates it still has not answered to.

Whether new or old thinking should prevail depends on the total good it will do for all people. In certain aspects of life, new ways of thinking has made life better for people, as in new agricultural techniques that provide more food for more people, or seat belts that save more lives. But in other aspects of life, older ways of thinking seem to make life better and happier for people. People often complain they get less and less for their dollar. Indeed, service and respect given to others has declined because of our desire for efficiency. This seems to have made more people less happy. For example, a salesperson who is indifferent to the consumer can get more work done, helping the company, but faces the problem of disgruntled consumers and lots of returned items. Likewise, the traditional town meeting, where everyones opinion was heard was time consuming, and would be even more so today, but this led to people being happier as they felt their opinions and interests were being looked out for. As a society, we have to decide if the need for efficiency and its bonuses outweigh the benefits gained from a slow, tedious, but more gratifying way of doing something.

Comment and Discussion

There is usually agreement among graders that level 6 essays stand out because they command attention. This essay demonstrates no special use of language. At times student 4 demonstrates awkwardness (e.g., the opening sentence). However, the strength of this essay is its strong development and its sophistication. The essay is replete with specific examples; student 4 seems to have a limitless fund of general knowledge to draw from. The apparently effortless referencing throughout the essay engenders confidence in the reader. Note, too, that student 4 has been felicitous in her choice of examples. Each example is effective, and each example later lends itself to the formulation of the explanatory principle.

The final paragraph is where the essay truly excels. Student 4 cites only a single explanatory principle. In most cases, the citation of a single principle would engender no special excitement in the reader. However, in this essay, the treatment of the principle stands out. Student 4 addresses "the total good" that would result from new ways of thinking or doing as being the concept people need when making a decision. This sentiment is utilitarianism, which is a well-known philosophy. The discussion that follows is superb. Student 4 provides a social critique of the twentieth century and successfully establishes the contradiction between efficiency and happiness, tapping in to one of the compelling issues of human existence. The final paragraph leaves the reader with the impression of having made acquaintance with a sophisticated and insightful person, which is an experience to cherish (especially at 40 essays per hour, the average scoring speed for MCAT graders).

Students may worry about the effect of factual errors on the scoring process. Be assured that factual errors are of little consequence. For example, this essay states that in the middle ages people believed "all the earth was supposedly composed of the four humors—fire, water, air and soil." This statement is incorrect. Student 4 probably meant to say that all matter was composed of four *elements*. (The humors were supposed fluids of the body, including blood, phlegm, choler, and black bile.) Does this error matter? Not at all. The point here is to encourage writers to simply bash through the assignment rather than getting hung up on trivial matters of absolute accuracy.

Student 5 (Score: 4)

We live in an evolving world. Things are forever changing around us. New ideas and technologies pop up all the time as a result of the demand for us humans to keep up with the world around us. The new ideas and ways of doing things are better then the old thinking and doing because new things are created to help us to better cope and survive in a new world. For example, as the population grows, there is greater demand for more land and more food. New technologies in agriculture allow farm lands to be continely used at greater efficiency. Synthetic fertilizers are made to keep the soil good for farming and new types of plants can be made to withstand and grow in changing environments. These advancements are much better and more productive then the old way of farming.

On the other hand, some things are better left alone. Sometimes in the race to always progress, things are made worse and it would be better to just stick to the old way of doing things. For example, we make new synthetic products to replace natural one's and the new ones are toxic. Artificial sweetner is a good example. People didn't want the calories of sugar, so artificial sweetners were made and now they are thought to cause cancer. So in trying to make new and better things, we only create more problems.

As creatures living in a changing world, we must create new things to keep up with the changes, but we should try to only change things that are necessities. Luxuries or the "extras" in life don't need to be tampered with. Besides, most things we do for enjoyment (and not necessity) are best in their natural state (for example, foods and the outdoors). If we try to alter them to something new and modern, we only take the chance of creating new problems and perhaps destroying what we already have.

Comment and Discussion

The comments and discussion about the essay written by student 4 emphasizes the upward sweep achieved at the end of the essay. In the essay written by student 5, the situation is reversed. This mediocre essay stumbles—not enough to fall out of the level 4 category, but only barely. The final paragraph begins with a windy generalization. Student 5 then attempts to draw a distinction between necessities and luxuries, which is a difficult task, especially without a specific example. The reader gets a sense that there could have been exciting development of this principle; however, the development is too slight. Instead of providing a useful example, student 5 attempts to establish a new formulation. Student 5 begins to discuss how things should be in their "natural state"; "foods and the outdoors" are listed, parenthetically, as examples. The word *natural* should be approached with great caution. What, exactly, is natural? In addition to semantic vagueness, the principle stated is poorly formed and unclear. The reader only gets a sense, not a complete understanding, of what student 5 is trying to convey.

The rest of the essay is stronger, but it also has flaws. Each of the first two paragraphs provides a specific example. Although one example per paragraph is adequate, a grader would probably prefer more than one example. To receive a higher score, an essay must have greater depth and complexity. Although each example in this essay is effective, the two examples together are not especially useful; it is easy to see how these examples led student 5 to the awkward response to the third writing task. Examples do not necessarily have to be parallel, but sometimes a more careful selection creates a stronger essay. If the writer had used examples of modern developments in farming, then perhaps he would have been able to write a stronger ending. If he had mentioned some unanticipated agricultural disaster that resulted from a technologic advancement (e.g., the construction of the Aswan Dam), then maybe he would have come up with a more coherent principle.

Student 5 is competent in his use of language and expression. However, there are signs that the writer is sometimes unclear or uncertain in his thinking. For example, in the first paragraph he states that "as the population grows, there is a greater demand for more land. . ." As real estate agents so cheerfully observe, "they ain't making any more land." As a reader, you may be able to understand perfectly well what student 5 meant. However, the grader should not have to pause because of momentary confusion. Also, student 5 could have used a better word to describe the deficiencies of artificial sweetener other than to call it "toxic." Also, note that there are several grammar, punctuation, and spelling mistakes.

Student 6 (Score: 2)

The author broadly states new ideas and ways of doing things are better than the old. This echos the American belief that we are always improving ourselves and our country. We are, after all, just begining to understand science. New materials are being found every day. For example plastics that do not burn are obviously better than flamible plastics in furniture. Computer and Medical science are improving year by year.

Some regions in the field of human endevors are not receptive to change. Religion acquires stability by actually resisting change. In addition, the author ignores cycles of changes in thinking and doing. Skirt length or heel height are always changing but not necessarily in "new" ways.

In a broad sense the author is quite correct. In *the Nature of Scientific Revolution* science is shown to progress in leaps, followed by periods of recursive improvements. The possibility of new ideas and ways must be included in our resorvoir of possible action. They offer us the ability to adapt to new demands. As a counter-example, if forced to choose between "new" and "old" with only "old ideas" and old "ways of doing" our society would crumble when faced with a new disaster. In that sense "new" ideas and ways provide a unique benefit that "old" ideas and ways cannot. Therefore "new" ideas and ways are acutually better.

Comment and Discussion

Essays that contain distortions of the writing tasks usually receive lower-half scores. This essay is a classic example of distorting the writing tasks. It should be obvious that the distortion occurs in the writer's handling of the third writing task. The third writing task requires the writer to synthesize or harmonize—to show how the opposite of a great truth is also a great truth. When a student handles the third writing task effectively, he is able to offer a wise suggestion for knowing when we should believe, follow, or act on a great truth and when we should believe, follow, or act on its opposite. Successfully addressing the third writing task is entirely different from simply compromising between the two truths proposed, and it is also different from simply opting for one of the truths. Student 6 "chooses sides" at the end of his discussion (which probably earned him the low score); he simply asserts that the new ideas and ways *are* better.

It is disappointing that the writer had a wrongheaded assertion, because he had enough material to write an effective essay. In fact, the reader gets the sense that the essay is a series of missed opportunities; the essay mirrors a more capable writer than it actually demonstrates. For example, student 6 mentions a promising lead in his second paragraph when he cites religion as an example of human endeavors that are not receptive to change. Unfortunately, the example is not developed. What if student 6 had explained that religious thought can often represent the highest stirring of the human heart, that its teachings provide ageless guidance to all who live? Not only would the second part of the essay have been much better, but student 6 would have had an opportunity to further discuss an interesting principle for the third writing task. The mention of skirt and heel lengths and the idea of cyclical change are both matters that would have made a stronger essay if they had been handled more effectively.

The reader can speculate about this writer's potential if he had a longer time period in which to work. Student 6 certainly has ideas, and surely he has a fund of knowledge. Consider the citation of a book title in the third paragraph. The reader knows that student 6 is somewhat well read. But what has it earned student 6? Although the book is cited briefly in example, there is insufficient development of its use in the essay. Also, although length of an essay is not a criterion for scoring MCAT Writing Samples, there can be no denying that a short essay is often a "symptom" of weakly developed discussions. The essay lacks development and distorts the third writing task. Also, note repeated errors in punctuation, grammar, and spelling. Observe all of these problems and avoid them.

TABLE 1. Approximate average percent of total questions answered correctly by examinees.

Exam	Verbal Reasoning	Physical Sciences	Biological Sciences
Columbia Review Practice MCAT	70%	59%	62%
1991 MCAT	85%	60%	60%
1994 MCAT	70%	60%	65%